Visual Pattern Analyzers

OXFORD PSYCHOLOGY SERIES

EDITORS

Donald E. Broadbent   Nicholas J. Mackintosh
Stephen Kosslyn   Endel Tulving
James L. McGaugh   Lawrence Weiskrantz

OXFORD PSYCHOLOGY SERIES NO. 16

Visual Pattern Analyzers

NORMA VAN SURDAM GRAHAM

Department of Psychology
Columbia University

OXFORD UNIVERSITY PRESS · New York
CLARENDON PRESS · Oxford
1989

Oxford University Press

Oxford   New York   Toronto
Delhi   Bombay   Calcutta   Madras   Karachi
Petaling Jaya   Singapore   Hong Kong   Tokyo
Nairobi   Dar es Salaam   Cape Town
Melbourne   Auckland

and associated companies in
Berlin   Ibadan

Copyright © 1989 by Oxford University Press, Inc.

Published by Oxford University Press, Inc.,
200 Madison Avenue, New York, New York 10016

Oxford is a registered trademark of Oxford University Press

Library of Congress Cataloging-in-Publication Data
Graham, Norma Van Surdam.
Visual pattern analyzers / Norma Van Surdam Graham.
     p.   cm. — (Oxford psychology series ; no. 16)
Bibliography: p.
Includes index.
ISBN 0-19-505154-8
1. Pattern perception. I. Title. II. Series.
QP491.G69   1989
152.1'423—dc19   88-34883   CIP

9 8 7 6 5 4 3 2 1
Printed in the United States of America
on acid-free paper

In memory of
Norma Van Surdam Keesler
Clyde C. Keesler
*who were partners in a
heavy-construction-equipment dealership
in Prospect Park, Pennsylvania*

and

Helen Tredway Graham
Evarts Ambrose Graham
*who were professors at the
Washington University School of Medicine
St. Louis, Missouri*

Preface

Visual perception can be described crudely as a two-part process: First, the visual system breaks the information in the visual stimulus into parts, and then second, the visual system puts the information back together again (not in its original form, however). Why should there be this analysis followed by a synthesis? The information in the visual stimulus as it impinges on the observer's eye (the retinal image or "proximal stimulus") is just a collection of points of light. The correspondences between the proximal stimulus and the important aspects of the world that is being perceived (the "distal stimulus") are far from straightforward, as the discussions of philosophers, visual scientists, and, more recently, computer scientists emphasize (e.g., see Hochberg 1978 and Marr 1982). Presumably, once the information in the proximal stimulus is analyzed into parts by the visual system's lower levels, it can be more easily reassembled by the visual system's higher levels to tell us what is where in the environment!

This book deals with many of the parts into which visual information is initially analyzed. Presumably, these are the parts that make economic and feasible the subsequent computation of "what is where." But just as with all the kings' men and Humpty Dumpty, current visual science knows much more about the parts than about the subsequent computations that put them back together again.

The parts that are the topic of this book are those relevant for patterns in space and time; that is, for discussions of shape and motion. Color and three-dimensionality are not discussed.

Our knowledge of these parts has come both from psychophysics and neurophysiology. This book's major topic is the psychophysical evidence—particularly that from experiments measuring human observers' ability to detect and identify near-threshold spatiotemporal patterns. Physiological "asides" are frequent in the book, however (see sections 1.4, 1.5, 1.6, 1.7, 3.6.1, 3.6.2, 3.7.8, 5.4.4, 8.7, 12.7, and 13.13), as the psychophysics and physiology have gone hand-in-hand.

Over the last quarter-century or so of such research an enormous amount has been learned. That information has been scattered over the pages of many different journals with many of the researchers themselves having little idea of how coherent the whole story has become. In fact, in the course of the eight years I spent writing this book, my original suspicions of chaos were replaced by a surprised sense of convergence and definitive conclusions. If one considers only near-threshold patterns, the results from different investigators using different methods turn out to agree remarkably well and add up to a consistent story of the low-level analyzers that exist in the human visual system. Organizing this material within a framework and making it part of a coherent story is the major aim of this book.

This book is primarily for readers with a very serious interest in visual perception or closely related fields. The prototypical reader might be a graduate student in vision or perception or an established researcher in another area of vision or perception. Much of the book (parts II through V on models of four kinds of psychophysical experiments) is just as applicable to people working in the psychophysics of audition, taste, or smell as it is to people working in vision.

On the other hand, the book does include a good deal of background material since people entering the field of pattern vision can come from medicine (ophthalmology), from biology (neurosciences, physiology), from engineering and physics (especially electrical and optical), from computer science, from experimental psychology, or from the arts (fine arts, film).

ORGANIZATION OF THE BOOK

As shown in the figure, the first part of the book provides background material about physiology and psychophysics (Chapter 1) and mathematics (Chapter 2). (Chapter 2 is more important for understanding Chapters 4, 5, 6, 12, and 13 than for the other chapters. Readers able to tolerate ambiguity could skim or omit Chapter 2.)

The next four parts discuss four kinds of psychophysical experiments that provide information about the parts into which the visual stimulus is analyzed: adaptation experiments (Chapter 3), summation experiments (Chapters 4, 5, and 6), uncertainty experiments (Chapters 7 and 8), and identification experiments (Chapters 9 and 10). For each kind of experiment, current explanations (more formally, models) of these experimental results are discussed at length. These models are illustrated using experimental results on the spatial-frequency dimension, but the general logic applies to experiments on other dimensions in pattern vision and in perception more generally. It is possible to read only the first chapter of each of these four parts (Chapters 3, 4, 7, and 9) with little loss of continuity.

The first chapter in the summation part (Chapter 4) along with the uncertainty and identification parts (Chapters 7 through 10) cover what is sometimes called *multidimensional signal-detection theory*. They could be read independently of the rest of the book quite easily.

The sixth part of the book summarizes results on all seventeen pattern-vision dimensions: spatial frequency, orientation, spatial position (2 dimensions), spatial extent (2 dimensions), spatial phase, temporal frequency (velocity), temporal position, temporal extent, temporal phase, direction of motion, degree of direction-selectivity, mean luminance, contrast, eye-of-origin, and degree of binocularity. Some readers might skip or skim the middle sections of the book

CHAPTERS **PARTS**

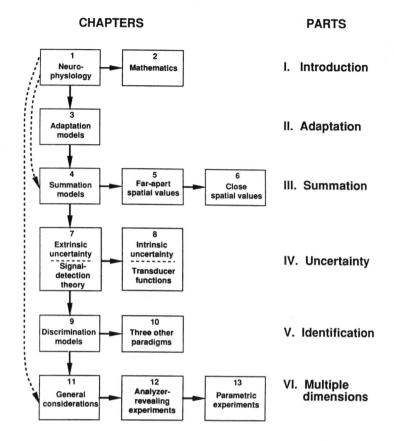

going directly from the introductory material to Chapter 11 (which discusses general issues of interpretation that arise when multiple dimensions are at issue) or even to Chapters 12 and 13, which summarize conclusions about analyzers on different pattern-vision dimensions (Chapter 12) and about parametric sensitivity on different pattern-vision dimensions (Chapter 13). The conclusions in Chapters 12 and 13, however, do depend on the theoretical framework outlined in the middle parts of the book. The final sections of Chapters 12 and 13 are lists of studies organized by both the primary and secondary dimensions studied. Only authors and dates are given in these lists, but the full references can be found in the bibliography.

An appendix at the end of the book lists the assumptions used in the models of Chapters 3 through 10 both in order of appearance and in groups according to function. There is an index of assumptions appearing before the topic index. A list of briefly defined symbols appears after the Table of Contents and the symbols also appear in the topic index (with Greek letters alphabetized immediately following their English equivalents).

ACKNOWLEDGMENTS

I thank Jacob Nachmias, Floyd Ratliff, Dorothea Jameson, Leo Hurvich, John Robson, and Fergus Campbell for introducing me to visual science—to its richness and complexity, to the vast amount that was known coupled with the vast amount that remained to be discovered, and (most importantly for me) to the increasingly sophisticated attempts to construct theories of the visual process and the challenge of trying to test these theories against the results of psychophysical and physiological experiments.

This book was begun during my sabbatical year in 1979–1980, funded by a James McKeen Cattell Fund Sabbatical Award. It was continued over subsequent years with substantial support from Columbia University. I am grateful to my friends, family, and colleagues who bore with me during all of it. I am particularly grateful to Jacob Nachmias, John Robson, James Thomas, Joyce Farrell, Mary Hayhoe, Donald Hood, Elizabeth Davis, Patricia Kramer, Neil Macmillan, Mark Georgeson, Stanley Klein, Anne Sutter, Asher Cohen, Anthony Movshon, Daniel Pollen, Robert Shapley, Herschel Leibowitz, Julian Hochberg, David R. Williams, Brian Wandell, and Andrew Watson—their critical readings of chapters and/or discussions of specific issues were a tremendous help.

New York   N.G.
November 1988

Contents

Part III. SUMMATION

4. Models for Far-Apart Values   131

5. Far-Apart Values on Spatial Dimensions   181

6. Close Values on Spatial Dimensions   212

Part IV. UNCERTAINTY

Part V. IDENTIFICATION

LIST OF SYMBOLS

c—intensity
cpd—cycles/degree of visual angle
c/deg—cycles/degree of visual angle
c/sec—cycles/second
Hz—cycles/second
M'—number of monitored analyzers
N'—number of analyzers
R—decision variable used by observer
R_i—output of the ith analyzer
S_i—sensitivity of the ith analyzer
S_{obs}—sensitivity of the observer
stim—stimulus
th—threshold (reciprocal of sensitivity S)
V—value on dimension of interest
V_i—value of ith simple stimulus

I
INTRODUCTION

1

Neurophysiology and Psychophysics

1.1 TWO THEMES—PATTERN VISION AND ANALYZERS

This book has two themes—pattern vision and analyzers. By *pattern* I mean a visual stimulus that varies only in time and two spatial dimensions. The third spatial dimension—depth—and also color are ignored, generally by being held constant throughout the comparisons made experimentally or theoretically. By *analyzer* I mean any entity sensitive to a range of values along some dimension of interest. Dimensions along which analyzers have been postulated include: in audition—temporal frequency (pitch) and several quantities important to speech (e.g., voice-onset time); in taste—quantities measuring chemical composition; in vision—wavelength (color), binocular disparity, orientation, spatial frequency (size), spatial position, and direction of motion. These last four dimensions, along with a number of others to be discussed, are the dimensions of visual patterns and of relevance here.

In many contexts, available evidence is insufficient to do more than suggest the existence of analyzers. In other contexts, the evidence constrains or at least suggests further properties of the analyzers. Generally, for example, analyzers sensitive to different values along the same dimension (but otherwise identical) are thought to act more or less in parallel. To delineate carefully what kind of evidence is sufficient for making what kind of statement about analyzers is a major concern of this book; it is as applicable to other dimensions as to those of pattern vision.

The kinds of evidence examined here are from psychophysical experiments using stimuli that are near their own detection thresholds. The detection threshold for a pattern is the lowest contrast—the lowest difference between the brightest and the darkest part of the pattern—at which an observer is able to discriminate between the pattern and the blank field. (A blank field is a stationary, spatially homogeneous field of light that has the same average luminance as the pattern.)

Even when only near-threshold patterns are considered, hundreds of experiments prove relevant. This large number is one reason why this book limits itself to near-threshold patterns. The major reason, however, is that the near-threshold experiments—guided and interpreted by theoretical work—have led to a clear, rigorous, and quantitative model of one stage of pattern vision. (See note 1.) This stage, which is presumably quite early in the stream of processing, consists of a set of analyzers with different ranges of sensitivities along certain dimensions. There is truly remarkable agreement across different near-threshold experimental paradigms and across different laboratories about which dimensions of pattern vision do and which dimensions do not have multiple analyzers in this stage.

To put it another way (but be warned that the following may be misleadingly strong), these near-threshold experiments have succeeded in uncovering the "primitives" or "alphabet" of an early-level process. They have told us, in effect, how the early processes decompose visual patterns into components.

As one would expect, this alphabet, or "set of primitives," or "decomposition," is less arbitrary than the ABC's of language; it is a systematic and sensible alphabet with a certain beauty. To uncover this alphabet—this set of primitives—investigators had to have some place to begin. The candidates for primitives suggested by nonmathematical intuition (e.g., lines and edges) turned out to be a step in the right direction. The addition of a certain amount of mathematical knowledge (described in the next chapter) did the trick.

In this enterprise, the mutual influence of neurophysiology and psychophysics was enormous and fruitful. We may now know not only *what* the primitives are but also *where* they are in the visual system. To describe the physiology in as much depth as the psychophysics is a prohibitively large task; but I have presented some relevant neurophysiology later in this chapter for its own sake and as a convenient introduction. And I could not resist inserting bits of physiology as asides throughout the book.

In addition to this lower level decomposition revealed by near-threshold experiments, higher level processes most certainly go on—the processes that decide which parts of the scene belong to which objects, for example. The neurophysiology of the last few years has revealed many visual areas higher in the stream of processing than the neurons that seem most like the analyzers in question here. (See further discussion later in this chapter.) This higher stages may well include higher level decompositions. If there is such higher level decomposition in any rigorous sense, our ordinary experience suggests that the primitives or alphabet of the highest level stages (those closest to the perceptions we are conscious of) are more like objects or parts of objects than like qualities such as colors or sizes or orientations. (For more discussion, see Biederman, 1985; Treisman, 1986; Treisman & Gormican, 1988.)

In any case, the existence of higher levels of processing leaves something of a mystery. Why are psychophysical experiments able to reveal the properties of the lower levels? Why, in particular, are near-threshold pattern-vision experiments able to reveal the properties of a set of relatively low-level analyzers? Are we being fooled? Is the quantitative agreement between the models and the results of these experiments a gigantic coincidence? I do not know a satisfactory solution to this mystery; see section 1.3.3 for further discussion.

1.2   ANALYZERS IN COLOR VISION AS AN EXAMPLE

Although this book is not about color vision, we will start with a simple model of color vision. This model in its general form is widely accepted, and it is an instructive counterexample to many wrong-headed statements that have been made about pattern analyzers. Starting with this model has the advantage that, since this book is not about color vision, we will not have to worry about the ways in which this model is not quite sufficient. (Introductions to and discussions of this model can be found in many places, including Boynton, 1979; Hurvich, 1981; and Hurvich and Jameson, 1957. The review by Jacobs, 1986, includes the history of the last quarter century.)

In this simple model of color vision there are two major stages of analyzers. A controversy that started in the middle of the last century between "trichromatic" theories of color vision (those by Young and Helmholz, among others) and "opponent-color theories" (by Hering) has resolved itself into these two-stage models of color vision. The first stage (upper left in Fig. 1.1) is the trichromatic stage. The physiological substrate for the three analyzers at this first stage is presumed to be three different photopigments (called here S, M, and L to stand for short, medium, and long wavelength, respectively). Each of these pigments is contained in a different type of retinal receptor (called a cone). Although each of the three pigments is sensitive to a broad range of wavelengths of light, the relative sensitivities of the three pigments to different wavelengths differ. Current estimates of the pigment sensitivity curves are shown in the upper right of

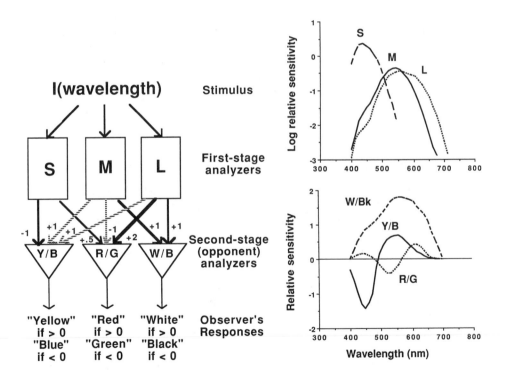

FIG. 1.1 A simple model of color vision consisting of two stages of analyzers (left) with the sensitivity of analyzers at each stage as a function of wavelength (right). S, short wavelength; M, medium wavelength; L, long wavelength. Y/B, yellow-blue; R/G, red-green; W/B, white-black.

Fig. 1.1. The output (at any point in time and space) of one of these analyzers (pigments) is representable as a single positive number.

The second stage of the model is the opponent-colors stage and again consists of three analyzers, called B/Y, R/G, and W/B (blue/yellow, red/green, and white/black, respectively). Each of these three opponent analyzer's outputs (at any point in time and space) is again a single number, but now this number can be either positive or negative. The output from an opponent analyzer equals a combination of the outputs from two or three of the first-stage analyzers. In many circumstances, the combination is approximately linear, that is, the output from a second-stage opponent analyzer equals the weighted sum of first-stage analyzers' outputs. The lower right of Fig. 1.1 shows a current estimate of the relative responsiveness of the three opponent analyzers to monochromatic stimuli in a dark surround. In the diagram on the left of Fig. 1.1, the small numbers next to each path from the first to the second stage indicate the relative weighting of that path. For example, the output of the R/G analyzer equals half the output of the S analyzer minus the output of the M analyzer plus twice the output of the L analyzer. As is discussed in more detail later, positive outputs from the opponent analyzers are associated with perceptions of red, yellow, or white and negative outputs with perceptions of green, blue, or black.

The physiological substrate of a second-stage opponent analyzer may be a neuron, perhaps in later stages of the retina or in the lateral geniculate nucleus, that combines the outputs from the three cone types appropriately. For example, a neuron that is a white/black analyzer might simply sum the outputs from a cone containing middle-wavelength pigment and from another cone containing long-wavelength pigment. (This example wiring diagram is probably much simpler than that for any real neuron—it ignores spatial organization—but it is not misleading for the current discussion.)

1.2.1 Color Matching and Color Appearance

Although there is now physiological evidence consistent with this simple model of color vision, the earliest and still the most compelling evidence for each stage of this model is psychophysical. According to this model, if two lights produce the same output from each of the three analyzers of the first stage, the observer will be unable to tell the two lights apart. In fact, it was the "trichromacy" evident in experiments where observers matched mixtures of wavelengths that first suggested a stage consisting of three independent analyzers (now presumed to be photopigments) responding linearly to combinations of wavelengths.

These three first-stage analyzers, however, cannot easily explain the color appearances of small homogeneous patches of light. The second, opponent-colors, analyzers can. Color appearance—particularly for small, stationary, homogeneous patches of light in a dark surround—can be subjectively analyzed into three perceptual components: degree of redness or greenness (where redness and greenness cannot coexist), degree of blueness or yellowness (similarly blueness and yellowness cannot coexist), and degree of whiteness. (The opposite of whiteness, blackness, is seen only when patches are surrounded by other bright patches. See note 2.) In fact, it is quite easy to get observers simply to say how much of each of the three pairs of percepts they see in a given patch (by rating on a scale from 0 to 100, for example). When the responses to different wavelengths of monochromatic light (all at the same intensity) are plotted, they look much like the drawing in the lower right of Fig. 1.1. Thus, magnitude of each perceptual component (as indicated by the observer's response) is assumed to be determined by the magnitude and direction of the response of the appropriate opponent-colors analyzer; in fact, it was these color appearances that originally suggested such a stage.

The commonly mentioned perceptual dimensions of brightness, saturation, and hue are a transformation of these three opponent-colors dimensions. Brightness is primarily determined by the amount of whiteness/blackness, saturation by the relative magnitudes of the other two compared with whiteness/blackness, and hue by redness/greenness and blueness/yellowness.

1.3 TWO CAUTIONS ABOUT ANALYZERS

Two points about analyzers in general are easily made from the color-vision example. First, more than one set of analyzers can exist on a single dimension— wavelength in this case. The analyzers suggested by one kind of experiment, therefore, do not necessarily coincide with the analyzers suggested by another kind of experiment. Notice how different the sensitivities of the first-stage and second-stage color analyzers are (right half of Fig. 1.1).

Second, the link between an observer's responses (presumably reflecting conscious percepts) and the analyzers' outputs can be of various kinds. The link between the opponent analyzers' outputs and color appearances is very simple: There is a one-to-one relationship between the magnitude of the output of an analyzer (e.g., R/G) and the magnitude of a given percept (redness or greenness) that the observer says is present. On the other hand, the link between the first-stage analyzers' (pigments') outputs and these color appearances would be quite complicated to state. The percept resulting from a particular magnitude of S analyzer output, for example, has no description independent of the magnitude of outputs by the M and L analyzers. In fact, the relationship between the first-stage analyzers' outputs and the observers' responses (percepts) cannot be described at all except by describing the second stage either explicitly or implicitly.

To put this point another way, to use multiple-analyzers models to explain visual phenomena (e.g., the observers' responses made in psychophysical experiments) requires more knowledge of the analyzers than just their outputs to all stimuli. Something must be assumed about the link between the analyzers' outputs and the observer's responses—that is, something must be known or assumed about the ways in which the analyzers' outputs are used by still higher order processes to produce the observer's responses.

1.4 TERMINOLOGY—RESPONSES VERSUS OUTPUTS

For the sake of clarity, the following entirely arbitrary convention is used here: The word *response* is reserved for observers, and the word *output* for analyzers and neurons.

1.5 MODELS OF NEAR-THRESHOLD PATTERN VISION—AN OVERVIEW

Most of the models suggested for near-threshold pattern vision and discussed in this book have the general form sketched in Fig. 1.2. They contain one stage of low-level analyzers. Only three of these analyzers are explicit in Fig. 1.2; the dashed lines indicate an indefinite number of others. The input to these analyzers is a visual pattern indicated by $L(x, y, t)$—luminance as a function of two spatial variables x and y and one temporal variable t. The form of the output from these analyzers—is it a single number, a function of time, a function of space and time?—is not indicated on the sketch, because it differs from one application to another.

The outputs from these analyzers determine the observer's responses by relatively simple rules that are indicated in Fig. 1.2 by a "decision stage." Three examples of rules are briefly described here. These rules [assumptions] and all other assumptions used in this book are listed by category and by sequential number in the appendix at the end of the book. Skimming this appendix at this point would provide further introduction to how the general model of Fig. 1.2

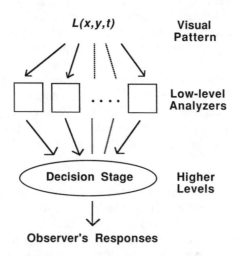

FIG. 1.2 A general framework for the models of pattern vision discussed here.

will be made more detailed in the book. Also there is an index of assumptions preceding the subject index.

1. *Maximum-output detection rule.* The most frequent decision rule we will meet in this book is the maximum-output detection rule. (In its usual form, this rule is applied to cases where the output from each analyzer can be represented as a single number.) This assumption says that an observer bases his or her response on the maximum of the outputs (i.e., on the peak output) from different analyzers. For example, in a yes-no detection experiment, the observer would respond, "Yes, a pattern is there," if the maximum of the analyzers' outputs were greater than some criterion; otherwise the observer would respond, "No, a pattern is not there."

2. *Sum-of-outputs detection rule.* Another possible assumption is the sum-of-outputs detection rule. It asserts that an observer bases a response in detection experiments on the sum of the outputs from different analyzers rather than on the maximum output.

3. *Concurrent identification rule.* For identification experiments, the decision rules will be more complicated. In what is perhaps the most complex experiment considered here (concurrent identification), the observer is asked whether each of several possible simple patterns is present in the stimulus (where none or all could actually be present). A possible decision rule in this case is: The observer says, "Yes, simple pattern 1 is present," if and only if the maximum output from all the analyzers sensitive to simple pattern 1 is above some criterion, and analogously for simple patterns 2, 3, and so on.

   The third decision rule assumes that the higher levels of processing can tell which output comes from which analyzer, whereas the preceding two decision rules assume only that higher levels use the magnitudes of the different outputs irrespective of which analyzer they come from. A common phrase (although not used in exactly the same way by all authors) for cases where higher levels of processing can tell which output comes from which analyzer is to say that the outputs are labeled (as if the output came upstream with a little label attached saying which analyzer it came from).

Other Characteristics. At one time or another in this book, we will consider other possible characteristics to add to the general framework of Fig. 1.2:

Is there inhibition among low-level analyzers?

Do individual analyzers desensitize (fatigue) after a period of being excited?

Is there variability (noisiness) in the outputs of different analyzers, and if so, what is its probability distribution? Is the variability in different analyzers' outputs correlated or independent?

Can the observer's response be based on the output from only a subset of analyzers?

Are all the analyzers revealed by the various kinds of near-threshold experimental paradigms at the same level (acting in parallel), or are there two or more levels of analyzers (or some other even more complicated organization of analyzers) being revealed?

1.5.1   Pattern and Color Vision Briefly Compared

In the color-vision model, the number of analyzers is very small. In the pattern-vision model, the number of analyzers is a good deal larger; indeed, the number of analyzers on any single dimension of pattern vision (e.g., spatial position) may be quite large.

In the color-vision model, there are two stages of analyzers; in the pattern-vision models discussed here, there is generally only one. Are these pattern analyzers more like the first-stage or the second-stage color analyzers? The answer depends on what properties are considered most important. That the pattern analyzers are usually nonopponent makes them more like the first-stage color analyzers than the second. On the other hand, the first-stage color analyzers (particularly M and L) have highly overlapping sensitivity functions (see upper right Fig. 1.1), whereas on most pattern dimensions having multiple analyzers (e.g., orientation), there are several effectively nonoverlapping ranges of values (e.g., several different orientations responded to by entirely different analyzers). The pattern analyzers' considerable degree of nonoverlap in sensitivity makes them quite different from the first-stage color analyzers.

The necessity for assumptions linking analyzers' outputs to observers' responses is frequently overlooked, particularly when assumptions are made implicitly, as they often have been in discussions of psychophysical experiments. Disagreement between a model and experimental results may be attributed to an error in the models' statements about the lower order analyzers, when the error actually lies in the (all too often implicit) assumption about the link between analyzers' outputs and observers' responses.

Component Percepts in Color. This latter problem is somewhat more acute in discussions of pattern vision than in those of color vision. For, in the case of color vision, there is some concensus about a set of component percepts. That is, most observers agree that the color appearance—at least of isolated small patches—can be subjectively analyzed into and completely described in terms of a small set of color appearances, namely red/green, blue/yellow, and black/white, as already discussed. Extending this analysis to the more complicated stimuli of everyday life requires at least some consideration of spatial relationships and produces some problems—for example, does brown really look like blackened orange? On the whole, however, even when the stimulus is a full visual scene, one can talk of analyzing the perceived color at any point into a few (maybe more than three and only approximately, but still quite well) basic perceptual components.

Of the assumptions linking analyzers' outputs to observers' responses that we will examine for pattern vision, the concurrent-identification one (briefly described previously) is the one most like the assumption for color vision. For it says that an observer will "see" (or, more strictly, will say that he or she sees) a particular simple component pattern if and only if the analyzer sensitive to that component responds enough, just as the color-vision assumption says that a person will "see" red if and only if the R/G analyzer is responding positively. However, in the case of pattern vision, there is no assertion that this assumption applies to all visual stimuli. It is meant only for the compound stimuli made up from a few potential components—all near their own detection thresholds—that appear in near-threshold concurrent identification experiments.

Lack of Component Percepts in Visual Patterns. In fact, no good candidate exists for a set of perceptual form components into which the perception of patterns can be broken down. If there is any higher level decomposition in pattern vision corresponding to our conscious perceptions, the vocabulary seems likely to be something like objects (or perhaps rather large parts of objects) rather than smaller components or features (cf. Biederman, 1985; Treisman, 1986). To put it another way, in the pattern-vision model of Fig. 1.2, much of what is important for full understanding of everyday pattern perception is lumped into the decision stage rather than into the low-level analyzers' stage.

The analyzers in pattern vision are presumably, however, a first step in allowing the visual system to see the objects in the scene. As suggested by the difficulties met in all attempts to think up procedures that could see objects in a scene (e.g., recent attempts to embody such procedures in computer programs include those by Frisby and Mayhew [1980], Marr [1982], and Ullman [1984]), such a computation is at best a multistage affair; thus it is little wonder that the outputs of the low-level analyzers are not represented in any straightforward way in the final perceived scene. (Hochberg [1978] has presented a compact but thorough and profusely illustrated overview of what is known about visual perception from the sensory to the cognitive end.) This does not imply, however, that the low-level analyzers are unimportant for everyday pattern perception. That would be like saying that the existence of three photopigments is unimportant for color perception.

1.5.2 About Simple Decision Rules and Near-Threshold Versus Suprathreshold Pattern Vision

In any case in this book that considers only near-threshold pattern vision, the question of component percepts is—for the most part—not relevant. The observer's responses in these near-threshold experiments are quite simple and, as it turns out, quite simple assumptions linking the outputs of low-level pattern analyzers to these responses prove adequate to predict the results quantitatively.

These simple assumptions are presumably adequate only because they are (perhaps fortuitously) good descriptions of what all the complicated higher level stages of pattern vision actually do in these simple situations. It is (or we can hope it is) as if the simplicity of the experimental situation has made all the higher level stages practically transparent. As mentioned earlier, why this should be so is something of a mystery. (See note 1.) Perhaps—for these simple tasks—the higher stages are able to act optimally, that is, to allow the observer to perform as well as possible. And optimal performance may be very well approximated by simple decision rules in at least some cases. (Optimality is discussed in sections 7.4, 9.4, 9.5, and 10.2.)

Suprathreshold Experiments. Although a number of experiments using visual patterns that are at contrasts far above their own detection thresholds have suggested the existence of analyzers, their results so far are either sketchy or else difficult to interpret in terms of a rigorous model. Considerable difficulty in interpreting the suprathreshold results come from the failures to replicate results across different laboratories or across different observers in the same laboratories. This lack of replicability may have a perfectly respectable source—observers may be able, once patterns are well above threshold, to perform what seems to be the same task in quite different ways. For example, when many analyzers are responding well above threshold, observers might make their decisions on the basis of the maximum output from some subset of mechanisms (and this subset may vary with observer). Or they could base their decisions on subtle aspects of the outputs considered as a function of the spatial positions of analyzers. For example, one observer might base a decision on how many different positions of analyzers were producing large outputs (on "how wide the bright bar looked"—see, for example, Field & Nachmias, 1984; Badcock, 1984a, 1984b; Nachmias & Rogowitz, 1983; Nachmias & Weber, 1975); another might base it on some other imperfectly correlated aspect. As the experiment progresses, particularly if the same discrimination is being repeatedly made, the observer may become more sophisticated about these subtle features, with consequent improvement in performance over a rather long time course. Such learning effects are indeed seen (for example, Fiorentini & Berardi, 1981; Sansbury, 1974; Swift & Smith, 1983).

No matter how respectable the cause of irreproducibility, it has slowed attempts to interpret results. And even with reproducible results (or results not yet known to be unreproducible), interpreting pattern vision experiments in terms of analyzers or any way at all will be difficult, since there are no fixed component percepts in pattern vision. Explanation of suprathreshold results will require much greater elaboration of the assumptions linking the low-level analyzers' outputs to observers' responses than the simple decision rules that have proved adequate for near-threshold experiments. To put it another way, explanation of suprathreshold results requires knowing a good deal more detail about stages of processing higher than the low-level analyzers.

In short, as a consequence of difficulties of replicability and interpretation, suprathreshold experiments have not yielded the quantity and quality of information about low-level analyzers that near-threshold experiments have.

1.6 NEUROPHYSIOLOGY AND PATTERN VISION

In the exploration of pattern vision, the mutual interplay between neurophysiology and psychophysics has been massive. Some neurophysiology is introduced here for its own sake, as an introduction to later concepts but perhaps primarily for the perspective it gives on the role of the visual pattern analyzers in perception. Much more complete reviews of visual neurophysiology can be found in Cowey, 1985; Enroth-Cugell and Robson, 1984; Lennie, 1980b; Robson, 1975, 1980, 1983; Shapley and Enroth-Cugell, 1984; Shapley and Lennie, 1985; Van Essen 1985; and Van Essen and Maunsell, 1983. These sources (at least) should be consulted before any of the following assertions about neurophysiology—many of which are undoubtedly oversimplified due to my lack of knowledge and this book's lack of space—are taken too seriously.

Isolating historical discoveries as done in the following, particularly when doing it partly in order to introduce concepts necessary for other purposes, produces a somewhat artificial view of the flow of history. For a delightful experience and some understanding of how much recent events have been foreshadowed by work in the last century, read Floyd Ratliff's (1965) book *Mach Bands,* which, organized around the work of the 19th-century scientist Mach, ranges widely over visual neurophysiology, psychophysics, and mathematical models. A brief and fascinating history of conceptual developments in the very early history of visual science—starting with the ancient Greeks and continuing through the centuries it took to discover the existence and basic properties of light and of the nervous system—can be found in the first chapter of Boynton (1979). Schiller's (1986) review of the last 25 years of visual neurophysiology also relates a good deal of the relevant history.

Establishing solid links between psychophysical results and possible physiological substrates is extremely difficult, and will not be attempted in this book. My personal policy is this: Whenever new neurophysiological results widen the universe of possible explanations or ways of understanding perception, I consider them, but I never try to use neurophysiology to rule out models (except in certain straightforward, even trivial ways when the physiology is truly completely understood). When in this book I put forward a possible physiological substrate for some entity in a psychophysical model (in particular, cells in area V1 as the substrate for the pattern analyzers), it should not be taken as a necessary aspect of the model. The following statement is true, however: No model suggested in this book to explain psychophysical results is too complicated to be consistent with known neurophysiological results. No matter how many peculiar psychophysical analyzers emerge, there are even more peculiar neurons.

1.6.1 *Visual Pathways in the Nervous System*

Four structures in the visual nervous system of humans are diagrammed in Fig. 1.3: eyes (E), superior colliculus (SC), lateral geniculate nucleus (LGN), and cortex (C). In our bilateral nervous system, each is actually a pair. The pathway

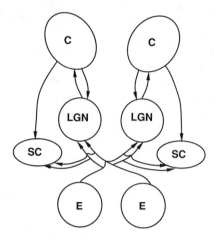

FIG. 1.3 Diagram of major pathways in the human visual system showing eyes (E), superior colliculus (SC), lateral geniculate nucleus (LGN), and cortex (C).

generally considered to be of most importance for pattern vision is that from the eye through the lateral geniculate nucleus to the cortex. The other major pathway, that from the eye to the superior colliculus (which also receives inputs directly from the cortex) may be of less direct importance to pattern vision; it is widely believed to be implicated in eye movements, however, which are certainly of importance in everyday pattern vision and may also be implicated in the initiation of other movements. Several structures not shown in Fig. 1.3 (several subdivisions of the pulvinar and a number of other thalamic and midbrain nuclei) are also heavily interconnected with the visual cortex.

The eye itself does a surprising amount of processing of visual stimuli and is sometimes described as a piece of brain moved out to a sense organ. The eye's retina contains five layers of different types of neurons, two of which will occasionally be mentioned here: the receptors (the cones and rods), which make up the first layer that directly absorbs the light, and the retinal ganglion cells, which make up the last layer, the layer that sends its outputs upstream in the so-called optic nerve. The five layers do extensive calculations on information received from the light before any message at all is sent upstream.

The optic nerve from each eye carries the outputs from the retinal ganglion cells upstream. It bifurcates, sending at least some outputs to each lateral geniculate nucleus and each superior colliculus. The lateral geniculate nucleus will figure little in the discussions in this book because, to a first approximation, it acts like a relay station rather than doing any further spatial or temporal processing of the stimulus. The cortex, however, will figure prominently in later physiological asides. And, for proper appreciation of the cortex as it has recently been revealed, a little further detail is needed.

First, in humans and other primates, a surprisingly large proportion of the full cerebral cortex is devoted to visual processing. One recent review (Van Essen,

1985) estimated this proportion at 24 to 40%. Second, much of this total volume is divided into areas that can be clearly distinguished from one another on several anatomical and physiological criteria. Although in the human only one distinct cortical visual area (striate or V1) had been confidently identified at the time of Van Essen's review, several converging techniques have verified that at least a dozen different such areas exist in the macaque, more precisely, 11 areas considered to be primarily or exclusively visual in function, 4 areas known to be polyfunctional but with a particularly strong visual component, 5 additional candidates for one or the other of these categories, and room in the cortex for at least a few more to be discovered. The number of identified visual areas in the macaque may thus reach two dozen or more. The human cortex is thought to have room for literally dozens of visual areas (Van Essen, 1985).

These areas seem—at least at present—to have quite organized relationships with one another. A possible hierarchy of these cortical visual areas has been inferred from the pattern of corticocortical connections; it is illustrated in Fig. 1.4 (Van Essen & Maunsell, 1983, for an introduction; Van Essen, 1985, for an extensive review). Present information strongly suggests that all connections between cortical areas are reciprocal, and the connections shown in Fig. 1.4 are to be interpreted that way.

The most extensively studied cortical visual area to date is area V1 (also known as the primary visual area, striate cortex, area 17). As mentioned earlier, it seems at present the most likely physiological substrate for the visual pattern analyzers discussed here. It is the area that receives inputs directly from the lateral geniculate nucleus, and is shown at the bottom of Fig. 1.4 as the lowest level in the hierarchy. Note that it has direct and reciprocal major projections with three other visual cortical areas (V2, V3, and MT). The areas V2 and MT (medial temporal but easier to encode as MT for motion) have recently been studied in some detail and will also be mentioned in physiological asides here.

About the other areas less is currently known, although inferotemporal cortex (PIT and AIT) has long been thought to be implicated in pattern and form vision: Lesions there impair performance in pattern discrimination and recognition. Individually these other areas will be mentioned only infrequently in this book. Emphasizing the fact of their existence seems very useful, however, in providing perspective on just what level of visual processing this book may be about.

The hierarchy shown in Fig. 1.4 is based primarily on anatomical considerations, but several pieces of physiological evidence suggest it corresponds to cortical function, with cells at successively higher levels in the hierarchy doing more complicated levels of information analysis. Areas at the same level in the hierarchy may perform different visual functions. Further, there may be several concurrent streams of processing going upward through this hierarchy. They are thought to be segregated as early as the lateral geniculate nucleus and then continue upward through several levels of the presumed cortical hierarchy. Roughly speaking, and available evidence will certainly not support a more precise statement, one stream seems very concerned with the processing of motion infor-

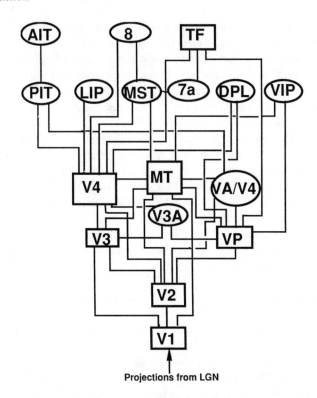

FIG. 1.4 A possible hierarchy of visual areas in the cortex of primates. Well-defined areas are indicated by boxes, less well-characterized areas by ellipses. Abbreviations in alphabetical order: AIT—anterior inferotemporal; DPL—dorsal prelunate; LIP—lateral intraparietal; LGN—lateral geniculate nucleus; MST—medial superior temporal; MT—middle temporal (also known as V5); PIT—posterior inferotemporal; TF—small area in temporal lobe; VA—ventral anterior; VIP—ventral intraparietal; VP—ventral posterior; V1—visual area 1; V2—visual area 2; V3—visual area 3; V4—visual area 4; 7a—in parietal cortex; 8—frontal eye field.

A stream of processing particularly concerned with motion perception may start with the magnocellular neurons in the LGN and continue upward through particular layers of V1 to MT and MST. Streams particularly concerned with form and color perception may start with the parvicellular neurons in the LGN and continue upward through particular parts of V1 to the areas V2, V4, PIT, and AIT. (Figure 7 of Van Essen [1985]; Copyright 1985; reprinted by permission.)

mation, one with form, and one with color (e.g., DeYoe and Van Essen 1988; Van Essen, 1985). The evidence for these streams is based on physiological recordings showing different patterns of selectivity for different neurons, a subject discussed extensively below. (Although there is no doubt that the neurons with different selectivities exist, the evidence for streams through several areas is scantier.)

In summary, the most likely physiological substrate for the visual pattern analyzers is the neurons of area V1 (and maybe V2). In the full stream of visual processing suggested by current physiological and anatomical knowledge, these neurons are someplace before the middle, and they may form something of a bottleneck in the processes important for shape and pattern perception.

1.6.2 Properties of Single Visual Neurons

In the earliest concepts of the visual nervous system, each single point of light on the retina initiated activity that was relayed essentially unchanged to higher levels in the nervous system. Thus the activity in, for example, the visual cortex of the brain was thought to be a point-by-point mapping of the stimulus reaching the retina. That map might be stretched and expanded, but was otherwise faithful.

Indeed, crude spatial mappings do exist. Neurons in one position in area V1 respond to light stimulating the fovea (the center of the retina); neurons at a nearby position in the same area respond to light stimulating the retina slightly to the left of the fovea, and so forth. These mappings are somewhat distorted, with the amount of area V1 receiving projections from any small retinal area being bigger the closer that area is to the fovea. This kind of distortion seems quite appropriate given how much better humans see detail presented in the fovea than in the periphery.

These crude spatial mappings, however, are only a small part of the story. Neurons, even at a single level of the nervous system, differ from one another in many spatial and temporal characteristics. For beginning this complicated and beautiful story, four investigators—Granit, Hartline, Hubel, and Wiesel— have won Nobel prizes in the last 25 years, and others might well have. A very brief review is given later in this chapter of the spatial and temporal characteristics of visual neurons and of how the discovery of these characteristics has influenced psychophysical theories and investigations (and vice versa). More details about these neurons and how they compare with the analyzers in psychophysical models will be given in physiological asides in later chapters.

The assertions, unless otherwise qualified, are based on work with the cat and the monkey, the higher animals on which most single-unit neurophysiology has been done. It is, in general, not possible to do the neurophysiology on humans, but one hopes to be able to generalize from these higher animals, particularly from primates. In any case, the more that is systematically known about the neurophysiology of higher animals, the greater the amount that can be learned from the small amount of electrophysiological recording possible on humans— during surgery, for example.

1.6.3 A Brief Mention of Sinusoids

A brief description of sinusoidal stimuli is given here (more is given in Chap. 2) to prepare for discussion of the responses of neurons to sinusoidal gratings.

A sinusoidal grating (e.g., Fig. 2.1) looks like a striped pattern with alternating, blurry, light and dark stripes. Its spatial frequency is the number of cycles (light-bar–dark-bar pairs) per unit distance, where distance is usually measured as degrees of visual angle. Thus the higher the spatial frequency, the narrower the stripes.

A sinusoidally flickering blank field is a homogeneous field getting brighter and dimmer repetitively. The repetition rate, that is, the number of light-dark cycles per unit time (usually seconds) is called the temporal frequency.

If a sinusoidal grating is drifted across the visual field (as if behind an opening or window) or if it is flickered, the temporal frequency is the number of light-dark cycles per unit time at any one point in the pattern.

The contrast of any pattern will be defined here to equal one half the difference between the lightest point and the darkest point divided by the mean luminance. Thus contrast can vary between 0 and 1 (or 0 and 100%).

1.7   SPATIAL CHARACTERISTICS OF VISUAL NEURONS

1.7.1   *Antagonism Between Excitation and Inhibition*

Soon after it became technically possible to record from single visual neurons, it was discovered that each neuron had a "receptive field," a rather extended region of the retina within which light stimulation elicits a response from the neuron (Hartline, 1938). One very common type of receptive-field organization (first reported by Kuffler [1953] in the cat and by Barlow [1953] in the frog) has come to be called a *center surround* or *concentric* organization and is represented in the upper left of Fig. 1.5. There are two sections to this kind of receptive field, one a circle and the other an annulus surrounding it. Light shining on one section (indicated by plus signs in Fig. 1.5) excites the neuron, causing an increase in its firing rate. Light shining in the other region (indicated by minus signs) inhibits the neuron, causing a decrease in its firing rate. The excitatory section can be either the center section (in which case the receptive field is often called an *on-center* or just *on* receptive field) or the surround. This receptive-field organization is the dominant one for primate retinal ganglion cells, but it also occurs in a few cortical cells.

Influence on and by Psychophysics. This antagonism between excitation and inhibition was early related to a number of perceptual phenomena, for example, the perceived appearance of Mach bands (the illusory light and dark stripes that an observer sees on either side of a slightly blurred edge between a dark and a light region). In fact, the existence of such antagonism was suggested on the basis of the perceptual results before the neurophysiology was known (see, e.g., Ratliff, 1965). Other perceptual results attributed to this antagonism include the "sensitization effect" of annuli on the thresholds for disks (Westheimer, 1965, 1967) and the dark appearance at the intersections of the white lines in the Hermann grid (Baumgartner, 1960).

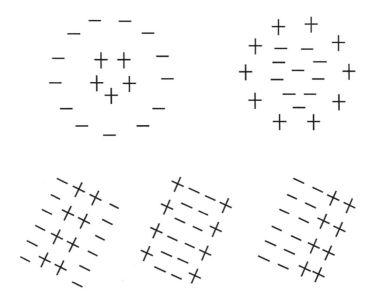

FIG. 1.5 Various kinds of receptive fields found for visual neurons. Plus signs (+) indicate regions in which light excites the neuron, minus signs (−) regions in which light inhibits the neuron.

1.7.2 Orientation Selectivity

Many cells in the lowest visual cortical areas (V1 and V2) of cat and monkey and presumably human—those cells called *simple cells* in the ground-breaking work of Hubel and Wiesel (1962, 1965, 1968, 1974, 1977)—have separate excitatory and inhibitory regions in their receptive fields, but these regions are not concentric. They have elongated receptive fields when mapped with spots of light, like those shown in Fig. 1.5 bottom. The elongated excitatory and inhibitory sections are usually arranged side by side. The fields may have even symmetry with either the excitatory or inhibitory section in the middle (left and middle sketches in bottom row of Fig. 1.5) or odd symmetry (right bottom sketch in Fig. 1.5) or in between. The overall orientation of the receptive fields can be vertical, horizontal, or anything in between (as in the oblique fields of Fig. 1.5).

As you might suppose, neurons with oriented receptive fields are most sensitive to lines or gratings when they are oriented at precisely the same angle as the receptive field. More particularly, in the case of these simple cortical neurons, the receptive field mapped with small spots permits qualitative prediction of the neuron's output to any other stimulus in an intuitively straightforward way: The more light that is falling in the excitatory section, the greater the neuron's output, whereas the more light that is falling in the inhibitory section, the less the neuron's output. In other words, the neuron acts as an adding and subtracting device. Technically, the neuron is, at least approximately, a linear system—a concept discussed in detail in Chap. 2. To convince yourself that the best orientation of a line or grating stimulus is parallel to the regions in the oriented receptive field, imagine lines or gratings of different orientations superimposed on one of the oriented receptive fields in Fig. 1.5 and roughly calculate how much excitation and inhibition is evoked. In fact, given the appropriate balance of excitation and inhibition, such neurons may not respond at all to lines or gratings at a perpendicular orientation.

In addition to these simple cells, cortical areas V1 and V2 contain the cells Hubel and Wiesel called *complex*. For a complex cell, a receptive field map either cannot be made with small spots of light or does not correctly predict outputs to other stimuli. (For a review of evidence relating the simple versus complex distinction to a linear- versus nonlinear-system distinction, see Shapley and Lennie, 1985). Although unlike simple cells in many ways, these complex cells also show orientation selectivity, the preferred orientation differing from cell to cell ranging over the full 360 degrees of a circle.

Both simple and complex cells also vary in their "orientation bandwidth," that is, in how wide a range of orientations they will respond to (e.g., De Valois, Yund, & Hepler, 1982).

Influence on Psychophysics. Very soon after the original Hubel and Wiesel studies, the existence of orientation-selective cortical cells was suggested as the basis for existing psychophysical results (e.g., the tilt aftereffect in which a line slightly tilted from the vertical looks even further from the vertical after a vertical line is viewed) and inspired new experiments using oriented stimuli (e.g., Andrews, 1967a, 1967b; Campbell & Kulikowski, 1966; Gilinsky, 1968; MacKay, 1957; McCollough, 1965; Sekuler, 1965). The portion of this work using near-threshold stimuli will be discussed at length later in this book. Thomas's (1986) paper is a brief history of the influence of neurophysiological findings on psychophysical studies of spatial vision from 1961 to 1986.

1.7.3   Size, or Spatial-Frequency, Selectivity

Although not emphasized in the original Hubel and Wiesel studies, later investigators have discovered that both simple and cortical cells have another important property. Not only are they selective for the orientation of a line or grating, but they are selective for the width of the line (or bars in the grating). (Early studies of this selectivity include those by Campbell, Cooper, and Enroth-Cugell, 1969, and by Maffei and Fiorentini, 1973.) This property is actually predictable from the properties of simple cortical cells as just described. For simple cells should respond best to a line when it is of approximately the same width as an excitatory section of the field (and positioned in that section); the cells may not respond at all to much wider lines and will respond much less to narrower lines. Similarly, they respond best to a sinusoidal grating when the widths of the bars match the widths of the individual regions in the receptive field; they will not respond to gratings of very different bar width. Since the spatial frequency of a grating is just the number of light-dark bar pairs per unit distance, this selectivity for bar width in gratings is often called spatial-frequency selectivity. As it happens, not only simple but also complex cells exhibit this spatial-frequency selectivity. More important than the selectivity of any single cell is the fact that different cortical cells (simple or complex) have very different preferred spatial frequencies, spanning the full range of visible spatial frequencies (for the species under consideration). Also, cells differ from one another in their spatial-frequency bandwidth, that is, in how wide a range of spatial frequencies they respond to well (see, e.g., De Valois, Albrecht, & Thorell, 1982; Foster, Gaska Nagler, & Pollen, 1985; Movshon, Thompson & Tolhurst, 1978c; Schiller, Finlay, & Volman, 1976c; Tolhurst & Thompson, 1981).

Influence on and by Psychophysics. Long before the spatial-frequency selectivity of individual cortical neurons was measured, the possible implications for perception of the existence of receptive fields with different sizes of excitatory regions was independently and simultaneously considered by at least three different groups of investigators. James Thomas and his colleagues at the University of California at Los Angeles used the variation in receptive-field size to explain a number of psychophysical results when the stimuli were different-sized disks (reviewed in Thomas, 1970). Allan Pantle and Robert Sekuler at Northwestern University, Evanston, Illinois, studied the psychophysical effect of adaptation to gratings of different spatial frequencies on the expectation that the greatest threshold elevation would occur when the adapting and test gratings were of the same spatial frequency, because then they would affect receptive fields of the same sizes (Pantle & Sekuler, 1968a). And a group of investigators working with John Robson, Fergus Campbell, and Colin Blakemore of Cambridge University, England, used the existence of receptive fields of different sizes to explain psychophysical sensitivity to compound stimuli containing sinusoidal gratings of different spatial frequencies, and also to explain the effect of adaptation to sinusoidal gratings of different spatial frequencies (e.g., Blakemore & Campbell, 1969; Campbell & Robson, 1964, 1968; Enroth-Cugell & Robson, 1966). The Cambridge group was the first to point out the potential usefulness of Fourier analysis (see Chap. 2) for understanding multiple analyzers selectively sensitive to different line widths (spatial frequencies). The Cambridge group also affords a particularly dramatic example of the interplay between psychophysics and neurophysiology, as these investigators collected both kinds of results themselves.

1.8 TEMPORAL CHARACTERISTICS OF VISUAL NEURONS

1.8.1 *Direction-of-Motion Selectivity*

Some visual neurons are strongly direction selective, responding well to a bar or grating moving in one direction but not responding at all to motion in the other direction. Found in the retina of many animals, including the cat, the gray squirrel, and the ground squirrel (but not the monkey), retinal directionally selective units have been most extensively studied in the rabbit, where a mechanism for producing this direction selectivity was proposed (Barlow, Hill, & Levick, 1964). Of more direct relevance to the psychophysical results, direction selectivity is present in cortical neurons of cats and monkeys and presumably humans (e.g., De Valois et al., 1982; Foster et al., 1985; Hubel & Wiesel, 1962, 1965, 1968, 1977; Tolhurst, Dean, & Thompson, 1981).

Distinctions have been made between several possible kinds of direction selectivity that may well underlie different psychophysical results. For some neurons (including many in V1 that project to MT), the preferred direction reverses if the light bar is replaced by a dark bar. Other neurons, however, including complex neurons in V1, show a stronger kind of direction selectivity, where the preferred direction of motion is the same for a light bar as for a dark bar.

A further clear distinction can be made with the aid of a compound stimulus composed of two superimposed gratings of different orientations seen moving behind an aperture (Movshon, Adelson, Gizzi, & Newsome, 1984). To a human observer, as long as the contrasts and spatial frequencies of the two gratings are rather similar, such a compound stimulus looks like a plaid and seems to move in the direction that each of the intersections between bars move in; let's call this the global direction of the pattern. (When each component grating is seen by itself, however, it seems to move in a direction perpendicular to the bars.) The question is how a neuron that is directionally selective when tested with single moving gratings responds to this compound pattern. Is its response based on the direction of the component gratings—that is, does it respond best when a component of the compound is moving in the originally preferred direction? Or is its response based on the global direction of the pattern—that is, does it respond best when the global direction of the pattern is in the originally preferred direction? By this criterion, some neurons (including many in V1) respond to the components and others (notably many in MT) to the global pattern direction.

Influence on and by Psychophysics. The existence of direction-selective neurons, along with an assumption that they show fatigue or desensitization after a period of excitation, early was used to explain several perceptual phenomena, notably the waterfall effect or motion aftereffect, in which, after a moving stimulus has been looked at for some time, a stationary stimulus appears to move in the opposite direction (Barlow & Hill, 1963), and direction-selective threshold elevation after adaptation to gratings (Sekuler & Ganz, 1963). Since then, a good deal of psychophysical work has continued to explore selectivity for direction of motion. The distinction between selectivity for global pattern direction and selectivity for component direction has been explored with human observers as well as with neurons. As previously mentioned, whenever the spatial frequencies, contrasts, and orientations of the two components are not too dissimilar, human observers perceive the suprathreshold compound pattern as a plaid moving in the global direction. Once the spatial frequencies, contrasts, or orientations of the two components are very different, however, the human observer sees the suprathreshold compound pattern as two separate gratings, each moving in a direction perpendicular to its own bars (Adelson & Movshon, 1982). The extensive work done with near-threshold stimuli moving in various directions will be presented in later chapters of this book.

1.8.2 Sustained Versus Transient Responses (Temporal-Frequency Selectivity)

At any given background level of illumination, some retinal ganglion cells respond better to stimulus transients (the onset and offset of stationary stimuli) than to maintained stationary stimuli, and such cells also respond quite well to stimuli of very high velocities. To put it another way, these cells respond somewhat better to high than to low temporal frequencies. Other neurons give more sustained responses throughout a stationary stimulus and do not respond well to stimuli moving at high velocities. That is, these cells seem to respond better to low than to high temporal frequencies. Cleland, Dubin, and Levick (1971) used the names *transient* and *sustained* to distinguish between these kinds of retinal ganglion cells in the cat. (As discussed below, these temporal differences among cells turn out to be highly correlated with a difference between linear and nonlinear behavior.)

In cat and primate cortex, some similar differences have been found between the temporal characteristics of cells in area V1 and those in area V2, with those in area V2 appearing more transient (Foster et al., 1985; Movshon et al., 1978c). These differences among cortical neurons in temporal characteristics—which can be described as differences in temporal-frequency selectivity (see Chap. 2)— are not as dramatic as the differences among cortical neurons in spatial-frequency selectivity.

Influence on Psychophysics. The initial emphasis on the distinction between sustained and transient retinal ganglion cells inspired an enormous amount of psychophysical work based on an hypothesized distinction between sustained (or pattern) and transient (or motion) analyzers (Breitmeyer & Ganz, 1976; Kulikowski & Tolhurst, 1973; Matin, 1975; Tolhurst, 1973; Weisstein, Ozog, & Szoc, 1975; to mention only a few of the early references). This psychophysical work in turn inspired more careful evaluation of the actual temporal differences among neurons (see Lennie, 1980b, for a review). As the years have passed, the nature of the possible psychophysical distinctions has become clearer, as has the fact that the sustained and transient retinal ganglion cells (in the cat) are not sufficiently analogous to the possible distinctions between psychophysical analyzers to be a likely physiological substrate for them. Instead, distinctions between concurrent streams of processing through the primate cortical hierarchy of Fig. 1.4 (in particular, between streams coming from the parvo- versus magnocellular divisions of the LGN) are often discussed in this context (see the paragraphs on direction-selectivity in Section 12.7.2).

1.9 OTHER CHARACTERISTICS OF VISUAL NEURONS

1.9.1 Dependence on Contrast

In general, the output of visual neurons increases as the contrast of the pattern increases. When a neuron's output (averaged across trials of the same stimulus) is plotted as a function of contrast, there is sometimes a threshold contrast below which no response is elicited from the neuron. Above this threshold (which may be zero), the average output increases linearly with contrast over quite a range of contrasts. Then, at high enough contrasts, the average output ceases to rise linearly with contrast but begins rapid compression to an asymptotic level (e.g., in the cortex of cat and monkey, Albrecht & Hamilton, 1982; Tolhurst, Movshon, & Thompson, 1981). The exact shape of this function varies a great deal from neuron to neuron.

There is also variation from neuron to neuron in whether positive contrasts (e.g., luminance increments on a background) or negative contrasts (e.g., luminance decrements on a background) lead to excitatory outputs.

1.9.2 Dependence on Mean Luminance

Visual neurons adapt to the prevailing average luminance level. As mean luminance increases, so does the difference that must exist between the peak and mean luminances of a pattern for that pattern to elicit a criterion-sized output from the neuron. Indeed, the necessary difference is approximately proportional to mean luminance (at high enough mean luminances). In other words, the necessary contrast—where contrast equals that difference divided by mean luminance—stays approximately constant. Furthermore, the time course of the neuron's output typically changes, becoming less sustained (more transient) as mean luminance increases. This light adaptation is visible in the outputs of retinal ganglion cells (reviewed in Shapley & Enroth-Cugell, 1984) and is reflected in the outputs of cortical cells.

In general, cortical neurons do not respond to blank stationary fields at all, and their outputs in general do not convey information about the mean luminance level (although see Bartlett and Doty, 1974, for a report of a subpopulation of cells that do).

1.9.3 Monocularity Versus Binocularity

Cortical cells also differ in whether they are responsive to the right eye, the left eye, or both (and if both, to what extent the eyes are equal). In the monkey there is a greater tendency for one eye to be dominant than in the cat (Hubel & Wiesel, 1962, 1968). (Cortical cells that are binocularly driven may also differ from each other with regard to what disparity they are most sensitive to, but depth per se is beyond the scope of this book and no more will be said.)

1.9.4 Linearity, Intracortical Inhibition, Variability, and Adaptability

Linearity or No? A linear system is one that, crudely speaking, just adds and subtracts inputs. (See Chap. 2 for more details.) A rigorous investigation of the linear behavior of visual neurons was first undertaken by Enroth-Cugell and Robson (1966), who discovered that they could use linearity to make a clear distinction between two types of cat retinal ganglion cells. Some of the cells they studied—the ones they called X cells—behave very much like linear systems in a number of situations (as long as the range of luminances remains relatively restricted). Y cells, on the other hand, do not act like linear systems (e.g., Hochstein & Shapley, 1976a, 1976b). A good introduction to and overview of work on the linearity of visual neurons can be found in Hochstein and Spitzer (1985) and in Shapley and Lennie (1985).

Intracortical Inhibition. The output of a cell to nonpreferred orientations, spatial frequencies, and directions may be lessened by inhibition from other cortical neurons and, indeed, this inhibition may be a major source of the selectivity shown by cortical neurons (e.g., Burr, Morrone, & Maffei, 1981; De Valois & Tootell, 1983; Foster et al., 1985; Morrone, Burr, & Maffei, 1982; Movshon et al., 1978c; Sillito, 1977; Sillito & Versiani, 1977).

Variability. A neuron's output to the same stimulus is not constant but varies from occasion to occasion, as has been noted by every physiological investigator and systematically investigated by a few (e.g., Barlow & Levick, 1969; Dean, 1981b; Tolhurst, Movshon, & Dean, 1983; Tolhurst, Movshon, & Thompson, 1981).

Adaptability. Cortical neurons are less sensitive to test patterns after a long presentation of an adapting pattern than they were before if the test and adapting stimulus are similar (Albrecht, Farrar, & Hamilton, 1984; Dean, 1983; Maffei, Fiorentini, & Bisti, 1973; Movshon & Lennie, 1979; Vautin & Berkley, 1977). This adaptation may help maintain differential sensitivity to changes in contrast around the prevailing background level of contrast (Albrecht et al., 1984; Ohzawa, Sclar, & Freeman, 1982). A potentially similar "contrast-gain" mechanism has been investigated thoroughly and described quantitatively in the retina of the cat (Shapley & Victor, 1978, 1979).

1.10 SOME TERMINOLOGY: ANALYZER, NEURON, MECHANISM, CHANNEL, AND ELEMENT

Analyzer. According to the definition being used here, an analyzer is simply something that is sensitive to a range of values along a dimension of interest. The analyzers that are used to explain the results of each kind of psychophysical experiment in subsequent chapters are specified in greater detail by listing the assumptions relevant in each place.

Neurons. The physiological substrate for an analyzer so generally defined might equally well be many things, including (a) a single neuron, or (b) an array of neurons that are homogeneous in some sense. For example, the neurons might all be sensitive to the same values on one or more dimensions of interest (e.g., orientation and spatial frequency), although they may be sensitive to different values on some other dimension (e.g., spatial position). So, for example, if you took all the neurons in V1 that had peak sensitivity for vertical orientations and 3 cycles per degree—no matter what their other properties were (e.g., no matter what spatial positions their receptive fields were centered at)—this array of neurons would serve as an analyzer on both the orientation and spatial-frequency dimensions.

To avoid using neurophysiological terms in the psychophysical models discussed throughout the rest of the book, some further terms to refer to entities in psychophysical models (without commitment to any particular physiology) will be defined here. In addition to analyzer, already introduced as the very general term, two further terms corresponding to a single neuron (mechanism) and to an array of neurons (channel) may be usefully defined.

Mechanism. A mechanism is the entity in a psychophysical model that is analogous to a single neuron. It is something that produces an output in response to a given stimulus, where the output is, in general, a function of time. Often, however, the output is considered to be a single number by taking the maximal instantaneous response, or integrating over a given time period, and so on.

Channel. It has often proved convenient to have a single word for a group of mechanisms where the group is usually homogeneous in some sense; the word *channel* will be so used here. The output of a channel to a visual pattern will not, in general, be a function only of time. For example, if you consider all mechanisms with peak sensitivity to the vertical orientation and to 3 cpd, the output of the channel is itself a group of outputs, each from one mechanism and each a function of time. If you simply number the mechanisms in the channel with an index ranging from 1 to N (the total number of mechanisms in the channel), the output of the channel can be expressed as a function of two dimensions— time and index number. Sometimes, however, those mechanisms may be systematically ordered along some other dimensions—for example, the two dimensions specifying the spatial position of the center of each mechanisms's receptive field. In that case, the output of the channel can be expressed as a function of time and two spatial dimensions. (A function giving the output of a channel at each point along relevant dimensions will sometimes be referred to below as an *output profile*.)

Frequently, a single number is extracted from the output profile and referred to as the *output of the channel*. The usual candidates for this single number are the largest value in the output profile—called the maximum or peak output— and the difference between the largest and smallest values—called the peak-trough or maximum-minimum difference.

Be warned that the term *channel* has been used in different ways in pattern vision and related areas. It has, for example, been occasionally used in the way the word *mechanism* is used here. More dangerously for our purposes, it has also been used to refer to a more elaborate concept, including not only a low-level analyzer but some assumptions about how the outputs of the analyzers determine perception or observers' responses.

Element. A final term for entities in psychophysical models will be useful in subsequent chapters and, for completeness' sake, it is introduced here. This is a term for a single mechanism at a single point in time (analogous to a single neuron at a single point in time). As it is the simplest, most elementary entity in the models discussed here, it will be called an *element.* The output of an element is always a single number.

1.11   FIVE PSYCHOPHYSICAL PARADIGMS

Five different kinds of psychophysical experiments using near-threshold patterns are covered in this book. Extensions of this list of experimental types to include some suprathreshold experiments can be found, for example in Braddick, Campbell, and Atkinson, 1978, and in Graham, 1981 (for pattern vision), in McBurney, 1978 (for taste), and in Treisman, 1986 (for pattern vision and object perception).

1.11.1   *Adaptation-Near-Threshold Paradigm*

An adaptation-near-threshold experiment measures the effect on an observer's detection thresholds of adapting to some other stimulus for an extended period (typically minutes). Typically, the adapting and test stimuli used in an experiment vary along some dimension of interest (e.g., wavelength, orientation, spatial frequency). A common result of such experiments is selective adaptation—that is, the greatest threshold elevation occurs for test stimuli that are identical to or very similar to the adapting stimulus, and lesser threshold elevation occurs whenever test and adapting stimuli are dissimilar. Selective adaptation is usually taken as evidence for the existence of multiple analyzers sensitive to different ranges along the dimension of interest (see Chap. 3).

Adaptation versus Masking Experiments. To clarify what is meant by the adaptation-near-threshold paradigm in this book and why it is included here although similar paradigms are excluded, some further comments seem useful.

The words *masking* and *adaptation* are sometimes used interchangeably to describe paradigms in which the presence of one stimulus (the masking or adapting stimulus) affects, usually detrimentally, the perception of another stimulus (the test stimulus). Here, however, I will use these terms to mean two different kinds of experiments, in order to keep track of a difference in procedure that seems crucial.

An *adaptation experiment* (the kind discussed in this book) will be one in which the test stimulus is presented after a relatively prolonged exposure (at least a number of seconds, usually minutes) of the adapting stimulus and after the adapting stimulus has itself been removed (preferably for some seconds).

A pure *masking experiment* is one in which the test stimulus and masking stimulus are of relatively short duration and are presented simultaneously or at least very close to simultaneously (within a few hundred milliseconds).

Effects in adaptation and masking experiments may well have different sources. The effects in adaptation experiments may involve relatively long-term changes in the properties of underlying analyzers. An easy example of such a long-term change is the bleaching of pigments in retinal receptors, a change often used to explain effects in color adaptation experiments. The effects in pure masking experiments, however, may not involve changes in the properties of underlying analyzers at all. These effects may come about instead because the outputs of the visual system to both the masking and the test stimulus are occurring simultaneously and the observer must, in some sense, disentangle the two to know how to respond to the test stimulus. Consider, for example, a masking experiment in which the observer's threshold for the test stimulus is being measured. Another way to view this experiment is that the minimal contrast at which the observer can discriminate between the mask and the mask-plus-test is being measured. Note that, once the masking stimulus is above its own detection threshold (as it almost always is), the observer is actually making a discrimination between two suprathreshold stimuli—the mask-plus-test combination versus the test alone. All such masking experiments are, therefore, suprathreshold experiments, and their interpretations encounter the difficulties that beset suprathreshold experiments in general. As a consequence, masking experiments are not included here. Mixed masking-plus-adaptation experiments, in which the interfering stimulus is on steadily both before, during, and after the short-duration test stimulus, are also not included except occasionally (in situations where no information from pure adaptation experiments is available).

Terminological Note. The words *adaptation* and *masking* are often used not only as names for experimental paradigms but also as names for the hypothesized processes that explain the effects measured in the experimental paradigms. The process that is referred to in Chap. 3 as "desensitization" or "fatigue," for example, is often called "adaptation."

1.11.2 Summation-Near-Threshold Paradigm

In summation-near-threshold experiments, the detection threshold for a compound stimulus—a stimulus containing two or more values along some dimension of interest (e.g., two lines at different orientations)—is compared with the detection thresholds for the component simple stimuli by themselves (e.g., each line by itself). Summation is said to occur if the threshold for the compound stimulus is less than the thresholds for both components (the observer's sensitivity to the compound is greater than sensitivity to either component). A typical result is to find that summation is greatest when the two values in the compound stimulus are close together on the dimension of interest, and that summation is less once the two values are far apart. Such value-selective summation is frequently taken as evidence for analyzers along the dimension of interest. (See Chap. 4.)

1.11.3   Uncertainty-Near-Threshold Paradigm

In uncertainty-near-threshold experiments, the detectability of a stimulus (typically a simple stimulus, that is, a stimulus containing only a single value on the dimension of interest) is measured both when the observer is certain as to which stimulus will be presented and when the observer is uncertain (typically because trials of many different stimuli are randomly intermixed). A typical result is that uncertainty causes a greater decrement in performance when the intermixed stimuli are far apart in value (e.g., of very different orientations) than when they are close together. Again this value-selective behavior can be taken as evidence for the existence of multiple analyzers. (See Chap. 7.)

1.11.4   Identification-Near-Threshold Paradigm

In identification-near-threshold experiments, the observer's ability to identify which of several near-threshold stimuli has been presented is measured. A number of rather different experiments, which have often been called by different names (e.g., discrimination, recognition), are being grouped together under this title: (a) forced-choice discrimination between two equally detectable stimuli, (b) identification of which of several simple stimuli was presented on a single-interval trial, (c) identification of which of several simple or compound stimuli were presented on a single-interval trial, (d) the 2 × 2 (two-by-two) paradigm in which each two-alternative forced-choice trial contains one blank and one pattern; the observer must say both which pattern it was (identification response) and which alternative was the pattern rather than the blank (detection response). Forced-choice discrimination is discussed in Chap. 9, the others in Chap. 10.

In many near-threshold identification experiments (and always in the 2 × 2 paradigm), the observer's ability to detect each pattern—that is, to discriminate each from a blank field—is measured simultaneously with the ability to identify which pattern it was.

Again, as with the first three paradigms, value-selective behavior is often observed. In particular, there is often more confusability among similar stimuli, or to put it the other way, better identifiability of dissimilar stimuli. This value-selective behavior is frequently taken as evidence for multiple analyzers along the dimension of interest. (See Chap. 9.)

1.11.5   Parametric-Contrast-Sensitivity Paradigm

In parametric-contrast-sensitivity experiments (Chap. 13), the observer's detection threshold is measured for simple patterns as a function of value along some dimension of interest.

Analyzer-Revealing Versus Parametric Paradigms. The first four paradigms—adaptation-near-threshold, summation-near-threshold, uncertainty-near-threshold, and identification-near-threshold—all differ from the last—parametric-contrast-sensitivity—in one very important respect. As we shall discuss in subsequent chapters, results from the first four can answer the question of whether multiple analyzers exist on a given dimension. That is, they are paradigms that can test between single-analyzer and multiple-analyzer models. The parametric paradigm, on the other hand, produces results that are guaranteed to be consistent with either single- or multiple-analyzer models. The results do, however, give further information about the dimension of interest, either by specifying the sensitivity of the single analyzer, if there is only one, or by specifying the overall sensitivity of the group of multiple analyzers.

1.11.6   Modified Paradigms Measuring Appearance Thresholds

Four of the preceding five paradigms (all but identification) measure an observer's ability to discriminate a pattern from a blank field (detection thresholds). A modified form of each of these four is sometimes used, however. Instead of measuring detection thresholds, a related kind of threshold—called *appearance thresholds* here—is measured. The claim is made that, in addition to setting detection thresholds indicating the minimum contrast at which anything other than a blank field is seen, observers can set thresholds using two other qualitatively different citeria. These two criteria are based on two different kinds of appearances that near-threshold patterns can have.

The initial observation, which is generally agreed on (van Nes, Koenderink, Nas, & Bouman, 1967; Kulikowski & Tohurst, 1973; Tolhurst, 1973; Tulunay-Keesey, 1972) is that patterns at detection threshold do have quite different appearances depending on their spatial and temporal frequencies, and these appearances are roughly of two sorts: a predominantly spatial appearance and a predominantly temporal appearance. In particular, gratings of high spatial frequency tend to appear stationary at threshold even when they are flickering, drifting, or turning on and off. Gratings of low spatial frequency appear more like what a naive person thinks they should—as a flickering grating or a stationary grating depending on their condition. Sometimes it is claimed that low-spatial-frequency gratings do not look like gratings at all, that is, their bars cannot be seen, only an appearance of temporal change can. At contrasts far enough above detection threshold, however, perceived appearances become "veridical" in the sense that a flickering, drifting, or on/off grating appears to be just what it is—a grating with distinct bars and distinct temporal change, no matter what its spatial and temporal frequency may be.

Agreement ceases to be universal when the further claim is made that observers can use two separate criteria—one a spatial (or pattern or sustained) criterion and the other a temporal (or motion or flicker or transient) criterion—and use them consistently. A number of studies have reported two kinds of thresholds, so the observers in these studies were obviously able to do the task (see reference lists in Chaps. 12 and 13). The criteria might not always have been exactly the same, however, even in these studies. Further, not all investigators have been able to get observers reliably to set something that might be called a spatial or pattern threshold for temporally modulated low spatial frequencies. M. Green (1980) (cf. also Watson & Nachmias, 1977) felt he had to settle for the overall detection threshold and a temporal-change (flicker) threshold when using gratings turning on and off at 8 cps. A final worry is that the measured sensitivities using these two criteria seem to differ from study to study (see Chap. 13). If too unstable, of course, these appearance thresholds will be of little use in revealing the mechanisms of pattern vision.

For the present, however, there continue to be many studies measuring such appearance thresholds, and they appear to be yielding some information. They are particularly crucial to theories of analyzers on a temporal-frequency dimension, theories that sometimes postulate two different kinds of analyzer (corresponding to the two different kinds of threshold).

1.12 SOME PRACTICAL MATTERS

This section describes some practical details of near-threshold pattern vision experiments. It can be skipped with little loss of continuity.

1.12.1 Generating the Stimulus

Since the early work of Schade (1948, 1956, 1958), sinusoidal gratings and related spatiotemporal patterns have typically been generated on the face of an oscilloscope or television or other display device using a cathode-ray tube (see section 13.12.1).

Keeping Mean Luminance Constant. On such displays, it is easy to keep the mean luminance constant while changing the type and contrast of pattern. Unless otherwise specified, all results discussed in this book for visual patterns were obtained in experiments where the mean luminance and hue of the visual display were constant throughout the experiment. Not only were all patterns at the same mean luminance, but the luminance and hue of the blank field occurring between patterns were the same as those of the pattern. This constant mean luminance means that the levels of adaptation in processes early in the visual system, at the receptors for example, may be constant throughout the experiment. (See note 1, but also see section 3.9 for discussion of the possible consequences of uneven early local adaptation.)

Traditional Optical Systems. Although it is possible to generate transparencies that produce good sinusoidal patterns when inserted into an optical system, it is not easy, and one needs a different transparency for each pattern. Further, changing the contrast of patterns with neutral-density filters, as is done in optical systems, also changes the mean luminance. Keeping mean luminance constant, therefore, requires a compensating source of luminance.

Most of the studies reported in this book, and almost all of the studies in which the stimuli were sinusoidal gratings, generated stimuli using cathode-ray displays. Those cases where the same results have been found using both oscilloscopes and optical systems are quite reassuring, since the possible artifacts introduced by the two systems are quite different.

1.12.2 Psychophysical Methods

Method of Adjustment. One common way of measuring detection thresholds is the method of adjustment. The observer simply adjusts (by pushing a button, turning a knob, or sometimes verbally instructing an experimenter) the contrast of the pattern until it is "at threshold" or "just visible." Often the pattern is on continuously during an adjustment, although sometimes short presentations of it are alternated with short presentations of a blank field. This method has the advantage of being quick and congenial to many observers. In one form, where the pattern is physically present at all times, this method has the disadvantage that the time course of stimulation is being controlled by the observer as he or she adjusts the contrast; some observers may introduce more rapid changes of contrasts than others. The method of adjustment also has the disadvantage of providing very little control over the observer's response criterion, either in the sense of the kind of quantitative criterion discussed by signal-detection theorists (see Chap. 7) or a qualitative criterion (for example, does an observer consider a vague sensation of something moving to be a blank field or a stationary grating?). For detection thresholds, observers are supposed to use any difference they can perceive between no stimulus and presence of stimulus in order to set threshold, but, particularly in the case of adjustment, it is difficult to be sure an observer has done so.

Forced-Choice Versus Single-Alternative Trials. The other psychophysical procedures that have been used to measure detection thresholds can almost all be classified by making two distinctions: (a) either forced-choice or single-alternative trials, and (b) either the method of constant stimuli or an adaptive method. A forced-choice trial presents the observer with two alternatives (often two intervals but sometimes two locations), one containing the stimulus (the pattern) and one not (a blank field of the same mean luminance). The observer is to indicate which alternative contains the stimulus.

A single-alternative trial presents either a stimulus (a pattern) or no stimulus (the blank). The observer says "yes" (or makes an equivalent response, e.g., pushes a designated button) to indicate a stimulus and says "no" to indicate the blank.

Method of Constant Stimuli Versus Adaptive Methods. In the method of constant stimuli, different contrasts of a given pattern are decided on beforehand and each is presented a given number of times, preferably in random order. Threshold is defined as that intensity leading to some criterion level of performance (e.g., either some proportion correct in forced-choice trials or some proportion of "yeses" in single-alternative trials).

In adaptive methods, the intensity of the stimulus (the contrast of the pattern) on a particular trial is determined by the observer's responses on previous trials. In the simplest staircase versions, the intensity is increased when the observer makes an error in a forced choice or says "no," and the intensity is decreased when the observer is correct several times in forced choices or says "yes." The intensities on different trials form a "staircase" going up and down around the threshold. Some reasonable rule for calculating threshold from this staircase of intensities is adopted. Lately, more sophisticated procedures have been developed, making better use of all the preceding responses (e.g., Watson & Pelli, 1983).

The use of methods other than adjustment may decrease the problem of understanding what response criterion an observer is using, but it does not eliminate it. Even in forced choice with feedback, two observers (or the same observer in different situations) may persist in making decisions based on different aspects of the perceptions or on some aspect related to a visual process other than the one the investigator wants to study.

Most near-threshold results do not seem to depend dramatically on psychophysical method except to the extent that different procedures intermix different numbers of stimuli, thus producing different conditions of uncertainty (the topic of Chap. 7). The absolute value of the thresholds may depend on the method, however, although the relationships among the thresholds seem stable. (See, for example, the comparison of psychophysical methods in Kelly and Savoie, 1973). Subtle effects have certainly not been ruled out.

Measuring Appearance Thresholds. Appearance thresholds are generally measured by the method of adjustment, or sometimes by the method of constant stimuli. Notice that, rigorously speaking in any case, there is no true forced-choice method for measuring these appearance thresholds. For there are no two stimulus alternatives that an experimenter can present to measure these thresholds where the experimenter can know beforehand that one alternative is correct and one is incorrect. If the choice is between a blank and a stimulus, for example, even when the stimulus is perfectly visible (above detection threshold), if it does not have the correct appearance the observer should not choose it. The situation is similar for any other two alternatives. Since the thresholds are defined to be the minimum contrast at which the observer perceives a particular appearance, only the observer (if anyone) can know for sure.

1.13 SUMMARY

Patterns are visual stimuli that vary only in two spatial dimensions and in time; color and depth are generally ignored here (except that color vision is used as an example to introduce some concepts early in this chapter).

An important and relatively low-level stage in pattern vision is now thought to be a set of multiple analyzers, each of which is sensitive to restricted ranges along various dimensions, for example, orientation and spatial frequency.

The primary topic of this book is the evidence for these analyzers and for their properties that comes from near-threshold psychophysical experiments. There is remarkable agreement across different near-threshold paradigms and across near-threshold experiments from different laboratories about which dimensions of pattern vision do and which do not have multiple analyzers at this relatively low-level stage.

A possible physiological substrate for these analyzers is cortical areas V1 and V2. In this chapter some of the relevant visual neurophysiology is briefly described to provide perspective on the psychophysical results in the rest of the book. Single cortical neurons are selectively sensitive along a number of dimensions, in particular orientation, spatial frequency, spatial position, and direction of motion.

Four near-threshold experimental paradigms capable of providing evidence for multiple analyzers will be discussed in this book and are briefly introduced here: adaptation's effect on threshold; summation at threshold; uncertainty effects at threshold; and identification of near-threshold stimuli. A fifth paradigm—parametric detection experiments—provides information about the sensitivity of the hypothetical analyzers but little evidence about their existence.

The patterns used in these experiments are typically generated on cathode-ray tubes. Thresholds are sometimes measured by a method of adjustment and sometimes by more rigorous forced-choice or yes-no procedures (either using a constant set of stimuli or an adaptive method).

Appearance thresholds—where the observer adjusts contrast until the pattern just has some desired appearance (as opposed to just being visible at all)—are also introduced in this chapter.

Notes

1. Using near-threshold stimuli reduces the problems of interpretation caused by the manifest nonlinearities in the visual system: early local light adaptation (reviewed in Shapley & Enroth-Cugell, 1984), perhaps a compressive nonlinearity at the outputs of the analyzers under consideration, and so forth.

2. Consistent with the observation that blackness is never seen in patches of light in a dark surround, examination of the connections in Fig. 1.1—meant to apply to the case of a dark surround—reveals that the output of the W/B analyzer there is always positive, because it simply sums positive numbers from M and L first-stage analyzers.

2

Some Mathematics

This chapter provides mathematical background about three kinds of functions and their properties: (a) sine waves (also called sinusoids or sinusoidal functions), (b) points (also called impulses or delta functions), and (c) patches of sine wave (also called windowed sinusoids and, in one special case, Gabor functions). These functions—taken to describe visual patterns and visual analyzers—play an important role in current investigations of pattern vision for reasons that I hope will become clear below. The last part of the chapter introduces linear systems. All of the material in this chapter is sketchy, but it should suffice for understanding much of the subsequent material in this book. Other introductions to much of this material can be found in Cornsweet, 1970, and Weisstein, 1980. Extended descriptions of this material can be found in books on Fourier analysis; five such are Bracewell, 1965; Gaskill, 1978; Jennison, 1961; Papoulis, 1962; and Stuart, 1961. This chapter can be skipped by those with appropriate background except for the section on dimensions of Gabor functions (section 2.3.4), which contains some idiosyncratic material.

2.1 SINUSOIDS AND FOURIER ANALYSIS

2.1.1 *Sinusoidal Gratings*

A sinusoidal grating is a visual stimulus that varies sinusoidally in one spatial dimension (top illustrations in Fig. 2.1). Such a grating is a one-dimensional pattern in the sense that the luminance varies along any line in one direction (in the horizontal direction in the figure—call it x) but is constant along any line in the perpendicular direction (vertical in the figure—call it y). When you plot luminance as a function of position along the dimension perpendicular to the bars, you get a sinusoidal function added to a constant luminance (top 2 rows of Fig. 2.2). A function that gives the luminance of a pattern on however many dimensions are relevant will be called a *luminance profile* of the pattern.

Formally, you can write the luminance profile of a sinusoidal grating as

$$L(x,y) = L_0[1 + m \cdot \cos(2\pi f x + \theta)] \tag{2.1}$$

where x—position—is on the horizontal axis in the sketches below the photographs, and $L(x)$—luminance—is on the vertical axis. The term L_0 is the constant to which the sinusoid is added and is the average of the luminance at all spatial positions, since the sinusoidal terms are above zero as often as they are

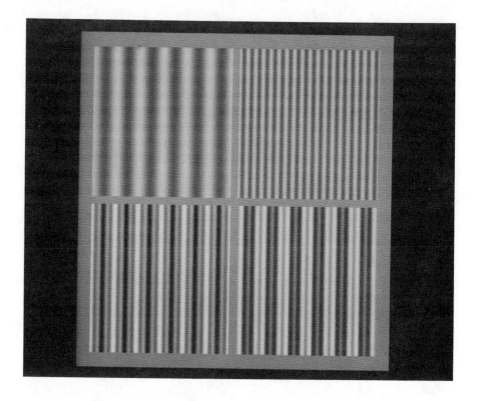

FIG. 2.1 Photographs of simple sinusoidal gratings (top) and compound gratings (bottom). Reproduction processes will have distorted these somewhat.

below zero. For simplicity in subsequent equations, a cosine rather than a sine appears above; its frequency is f, its phase is θ.

Spatial Frequency. For simple sinusoidal gratings like those in Fig. 2.1, it is very easy to understand what spatial frequency is. It is simply the frequency f with which the sinusoid repeats itself across the pattern. For example, in the middle row of Fig. 2.2, f is three times per unit of distance on the horizontal axis. The unit of distance used most often is a degree of visual angle. We will abbreviate cycles per degree of visual angle as either cpd or c/deg.

Degrees of Visual Angle. Something having a width of 1 cm at a distance of 57 cm from the eye subtends an angle of 1 degree at the eye, that is, has a width of 1 degree of visual angle. A person's thumb at arm length typically subtends 1 or 2 degrees of visual angle.

Spatial Phase. The parameter θ in Eq. 2.1 specifies the spatial phase of the pattern. Notice that in the top drawings of Fig. 2.2 the sinusoid is placed so that its peak is centered over zero (its value is maximal at $x = 0$). This phase is known as "cosine" phase and the phase parameter θ equals 0.

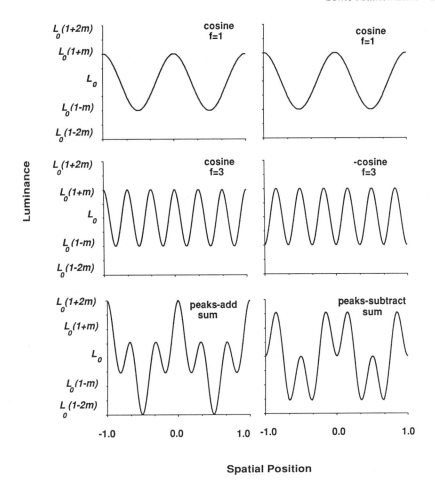

Spatial Position

FIG. 2.2 Luminance profiles of simple sinusoidal gratings (top and middle) and compound gratings (bottom). The profiles in the top row here correspond to the top left photograph of Fig. 2.1; those in the middle row here correspond to the top right of Fig. 2.1; and those in the bottom left and right here correspond to the bottom left and right, respectively, of Fig. 2.1.

If the pattern were displaced one quarter cycle to the right (making $\theta = -\pi/2$ radians, or -90 degrees), the cosinusoid would be crossing zero at $x = 0$ (the luminance would be crossing the average luminance L_0) and increasing from left to right. This phase is known as "sine" phase. Other positions or phases of the pattern do not have conventional names, but can be expressed as values of the phase parameter θ.

Amplitude and Contrast. The sinusoidal oscillation in Eq. 2.1 and the top two rows of Fig. 2.2 reaches a maximum luminance of $L_0 (1 + m)$ at the brightest points and drops to a minimum luminance of $L_0 (1 - m)$ at the darkest points, making a difference of $2L_0 m$. This quantity is called the *peak-trough amplitude;* one half this quantity is $L_0 m$ and is called the *amplitude* or *modulation depth.*

As mentioned earlier, the contrast of a pattern will be defined here as one half the difference between the maximum and minimum luminance divided by the mean luminance; thus contrast equals m in Eq. 2.1.

Contrast is more commonly used than amplitude, probably because thresholds measured in terms of it are often independent of mean luminance in the photopic range. (See Chap. 13.)

Spatial Extent. The sinusoidal gratings illustrated in Fig. 2.1 and 2.2 are truncated; Eq. 2.1 ought to be modified to read that it is only valid for values of x in a limited range.

An untruncated sinusoid—which would extend infinitely far on both the left and right sides—is unrealistic, of course, for a visual pattern. Even if a pattern could be infinitely wide, the eye would receive light from only a finite portion of it.

2.1.2   Compound Sinusoidal Gratings

Stimuli containing two sinusoidal components (one three times the spatial frequency of the other) are shown in the bottom half of Fig. 2.1; sketches of the luminance profiles are at the bottom of Fig. 2.2. The luminance profile of each of these compound-grating patterns is the sum of three functions: (a) a constant L_0, which equals the mean intensity of the pattern, (b) the lower spatial-frequency sinusoid from the upper left photograph (the luminance profile in the top row of Fig. 2.2), and (c) the higher spatial-frequency sinusoid from the upper right photograph of Fig. 2.1 (the luminance profile in the middle rows of Fig. 2.2). (When functions are added, it is their values at each point that are added.)

The difference between the two compound gratings in the bottom of Fig. 2.1 is the relative phase of the two simple sinusoidal components. In the compound grating on the left, the brightest points of the two sinusoidal components juxtapose as shown in the left column of Fig. 2.2. In the one on the bottom right of Fig. 2.1, a brightest point of the lower spatial-frequency (wider bar) grating is juxtaposed with a darkest point of the higher spatial-frequency (narrower bar) grating as shown in the right column of Fig. 2.2.

A compound grating is said to contain the spatial frequencies of the sinusoidal components of which it is composed.

2.1.3   Fourier Analysis

Jean Baptiste Fourier, a French physicist and mathematician (1768–1830), discovered a mathematical truth that has had far-reaching consequences outside mathematics. Glossing over the technical fine points, he discovered that any function at all is equal to the sum (or integral if the function is not periodic) of sinusoidal functions of various frequencies, amplitudes, and phases.

To restate this very important mathematical fact in other words: Any function can be decomposed into sinusoidal components. This decomposition and the associated mathematical techniques are often called Fourier analysis in honor of their inventor.

In general, therefore, any one-dimensional visual pattern is equal to the sum (or integral) of a number of sinusoidal components (plus a constant mean luminance). This sinusoidal components will differ one from another in spatial frequency, amplitude, and spatial phase (but they will all have the orientation of the original one-dimensional pattern). The original pattern is said to contain the spatial frequencies of all the sinusoids into which its luminance profile decomposes. This is an unambiguous definition of what spatial frequencies a pattern contains, for there is one and only one combination of sinusoids of different spatial frequencies that can be added together to form any given one-dimensional function (e.g., the luminance profile of any one-dimensional pattern). Or, as mathematicians say, the Fourier decomposition of any function is unique.

A demonstration of how a square-wave grating is decomposed into sinusoids can be found in Cornsweet, 1970 (Figs. 12.2 and 12.3).

Fourier Transform. Calculating how much of each frequency of sinusoid (and at what phase) you need to add (or integrate) together to equal the original function is known as calculating the Fourier transform of the original function. The Fourier transform is a function of frequency (which we will call f), and for each frequency it gives two numbers: the amplitude of the sinusoid at that frequency and the phase of the sinusoid at that frequency. (One can combine these two numbers into a single complex number if one wishes.) See the appendix, section 2.10, for more details.

If you consider just the amplitude as a function of frequency (how much of each frequency of sinusoid you need to add up to form the original function), you may call it the *amplitude spectrum* or the *amplitude characteristic* of the Fourier transform. If you consider just the phase as a function of frequency (what phase each frequency of sinusoid needs to be in) you may refer to the *phase spectrum* or *phase characteristic.* (If the "spectrum" is referred to, the amplitude spectrum or its square—the *power spectrum*—is generally meant.)

As an example, let's describe the Fourier transform of the peaks-subtract compound grating illustrated in the lower right of Fig. 2.1 and Fig. 2.2, assuming for the moment that it is infinite in extent and the illustration shows only a piece of it. The amplitude characteristic of the compound grating's Fourier transform is zero everywhere except at three spatial frequencies. When the spatial frequency equals 1 or 3 cpd, the amplitude characteristic equals m (both the sinusoidal components are drawn as having an amplitude m). The phase parameter θ at both 1 and 3 cpd equals $-\pi/2$. When the spatial frequency equals 0 cpd, the amplitude characteristic of the compound grating's Fourier transform equals L_0 (the average value). (This compound at 0 cpd is often called the DC component, by analogy with electric circuits.)

The Fourier Transform of a Constant—a DC Term. Why does the mean luminance term (the constant as a function of spatial position) appear at a frequency of 0? You can think of it this way: The lower the spatial frequency of a sinusoid, the slower the rate at which luminance changes as a function of position. And for a constant that rate is zero.

Symbols. If the original function is called $L(x)$, its Fourier transform is often called $\overline{L}(f)$. The same letter is used but a bar is placed over it and the argument x is replaced with argument f, indicating frequency.

Inverse Fourier Transform. To calculate the original function from its Fourier transform is equivalent to putting the sinusoidal components back together again to form the original function; it is known as taking the inverse Fourier transform. See the appendix to this chapter, section 2.10, for equations.

Effect of Limited Extent on Fourier Transform. As just mentioned, the gratings shown in Fig. 2.1 are of limited rather than infinite extent. The Fourier transform of a sinusoid of limited extent is presented in the section on Gabor functions.

2.1.4   Orientation and Two-Dimensional Fourier Transforms

The photographs in Fig. 2.1 show vertical gratings. The gratings could, of course, be rotated into other orientations. We will specify the orientation of a grating in degrees of rotation relative to vertical (where counterclockwise is positive) and use the symbol ρ for it. Notice that orientation of a sinusoidal grating goes only through 180 distinct degrees, since rotating a grating by 180 degrees transforms it back into its original orientation.

As it turns out, any two-dimensional pattern (a stimulus having luminance varying in both the x and the y direction) can be formed by summing up simple sinusoidal gratings like that shown in Fig. 2.1, as long as not only their spatial frequencies but also their orientations are allowed to vary.

And—a generalization of what was said before in the context of one-dimensional functions about Fourier decompositions being unique—there is only one combination of sinusoidal gratings of different orientations and spatial frequencies that will form a given two-dimensional pattern. For example, suppose you have a pattern that you know is the sum of (a) a vertical grating of 3 cpd having contrast 1.5% and in sine phase at the fixation point, (b) a horizontal grating of 7 cpd having contrast 4% and in cosine phase at the fixation point, (c) a grating rotated 10 degrees clockwise from vertical of frequency 8 cpd having a contrast of 2% and in cosine phase at the fixation point, and (d) a constant intensity term. You might wonder if some other combination of orientations and spatial frequencies (in whatever amplitudes and phases were necessary) might combine to give the same pattern. The answer is no. (See, for example, Bracewell, 1965, Chap. 12.)

Two-Dimensional Fourier Transform. A function of two variables (e.g., $L[x,y]$ has a Fourier transform that is a function of two variables as well. These latter two variables can be taken to equal the spatial frequency f_S (the number of cycles per unit distance in the direction perpendicular to the bars) and orientation ρ (the degrees of rotation from vertical) of a sinusoidal component. Then the amplitude characteristic of the two-dimensional Fourier transform at any particular pair (f_S, ρ) will tell you how much of a sinusoid at that spatial frequency and orientation you would need to use in adding up sinusoids to form the original function, and the phase characteristic will tell you in what phase that sinusoid will need to be.

Horizontal and Vertical Frequency. Rather than expressing these two variables as spatial frequency and orientation, it is often more convenient (although less intuitively appealing) to express them as "horizontal" and "vertical" spatial frequencies f_x and f_y—which are the frequency variables corresponding to the x and y of the original function. The relationship between the pair of variables f_S and ρ (spatial frequency and orientation) and the pair f_x and f_y (horizontal and vertical spatial frequencies) is straightforward: Spatial frequency and orientation are the polar coordinates (spatial frequency being the radial and orientation the angular coordinate) corresponding to Cartesian coordinates f_x and f_y. Suppose, for example, you consider a sinusoidal component having a spatial frequency of 3 c/deg and an orientation of 45 degrees. You transform these polar coordinates (a radius of 3 and an angle of 45 degrees) back into Cartesian coordinates (both horizontal and vertical equal 2.12 c/deg). To convert from (f_x, f_y) to (f_S, ρ), or vice versa:

$$\rho = \arctan\frac{f_y}{f_x} \quad \text{and} \quad f_S = (f_x^2 + f_y^2)^{1/2}$$
$$f_y = f_S \cdot \sin\rho \quad \text{and} \quad f_x = f_S \cdot \cos\rho \tag{2.2}$$

For gratings like those in Fig. 2.1, which are called vertical, the direction in which the luminance varies is horizontal. Thus, the horizontal spatial frequency (f_x) is equal to the spatial frequency perpendicular to the bars (f_S), and the vertical spatial frequency equals zero. In general, for any grating the horizontal spatial frequency is the frequency along any horizontal line and the vertical spatial frequency is the frequency along any vertical line.

2.1.5 Temporal Sinusoidal Stimuli

Flickering Spatially Homogeneous Fields. Consider taking a spatially homogeneous stimulus (ideally a "ganzfeld" that illuminates the whole retina uniformly at any one moment) and changing its luminance sinusoidally in time. The luminance at any point on the retina could then be expressed as the following function of time, a function analogous to that in Eq. 2.1 for a static stationary grating:

$$L(t) = L_0[1 + m \cdot \sin(2\pi f_T + \theta_T)]$$

where L_0 = mean luminance (averaged over time and/or over space)
m = modulation depth
f_T = temporal frequency (number of cycles of flicker per unit time)
θ_T = temporal phase

Drifting Gratings. Suppose first that an infinitely extended sinusoidal grating (like the infinite extension of that in the top of Fig. 2.1) is set drifting from left to right at a constant velocity of 2 units of distance per unit time. Imagine what such a pattern would look like. Each bar would be drifting from left to right; at any one point the luminance would be modulating sinusoidally in time as the bars drifted over it. Since there are three light-dark cycles in the grating per unit of distance, and since the grating is moving at a velocity of 2 units of distance per unit time, 6 light-dark cycles would move over any point per unit of time. Therefore, the temporal frequency at any point in space would be just 6 cycles per unit time. More generally, velocity times spatial frequency gives temporal frequency.

The luminance profile for a drifting grating can be represented by the following equation (setting the spatial and temporal phase terms equal to zero for simplicity):

$$L(x, t) = L_0\{1 + m \cdot \sin[2\pi(f_S \cdot x - f_T \cdot t)]\} \tag{2.3}$$

where f_S is the spatial frequency, f_T is the temporal frequency, and the velocity is given by f_T divided by f_S. Given the usual conventions such that both f_S and f_T are positive numbers and x increases from left to right, this equation gives rightward motion at a constant velocity.

Temporal frequency is usually given in cycles per second, abbreviated c/sec or Hz.

Flickering (Counterphase) Gratings. Another way of introducing sinusoidal temporal variation is to flicker a grating in the following fashion (often known as sinusoidal counterphase modulation): The spatial boundaries between the bright bars and the dark bars (the positions x at which $L[x, t]$ equals L_0) stay in the same place. However, the positions that are the brightest positions at one time will be the darkest positions one half of a temporal cycle later; the positions that are the darkest positions at the first time will be the brightest positions at the later time. Further, the change from bright to dark to bright that occurs at almost all positions (all except the spatial boundaries) occurs as a sinusoidal function of time.

The luminance profile for such a flickering grating can be represented by the following equation, where the symbols have the same meaning they had for the preceding equation:

$$L(x, t) = L_0[1 + m \cdot \sin(2\pi f_T t + \theta_T) \sin(2\pi f_S x + \theta_S)] \tag{2.4}$$

Notice that this equation could have been obtained from Eq. 2.1 for a stationary sinusoidal grating by replacing m in that equation with m multiplied by a sinusoidal function of time.

Notice further that there is no ambiguity in the spatial or temporal frequency definitions for drifting or flickering gratings—that is, the temporal frequency is the same at every spatial position, and the spatial frequency is the same at every point in time.

Flicker Is the Sum of Drifts. There is a mathematical relationship between flickering and drifting gratings that will turn out to be important in a number of places. Any flickering grating is the sum of two drifting gratings of the same temporal frequency but opposite direction of movement. (There is a nice figure demonstrating this summation in Sekuler, Pantle, and Levinson, 1978; the somewhat more complicated decomposition of gratings turning abruptly on and off is also illustrated there.) The overall contrast of the flickering grating is twice that of either drifting component. For example, a vertical grating of spatial frequency 10 cpd that is flickering at 3 cps and is of contrast 8% is equal to the sum of two vertical gratings, both of 10 cpd and 4% contrast, where one is drifting leftward at the velocity of 3 cps and the other is drifting rightward at the same velocity.

To put it another way: If you take Eq. 2.3 for a rightward drifting grating and add to it a second equation just like it except that the minus sign has been changed to a plus sign to give leftward motion, and if you then add the two equations together (and simplify the result), you will get Eq. 2.4 except that the modulation will be doubled ($2m$ rather than m as in Eq. 2.4).

Drift Is the Sum of Flickers. Conversely, a drifting grating is equal to the sum of two flickering gratings (e.g., Kelly 1985a), although that fact has played a smaller role in discussions of pattern vision.

2.1.6 Spatiotemporal Patterns and Three-Dimensional Fourier Analysis

Any spatiotemporal pattern can be represented as its luminance profile $L(x, y, t)$, which is a function of three dimensions (two spatial dimensions and one temporal dimension). In a straightforward extension of facts about one- and two-dimensional functions, any three-dimensional function can also be subjected to Fourier analysis, that is, uniquely decomposed into sinusoidal components. This mathematical fact translates back into visual patterns as follows: Any spatiotemporal pattern is equal to the sum of drifting sinusoidal gratings of different spatial frequencies, orientations, temporal frequencies (equivalently, velocities), and directions of drift.

Further, this decomposition is unique. That is, there is one and only one set of drifting-grating components that equals any particular spatiotemporal pattern. And this decomposition can be calculated in a straightforward way, by computing the three-dimensional Fourier transform.

2.1.7 Some History

Sinusoidal stimuli are very useful in the investigation of electrical networks and optical systems, because the latter are (at least approximately) translation-invariant and linear systems. (See section 2.6.) Consequently, use of sinusoids and Fourier analysis had become commonplace in several fields, including electrical engineering and optics. It was their use in these other fields that led to their use in both psychophysical and physiological studies of vision.

The first sinusoidal stimuli to make their appearance in visual science seem to have been the sinusoidally flickering spatially homogeneous stimuli used by Ives (1922a, 1922b). He found the highest temporal frequency at which a human observer could just tell that the stimulus was flickering rather than steady. DeLange (1952, 1954, 1958) was the first to measure what have come to be called temporal contrast sensitivity functions—that is, an observer's sensitivity as a function of temporal frequency for sinusoidal stimuli of many temporal frequencies. And several investigators soon measured the temporal contrast sensitivity functions of neurons using temporal sinusoidal stimuli (e.g., Enroth-Cugell, 1952; Knight, Toyoda, & Dodge, 1970).

Spatial sinusoids were not commonly used as visual stimuli quite as early as temporal sinusoids, perhaps due to greater difficulty in generating the stimuli. The use of spatial sinusoids in psychophysics seems to have begun with the studies of Schade (1948, 1958). Schade was followed within another decade by many other investigators—including, for example, Bryngdahl (1964), Campbell and Kulikowski (1966), Campbell and Robson (1964, 1968), Davidson (1968), DePalma and Lowry (1962), Green and Campbell (1965), Kelly (1966), van Nes and Bouman (1967), Patel (1966), and Watanabe, Mori, Nagata, and Hiwatashi (1968).

Stimuli varying sinusoidally in both time and space—flickering or drifting gratings—were soon used both in psychophysics (e.g., Kelly, 1966; van Nes, 1968; van Nes, Koenderink, Nas, & Bouman, 1967; Robson, 1966) and in neurophysiology (e.g., Enroth-Cugell & Robson, 1966). Ratliff's 1965 book on Mach bands contained a small section on results using sinusoidal stimuli; Cornsweet's 1970 book contained a large section. Since then, the use of sinusoidal stimuli has become commonplace.

2.2   LINES AND POINTS AND IMPULSES (DELTA FUNCTIONS)

Another way of decomposing patterns into component parts is to use components that are lines (in the case of one-dimensional spatial patterns), points (in the case of two-dimensional spatial patterns), or points of light flashed on just for a moment (in the case of spatiotemporal patterns). Thus, for example, the one-dimensional pattern in the upper left of Fig. 2.1 can be described as the sum (or integral) of many vertical lines of light. (A vertical line has luminance equal to zero everywhere except along a vertical line, and along that line its luminance is constant.) For the pattern in the upper left of Fig. 2.1 the component line at position 0 has a luminance equal to L_0, the line at position 0.25 has a luminance equal to $(L_0 + m)$, the line at position 0.50 has a luminance equal to L_0, the line at position 0.75 has a luminance equal to $(L_0 - m)$, and so forth throughout an (infinite) list of lines at all positions, with $L(x)$ being the luminance of the line at position x.

Similarly, a two-dimensional pattern (one that varies in luminance along both horizontal and vertical lines, for example) cannot be decomposed into horizontal or vertical lines, but it can easily be decomposed into points of light that are zero everywhere except at a single position. If you consider an (infinite) list of points at all positions (x, y) where the point at position (x, y) has a luminance equal to $L(x, y)$—that is, has a luminance equal to the luminance of the pattern under consideration—and if you then sum up all the points in this list, you get back the original pattern.

And finally, a spatiotemporal pattern (one that varies in luminance along both spatial directions and also the temporal dimension) can be decomposed into instantaneous points of light, where an instantaneous point of light is a stimulus that is zero everywhere and at all moments except at one position and at a particular instant. The instantaneous point of light at position (x, y) and time t has to have luminance equal to the luminance of the original pattern at that point and time, that is, $L(x, y, t)$.

To capture mathematically these ideas of a line, of a point, or of a point flashed on for just an instant turns out to be a little tricky. For the ideas imply the existence of a definite amount of light (more generally, energy) but concentrated all in an infinitely thin line, in an infinitely small point, or at a single instant at a single point. The formalization of this idea is called a *delta function* or an *impulse*. Mathematically speaking, delta functions require a generalization of the usual definitions of functions (and consequent generalizations of derivatives and integrals). Standard textbooks (e.g., Bracewell, 1965) deal with this topic. Here readers who are not familiar with the mathematics of delta functions can get along on their intuitions about points (as in fact the earliest scientists to use delta functions undoubtedly did before the mathematicians had clarified the concept). Indeed, section 2.2.1 giving formal symbols can be skipped with little effect on understanding the rest of this book.

2.2.1 Delta Functions (Impulses)

One-Dimensional Case. For the one-dimensional case, we start with a line centered at point zero and having an energy equal to 1, that is,

$$\delta(x) = 1 \quad \text{for } x = 0$$
$$= 0 \quad \text{everywhere else} \tag{2.5}$$

where the integral (or area under the function, or intuitively, the energy or amount of light in the function) is given by

$$\int_a^b \delta(x) \, dx = 1 \quad \text{if} \quad a < 0 < b$$
$$= 0 \quad \text{otherwise} \tag{2.6}$$

(If delta functions were ordinary functions, this integral would always equal 0.0.)

To represent a line centered someplace other than at zero and/or of energy equaling something other than 1, we simply horizontally translate the above function to the desired position and multiply its height by the desired energy;

for example, a line of energy 10 at position 3.5 is represented by

$$10 \cdot \delta(x - 3.5)$$

More abstractly,

$$\delta(y - x) = 1 \qquad \text{when } y = x$$
$$= 0 \qquad \text{otherwise}$$

Now to represent the one-dimensional pattern $L(x)$ as the sum (more rigorously, integral) of lines at all different positions (where each line is of the appropriate luminance), one can write

$$L(x) = \int_{-\infty}^{+\infty} L(y) \cdot \delta(y - x) \, dy \qquad (2.7)$$

To work with two- and three-dimensional patterns, one just extends the above to use two- and three-dimensional delta functions that are zero everywhere except at $(0, 0)$ (in the two-dimensional case) and at $(0, 0, 0)$ (in the three-dimensional case).

2.2.2   Some History

Thinking of any visual pattern as the sum of many points of light and using points of light as visual stimuli antedated sinusoidal stimuli by many years, indeed by centuries. See, for example, the discussions of sensations and structuralism in Hochberg, 1978.

2.2.3   The Decomposition of a Sinusoid Into Delta Functions

The decomposition of a sinusoidal function (e.g., the luminance profile of a one-dimensional sinusoidal grating) into delta functions (e.g., the luminance profiles of lines) is straightforward and intuitively appealing, and was, in fact, the example at the beginning of section 2.2. In symbols, the decomposition is given by Eq. 2.7, with $L(x)$ given by Eq. 2.1.

2.2.4   The Decomposition of a Delta Function Into Sinusoids

The decomposition of a delta function (e.g., the luminance profile of a line) into sinusoidal functions (e.g., the luminance profiles of one-dimensional sinusoidal gratings) is less intuitively appealing. Figure 2.3 attempts to provide some insight into this decomposition by showing the luminance profiles of a line (top row) and several of the sinusoids into which that line decomposes, that is, several of the sinusoids that sum up to equal that line. In general, a delta function is the sum (or the integral if one considers positions from minus to plus infinity) of sinusoids of all possible frequencies; all the component sinusoids have identical amplitude, and all are in the phase that puts a peak at the position of the

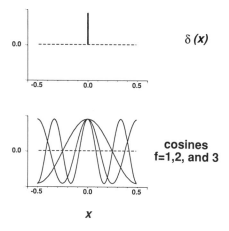

FIG. 2.3 A delta function centered at 0 and three of the sinusoids that would need to be added together to form the delta.

line. Since all the sinusoids have their peaks at that same position, their sum (or integral) will be nonzero at that position. At every other position, however, they will sum (integrate) to zero, because the sinusoids of different frequencies cancel each other out at every other position.

To put it in other words, a delta function's amplitude spectrum (the amplitude characteristic of the Fourier transform of a delta function) is 1 at all frequencies. The phase characteristic specifies that the peaks of all the sinusoids should superimpose at the position where the delta function is not zero; when that position is zero (as in Fig. 2.3), $\theta = 0$ for all frequencies.

There is an interesting trade-off between frequency and position illustrated at the extremes by sinusoidal and delta functions. Notice that a sinusoid is infinitely extended on the position dimension (is nonzero at positions ranging from minus infinity to plus infinity) but is completely localized on the frequency dimension (its spectrum is nonzero at only one frequency—that is, a sinusoid contains only one frequency). Similarly but oppositely, a line is infinitely extended on the frequency dimension (its spectrum is nonzero for frequencies ranging from minus infinity to plus infinity) but is completely localized on the position dimension. Thus perfect localization on either the position or frequency dimension implies infinite extension on the other of the two dimensions.

2.3 WINDOWED SINE WAVES—GABOR FUNCTIONS

The third kind of function is a full sine wave as "seen through a window," but it may be a window with gradual edges. Such a windowed sine wave (bottom row Fig. 2.4) is just a sine wave (top row Fig. 2.4) multiplied by some "window" function that goes to zero outside a limited area (middle row Fig. 2.4). For most

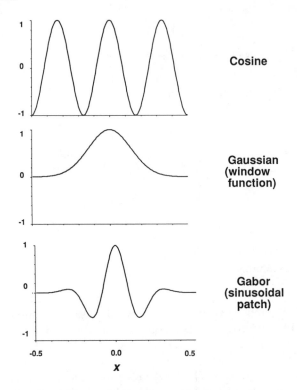

FIG. 2.4 A sine function (of frequency 3 cycles per unit distance, in cosine phase), a Gaussian window function (with half-height full-width equal to 0.32 units of distance), and their product—a Gabor function.

of our purposes, the exact shape of the window functions will not be crucial as long as the window's edges are not too abrupt.

2.3.1   Gabor Functions

When the window function is Gaussian (as it is in Fig. 2.4) the associated mathematics are particularly simple. (Some readers may know the Gaussian function best as the bell-shaped curve of statistics, that is, the probability density function for the normal distribution.) We will call such a windowed sinusoid a *Gabor function* in honor of D. Gabor, who pointed out the advantages of such functions for communication (Gabor, 1946). These functions have also been called *elementary Gaussian signals* or just *elementary signals*. In symbols, a Gabor function (of *x*) can be written

$$m \cdot \exp\left[\frac{-2.77(x - x_0)^2}{W_X^2}\right] \cdot \cos[2\pi f_S(x - x_0) + \theta_S] \qquad (2.8)$$

where x_0 = center position
W_X = full width at half height
m = height of Gaussian window
f_S = frequency of sinusoid
θ_S = phase of sinusoid with respect to center of Gaussian window
m = overall amplitude of Gabor function

(The constant 2.77 is used to make the measure of width W be the full width at half height. See Table 2.1 and later discussion.)

Sinusoidal and Delta Functions Are Extreme Gabor Functions. Notice that, as the width W_X of the Gaussian function gets larger and larger (while the other parameters—particularly f_S—stay constant), the Gabor function becomes more and more like a sinusoidal function. Conversely, as the Gaussian function's width gets smaller and smaller, the Gabor function becomes more and more like a delta function. Technically, therefore, the full family of Gabor functions includes sinusoidal and delta functions. When we talk about Gabor functions, however, we will usually be talking about Gabor functions in a middling range, where they are definitely neither infinitely extended sinusoids nor perfectly localized delta functions.

Different Measures of Gaussian Functions' Width. One of the bothersome things in dealing with Gaussian and Gabor functions is that different groups of people tend to use different measures of width for Gaussian functions. A number of the popular ones are indicated in Fig. 2.5, and the relationships between them are summarized in Table 2.1. The equations in the text will use W, the full width at half height. It is about one fifth larger than 2 standard deviations (2σ) and slightly smaller than the equivalent bandwidth (the area under a function divided by the function's maximum height, denoted by Q here).

TABLE 2.1. Relationships among Four Measures of a Gaussian Function's Width.

	Q	W	a	σ
Q	$Q = Q$	$Q = 0.5\sqrt{\pi (\ln 2)}\, W$ $= 1.064W$	$Q = \sqrt{\pi}\, a$ $= 1.77a$	$Q = \sqrt{2\pi}\, \sigma$ $= 2.51\sigma$
W	$W = 2\sqrt{(\ln 2)/\pi}\, Q$ $= 0.940Q$	$W = W$	$W = 2\sqrt{\ln 2}\, a$ $= 1.665a$	$W = 2\sqrt{2 \ln 2}\, \sigma$ $= 2.35\sigma$
a	$a = Q/\sqrt{\pi}$ $= 0.564Q$	$a = W/(2\sqrt{\ln 2})$ $= 0.601W$	$a = a$	$a = \sqrt{2}\, \sigma$ $= 1.414\sigma$
σ	$\sigma = Q/\sqrt{2\pi}$ $= 0.399Q$	$\sigma = W/2\sqrt{2 \ln 2}$ $= 0.425W$	$\sigma = a/\sqrt{2}$ $= 0.707a$	$\sigma = \sigma$

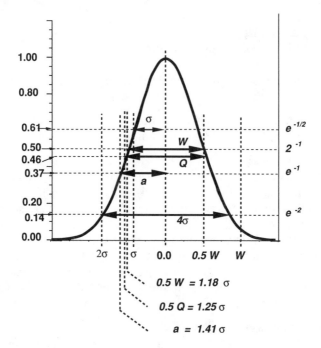

FIG. 2.5 Diagram illustrating relationship of some alternative measures of widths of Gaussian functions: a is the $(1/e)$ half width; σ is the standard deviation; W is the half amplitude, full width; and Q is the equivalent width (the area divided by the peak height). See Table 2.2 for equations.

Fourier Transform of a Gaussian Function. The amplitude characteristic of the Fourier transform of a Gaussian function is itself another Gaussian function (see section 2.10.6) centered at a frequency of zero. Its width on the frequency axis is inversely proportional to the width of the original Gaussian function. Table 2.2 summarizes the relations between the width of a Gaussian function and the width of its Fourier transform.

Fourier Transform of a Gabor Function. In the typical case, the amplitude spectrum of the Fourier transform of a Gabor function is almost exactly a Gaussian function of (positive) spatial frequency; this function is centered at the spatial frequency of the sinusoid f_S. (See section 2.10.7 for more details.) An example of a Gabor function and its amplitude characteristic will be shown later in Fig. 6.9.

Table 2.3 shows the relationship between the number of cycles in a patch at half height (left column) or within 2 standard deviations of the center (second to left column) and the octave bandwidth of the Fourier transform of the patch at half height (right column) and the ratio of the frequency bandwidth to the best frequency (second to right column).

TABLE 2.2. Relationships Between a Gaussian Function and Its Fourier Transform Expressed Using Four Different Measures of Width.[a]

Measure of Width	$L(x)$	$\overline{L}(f)$	Width of $\overline{L}(f)$	$\overline{L}(0)$
Equivalent bandwidth Q	$e^{-\pi(x/Q_X)2}$	$\overline{L}(0)e^{-\pi(f/Q_F)2}$	$Q_F = \dfrac{1}{Q_X}$	Q_X
Half-height full-width W	$e^{-4\ln 2(x/W_X)2}$	$\overline{L}(0)e^{-4\ln 2(f/W_F)2}$	$W_F = \dfrac{4\ln 2}{\pi W_X}$ $= \dfrac{0.8825}{W_X}$	$\dfrac{\sqrt{\pi}\,W_X}{2\sqrt{\ln 2}} = 1.065 W_X$
$(1/e)$ − half-width a	$e^{-(x/a_X)2}$	$\overline{L}(0)e^{-(f/a_F)2}$	$a_F = \dfrac{1}{\pi a_X}$ $= \dfrac{0.318}{a_X}$	$\sqrt{\pi}\,a_X = 1.772 a_X$
Standard deviation σ	$e^{-1/2(x/\sigma_X)2}$	$\overline{L}(0)e^{-1/2(f/\sigma_F)2}$	$\sigma_F = \dfrac{1}{2\pi\sigma_X}$ $= \dfrac{0.159}{\sigma_X}$	$\sqrt{2\pi}\,\sigma_X = 2.507\sigma_X$

[a] The width of the original Gaussian function is subscripted X. The width of the its Fourier transform is subscripted F.

2.3.2 Decomposition Into Gabor Functions

Any one-dimensional function can be decomposed into Gabor functions (equals the sum of Gabor functions), just as it can be decomposed into sinusoids or delta functions. In fact, the decomposition into Gabor functions is much like that into sinusoids except that the decomposition is done separately in each local region of space and/or time. (Such a decomposition is sometimes called *piecewise Fourier analysis,* and can be done with window functions other than Gaussian.) A good deal is known about the existence and uniqueness of decompositions into Gabor functions (e.g., Gabor, 1946; Geisler & Hamilton, 1984; Lerner, 1961; Marcelja, 1980).

2.3.3 Sinusoidal Patches (Gabor Patches)

One of our uses for windowed sinusoids (in particular, Gabor functions) will be in the description of certain visual stimuli that we will call *sinusoidal patches* or

TABLE 2.3. Relationship Between Number of Cycles in a
Gabor Function and Width of Its Fourier Transform.

Number of Cycles		Frequency Bandwidth	
At Half-Height $= W_x f_s$	Within $\pm 2\sigma$ of Center x_0	Proportional W_F/f_s	Octave Bandwidth[a]
8.82	14.99	0.10	0.145
4.41	8.67	0.20	0.291
2.94	5.00	0.30	0.438
2.21	3.76	0.40	0.587
1.76	2.99	0.50	0.739
1.47	2.50	0.60	0.893
1.26	2.14	0.70	1.06
1.11	1.89	0.80	1.23
0.98	1.67	0.90	1.39
0.88	1.50	1.00	1.59
0.80	1.36	1.10	1.79
0.735	1.25	1.20	2.00
5.10	8.67	0.173	0.25
2.57	4.37	0.343	0.50
1.74	2.95	0.508	0.75
1.32	2.25	0.667	1.00
1.08	1.84	0.816	1.25
0.924	1.57	0.955	1.5
0.815	1.39	1.08	1.75
0.735	1.25	1.20	2.00

[a] The octave bandwidth equals $\log_2 \dfrac{f_S + (W_F/2)}{f_S - (W_F/2)}$

sometimes *Gabor patches*. Examples of (stationary) Gabor-patch visual stimuli
are shown in Fig. 2.6. At any moment in time, a Gabor-patch stimulus looks
like a fuzzy-edged circle or ellipse containing alternating dark and light fuzzy-
edged stripes. The spatial luminance profile along any line perpendicular to the
stripes—the luminance as a function of spatial position along that line at any
particular point in time—is a mean-luminance term plus a Gabor function (or
more generally, plus some windowed sinusoid). Along any line parallel to the
stripes, the spatial luminance profile is a mean-luminance term plus a window
function; this parallel window function may have the same width as the perpendicular window function, in which case the patch looks circular, or it may not,
in which case the patch looks elliptical.

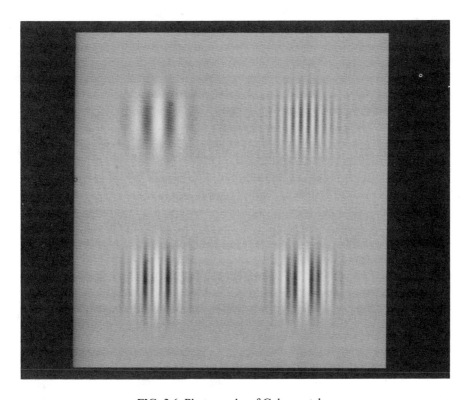

FIG. 2.6 Photographs of Gabor patches.

Overall, therefore, the luminance profile $L(x, y, t)$ of a vertically oriented Gabor patch (that is stationary in time) can be written as

$$L(x, y, t) = L_0 \left\{ 1 + m \right.$$

$$\cdot \exp \left[\frac{-2.77(x - x_0)^2}{W_X^2} \right] \exp \left[\frac{-2.77(y - y_0)^2}{W_Y^2} \right]$$

$$\left. \cdot \cos[2\pi f_S(x - x_0) + \theta_S] \right\} \tag{2.9}$$

where W_Y is the width of the window parallel to the stripes, y_0 is its center, and the other symbols have the same meaning as in Eq. 2.8.

Temporal variation in sinusoidal patches can be introduced by either drifting the sinusoidal grating behind the window (Eq. 2.3) or flickering it sinusoidally (counterphase modulation, Eq. 2.4); and the overall time course of the stimulus can be expressed by multiplying it by a temporal window function. The equation for a flickering vertically oriented Gabor patch is, therefore,

$$L(x, y, t) = L_0 \left\{ 1 + m \cdot \exp\left[\frac{-2.77(t - t_0)^2}{W_T}\right]\right.$$

$$\cdot \exp\left[\frac{-2.77(x - x_0)^2}{W_X^2}\right] \exp\left[\frac{-2.77(y - y_0)^2}{W_Y^2}\right]$$

$$\left. \cdot \cos[2\pi f_S(x - x_0) + \tau_S]\cos[2\pi f_T(t - t_0) + \theta_T]\right\} \quad (2.10)$$

where W_T = width of temporal window
   t_0 = center of temporal window
   f_T = frequency of temporal flicker
   θ_T = phase of temporal flicker with respect to temporal window

(The other symbols have the meanings in Eq. 2.9.)
   You could also write

$$\text{PATCH}(x, y, t) = L_0[1$$

$$+ m \cdot \text{WINDOW}(x, y, t) \cdot \text{GRATING}(x, y, t)] \quad (2.11)$$

where PATCH replaces $L(x, y, t)$ and WINDOW is the window "through which" the infinitely extended GRATING is viewed. More precisely, for the Gabor patch of Eq. 2.10, WINDOW(x, y, t) is the product of the three Gaussian functions (the three exponential terms) in Eq. 2.10 and GRATING(x, y, t) is the product of the two cosine terms at the end of Eq. 2.10. (Notice that the mean luminance term L_0 and the contrast term m have been separated from the window and the sinusoidal terms. GRATING now is a function that goes above and below zero.)

An equation for a drifting Gabor patch would be much the same as Eq. 2.10 except that the product of cosine terms representing the flickering grating would be replaced by an expression like that in Eq. 2.3 for a drifting grating.

As Descriptions of Weighting Functions. In addition to their description of visual stimuli, Gabor-patch functions like those in the above equations will turn out to be useful to us in a rather different capacity—as descriptions of the spatiotemporal weighting functions (receptive fields) of real neurons and of mechanisms in psychophysical models. In that case, however, the mean luminance term would almost always be dropped (since a typical neuron has zero sensitivity outside a limited area), and one would get only the product of the window function and the sinusoidal modulation. More of that later.

2.3.4   *Fifteen Dimensions of Sinusoidal Patches*

If one counts the parameters in Eq. 2.10 for a flickering sinusoidal patch, one finds 12; several others are hidden in the presentation of Eq. 2.10. Varying any one of these parameters defines a dimension.

Seven Spatial Dimensions. Seven of these dimensions are spatial; they are illustrated in Fig. 2.7. Four of these dimensions are illustrated in the left column by luminance profiles in the direction perpendicular to the stripes in Gabor patches. Three are illustrated in the right column by two-dimensional maps of Gabor patches in which a plus indicates a value greater than the mean L_0 and a minus a value less than the mean L_0. Two otherwise identical Gabor patches can differ in spatial frequency (f_S), orientation, horizontal spatial position (x_0), vertical spatial position (y_0), horizontal spatial extent (W_x), vertical spatial extent (W_y), and spatial phase or symmetry (θ_S).

No parameter for orientation appeared in Eq. 2.10. To write an equation that allows for nonvertical gratings, one would allow for a rotation of the (x, y) axes by an angle ρ corresponding to the desired orientation.

The values used on each dimension will usually be in retinal coordinates (e.g., cycles per degree of visual angle) rather than in world coordinates (e.g., cycles

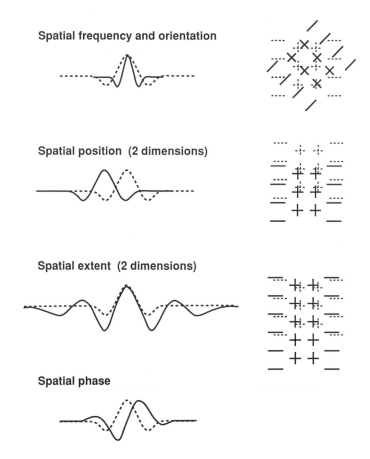

Spatial frequency and orientation

Spatial position (2 dimensions)

Spatial extent (2 dimensions)

Spatial phase

FIG. 2.7 Seven spatial dimensions along which Gabor patches can differ.

per centimeter), because retinal value seems to be the important determiner for experimental results using near-threshold visual patterns.

Remember that aperiodic stimuli (e.g., lines or disks) can be represented as a 0-cpd spatial sinusoid (which is equivalent to a constant function) multiplied by a window function. (The spatial window functions used in experiments with aperiodic stimuli have been more frequently rectangular than Gaussian, however.) When such aperiodic stimuli are varied in width or height, they are equivalent to 0-cpd sinusoidal patches varied in spatial extent.

Variation in the spatial-phase parameter produces spatial luminance profiles of different symmetries. An even-symmetric and an odd-symmetric one (corresponding to $\theta = 0$ and $-\pi/2$, respectively) are shown in Fig. 2.7. Any other spatial phase (symmetry) of sinusoidal patch can be formed as a weighted sum of the two spatial phases shown here (or almost any other two given phases). Only two truly independent values along this spatial-phase dimension exist, therefore.

Five Temporal Dimensions. Four temporal dimensions are straightforwardly analogous to spatial dimensions. Two otherwise-identical sinusoidal patches—which are represented in the first four rows of Fig. 2.8 by their temporal luminance profiles—can have temporal luminance profiles that differ in temporal frequency (f_T), temporal position (t_0—relative to the beginning of trials would be more useful than relative to some absolute zero in history), temporal extent (W_T), and temporal phase or symmetry (θ_T).

For drifting gratings this last dimension is not relevant, or, more precisely, it is inextricably confused with spatial phase. The fifth temporal dimension—direction of motion—is relevant for drifting gratings. For a sinusoidal grating of infinite spatial extent (both parallel and perpendicular to the bars)—such as the sinusoidal grating drifting "behind the window" in a sinusoidal patch—there are only two distinct directions of motion (those indicated by the arrows). (See section 11.6.4 for further discussion.)

Three Miscellaneous Dimensions. Figure 2.9 shows three other dimensions on which values must be given in order to specify completely a sinusoidal-patch stimulus. The first two of these are represented by parameters in Eq. 2.10: contrast (m) and mean luminance (L_0).

The third miscellaneous dimension we have not mentioned before—it is simply which *eye* the sinusoidal patch stimulates. If a patch stimulates both eyes, it will be said to be a compound stimulus on this dimension. As mentioned earlier, we are not considering depth in this book, and thus differences in depth, which would produce differences in the binocular disparity of the patches in two eyes, will not be considered here.

2.3.5   *Some History, and Other Kinds of Function*

To use Gabor patches (or any kind of soft-edged sinusoidal patches) as visual stimuli requires fancier electronics than just sinusoidal gratings that fill up a cathode-ray-tube screen (e.g., John Robson's display used in Graham, Robson,

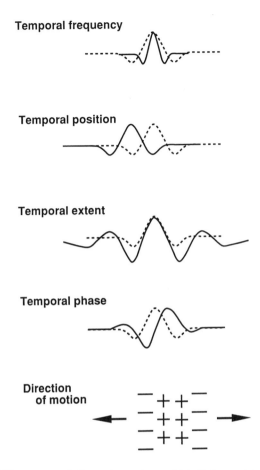

Temporal frequency

Temporal position

Temporal extent

Temporal phase

Direction of motion

FIG. 2.8 Five temporal dimensions along which Gabor patches can differ.

and Nachmias, 1978; Watson & Robson, 1981). The desirability of Gabor patches as stimuli is closely related to the fact that they are good descriptions of neurons' and mechansims' spatiotemporal weighting functions and that their mathematical properties might have implications for visual processing (Bossomaier & Snyder, 1986; Daugman, 1984, 1985; Jones & Palmer 1987a, 1987b; Jones, Stepnoski, & Palmer, 1987; Kulikowki & Bishop, 1981; Kulikowski, Marcelja, & Bishop, 1982; Marcelja, 1980; Pollen, Foster, & Gaska, 1985; Watson, 1983; Webster & DeValois, 1985).

Several other kinds of functions have been used instead of Gabor functions. In one dimension, a difference between two Gaussian functions (a narrow excitatory one and a broad inhibitory one) looks very like a Gabor function containing 1.5 cycles or so. Such difference-of-Gaussians (sometimes called DOGs) have been used in discussing the interplay between excitation and inhibition in retinal ganglion cells (e.g., Enroth-Cugell & Robson, 1984; Frishman, Freeman, Troy, Schweitzer-Tong, & Enroth-Cugell, 1987; Linsenmeier, Frishman, Jakiela, &

Contrast

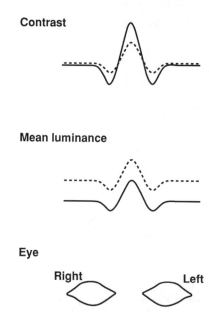

Mean luminance

Eye

Right   **Left**

FIG. 2.9 Three miscellaneous dimensions along which Gabor patches can differ.

Enroth-Cugell, 1982; Rodieck 1965; Rodieck & Stone, 1965) and also in psycho-physical models (especially by Hugh Wilson and his colleagues). The use of several adjacent concentric DOGs to form an oriented patch as a model of simple cortical cells' receptive fields has been explored (e.g., Daugman, 1980; Hawken & Parker, 1987; Rose, 1979; Soodak, 1986). A Gaussian-derivative model for oriented receptive fields is very much like a two-dimensional Gabor function (Webster & DeValois, 1985; Young, 1987). Another related function (only for nonorientation-selective concentric weighting functions, however) is the Laplacian operator (Marr, 1982; Marr & Hildreth, 1980). Cauchy functions have several advantages in describing the Fourier transform spectrum of analyzers on the spatial-frequency dimension (Klein & Levi, 1985). Hermite functions (Hermite polynomials multiplied by Gaussian windows) closely resemble Gabor functions but may be more tractable for some analytic work (Alan L. Stewart, personal communication, 1988).

2.4   THE FOURIER TRANSFORM OF A SINUSOIDAL PATCH

2.4.1   *The Amplitude Spectrum of a Gabor Patch*

Let's consider the amplitude spectrum (that is, the amplitude characteristic of the Fourier transform) of a Gabor patch of drifting sinusoidal grating. We will use 7 of the 15 eight parameters in Figs. 2.7, 2.8, and 2.9. The drifting sinusoid has spatial frequency f_S and temporal frequency f_T. For the moment we will assume it has a vertical orientation (nonvertical orientations are considered below) so ρ will not appear in the equation. It's three Gaussian windows have full widths at half height of W_X (also called W_{PERP} because it is the window perpendicular to the bars), W_Y (also called W_{PRLL} because it is the window parallel to the bars), and W_T (the temporal window). The mean luminance and contrast of the patch are L_0 and m, respectively. The spatial parameters of such a patch are illustrated in Fig. 2.10 left.

Let me emphasize that the spatial and temporal phases, direction-of-motion the center positions of the Gaussian windows do not affect the amplitude characteristic of the Fourier transform; they affect only the phase characteristic and thus are not discussed here. The eye dimension is not represented in the Fourier transform at all.

The amplitude characteristic of the Fourier transform of the vertical Gabor patch of drifting grating is sketched in Fig. 2.10 right and is

$$|\overline{\text{PATCH}}(f_x, f_y, f_t)|$$

$$= mL_0 W_X W_Y W_T \exp\left\{-2.77\left(\frac{(f_x - f_S)^2}{W_{\text{FX}}^2} + \frac{(f_y - 0)^2}{W_{\text{FY}}^2} + \frac{(f_t - f_T)^2}{W_{\text{FT}}^2}\right)\right\}$$

$$+ mL_0 W_X W_Y W_T \exp\left\{-2.77\left(\frac{(f_x + f_S)^2}{W_{\text{FX}}^2} + \frac{(f_y + 0)^2}{W_{\text{FY}}^2} + \frac{(f_t + f_T)^2}{W_{\text{FT}}^2}\right)\right\} \qquad (2.12)$$

$$+ L_0\delta(f_x, f_y, f_t)$$

where W_{FX}, W_{FY}, and W_{FT} equal 0.8825 divided by W_X, W_Y, and W_T, respectively (as in Table 2.2 second row).

The first two terms in the amplitude characteristic are three-dimensional

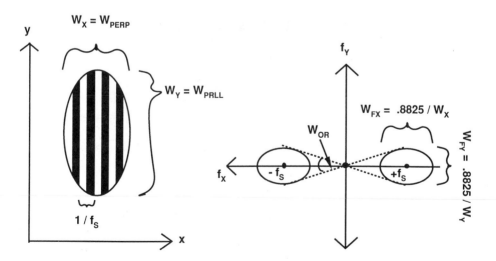

FIG. 2.10 A vertical Gabor patch (indicated by sketch on left) and its Fourier spectrum (right).

Gaussian functions centered at positive (f_S, 0, f_T) and at negative ($-f_S$, 0, $-f_T$) frequencies. These two terms are illustrated in the right half of Fig. 2.10 by ellipses drawn at the point where their amplitude has decreased to half its maximum. Only the two spatial-frequency dimensions are shown. (You can consider the righthand and lefthand three-dimensional Gaussian functions to have been projected onto the same plane from their positions in the $f_t = f_T$ and $f_t = -f_T$ planes, respectively; alternately you can view the drawing in Fig. 2.10 right as the spectrum of a stationary grating where $f_T = 0$.) The widths of each of the Gaussian functions in the amplitude characteristic are inversely proportional to the widths of the Gaussian windows on the original dimensions.

DC Term. The third term in Eq. 2.12 is a delta function of height L_0 positioned at the origin (at the point where all three frequencies equal zero). This delta function results from the space- and time-average constant L_0 and disappears, of course, when that constant is zero (which it can never be for any pattern other than a completely dark visual field). The delta function is illustrated as a solid circle at the origin in Fig. 2.10 right.

Nonvertical Orientations. If the orientation of the Gabor patch was not vertical but was rotated ρ degrees counterclockwise from vertical (left half Fig. 2.11), then the Fourier transform would be identical to that of the vertical grating but rotated ρ degrees counterclockwise (right half Fig. 2.11). This changes the center of the rightmost Gaussian function, for example, from (f_S, 0, f_T) to ($f_S \cos \rho$, $f_S \sin \rho$, f_T) by Eq. 2.2.

One might also consider the case (not illustrated) where the sinusoid in the Gabor patch was rotated ρ degrees from the vertical but the window functions remained aligned with the x and the y axes. Then the center position of the three-dimensional Gaussian functions in the amplitude spectrum would be moved as in Fig. 2.11, but their axes would remain parallel to the f_x and f_y axes.

Extension to Flickering Grating. The amplitude spectrum of a flickering grating contains four three-dimensional Gaussian functions: the two in Eq. 2.12 (but each at half the amplitude they are there) plus an analogous two centered at (f_S, 0, $-f_T$) and ($-f_S$, 0, $+f_T$) which, by themselves, compose the amplitude spectrum of a leftward drifting grating.

Some Technical Comments. The derivation of Eq. 2.12 is sketched in section 2.10.7. The constant of inverse proportionality between widths of the Gabor-patch windows and widths in its amplitude spectrum depends on which measure of Gaussian width you use. Several possibilities are given in Table 2.2.

We are going to ignore negative frequencies in the text much of the time, as they are difficult to justify intuitively and they can be ignored without serious effect. However, one has to be a bit careful about constants. For example, when adding up sinusoids to form a Gabor patch, how much do you need to add of the sinusoid having some particular set of frequencies (e.g., spatial frequency = 3 c/deg, orientation = 10 degrees rotation clockwise, temporal frequency = 7 c/sec)? The answer is TWICE the amplitude characteristic of the Gabor's patch

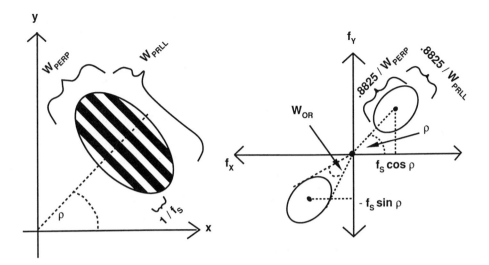

FIG. 2.11 The same patch of Fig. 2.10 but rotated 45 degrees counterclockwise (left) and its Fourier spectrum (right).

Fourier transform at those frequencies (e.g., at 3 c/deg, 10 degrees of rotation, and 7 c/sec). Or, to put it another way, you would have to add the amplitudes at the positive (e.g., 3, 10, 7) and the negative (e.g., -3, -10, -7) frequencies. These amplitudes are always identical. See section 2.10.2 for more details.

In the case where the spatial frequency is neither zero nor large (as we assumed for Figs 2.10 and 2.11) but is small relative to the spatial-frequency bandwidth (so there are very few cycles in that patch), then the two three-dimensional Gaussian functions in the amplitude spectrum of the Gabor patch would overlap to some extent and thus the amplitude characteristic at frequencies around the origin would receive contributions from both Gaussian functions and not be exactly Gaussian-function shaped. An analogous comment applies to temporal frequency.

2.4.2 Properties of a Multiple-Region Oriented Patch and Properties of Its Amplitude Spectrum

The relationship between properties of a multiple-region oriented patch (e.g., a Gabor patch) and properties of its Fourier transform will be important in later chapters where sinusoidal-patch functions are used both as descriptions of visual stimuli and as descriptions of mechanisms' weighting functions (or, speaking physiologically, of cortical neurons' receptive fields). Table 2.4 summarizes relationships between the amplitude spectrum (top row and left column labels) and properties of the original sinusoidal-patch function (interior of table). The entries in parentheses give the relationships for the Gabor patch in symbols;

TABLE 2.4. Relationships Between Properties of a Multiple-Region Oriented Patch Function (Entries in the Table) and Properties of Its Fourier Transform (Best Value and Bandwidth on Each of Three Dimensions).

Dimension	Best Value on Dimension[a]	Bandwidth on Dimension
Spatial frequency	Reciprocal of width of positive plus negative region in patch (f_S)	Inversely proportional to width of spatial window perpendicular to bars $\left(W_{FS} = \dfrac{0.8825}{W_{PERP}} \right)$
Orientation	Orientation of regions in patch (ρ)	If small, inversely proportional to width of spatial window parallel to bars times best frequency $\left(W_{OR} = \dfrac{0.8825}{W_{PRLL} \cdot f_S} \right)$
Temporal frequency	Reciprocal of duration of positive plus negative phase at any location (f_T)	Inversely proportional to temporal window width $\left(W_{FT} = \dfrac{0.8825}{W_T} \right)$

[a] Symbols for a Gabor patch are enclosed in parentheses.

qualitatively, however, as indicated by the words, the results hold for any kind of oriented multilobed function.

Best Values. The best spatial frequency is the spatial frequency at which the amplitude spectrum is maximal. It is approximately equal to the "spatial frequency" in the original patch, that is, to 1 divided by the sum of the widths of a positive plus negative region. (This reciprocal equals f_S—the spatial frequency of the sinusoid—in the case of a Gabor patch, and the best frequency is exactly equal to it.)

The best orientation is approximately equal to the orientation of the patch (assuming that the window functions are aligned with the orientation of the individual regions).

The best temporal frequency is approximately equal to the reciprocal of the total duration of a positive plus a negative temporal phase (exactly for Gabor patches). See Chapter 12 note 2 for a discussion of the case where there is no negative phase.

I have been assuming in the last few statements that the best value on one dimension (e.g., orientation) does not depend on values on the other dimensions (e.g., spatial frequency and temporal frequency). Although this kind of separability (and separability of bandwidths as well) in the amplitude spectrum holds for many kinds of patch functions at least approximately (Gabor patches exactly), there are some oriented multilobed patches for which it does not. (See Daugman, 1980, for a discussion of these issues in the context of spatial frequency and orientation and cortical neurons.)

Bandwidths. The spatial-frequency bandwidth of multiple-region patches is approximately proportional to the reciprocal of the spatial extent of the patch perpendicular to the bars (exactly for Gabor patches). That is, the greater that extent (the more positive-negative cycles there are), the narrower the bandwidth. Figure 2.12 shows an example of this relationship in the same format as the previous two figures. The patch in the middle row has greater spatial extent perpendicular to the bars than does that in the top row, and proportionally smaller

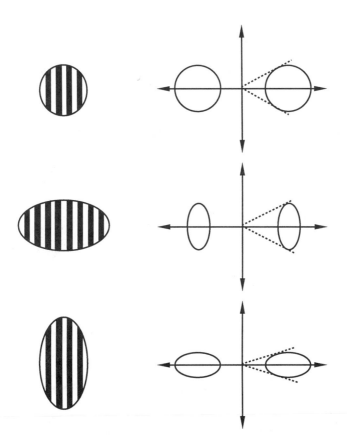

FIG. 2.12 The effect of changing either the spatial extent perpendicular to the bars (middle row) or the spatial extent parallel to the bars (bottom row) on the spectrum of the Gabor patch (right column). (Adapted from Daugman, 1985.)

spatial-frequency bandwidth. For Gabor patches using the half-peak full-bandwidth measure, the spatial-frequency bandwidth W_{FS} is $0.8825/W_{PERP}$. Table 2.2 gives the relationship for other measures of bandwidth.

If spatial extent is expressed in number of cycles (regardless of the spatial frequency of the sinusoid in the patch), then the ratio of the spatial-frequency bandwidth to the best spatial frequency does not depend on the spatial frequency of the sinusoid in the patch; equivalently, the bandwidth on a logarithmic frequency axis and the bandwidth in octaves do not depend on the spatial frequency of the sinusoid in the patch. (An octave is a factor of 2. To say that something is one-octave wide means that its upper limit is two times its lower limit. To say that something is x octaves wide means that its upper limit divided by its lower limit = 2^x.) Table 2.3 gives quantitative examples of the octave bandwidths implied by spatial extents measured in numbers of cycles.

If spatial extent is expressed in units of distance (e.g., degrees of visual angle), then it is the frequency bandwidth in cycles per degree that is determined independent of the frequency of the sinusoid. For example, $W_S = 1$ degree implies that $W_{FS} = 0.88$ c/deg regardless of the value of f_S.

Exactly analogously, temporal-frequency bandwidth depends on temporal extent; Table 2.3 applies to the temporal Gabor function (the temporal window multiplied by the temporal sinusoid) as well as to the spatial.

The orientation bandwidth is slightly more difficult to deal with, although the relationships are much the same. It is usually expressed in terms of the angle at the origin that is spanned by one of the Gaussian functions in the amplitude spectrum (see Figs. 2.10, 2.11, and 2.12). We will use full bandwidth at half height—which we will call W_{OR}. It is approximately inversely proportional to W_{PRLL}—the spatial extent of the patch in the direction parallel to the bars (measured in units of distance). In the case of Gabor patches and for small orientation bandwidths, where the sine of an angle is approximately equal to the angle, W_{OR} is approximately equal to $0.8825/(W_{PRLL} \cdot f_S)$. And, therefore, the larger the spatial extent parallel to the bars (for a given spatial frequency), the smaller the orientation bandwidth, as shown in Fig. 2.12 (bottom versus top row).

A slightly different way of describing these relationships between spatial extents and spatial-frequency and orientation bandwidths can be found in Section 12.2.3.

2.4.3   Aperiodic Functions

A spatially aperiodic patch (e.g., the luminance profile of a disk of light, or the receptive field of a neuron that has only an excitatory region) can be described by a constant function (the function that is constant at all spatial positions—that is, a sine wave of zero spatial frequency) multiplied by the window functions. Similarly, a temporally aperiodic stimulus can be described as a constant function (constant at all temporal positions, that is, a sine wave of zero temporal frequency) multiplied by the window functions.

The amplitude spectrum of such an aperiodic stimulus will be like that described above for Gabor patches in general, except that f_S (or f_T) will equal zero. When $f_S = 0$, the amplitude spectrum projected onto the spatial-frequency plane (the plane where $f_t = 0$) would only contain a single Gaussian function, centered at the origin. The two Gaussian functions in Fig. 2.10 or 2.11, for example, would have moved together and be superimposed at the origin. When $f_T = 0$, the two Gaussian functions would both be centered at $f_T = 0$, so that the spectrum projected onto the temporal-frequency axis (when both f_x and $f_y = 0$) would show only one Gaussian function.

Thus the best spatial frequency for spatially aperiodic stimuli is 0 c/deg. Strictly speaking, the best orientation (the angular coordinate at $f_S = 0$) is indeterminate. One could instead define the best orientation as the orientation at which the amplitude spectrum (considered as a function of orientation) for any fixed nonzero spatial frequency is maximal. This orientation is determined by the relative lengths of the two spatial window functions. It will be indeterminate if both spatial window functions are identical since the amplitude spectrum is then circularly symmetric.

For temporally aperiodic stimuli, the best temporal frequency is at 0 cps.

For a spatially or temporally aperiodic patch, the spectrum as a function of spatial or temporal frequency is highest at zero and then decreases. Thus one does not always speak of a bandwidth for the spectrum (in octaves, the bandwidth would be infinity). One usually says instead that the spectrum is "low pass." However, the width of this low-pass spectrum (the spatial or temporal frequency at which the amplitude has decreased to one half, for example) is still at issue, and again, the larger the spatial extent, the narrower the width of the spectrum. Orientation bandwidth can be defined for any fixed non-zero spatial frequency (unless both spatial windows are identical) but will vary greatly with spatial frequency.

2.4.4 Non-Gaussian Window Functions

Any multiple-region oriented patch in which the widths of the positive and negative regions are approximately equal can be well described as a sinusoid (stationary, flickering, or drifting) multiplied by window functions. And, to a good approximation, the relationships shown in Table 2.4 still hold.

More precisely, if one or more of the three window functions of a patch is not Gaussian, the amplitude spectrum of the patch will not contain three-dimensional Gaussian functions. For a vertical drifting-rightward sinusoid under any other kind of window, for example, the patch would still have two "mounds," but the shape of the mounds along one or more dimensions would not be Gaussian but would be the shape of the spectrum of the non-Gaussian window. The mounds would still be at positions (f_S, 0, f_T) and ($-f_S$, 0, $-f_T$), and the widths would be inversely proportional to the widths of the window function. See appendix to this chapter and Eq. 2.39.

If the window function is smooth and roughly mound shaped like the Gaussian function, it will for all practical purposes (and all our purposes in this book) act just like a Gaussian window.

Rectangular window functions, however, need some further discussion. Rectangular window functions are of uniform height over some range of positions and are zero outside that range. They are used in describing the luminance profiles of many aperiodic stimuli (bars, disks, lines) and of grating stimuli having sharp spatial edges and/or abrupt onsets and offsets. The Fourier transform of a rectangular function contains not only a central "mound" (much like the mound in the transform of a Gaussian function) but has subsidiary mounds at higher frequencies. (See any standard text.) Thus, the spectrum of a patch with sharp spatial or temporal edges will contain not only the mounds at the frequencies f_S and f_T (much like the mounds if the window were Gaussian of about the same effective width) but also subsidiary mounds at frequencies quite far from the nominal frequencies of the patch.

2.4.5 The Phase Characteristic

The job of the phase characteristic of the Fourier transform is to keep track of the original position of the window—x_0, y_0, and t_0—and of the spatial and temporal phase and the direction of motion—what the sinusoid is doing at position (x_0, y_0) and time (t_0). Then the sinusoids into which the patch decomposes are lined up appropriately.

For example, if the patch has odd spatial symmetry (say a positive region to the right and a negative region to the left of center), all of the spatial sinusoids that the odd-symmetric function decomposes into must have their zero crossings located at the spatial center. If the patch has even spatial symmetry (say a positive region at the center flanked by negative regions), all the sinusoids must have their peaks at the center. (Patches with intermediate symmetries—intermediate phases—can be represented as the sum of an even and odd patch.)

2.4.6 Uncertainty Relation (Trade-off Between Localization in Position and in Frequency)

While a delta function is completely localized on a position dimension and completely spread out on the corresponding frequency dimension (and vice versa for a sine function), the less extreme members of the Gabor family are somewhat localized on both the position and the frequency dimensions. There is a theoretical limit to how well localized a function can be on both position and frequency dimensions simultaneously (by one mathematically tractable measure of localization). As it happens, one-dimensional Gabor functions (Gabor, 1946) and two-dimensional Gabor patches (the two spatial dimensions—Daugman, 1985) have been shown to attain this theoretical limit. Whether this particular measure of localization is of significance to visual processing remains to be understood. And reaching this limit with respect to linear frequency is not the same as reaching it with respect to logarithmic frequency (Klein & Levi, 1985).

2.5 LINEAR SYSTEMS AND POINTS

In some, but far from all, of the models we will look at in subsequent chapters, the properties of individual analyzers can be specified in enough detail that the concepts of "linear systems," "weighting functions," and "impulse-response functions" will be necessary. In some other cases, understanding these concepts makes certain explanations easier, because it makes generating examples and counterexamples easier. Consequently, the concepts will be very briefly introduced here, I hope well enough that a reader can follow the discussions in subsequent chapters. Lengthier definitions and discussions can be found in many books (e.g., Bracewell, 1965; Papoulis, 1962).

2.5.1 The Superposition and Multiplication Properties

A linear system is an entity having inputs and outputs that obey two rules—called the *superposition property* and the *multiplication property* here.

The superposition property can be stated in a slightly cryptic but easy-to-memorize fashion as: "The output to a sum is the sum of the outputs."

Less cryptically, consider the output of a linear system to a compound input (a compound input is an input that is the sum of two or more components). Also consider the two or more outputs generated when the system responds to each component by itself. Then, the superposition property says that the output to the compound input equals the sum of the outputs to the components.

Notice that, implicit in the superposition property above, is the notion that it makes sense to talk about adding inputs and about adding outputs.

To define a linear system rigorously, one must also use the multiplication property: the output to a constant times a function equals that constant times the output to the function. (The superposition property will imply this multiplication property for rational constants—twice a function is the same as a compound made up of two identical functions—but cannot be stretched to imply it for irrational numbers.)

2.5.2 Examples of Linear Systems

Single-Number Outputs. As mentioned above, certain neurons (for example, the X retinal ganglion cells) do act quite like linear systems (under certain constraints, e.g., the mean luminance is kept constant). To make this statement some care is necessary in defining the neuron's output. One good (from this point of view) definition of the output of the neuron is the maximum instantaneous firing rate in response to a pattern minus the baseline firing rate in response to a steady blank field at that same mean luminance as the pattern. According to this definition, the output of the neuron can be represented as a single number. Then the output of an X cell to, for example, two points of light will equal the sum of its outputs to each of the two points by itself (assuming the points are not so bright as to change the mean luminance by enough to produce light adapatation—a highly nonlinear process). A similar computation would give its output to any other compound visual pattern, for example, to a stationary compound grating containing two components at different spatial frequencies.

Outputs That Are Functions of Time. Another useful definition of the neuron's output is the whole function giving the instantaneous firing rate as a function of time (again minus the baseline rate). Addition of two such outputs is defined in the straightforward way by adding, for each point in time, the two numbers from the two individual outputs. According to this definition also, the output of an X cell to a pair of points (or to a compound grating containing two sinusoidal components) equals the sum of the outputs to each point by itself (or to each sinusoidal component by itself). (Remember in such discussions the mean luminance is always assumed to be held constant, and a steady blank field at that mean luminance is equivalent to zero input.)

Outputs That Are Functions of Space (e.g., Arrays of Neurons or Mechanisms). Now consider an array of X cells rather than just a single one. These cells are assumed to have receptive fields heavily overlapping and scattered all over the visual field. Then the whole array can be considered a linear system where the output at a particular (x, y) or (x, y, t) is just the output (or the output at time t) of the X cell having its receptive field centered at (x, y). The sum of two such outputs is gotten simply by adding, for each point in space (and time), the two numbers from the individual outputs. (Again, output equals firing rate minus baseline rate.) Since each X cell is assumed to be a linear system, the array of X cells is a linear system also. Note that in this final example, both the input (the visual stimulus) and the output (from the neural array) are represented as functions of three dimensions (x, y, t).

2.5.3 Weighting Functions

For a Linear System with Single-Number Outputs. Consider any one of the receptive fields in Fig. 1.5 and assume the neuron or mechanism possessing that receptive field is a linear system. Rather than roughly plotting the receptive field in the manner shown, however, one could precisely measure the magnitude of the output of the neuron to a point of light at a given intensity when the point was in many different spatial positions.

A plot of the magnitude of output (with baseline rate subtracted) as a function of position (x, y) gives a *weighting function*. Let's call this function $w(x, y)$.

Alternately, one could vary the intensity of the point of light at each position until one found the intensity producing a given size of output. If the neuron or mechanism is a linear system—as we have been assuming—the reciprocal of this intensity will be exactly proportional to the magnitude of output found by the first procedure. Thus a plot of the reciprocal of the intensity versus spatial position will again yield the weighting function. This second measurement is often called the *sensitivity profile* of a neuron's receptive field.

Using the Weighting Function to Compute the Output to Any Input. For a linear system with a single-number output, the output to any input can be computed easily, as shown in the following equation for the two-dimensional case:

$$R = \int_{-\infty}^{+\infty} L(x, y)w(x, y) \, dx \, dy \tag{2.13}$$

In words, simply multiply the input by the weighting function (in other words, "weight" the input by the weighting function) and then add (or, in the general case, integrate) over all positions.

If it is not obvious to you why this procedure works, consider the following: (a) Any input can be considered to be the sum of many points (many delta functions). See section 2.2. (b) The linear system's output to the original input equals the sum of the outputs to the individual points (by the superposition property). (c) The output to any one of these points equals the point's intensity multiplied by the value of the weighting function at the point's position. (After all, the weighting function was generated in the first place by taking the output to points all at the same intensity but at different positions.)

Of a Homogeneous Array. Consider an array of many neurons or mechanisms, all having identical properties (e.g., size and shape of receptive field, temporal characteristics) except that their receptive fields are in different positions on the retina. Suppose there are so many neurons or mechanisms that there is, for all practical purposes, a different receptive field centered at each point in the visual field. Let the output of this array be a function of two dimensions (x, y) where the response at any point (x, y) is the output of the neuron or mechanism having a receptive field centered at (x, y). Assume that the array is a linear system because each neuron or mechanism is.

In this homogeneous array the weighting functions of all the neurons or mechanisms are identical except for translation. This weighting function—strictly speaking, the weighting function centered at zero—is called the *weighting function of the array.* The output of the homogeneous array at point (x_0, y_0)—which is the output of the neuron or mechanism having receptive field centered at point (x_0, y_0)—can thus be calculated from the luminance profile and the weighting function by the following generalization of Eq. 2.13:

$$R(x_0, y_0) = \int_{-\infty}^{+\infty} L(x, y)w(x - x_0, y - y_0) \, dx \, dy \tag{2.14}$$

One can easily generalize to three dimensions

$$R(x, y, t) = \int_{-\infty}^{+\infty} L(x, y, t)w(x - x_0, y - y_0, t - t_0) \, dx \, dy \, dt \quad (2.15)$$

A Terminological Caution. Strictly speaking, one should reserve the phase *weighting function* for use with linear systems. In the following chapters, however, it will occasionally be used more loosely to represent the responses to points of light even if the neuron or entity under discussion is not strictly linear.

2.5.4   Impulse-Response Functions

For linear systems having outputs that are functions of at least one variable, it is useful to define another function that is closely related to the weighting function—the impulse-response function.

Of Homogeneous Arrays. For ease in introducing the impulse-response function, let us again ignore the temporal dimension for a moment and consider a homogeneous array of neurons, as described above. The weighting function specifies how much the output at one position (the output of one neuron or mechanism in the array) is affected by points of light at a number of different positions. Suppose one considers instead how the outputs at a number of different positions are affected by a point of light at one position. The function corresponding to this second alternative is known as the impulse-response function, since it is the response to an impulse (to a single point of light in this case). Here we will call the impulse-response function $h(x, y)$ when the impulse is stimulating the point $(0, 0)$. When the impulse is translated to another point (x_1, y_1) the output will be translated accordingly to give an output $h(x - x_1, y - y_1)$.

Further, there is a very simple relationship between the weighting function and the impulse-response function: namely, $w(x) = h(-x)$. In words, one is just a left-right reversal of the other. This relationship is illustrated in Fig. 2.13 for a linear system having one-dimensional inputs and outputs. The top row shows the weighting functions for six different neurons having receptive fields centered at the positions indicated by vertical lines. The middle row shows an impulse of light stimulating position 3. The bottom row shows—as the labeled points on the curve—the outputs of all six neurons to that impulse as well as the complete impulse-response curve.

To discuss linear systems having two-dimensional inputs and outputs, let's consider a particular example. Consider an impulse of light (having one unit of intensity) at position $(0, 0)$ and consider a neuron or mechanism having a weighting function centered 2 units to the right ($x = +2$) and 3 units below ($y = -3$) that impulse of light. Either the impulse-response function or the weighting function can be used to compute that neuron's output to the point of light.

Since the light impulse is at the origin in this example, the value of the impulse-response function h at position (x, y) directly gives you the output of the neuron having weighting function at position (x, y). Thus, since the neuron

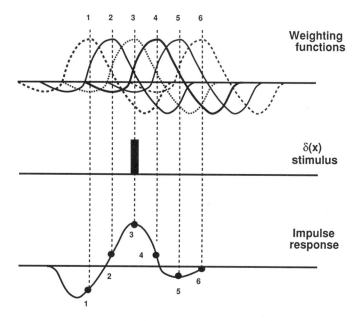

FIG. 2.13 The weighting functions of six mechanisms are shown in the top row. The vertical lines show their centered positions. An impulse is shown in the second row. The response of the six mechanisms to that impulse are shown by the numbered points in the bottom row; the continuous line drawn between those points illustrates the impulse-response function of the whole system.

we are using in this example is 2 units to the right and 3 units down $(+2, -3)$, its output equals $h(+2, -3)$.

This neuron's output can also be calculated by noticing that the impulse of light is 2 units to the left of (-2) and 3 units above $(+3)$ the center of the neuron's receptive field. Therefore, the intensity of that impulse—which is 1 unit by definition—can be multiplied by the value of the weighting function 2 units to the left and 3 units to the top—$w(-2, +3)$—to give the neuron's output. Thus, the neuron's output equals $w(-2, +3)$.

Putting these two facts together gives: $w(-2, +3) = h(+2, -3)$. More generally,

$$w(x, y) = h(-x, -y) \qquad (2.16)$$

Substituting into Eq. 2.14 then gives you

$$R(x_0, y_0) = \int_{-\infty}^{+\infty} L(x, y)h(x_0 - x, y_0 - y)\, dx\, dy \qquad (2.17)$$

Notice that this equation has the same form as Eq. 2.14 for the weighting function except for the left-right reversals in going from w to h.

Convolutions. When two functions L and h are combined as in Eq. 2.17, they are said to be convolved, and the resulting function R is said to be the convolution of the two. Convolutions play an important role in the formalisms of linear-systems analysis. Using $*$ for convolution, Eq. 2.17 can be written $R = L * h$.

Of Spatiotemporal Arrays. More generally, if one considers a three-dimensional (e.g., both spatial dimensions and one temporal dimension) translation-invariant linear system

$$w(x, y, t) = h(-x, -y, -t) \tag{2.18}$$

By a straightforward extension of Eq. 2.17 one can compute the response of such a linear system to any stimulus $L(x, y, t)$ by convolving the three-dimensional functions L and h, that is,

$$R(x_0, y_0, t_0) = \int_{-\infty}^{+\infty} L(x, y, t)h(x_0 - x, y_0 - y, t_0 - t) \, dx \, dy = L * h \tag{2.19}$$

2.6   LINEAR SYSTEMS AND SINES

Sinusoidal stimuli are particularly useful in studying linear systems. For, as mentioned earlier, any stimulus can be considered to be the sum (or more generally integral) of sinusoids. And the output of a linear system to a sum is just the sum of the outputs. Hence, if the output of a linear system to all sinusoids (varying on whatever dimensions are under consideration) is known, its output to any stimulus whatsoever (which varies on those same dimensions) is known.

2.6.1   *When the Output to a Sine Is a Sine (Translation Invariance)*

A further simplification occurs for certain kinds of linear systems, in particular translation-invariant ones like the homogeneous array of neurons discussed above. Then the output to any sinusoidal input is a sinusoid of the same frequency (or frequencies in the multidimensional case). (I know of no intuitively appealing proof of this fact. But a few trial calculations with homogeneous arrays of receptive fields simplified to one dimension may help convince you of its truth.) Thus, to know the output of a translation-invariant system to a sinusoid of frequency f, we just need to know two numbers: the factor by which the system multiplies the amplitude of the sine and the amount by which the system shifts the phase. You can combine these numbers into a single complex number that we will call $S(f)$, where the absolute value (amplitude, modulus) of the complex number—$|S(f)|$—and its phase (argument, polar angle)—ph $S(f)$—are the two numbers, respectively. Because it specifies how the system "transfers" an input of frequency f into an output, this function $S(f)$ is sometimes called the *transfer function of the system.*

2.6.2 *The Output to an Arbitrary Stimulus*

Now we will decompose an arbitrary one-dimensional stimulus $L(x)$ into sinusoidal components, calculate the output of the translation-invariant linear system to each of those components (using the transfer function just defined), and then add up those component outputs to find the full output $R(x)$.

Consider the component sinusoid at frequency f in the input $L(x)$. The amplitude of this input sinusoid is $|\overline{L}(f)|$—the Fourier spectrum of the input luminance profile at the frequency in question—and its phase is ph $\overline{L}(f)$. We know the output to this sinusoid by itself would be a sinusoid of frequency f, and we know also that this is the only sinusoid of frequency f in the full output $R(x)$. Hence, the amplitude of the output sinusoid at frequency f can be written $|\overline{R}(f)|$—the Fourier spectrum of the output at the frequency in question—and its phase can be written ph $\overline{R}(f)$. We know finally that the output and input amplitudes are in the ratio given the amplitude of the transfer function $|S(f)|$ and the output and input phases are shifted by the constant ph $S(f)$. In short,

$$|\overline{R}(f)| = |\overline{L}(f)| \cdot |S(f)|$$

$$\text{ph } \overline{R}(f) = \text{ph } \overline{L}(f) + \text{ph } S(f)$$

These last two equations can be combined to read

$$\overline{R}(f) = \overline{L}(f) \cdot S(f) \tag{2.20}$$

(Remember that the multiplication of two complex numbers is equivalent to multiplying their amplitudes and adding their phases.) This last equation is true for any translation-invariant linear system—where $S(f)$ is its transfer function—and any input $L(x)$.

If one carries out the above procedure for every frequency f, one will have calculated the full Fourier transform $R(f)$. To find out what the output $R(x)$ is, one calculates the "inverse Fourier transform" of $\overline{R}(f)$, which is equivalent to adding (integrating) sinusoids with amplitudes and phases specified by $\overline{R}(f)$ as discussed in section 2.10.2.

Three Dimensional. These relationships generalize straightforwardly to more dimensions. The three-dimensional output $R(x, y, t)$ of a translation-invariant (on all three dimensions) linear system in response to an arbitrary pattern $L(x, y, t)$ can be found by calculating

$$\overline{R}(f_x, f_y, f_t) = \overline{L}(f_x, f_y, f_t) \cdot \overline{h}(f_x, f_y, f_t) \tag{2.21}$$

(which is equivalent to multiplying the amplitudes and adding the phases) and then performing an inverse Fourier transform.

One could also have found the output $R(x, y, t)$ by using Eq. 2.19. But it is often easier on the computer (because of the existence of Fast Fourier Transforms) or on one's intuitions to use the Fourier transforms instead. Since the two methods are totally equivalent in their output, however, it is only a question of ease.

2.6.3   *The Fourier Transform of the Impulse Response Is the Transfer Function*

As it turns out, the transfer function $S(f)$ of a translation-invariant linear system equals the Fourier transform of the impulse response $\overline{h}(f)$. Why should this be so? An impulse at zero contains sinusoids at all frequencies, all at an amplitude of 1 unit and all at a phase of 0. (See section 2.2.4.) Therefore, the output of the system to that impulse contains the outputs to all those sinusoids; their amplitudes in the output equal the factors by which the system multiplies by the input at each frequency (because the input amplitudes were all 1) and their phases equal the constants by which the system shifts the phase (because the input phases were all 0). In symbols, one can write the proof as follows, remembering that the impulse response $h(x)$ is the output to $\delta(x)$, the impulse at position 0. Hence, by Eq. 2.20

$$\overline{h}(f) = S(f) \cdot \overline{\delta}(f),$$

and (see sections 2.2.4 and 2.10.5)

$$\overline{\delta}(f) = 1$$

Hence

$$\overline{h}(f) = S(f) \tag{2.22}$$

This proof can be generalized to more dimensions straightforwardly. For three dimensions, one finds that

$$\overline{h}(f_x, f_y, f_t) = S(f_x, f_y, f_t) \tag{2.23}$$

Since the weighting function is just the left-right reversal of the impulse-response function, that is, $w(x, y, t) = h(-x, -y, -t)$ the Fourier transform of the weighting function is also very closely related to the system's transfer function. Its amplitude characteristic is the same in fact; only some systematic phase changes to keep track of the left-right reversal distinguish it. Specifically, the Fourier transform of the weighting function is the complex conjugate of the Fourier transform of the impulse-response function.

   Therefore, the Fourier transform of either the impulse response or the weighting function tells how a translation-invariant linear system will respond to sinusoids of different frequencies. In the visual system, the weighting functions of many mechanisms (either physiological neurons or entities in psychophysical models) are multiple-region oriented patches and are probably well described as Gabor-patch functions. Hence the relationships between properties of such functions and properties of their Fourier transforms (summarized in Table 2.4) will be useful not only in discussions of visual patterns—where those relationships allow one to relate the luminance profile of a visual pattern to how much of various sinusoids are "contained in" the pattern—but also in discussions of visual analyzers—where those same relationships tell how well an analyzer responds to sinusoids of different frequencies.

For example, an array of linear mechanisms with multiple-region oriented weighting functions responds best when the spatial frequency of a grating is such that one bar of the grating is the same size as one region in the weighting function and when the orientation of the grating is such as to line up the grating with the regions in the weighting function. Further, the bandwidth of spatial frequencies responded to by a mechanism is inversely proportional to the spatial extent of the patch perpendicular to the bars (to the number of regions) (an attempt to demonstrate intuitively why this should be so is given in Graham, 1980.) And so forth through Table 2.4.

2.6.4   Series of Linear Systems

Consider a series of linear systems where the output of the first is the input to the second, and so on. To find the output of the last system in the series, you would (a) multiply the input's Fourier transform by the first system's transfer function to get the Fourier transform of the first system's output, (b) multiply that by the transfer function of the second system to get the Fourier transform of the second system's output, and so on.

This convenient fact, however, has a consequence that is sometimes unpleasant. If science has access only to the initial input and the final output of a series of linear systems, there is no way the individual systems in the series can ever be disentangled from one another. For they always act precisely like an infinite number of other series (for example, like a single linear system having a transfer function equal to the product of those in the series).

2.6.5   Reductions to Lower Dimensionality

In many places throughout this book we will be considering stimuli varying on only one or two of the three possible dimensions. For example, a stationary sinusoidal grating varies only on one dimension, the spatial dimension perpendicular to the bars. And a flickering homogeneous field varies only on the temporal dimension. In such cases, we can restrict our view and consider luminance profiles, weighting functions, impulse-response functions, Fourier transforms, on only one or two dimensions (as we have been doing).

In general, no confusion will result from so doing. Trouble can result, however, if one flips back and forth carelessly from an original higher dimensional function (e.g., the two-dimensional weighting function corresponding to a neuron's receptive field) to a lower order function (the one-dimensional weighting function for predicting this neuron's responses to sinusoidal gratings of different spatial frequency). For the lower dimensional function is not always simply a cut across the original higher dimensional function. Suppose you wanted the one-spatial-dimensional weighting function that tells how the neuron would respond to long vertical lines placed at each position on a horizontal line (this is the one-dimensional function we have been considering). Then this one-dimensional weighting function needs to be calculated by integrating the original higher dimensional function along the vertical dimension.

Sometimes the lower dimensional function is just a cut across the higher dimensional function, however. For example, suppose you wished to know how the neuron would respond to a point placed at different positions along that horizontal line; this latter is a one-dimensional cut through the original higher dimensional weighting function.

2.7   HOW STIMULUS DECOMPOSITIONS ARE USEFUL

Let's return here to the question of why sinusoidal stimuli are useful in studying pattern vision. Initially their use in visual science was inspired by their use in investigations of translation-invariant linear systems (electrical networks, optics). As will be discussed in detail in subsequent chapters, however, the visual system, even the restricted parts of it important for the early-level processing of patterns, cannot be modeled as a single, translation-invariant linear system. And, indeed, even the individual analyzers may not be linear systems. In spite of this, the popularity of sinusoidal stimuli only increases. Assuming this increase is a result of more than fad and fashion, investigators must be finding these stimuli useful. One naturally wonders why. In general, I think there are at least three kinds of reasons why decompositions of stimuli into restricted sets of component stimuli (sinusoids, for example, as well as points or Gabor patches) and the resulting use of these components as stimuli in their own right are useful in the investigation of the visual system.

2.7.1   *The Investigator*

The first kind of reason results from the cognitive psychology of the investigator. A stimulus decomposition may be useful simply because it is different from any way of thinking about stimuli that investigators have used before. In emphasizing different aspects of the stimulus and of the processing of the stimulus, its novelty may give new clues to the human investigator who is trying to unravel the sensory process. Certainly sinusoidal stimuli, when they were introduced, had this novelty, being in at least one sense about as different from the historically earlier points as is possible.

2.7.2   *Mathematics*

The second kind of reason stems from mathematics. Some kinds of stimuli may just allow one more easily to do mathematics. Knowing the output of the system to some set of component stimuli may be sufficient—given the current state of mathematical knowledge—to easily calculate its output to any arbitrary stimulus. (As just discussed, this is true for sinusoidal stimuli and linear-translation invariant systems.) Using the components as stimuli would then allow the investigator to understand and predict the system's outputs to any arbitrary stimulus.

Even though the visual system is certainly not a single linear system, people have not given up the idea that the early-level analyzers may be linear systems in parallel. If so, knowing the output of any one of these multiple analyzers to sinusoids would allow one to calculate its output to anything else. Thus some investigators continue to try to use sinusoidal stimuli to characterize the outputs of each of multiple analyzers. Point stimuli could also be used for this purpose, and of course have been. But sinusoids have the following advantage over point stimuli, particularly in psychophysics. The form of a linear translation-invariant system's output to a sinusoid is known to be a sinusoid (section 2.6.1) and therefore only two numbers (amplitude and phase) need to be measured to specify the complete output. The form of such a system's output to a point, on the other hand, is quite arbitrary. Particularly in psychophysics, it is difficult to devise ways to measure very many numbers at once.

There are other somewhat different ways in which mathematics may suggest the use of certain stimuli. For example, given the current state of mathematical knowledge, some investigators find sinusoidal stimuli very useful in the investigation of nonlinear systems (even though the response of such systems to an arbitrary stimulus cannot be directly computed from their response to sinusoids) because it is possible to calculate the expected output of various nonlinear models to sinusoidal (and related) stimuli and thereby to test such models (e.g., Shapley & Victor, 1978; Spitzer & Hochstein, 1985a, 1985b; Victor & Shapley, 1979a, 1979b).

2.7.3 The Structure of the Visual System

The third reason comes from the visual system itself. A stimulus decomposition can be useful because it corresponds to a decomposition that is actually performed by the sensory-perceptual system under study. There might be, for example, analyzers each of which responded to only one of the stimulus components. Then the stimulus components might be said to be the "natural units" for some important stage of processing done by the system, and use of one of these components as a stimulus might isolate a single analyzer (that is, cause only a single analyzer to respond). The structuralists hoped, for example, that by studying the perceived appearance of points of light in isolation, they could understand and describe the appearance of any visual stimulus. They hoped, that is, that the perceived appearance of any stimulus was some simple combination of the perceived appearances of individual points, as it might be if the visual system did a decomposition into points at some important stage of its processing and then acted on the points individually. (See Chaps. 3 and 4 in Hochberg, 1978, for a discussion of this point of view.) The discovery that the appearance of a visual stimulus cannot be straightforwardly predicted from the appearance of individual points frustrated this hope in its most ambitious form. Note well, however, that the visual system does do something like a decomposition into points at the earliest stage of processing, since individual receptors (rods and cones) respond primarily to light within a very small area. This receptor level is not very directly linked to perception, however.

The more recent proposal that the visual system contains spatial-frequency analyzers (that is, multiple analyzers acting in parallel, each of which is sensitive to a different range of spatial frequency and orientation) might, in its extreme form (not in its original form), be paraphrased as saying that the visual system does a decomposition into spatial sinusoids, or in other words, that the visual system does a Fourier analysis. (The output of an analyzer would then be proportional to the amplitude of a particular sinusoidal component in the two-dimensional Fourier decomposition.) Although the evidence reviewed later in this book demonstrates that nothing this extreme is true, analyzers do seem to exist that are selectively sensitive to different ranges of spatial frequency and orientation. These ranges are rather broad, as would be expected from analyzers like the neurons described above having receptive fields containing several excitatory and inhibitory regions of limited length. Thus, it would be incorrect to say the visual system does a decomposition into sinusoids.

Even though the analyzers respond to a broad range of spatial frequency and orientation, however, sinusoidal stimuli may have a decided advantage over points or disks of light in the isolating of an individual analyzer. For individual analyzers seem to be sensitive only to intermediate spatial frequencies and completely insensitive to much higher or lower spatial frequencies. Thus, a given sinusoidal grating will stimulate some sizes of analyzers (those with peak sensitivities near the spatial frequency and orientation of the grating) but will not stimulate the other sizes at all. (See discussion of advantages of sinusoidal gratings as visual stimuli in neurophysiology on page 257 of Enroth-Cugell and Robson, 1984.)

With aperiodic stimuli (circles or disks of lights, or bars, or lines), this kind of clean isolation of different sizes could not happen. Individual analyzers (neurons or mechanisms) are not sensitive to intermediate sizes of aperiodic stimuli, with sensitivity falling to zero for smaller or larger sizes. Rather, they seem to be sensitive to all sizes of aperiodic stimuli smaller than a given size (corresponding to the size of their receptive or weighting function excitatory region—as long as the stimulus is located within the appropriate region of the visual field). A given disk or bar of light, therefore, will cause a large set of analyzers to respond—all those having center sizes greater than the width of the disk or bar. Different diameters of disks or different widths of bars of light, therefore, cannot isolate different sizes of receptive field as well as different spatial frequencies of sinusoidal grating can.

Certain aperiodic stimuli, in particular points and disks of light, do have one advantage over sinusoidal gratings, however, They can isolate analyzers (neurons, mechanisms) sensitive to different spatial positions much better than wide-field sinusoidal gratings can.

And, consequently, the third kind of stimulus—Gabor patches—may prove to be the best kind of stimulus for isolating individual analyzers in pattern vision. That is, it may do the best job of stimulating a single mechanism a great deal while stimulating most other mechanisms much less or not at all.

Why the visual system contains analyzers that decompose the stimulus into windowed sine-waves (e.g., Gabor patches) is a related question. An interesting class of possible answers (carefully considered by Field, 1987) is that the visual stimuli we encounter in everyday life are well represented (in any one of a number of possible senses) by a code based on a decomposition into Gabor patches.

2.8 SELECTIVITY OF ANALYZERS

The 15 dimensions used to characterize Gabor-patch stimuli (Figs. 2.7 through 2.9) are also dimensions along which visual analyzers (e.g., single neurons) might be selectively sensitive. Indeed, many of these are the dimensions along which neurons are known to differ in selectivity, as we discussed earlier. In Chapters 11 through 13 we will discuss all these dimensions plus 2 more closely related ones (see section 11.6) and the evidence for (or against) the existence of analyzers selectively sensitive on each of them. (Of course, neurons or analyzers must have many other properties as well, and therefore neurons or analyzers might differ from one another in many other ways. Some of these will be mentioned from time to time.)

Here I will make just one more comment about the spatial dimensions, because summation experiments on these dimensions (and on the interrelationships among these dimensions) will be the subject of Chapters 5 and 6. To obtain selective analyzers on the seven spatial dimensions, it is sufficient to have mechanisms (e.g., single neurons) that are linear systems and to have Gabor-type spatial weighting functions. Then the drawings in Fig. 2.7 can be reinterpreted as representations of the mechanisms' spatial weighting functions. Mechanisms having weighting functions that differ along any one of the seven spatial dimensions (e.g., spatial frequency as in the upper left of Fig. 2.7) would differ in their sensitivity to patterns that vary along that dimension (gratings of different spatial frequency, for example). The mechanisms might also, however, differ in sensitivity to patterns that vary along some other dimension as well (e.g., spatial position; see Chaps. 5, 6, and 11 for more discussion of these interdependencies).

Note that visual analyzers that are NOT linear systems might also be selectively sensitive to patterns that vary along any of these seven spatial dimensions. For much of this book, in fact, it will turn out that the linearity is not at issue.

2.9 SUMMARY

Stationary points, stationary lines, and instantaneous presentations of points or lines are examples of visual stimuli that can be described by *delta* or *impulse* functions.

Sinusoidal functions are used in the description of stationary sinusoidal gratings (which look like blurry striped patterns) and moving and flickering sinusoidal gratings.

Any visual pattern can be decomposed into (considered to be the sum of) many different instantaneous points of light.

More difficult to understand intuitively, any visual pattern can also be decomposed into sinusoidal components (Fourier analysis).

Sinusoidal functions and points (impulses or delta functions) are—at least in one important sense—as different from one another as two functions can get. A sinusoidal function is completely spread out in position (continues to take on nonzero values from minus infinity to plus infinity) but completely localized in frequency (contains only one frequency). Conversely, an impulse is completely localized in position but completely spread out in frequency (contains equal amounts of sinusoids of all possible frequencies).

Just the fact that sinusoids (a relatively new kind of visual stimulus) are so different from points (an old kind of visual stimulus) seems to contribute to their usefulness in the study of vision.

A compromise between these two functions is a *windowed sinusoid,* where a sinusoid is multiplied by a window function that is zero outside some limited range of spatial positions. A particularly easy to work with kind of windowed sinusoid is a Gabor function—a Gaussian function multiplied by a sinusoid.

These windowed sinusoidal stimuli may be useful because they do the best job possible of isolating the single visual analyzers at a relatively low level in the visual system. By "isolating a single analyzer" I mean causing it to respond a great deal while causing little response in other analyzers.

One can identify 15 different dimensions on which two-dimensional windowed sinusoidal functions may differ. Seven are spatial dimensions: spatial frequency, spatial orientation, spatial position (two dimensions), spatial extent (two dimensions), and spatial phase. Five are temporal dimensions: temporal frequency, temporal position, temporal extent, temporal phase, and direction of motion (this last is really a hybrid spatiotemporal dimension). Three are miscellaneous dimensions: mean luminance, contrast, and eye of origin.

These 15 dimensions form a useful classification system. They serve to classify many experiments in terms of (a) the dimensions on which the visual stimuli used in the experiment have varied (even aperiodic stimuli fit rather well into the classification), and/or (b) the dimensions on which the experiments' results have suggested the existence of multiple visual analyzers. Two more dimensions are introduced in Chapter 11.

A linear system's output to a compound stimulus is the sum of its outputs to the component stimuli presented by themselves or, more briefly, the output to a sum is the sum of the outputs.

In the study of linear systems, sinusoidal components are particularly useful because the output of a linear system to a sinusoid is again a sinusoid of the same frequency.

This and other convenient mathematical facts have probably also contributed to the usefulness of sinusoidal stimuli in the study of visual processes.

2.10 APPENDIX. FOURIER TRANSFORMS OF SINUSOIDAL, DELTA, GAUSSIAN, AND GABOR FUNCTIONS

2.10.1 *The Fourier Transform (Fourier Analysis)*

The Fourier transform of any function $L(x)$ is given by

$$\overline{L}(f) = \int_{-\infty}^{+\infty} L(x)\exp(-i2\pi fx)\, dx \qquad (2.24)$$

where the Fourier transform is defined for both positiive and negative values of frequency f. Negative frequencies seem mysterious, but one's intuitions seldom go astray by ignoring them as long as one's equations keep track of them.

In general, the value of the Fourier transform is a complex number. When expressed in polar coordinates in the complex plane, its length (absolute value, modulus) gives the amplitude characteristic of the transform and can be written as $|\overline{L}(f)|$. And its angle with the horizontal axis (argument, polar angle) gives the phase characteristic, which we will write as ph $\overline{L}(f)$. Thus,

$$\overline{L}(f) = |\overline{L}(f)|\exp[i \cdot \text{ph } \overline{L}(f)] \qquad (2.25)$$

If $L(x)$ is a real-valued function (as it always will be in our applications), then its Fourier transform always has the following properties:

$$|\overline{L}(f)| = |\overline{L}(-f)| \qquad \text{ph } \overline{L}(f) = -\text{ph } \overline{L}(-f) \qquad (2.26)$$

That is, $\overline{L}(f)$ is the complex conjugate of $\overline{L}(-f)$.

This can easily be extended to more dimensions. The Fourier transform of a function $L(x, y, t)$ is given by

$$\overline{L}(f_x, f_y, f_t) = \int_{-\infty}^{+\infty} L(x, y, t)\exp[-i2\pi(f_x x + f_y y + f_t t)]\, dxdydt \qquad (2.27)$$

2.10.2 *The Inverse Fourier Transform (Fourier Synthesis)*

One can obtain the original function from the Fourier transform very similarly (known as taking the inverse Fourier transform):

$$L(x) = \int_{-\infty}^{+\infty} \overline{L}(f)\exp(+i2\pi fx)\, df \qquad (2.28)$$

This formula can be generalized to more dimensions just as the previous one was.

This last formula represents the synthesis of the original function $L(x)$ from sinusoidal components; you may see this synthesis more clearly if the complex exponential is replaced with ordinary cosine functions, as is done next. Notice that now the integration is taken only over positive frequencies (and zero):

$$L(x) = \int_0^{+\infty} 2|\overline{L}(f)|\cos[2\pi fx + \text{ph } \overline{L}(f)] \, df \qquad (2.29)$$

In words, to form $L(x)$ by adding up cosines of different frequencies, the amplitude of the cosine of frequency f must be twice the amplitude characteristic of its Fourier transform at that frequency, and the phase of that cosine must equal the phase characteristic of the Fourier transform at that frequency.

Rather than representing the two pieces of information in a Fourier transform at frequency f as the amplitude and phase of a single sinusoidal modulation, people sometimes use two amplitudes instead. These two are the amplitudes of two sinusoidal modulations at frequency f; one of these modulations is in cosine phase and the other is in sine phase (i.e., the two amplitudes are the amplitudes of a cosine and of a sine). Standard textbooks, for example, Bracewell, 1965, discuss both these representations.

In the following, a number of general theorems of Fourier analysis are invoked to explain specific results. Such general statements are preceded by a ★ for emphasis.

2.10.3   *The Fourier Transform of a Cosine*

The Fourier transform of $\cos(2\pi f_S x + \theta_S)$ is

$$\tfrac{1}{2}\exp(i\theta_S)\delta(f - f_S) + \tfrac{1}{2}\exp(-i\theta_S)\delta(f + f_S)$$

That is, it is a pair of delta functions both of amplitude $\tfrac{1}{2}$. The one at $+f_S$ has phase $+\theta_S$ and the one at $-f_S$ has phase $-\theta_S$.

2.10.4   *The Fourier Transform of Flickering and Drifting Sinusoids*

The following function (which is the modulated term in Eq. 2.4 for a flickering vertical grating)

$$M(x, y, t) = \cos(2\pi f_S x + \theta_S) \cdot \cos(2\pi f_T t + \theta_T)$$

is "separable," that is, it is a function of three variables (x, y, and t) but equals the product of three functions of one variable each. (The functions for x and t are obvious in the equation and are cosines. The function for y is equal to 1.0 at all values of y.) ★The Fourier transform of a separable function is the product of the Fourier transforms of its individual factors. Hence the Fourier transform of the above is a product of two Fourier transforms like that in section 2.10.3 for cosines and of a third Fourier transform—that of a constant function. ★The Fourier transform of a constant function is just a delta function positioned at a frequency of zero and of height equal to the constant.

Therefore, multiplying these three Fourier transforms (and substituting a three-dimensional delta function for each of the products of three delta functions), the transform of the flickering vertical sinusoid is

$$\overline{M}(f_x, f_y, f_t) = \text{¼} \exp[i(\theta_S + \theta_T)\delta(f_x - f_S, f_y, f_t - f_T)]$$
$$+ \text{¼} \exp[i(\theta_S + \theta_T)\delta(f_x + f_S, f_y, f_t + f_T)] \qquad (2.30)$$
$$+ \text{¼} \exp[i(\theta_S - \theta_T)\delta(f_x + f_S, f_y, f_t - f_T)]$$
$$+ \text{¼} \exp(i(\theta_S - \theta_T)\delta(f_x - f_S, f_y, f_t + f_T)]$$

Thus, the Fourier transform of a flickering sinusoid is a quadruple of two-dimensional delta functions each of amplitude ¼. Consider the first pair of delta functions in the above expression. Notice that these delta functions have their nonzero value either when f_x and f_t are both negative or when they are both positive (and also they both are characterized by the same phase, which equals the sum of the spatial and temporal phases). This pair is, in fact, the Fourier transform of a rightward-moving drifting sinusoid. (See Eq. 2.3, except the amplitude is halved here.) For the other pair of delta functions, one frequency is positive and the other is negative and both have the same phase, which equals the spatial phase minus the temporal phase. This is the Fourier transform of the leftward-drifting component (again at half amplitude) of the flickering sinusoid.

The Fourier transform for a flickering or drifting grating of some orientation other than vertical would be obtained by rotating the Fourier transform above for a vertical grating by the appropriate amount. (★If one function is identical to a second function except that the first has been rotated from the second by an angle ρ in the (x, y) plane, then the Fourier transform of the first is identical to the Fourier transform of the second except that the first Fourier transform is rotated from the second by an angle ρ in the (f_x, f_y) plane.)

2.10.5 The Fourier Transform of a Delta Function

The Fourier transform of a delta function $\delta(x - x_0)$ is

$$\exp(-i2\pi f x_0) = \cos(2\pi f x_0) + i \cdot \sin(2\pi f x_0) \qquad (2.31)$$

This Fourier transform has amplitude 1 at all frequencies. Its phase depends on x_0 and embodies the fact that all the cosines are lined up with their peaks at x_0.

2.10.6 The Fourier Transform of a Gaussian Function

The Fourier transform of a Gaussian function is a Gaussian function. In particular, consider the Gaussian function centered at 0 with height equal to 1 and an area underneath it equal to 1.0. The formula for that Gaussian is

$$\exp(-\pi \cdot x^2) \qquad (2.32)$$

The Fourier transform turns out to be of exactly the same form, that is

$$\exp(-\pi \cdot f^2) \qquad (2.33)$$

More generally, the width of the Fourier transform is inversely proportional to the width of the original function. The constant of proportionality depends on what measure of width is being used. See Table 2.2 for some examples (all of which can be derived from the preceding relationships by standard theorems). The measure of width of the original function is subscripted S, and that of the Fourier transform is subscripted F. When the equivalent-width measure is used, the width of the Fourier transform is exactly equal to 1 divided by the width of the original function. When W—the full width at half height is used—this reciprocity does not quite hold, although it is close.

The Fourier transform of a Gaussian function is always centered at 0 cpd (whether or not the original Gaussian function was), and its height is therefore its value at 0 cpd. Its value there (as is true for all Fourier transforms) is simply the area under the original function. See Table 2.2 for the areas under several alternative formulas of the Gaussian function.

When the original Gaussian function is centered at zero as in Eq. 2.32, the phase characteristic is zero at all frequencies. ★If any function is translated to another spatial position, say x_0, its Fourier transform is multiplied by $\exp(-i2\pi f x_0)$. This leaves the amplitude characteristic unchanged but contributes a phase term proportional to frequency. (In the case of the Gaussian, this reflects the fact that now all the cosinusoids have to be lined up with their peaks at position x_0 rather than at the origin.) As another example of these relationships, let's take the Gaussian function specified by a full width at half height of W_X, a height of 1, and centered at x_0:

$$\exp\left[\frac{-2.77(x - x_0)^2}{W_X^2}\right] \tag{2.34}$$

Then its Fourier transform is

$$1.065\, W_X \exp(-i2\pi f x_0)\exp\left(\frac{-2.77f^2}{W_F^2}\right) \tag{2.35}$$

where W_F is equal to $0.8825/W_X$.

2.10.7 The Fourier Transform of a Gabor Patch

It will be convenient to slightly rearrange Eq. 2.12 for a Gabor patch into

$$\text{PATCH}(x, y, t) = L_0$$

$$+ m \cdot L_0 \cdot \text{WINDOW}(x, y, t) \cdot \text{GRATING}(x, y, t) \tag{2.36}$$

Let a line over the name of a function represent the Fourier transform of that function. Then

$$\overline{\text{PATCH}}(f_x, f_y, f_t) = L_0\delta(f_x, f_y, f_t)$$

$$+ m \cdot L_0 \cdot \overline{\text{WINDOW}}(f_x, f_y, f_t) * \overline{\text{GRATING}}(f_x, f_y, f_t) \tag{2.37}$$

where * indicates convolution. (See discussion of Eq. 2.17 for definition of convolution.) This expression follows from standard theorems of Fourier analysis: ★The Fourier transform of the product of two functions (in particular, WINDOW and GRATING) is just the convolution of the Fourier transforms of the two functions; ★the Fourier transform of the sum of two functions is the sum of their individual Fourier transforms; ★the Fourier transform of a constant times a function is that constant times the Fourier transform of the function; and the Fourier transform of a constant was discussed above.

We will first discuss the case of a vertical patch. WINDOW(x, y, t) in Eq. 2.10 is separable, a product of three Gaussian functions where each is a function of only one of the variables. Therefore, its Fourier transform is the product of three one-dimensional Fourier transforms. In particular, for the three-dimensional Gaussian window of Eq. 2.10, the Fourier transform is

$$\overline{\text{WINDOW}}(f_x, f_y, f_t) = 1.065 W_X W_Y W_T \cdot \exp[-i2\pi(f_x x_0$$

$$+ f_y y_0 + f_t t_0)] \cdot \exp\left[-2.77\left(\frac{f_x^2}{W_{FX}^2} + \frac{f_y^2}{W_{FY}^2} + \frac{f_t^2}{W_{FT}^2}\right)\right] \quad (2.38)$$

where the widths on the frequency dimensions (W_{FX}, W_{FY}, W_{FT}) are equal to 0.8825 divided by the widths on the original dimensions (W_X, W_Y, W_T, respectively). Thus the Fourier transform of the window function is a three-dimensional Gaussian function centered at $(0, 0, 0)$ with widths on the three frequency dimensions inversely proportional to the widths on the three original dimensions. (Remember that the complex exponential term that multiplies each Gaussian function in the above transform has amplitude 1.0 at all frequencies and is just keeping track of phases in the case that the original Gaussian window was not centered at $[0, 0, 0]$.)

We need the convolution between this Fourier transform and the Fourier transform of GRATING. Remember that the latter is either a pair (for drifting) or a quadruple (for flickering as in Eq. 2.30) of delta functions centered at various versions of the triplet of frequencies ($\pm f_S$, 0, $\pm f_T$) describing the grating. This convolution between a pair (or quadruple) of delta functions and a three-dimensional Gaussian function centered at $(0, 0, 0)$ results in either a pair (or a quadruple) of three-dimensional Gaussian functions where each three-dimensional Gaussian function in the result is centered at a position occupied by a delta function in the Fourier transform of GRATING.

For example, for a Gabor patch containing a rightward-drifting grating (we are still talking about the vertical case).

$$\overline{\text{GRATING}} * \overline{\text{WINDOW}}(f_x, f_y, f_t) \quad (2.39)$$

$$= \frac{1}{2} \exp[i(\theta_S + \theta_T)]\overline{\text{WINDOW}}(f_x - f_S, f_y, f_t - f_T)$$

$$+ \frac{1}{2} \exp[i(\theta_S + \theta_T)]\overline{\text{WINDOW}}(f_x + f_S, f_y, f_t + f_T)$$

To finish the derivation of the Fourier transform of the Gabor patch we need only to multiply the pair or quadruple of three-dimensional Gaussian functions by $m \cdot L_0$ and to add $L_0 \cdot \delta(f_x, f_y, f_t)$, the delta function centered at $(0, 0, 0)$ that is the Fourier transform of the constant term L_0.

For nonvertical patches, see Fig. 2.10 versus Fig. 2.11 in the text.

If the center positions of the three-dimensional Gaussian functions are far from the origin relative to their widths (as they will be if there are several cycles of the spatial and temporal modulation within the patch), they will not overlap with each other to any significant extent. Then the amplitude characteristic along each frequency dimension will be almost exactly a Gaussian function where the Gaussian functions are centered at the nominal frequencies (the values $\pm f_s$, 0, and $\pm f_t$).

If the center positions are closer to the origin (if the number of spatial or temporal cycles is small), the two three-dimensional Gaussian functions overlap and interact. In this case, if the original Gabor patch had spatial odd symmetry (θ_S is $-\pi/2$), for example, the two three-dimensional Gaussian functions are of equal amplitude but exactly opposite phases (180 degrees different in phase). Therefore, since they are the same distance from the origin, they cancel out at the origin (but not at other places), leaving only the L_0 delta function to contribute to the amplitude characteristic there. (The space and time average of the Gabor patch exactly equals L_0.) If, however, the original Gabor patch has spatial even symmetry ($\theta_S = 0$) with a positive-going region in the middle, the two three-dimensional Gaussian functions are both real valued and positive and, if they are not truly zero at the origin, they will add up to something greater than zero there, contributing to the DC term. The original Gabor patch has a space and time average that is somewhat higher than L_0.

II
ADAPTATION

3

Models of Selective Effects

3.1 A TYPICAL ADAPTATION EXPERIMENT

In a typical adaptation experiment, an observer first looks for several minutes at an adapting stimulus, for example, at the grating in the upper left part of Fig. 2.1. When the adapting stimulus is a stationary pattern, as in this case, the observer should move his or her eyes systematically throughout the central region of the pattern to avoid the formation of "conventional afterimages," which are presumed to arise at a different level of the visual system than the analyzers of interest. (See section 3.9 for more about the problem of conventional afterimages.)

The observer then makes a judgment about a relatively brief test stimulus (a grating of the same or different spatial frequency, for example), perhaps adjusting its contrast until it is just discriminably different from a blank field.

Then follows another brief period (perhaps 10 seconds) of readaptation to the adapting stimulus, followed by another presentation of the same or a different test stimulus, and so forth. In this way, thresholds for a number of different test stimuli would be measured. Then the adapting stimulus might be changed and the whole procedure repeated.

Thresholds would also be measured "before adaptation" or "in the absence of adaptation," or more precisely while the observer is in a "neutral state of adaptation." The preferred procedure would be to measure these thresholds using precisely the same procedure as that used for measuring the thresholds after an adapting stimulus but, in place of the adapting stimulus, using an appropriate neutral stimulus (in this example, a blank field at the same mean luminance as the adapting and test gratings would be appropriate).

Possible results of an adaptation experiment—one that shows selective adaptation—are illustrated in Fig. 3.1. The value V_T of a test stimulus along the dimension of interest (e.g., spatial frequency, orientation, wavelength, auditory frequency) is plotted along the horizontal axis. The solid line in the upper panel shows the observer's sensitivity S_{obs} (plotted logarithmically on the left vertical axis), or equivalently, threshold th_{obs} (plotted logarithmically on the right vertical axis) in a neutral state of adaptation. The dotted line shows sensitivity after adaptation. After adaptation, the observer's sensitivity is decreased for test stimuli having values at or near the value of the adapting stimulus but is unchanged for test stimuli far from the adapting value. The bottom panel of Fig. 3.1 shows the vertical distance (on an expanded scale) between the two curves from the top panel of Fig. 3.1. This distance is a difference between logarithmic sensitivities (thresholds) and thus is equivalent to the logarithm of the ratio of the una-

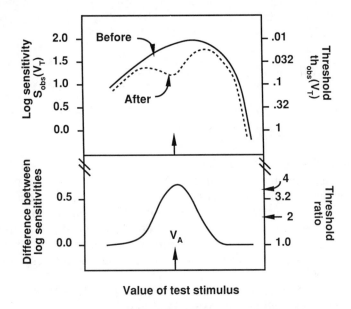

FIG. 3.1 Typical results of selective-adaptation experiments.

dapted to the adapted sensitivity (or the ratio of the adapted to the unadapted threshold).

About Symbols and Definitions. The use of multiletter symbols, as in "th" for threshold and "obs" for observer, is somewhat unconventional. Its advantage is that it allows use of symbols of great suggestive power while avoiding duplication when many symbols are needed. Its disadvantage is possible confusion with multiplication; for example, "th" might also mean t multiplied by h if those single letters were also used as symbols. This problem can be avoided by always using a dot between two symbols when multiplication is intended (single symbols are also conventionally italicized). Thus "$t \cdot h$" would denote t multiplied by h.

How the psychophysical threshold of a stimulus is defined depends on the psychophysical method. In the method of adjustment, the intensity chosen by the subject is said to be the threshold intensity. In a two-alternative forced-choice method, each trial contains two intervals—one having the stimulus and one having a neutral (blank, noise) stimulus. The observer has to say which interval has the stimulus. Threshold is often defined as that intensity producing 75% correct answers. Other percentages are occasionally used.

3.1.1   *Spatial-Frequency Selective Adaptation*

The earliest adaptation experiments on the spatial-frequency dimension were those of Blakemore and Campbell (1969) using sinusiodal gratings, and of Pantle and Sekuler (1968a) using square-wave gratings. Many replications and variations have been done since. (References to many of these are given in Chap. 12.) Results from three are shown in Fig. 3.2, which is plotted in the same way as the bottom of Fig. 3.1 except that adapting spatial frequency rather than test frequency is plotted for the top graph and the vertical axis is labeled as "log threshold elevation." (Logarithms have base 10 as is conventional in visual science.) In all these results, the maximal threshold elevation occurs when the adapting and test sinusoidal gratings have equal or close spatial frequencies. Spatial frequencies differing from the adapting frequency by a factor of about 2 show no threshold elevation and may even show facilitation. This facilitation—which so far has only been demonstrated with the method of adjustment—may be the result of changes in processing at a much higher stage than the analyzers of interest here (due to what might be considered a cognitive response bias). If not, however, this facilitation after adaptation has important theoretical ramifications that will be discussed in the latter part of this chapter.

To demonstrate true selective adaptation, one needs to collect several curves (see Fig. 3.2 top and middle), a point that is sometimes overlooked. For if only one curve is collected (only one adapting or one test stimulus is used), even though it shows a peaked shape, the curves from all other stimuli might peak at the same place. This result, although uncommon, occurs in some contexts (it may occur when temporal frequency is varied; see Chap. 12).

3.1.2 Preview of Rest of Chapter

Four classes of explanation of selective-adaptation effects are examined in this chapter. The first and most extensively discussed class is based on a notion of fatigue or desensitization of analyzers; this class is widespread in explanations of selective-adaptation effects throughout sensory and perceptual systems. The second and third classes postulate inhibition among analyzers—the second inhibition with fatigue and the third inhibition only. The fourth explanation—one based on local point-by-point adaptation effects (afterimages)—is an example of attempts to explain selective-adaptation effects on one dimension (in this case, spatial frequency) with analyzers that are not selective on that dimension but are selective on another (spatial position in this case).

3.2 A SIMPLE FATIGUE MODEL

The basic idea of fatigue models is this: Suppose there are multiple analyzers sensitive to different ranges along the dimension of interest and that an analyzer becomes less sensitive (becomes desensitized or fatigued) after a period of being excited. According to this notion, any analyzer that is sensitive to the adapting stimulus would be desensitized after adaptation, but other analyzers would be unchanged. When the test and adapting stimuli are very dissimilar (very far apart on the dimension of interest), no analyzer responds to both. Then analyz-

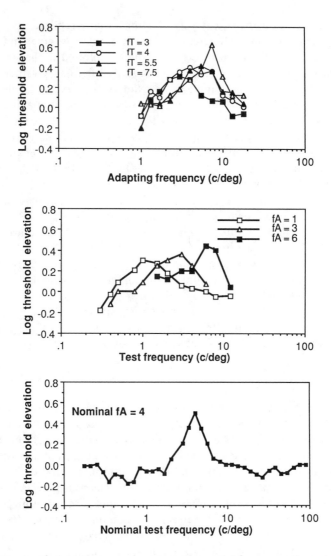

FIG. 3.2 Results of adaptation experiments on the spatial-frequency dimension. Threshold after adaptation divided by threshold before adaptation is plotted on a vertical logarithmic scale; spatial frequency of adapting stimulus (top panel) or of test frequency (middle and bottom panels) is plotted on a horizontal logarithmic axis. The test (top panel) or adapting (middle panel) frequencies are given in the insets. The bottom panel shows average results from many sessions using different adapting frequencies between 0.84 and 13.45 c/deg. The data have been shifted to always plot the adapting frequency at 4 c/deg. (That is, each test frequency was divided by the adapting frequency and then multiplied by 4.) (Top, middle, and bottom panels show results replotted from Graham, 1972; Kelly and Burbeck, 1980; and De Valois, 1977b, respectively.)

ers that respond to the test stimulus would not be affected by the adapting stimulus, and the observer's threshold for the test stimulus would remain unchanged. When the test and adapting stimuli are similar, however, some analyzer (or analyzers) responds to both; and hence at least some analyzer (or analyzers) sensitive to the test stimulus would have been desensitized by the adapting stimulus. The observer's threshold for the test stimulus would therefore be elevated by the adapting stimulus.

Elaborating the basic idea of desensitization or fatigue is not completely straightforward. Many possible versions of such an explanation exist. In this section we will look at one common fatigue model in detail and then examine its implications and the ways it can be tested. This specific model may be familiar to some readers, as it is a simplification of the model (given in section 3.3) that Stiles used to account elegantly and quantitatively for the results of experiments on selective adaptation along the wavelength (color) dimension (see, for example, Stiles, 1967). It is this simpler version of a fatigue model that, explicitly or implicitly, seems to lurk behind many qualitative discussions of selective-adaptation effects and some discussions of masking effects.

To avoid possible confusion, let me explicitly mention that in Stiles's experiments the "adapting" stimulus (a steady monochromatic field) was not only on for a long time before the test stimulus (another steady monochromatic light) but also remained on during the test stimulus. In the pattern-adaptation experiments considered here, however, the adapting pattern was always turned off (leaving a blank field at the same mean luminance) before the test pattern was turned on (as discussed in section 1.11.1).

Terminological Cautions—Fatigue, Analyzer. Fatigue is used here simply as a short name for desensitization resulting from previous excitation, and it is not meant to imply any other properties. In particular it is not meant to imply an extremely long time course.

In explaining the results of selective-adaptation experiments with gratings of different spatial frequencies, one could take an analyzer in the following models to be either an individual mechanism (for which the physiological substrate might be a single neuron) or a spatial-frequency channel (for which the physiological substrate might be an array of neurons all tuned to the same spatial frequency but having receptive fields at different spatial positions). Either form (or something else entirely) could have the properties embodied in the following assumptions. It is the properties in the assumptions, rather than any potential physiological substrate, that should be taken as defining the model.

3.2.1 *Conventions about Assumptions*

This simple fatigue model can be expressed as five assumptions (discussed in subsequent subsections). How finely one subdivides assumptions is a matter of personal preference, or of the particular use for the model, and of convenience in exposition. For example, the first three assumptions that follow—which are about properties of individual analyzers—can be collapsed into two "displacement rules" (as Stiles did) or even into a single assumption. For our future use, however, it will be more convenient to have all three.

Beginning with this chapter, assumptions that are stated formally in this book are numbered in sequential order and given a short name. All of the assumptions in the book are gathered into an appendix at the end of the book for ready reference. There they are listed in two ways—in groups according to their function in multiple-analyzer models, and sequentially according to number in the text. (Preceding the subject index there is an index of assumptions.)

3.2.2 An Analyzer's Transducer Function

Suppose you have determined an analyzer's sensitivity (the reciprocal of its threshold) for two stimuli (e.g., gratings of two different spatial frequencies). Suppose you now present those two stimuli at intensities seven times the analyzer's threshold intensity. A priori, the analyzer may respond differently to the two stimuli now they are at seven times threshold intensity. According to the first assumption we will make, however, the analyzer's outputs must be identical, although not necessarily seven times the output to the threshold intensity.

Assumption 1. Intensity-Sensitivity Product. *An analyzer's output to a stimulus is a function of the product of its sensitivity for that stimulus (the reciprocal of its threshold for that stimulus) and the stimulus intensity.*

You could also say that an analyzer's output to a stimulus is a function of the ratio of the stimulus intensity to the analyzer's threshold for that stimulus. This property has been called the *stability hypothesis* (Maloney & Wandell, 1984) and was introduced by Stiles (1939) in defining analyzers for color.

Graphically, Assumption 1 can be illustrated easily if the output of an analyzer can be represented as a single number. Strictly speaking, this latter assumption is not necessary for our application to selective-adaptation experiments, but it makes explanation easier and has, in fact, been used in all applications of this model to be mentioned. Then you can plot intensity-output curves (like the three in Fig. 3.3) showing the analyzer's output as a function of stimulus intensity on a logarithmic horizontal axis. The letter c (for contrast) will be used for intensity, to save the letter i for indexing subscripts. Contrast is the intensity dimension of primary interest in this book. According to Assumption 1, an analyzer's intensity-output curves for different stimuli will simply be horizontal translations of each other on the logarithmic intensity axis, as shown in the three curves in Fig. 3.3. To see why, consider choosing a pair of points—one on each of two intensity-output curves—having the same vertical coordinate. The horizontal coordinates of those two points give the intensities necessary for two different test stimuli to produce the same analyzer output. According to Assumption 1, these two intensities will always be in the same ratio no matter what vertical coordinate (output magnitude) is chosen. Hence the horizontal distance separating the logarithms of these two stimulus intensities will always be the

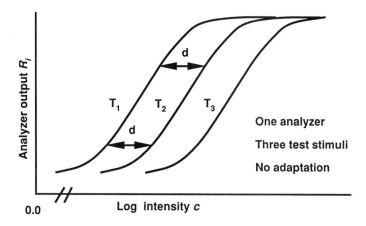

FIG. 3.3 Illustration of Assumption 1 that an analyzer's output is a function of its sensitivity times stimulus intensity.

same. (The fact that equal ratios on the original scale correspond to equal distances on a logarithmic scale is a consequence of the most fundamental property of logarithms. Practically speaking, it allows easy graphical representations of many relationships common in the study of sensory and perceptual systems.)

Readers lacking a taste for algebra may skip this paragraph (as well as later paragraphs giving the other assumptions in equation form) with little loss of continuity. In symbols, Assumption 1 can be written: A function f_i exists such that the

$$R_i(\text{stim}) = f_i[S_i(\text{stim}) \cdot c(\text{stim})]$$

where R_i—the analyzer's output—may in this case be more than a single number. Indeed it may be a set of random variables (a set of numbers each of which may vary from presentation to presentation of the same stimulus). Then the function f_i just needs to be defined appropriately, with its domain being the real numbers and its co-domain being the appropriate entity for R_i.

Whether the output of an analyzer is a direct effect of stimuli on the analyzer or due to interactions among analyzers is irrelevant for this model as long as the analyzer's output obeys Assumption 1.

3.2.3 Stiles's Vertical Displacement Rule for Different Test Stimuli

Figure 3.4 illustrates the next assumption graphically by showing functions giving three analyzers' sensitivities to different values along the dimension of interest both before (left panel) and after (right panel) adaptation. Sensitivity (or equivalently, threshold) is plotted logarithmically on the vertical axis. Notice that the sensitivity function for an individual analyzer on a logarithmic vertical axis is simply translated downward by adaptation. If, for example, an analyzer's

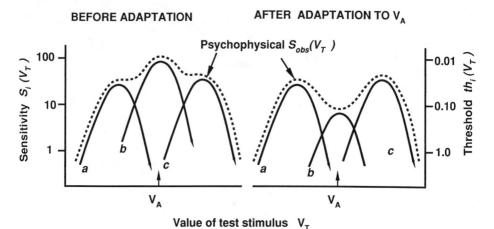

FIG. 3.4 Illustration of Assumption 2 that adaptation elevates an analyzer's threshold by the same factor for all test stimuli.

threshold for a grating of 3 cpd has been raised by a factor of 1.5, so will its threshold be raised for every other spatial frequency. Or

Assumption 2. Same Factor for All Test Stimuli.   *After adaptation to an adapting stimulus, a given analyzer's threshold (equivalently, its reciprocal—sensitivity) is assumed to change by the same multiplicative factor for all test stimuli.*

Figure 3.5 shows a graphical illustration of this assumption using what are sometimes called *tvi curves* (threshold-versus-intensity curves). Each tvi curve shows the threshold of a particular analyzer for a particular test stimulus after adapting to various intensities (plotted logarithmically on the horizontal axis) of a particular adapting stimulus. The three curves in Fig. 3.5 are for three different test stimuli. Since the ratio of an analyzer's thresholds for two test stimuli (the distance between the thresholds on the logarithmic vertical scale in Fig. 3.5) is assumed to be the same no matter what the intensity of the adapting stimulus, an analyzer's tvi curves for any two test stimuli (with the same adapting stimulus) must simply be vertical translations of each other, as shown in Fig. 3.5.

Algebraic Statement. Alternately, Assumption 2 can be expressed algebraically. Let

$$S_i(V_T; V_A, c_A) \quad \text{and} \quad \text{th}_i(V_T; V_A, c_A)$$

be the ith analyzer's sensitivity and threshold, respectively, for a test stimulus that has value (or values) V_T on the dimension of interest after adaptation to an adapting stimulus having intensity c_A and value (or values) V_A. Zeros will be used in place of both V_A and c_A when the adapting stimulus is the neutral stimulus (a homogeneous blank field at the same mean luminance as the stimuli in

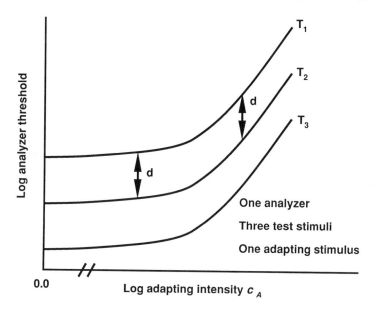

FIG. 3.5 Illustration of Assumption 2 in the form of Stiles's vertical-displacement rule for threshold-versus-intensity (tvi) curves.

the case of pattern vision). Then, Assumption 2 says that the amount of sensitivity loss does NOT depend on the test stimulus (on V_T), although it may depend on the analyzer (on i) and on the adapting stimulus (on V_A and c_A). Thus, there is a function k depending on i, V_A, and c_A (but not on V_T) such that

$$\frac{S_i(V_T; V_A, c_A)}{S_i(V_T; 0, 0)} = \frac{\text{th}_i(V_T; 0, 0)}{\text{th}_i(V_T; V_A, c_A)} = k_i(V_A, c_A)$$

In what follows, the leftmost term is called *sensitivity loss* and the middle term is called *threshold elevation*. They are, by definition of sensitivity, always equivalent. What this assumption says is that they are independent of test stimuli.

3.2.4 Stiles's Horizontal Displacement Rule for Different Adapting Stimuli

The third assumption of the simple fatigue model guarantees that, if two adapting stimuli lead to identical outputs from a given analyzer, they will lead to identical sensitivity losses in that analyzer. Or,

Assumption 3. Sensitivity Loss Depends Only on Output to Adapting Stimulus. *An analyzer's loss of sensitivity after adaptation is assumed to depend only on the analyzer's output to that adapting stimulus, not on any other characteristic of the adapting stimulus.*

Algebraically, therefore,

$$\frac{S_i(V_T; 0, 0)}{S_i(V_T; V_A, c_A)} = h_{i,T}[R_i(V_A, c_A)]$$

where h is the function giving the desensitization of the ith analyzer for test stimulus T and depends only on the output of the ith analyzer to the adapting stimulus, not on any other characteristics of the adapting stimulus. That is:

Horizontal Displacement Rule. Assumption 3 says that an analyzer's sensitivity loss for a given test stimulus is a function (called h) only of the analyzer's output to the adapting stimulus. But Assumption 1 says that the analyzer's output to the adapting stimulus is a function (called f) only of the product of its sensitivity times the intensity of the adapting stimulus. Together, therefore, these assumptions say that an analyzer's sensitivity loss after adaptation is a function only of its sensitivity to the adapting stimulus times the intensity of the adapting stimulus, or

$$\frac{S_i(V_T; 0, 0)}{S_i(V_T; V_A, c_A)} = h_{i,T}\{f_i[c \cdot S_i(V_A; 0, 0)]\}$$

Consequently when, as in Fig. 3.6, threshold elevation for a particular test stimulus is plotted against logarithmic adapting stimulus intensity, the curves for different adapting stimuli will be horizontal translations of one another. This combined assumption is the second of Stiles's displacement rules.

Combination of First Three Assumptions. All three assumptions can be combined into one equation: For each analyzer i, there is a function g_i such that

$$\frac{S_i(V_T; 0, 0)}{S_i(V_T; V_A, c_A)} = g_i[c \cdot S_i(V_A; 0, 0)]$$

where

$$g_i(\text{stim}) = h_{i,T}[f_i(\text{stim})]$$

Note that the function g_i relating sensitivity loss to the product of sensitivity times intensity may be different for different analyzers, but it does NOT depend on the test stimulus or on any properties of the adapting stimulus except its contrast and the analyzer's sensitivity to it.

3.2.5 *Assumption about the Observer's Response*

The following simple assumption turns out to be very useful: The observer's threshold for a given test stimulus is exactly equal to the threshold of whichever single analyzer (of all the analyzers) is most sensitive to that test stimulus. Graphically, therefore, the psychophysical contrast sensitivity function is

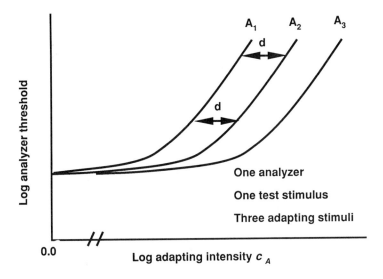

FIG. 3.6 Illustration of Assumptions 1 and 3 in the form of Stiles's horizontal-displacement rule for threshold-versus-intensity (tvi) curves.

assumed to equal the envelope of the sensitivity functions of the individual analyzers. To state it formally:

Assumption 4. Most Sensitive Analyzer Rule. *The observer's sensitivity to a stimulus is equal to the sensitivity of the one analyzer that, of all analyzers, is most sensitive to that stimulus.*

In subsequent chapters we will discard this most sensitive analyzer rule as being not quite correct. For the time being, however, we will ignore its relatively minor defects, because its simplicity is a great advantage.

3.2.6 Assuming That Adaptation Does Not Affect Which Analyzer Is Most Sensitive

This fatigue model is particularly easy to deal with if one further assumption can be used:

Assumption 5. Same Most Sensitive Analyzer. *The analyzer that is the most sensitive for a given test stimulus prior to any adaptation is still the most sensitive for that test stimulus after adaptation to any adapting stimulus whatsoever.*

Simple Fatigue Model. By the "simple fatigue model" we will mean the five assumptions just given. On this model—no matter what the condition of adaptation—the psychophysical threshold for a particular test stimulus will always equal the threshold of one particular analyzer. For a given test stimulus, therefore, the psychophysical tvi curves (the observer's threshold versus log adapting intensity) for different adapting stimuli will be exactly the same as that one particular analyzer's tvi curves. The psychophysical tvi curves will, therefore, obey Stiles's horizontal-displacement rule.

3.2.7   Some tvi Curves From Spatial-Frequency Adaptation Experiments

Using sinusoidal gratings varying in spatial frequency, psychophysical tvi curves (threshold-versus-log adapting contrast) have been measured for the same test frequency with a number of different adapting frequencies. The curves have not always turned out to be horizontal translations of one another, as we will see. One investigation, however, did find horizontally translated curves (Swift & Smith, 1982). The results for two subjects with a test grating of 4 c/deg and various adapting frequencies are shown in Fig. 3.7. The solid curves drawn on the figures are not horizontal translations of each other, but are best fit functions of a particular form in which the slope of the righthand segment and the point at which the bend occurred were allowed to vary to get the best fit. As can be seen, the fitted functions in general have very similar righthand slopes (0.3 on the

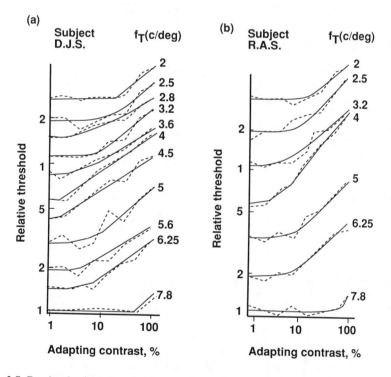

FIG. 3.7 Psychophysical threshold-versus-intensity (tvi) curves for spatial-frequency adaptation. (From Fig. 6 of Swift & Smith, 1982; used by permission.)

average) and so are quite close to being horizontal translations. Curves with identical slopes would fit the results quite well.

3.2.8 Measuring an Analyzer's Sensitivity Function (Bandwidth)

According to the simple fatigue model, it is straightforward to measure an analyzer's bandwidth, or more completely, to measure the sensitivity of an analyzer to different values along the dimension of interest. Simply measure the psychophysical tvi curves for a single test stimulus and a number of adapting stimuli of different values along the dimension of interest. The horizontal displacements between two tvi curves for two adapting stimuli give the logarithm of the ratio of the single analyzer's sensitivity to these two adapting values.

This procedure was followed for the results shown in Fig. 3.7. The point at which the bend occurs in the fitted functions of Fig. 3.7 was taken as a measure of the horizontal displacement between tvi curves and used to calculate the sensitivity of the presumed underlying analyzer. The resulting sensitivity functions had half amplitude full bandwidths that were definitively less than an octave wide and perhaps as narrow as half an octave (Swift & Smith, 1982).

Equivalent Contrast Transformation. If the psychophysical tvi curves are horizontal translations of one another (if the simple fatigue model holds, for example), then the full tvi curve has only to be measured for one adapting stimulus. For the other adapting stimulus, using a single adapting contrast will be sufficient. The one fully measured tvi curve is simply horizontally translated until it goes through the one measured point for any other adapting stimulus. This is one way of presenting the basic idea behind the "equivalent contrast transformation" introduced by Blakemore and Nachmias (1971) and used several times since. If, however, the full tvi curves are not horizontal translations of each other, the meaning of the plot of equivalent contrasts is not clear, as Georgeson and Harris (1984) demonstrated for their results (described later).

Cautions about Estimating Bandwidths from the Simple Fatigue Model. Note that the vertical distances between tvi curves (e.g., Fig. 3.7) are not in general the same as the horizontal distance between the curves. They are the same only when the slope is 1. According to the simple fatigue model, the horizontal distances—not the vertical distances—give the relative sensitivities of the one analyzer determining psychophysical threshold to the different adapting stimuli. Plotting threshold (or threshold elevation) for one test stimulus after adaptation to each of many stimuli (where the intensities of all the adapting stimuli are the same although their values are different, e.g., Fig. 3.2, top) results in a plot reflecting vertical, not horizontal, displacements, and so does not give an analyzer's sensitivity function unless further transformation is done to correct for the actual slope.

If the fatigue model is correct, adaptation to one value and testing at many values (as was done for the middle and bottom parts of Fig. 3.2) will give information about the effect of one adapting stimulus on many different analyzers.

Only if different analyzers have identical sensitivity functions (except for translation to a different preferred value) can one reason from such results to the properties of an individual analyzer (on these assumptions).

3.3   THE GENERAL STILES MODEL

The simple fatigue model might be the end of our story except for two problems. One is a logical problem: The same most sensitive analyzer assumption (Assumption 5) is, in general, inconsistent with the first four assumptions of the simple fatigue model. The other is an empirical problem: The results of many pattern-adaptation studies do not produce horizontally translatable tvi curves for different adapting stimuli. We will look at consequences of the logical problem in this section and return to the empirical results in section 3.4.

3.3.1   When the Most Sensitive Analyzer Changes after Adaptation

Assumption 5 will, in general, be inconsistent with the first four assumptions because adaptation can reduce the sensitivity of what was originally the most sensitive analyzer (for a given test stimulus) by so much that a second analyzer becomes the most sensitive (for that test stimulus). This possibility occurs in Fig. 3.4, in fact. Take note of the range of test values for which the middle analyzer b was the most sensitive analyzer before adaptation (left half of figure). After adaptation (right half of figure), however, analyzer a or c became the most sensitive for many of those test values. Dropping Assumption 5 and leaving the first four assumptions gets us back to the general Stiles adaptation model. To make it explicit that we are dropping this assumption let us substitute the following:

Assumption 6. Most Sensitive Analyzer May Change.

Fig. 3.8 makes this same point but uses tvi curves from several different analyzers for a single test stimulus and a single adapting stimulus. In this example, three analyzers (a, b, and c) are somewhat sensitive to the test stimulus, with c being the most sensitive in the unadapted state. Analyzer c is also much more sensitive to the adapting stimulus than the other analyzers, however, and hence begins to be adapted at lower adapting intensities than the others, that is, the bend in its tvi curve occurs further to the left. As a result, after adaptation to medium adapting intensities, analyzer b is the most sensitive analyzer to the test stimulus. And after adaptation to higher adapting intensities still, analyzer a is the most sensitive. The observer's threshold curve (dashed line) will be the lower envelope of the individual analyzer's curves (by the most sensitive analyzer rule, Assumption 4).

The bottom of Fig. 3.8 shows the same psychophysical curve as that in the top panel plus a second psychophysical curve for a second adapting value (with the same test value). The portions of each psychophysical curve belonging to a

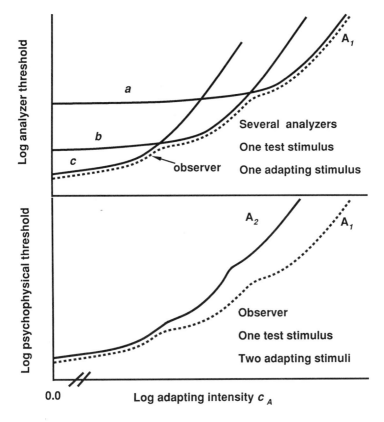

FIG. 3.8 Illustration of threshold-versus-intensity (tvi) curves predicted by general Stiles model.

single analyzer are just horizontal translations of each other (by the horizontal displacement rule of Assumptions 1 and 3). Analyzers a and b in this example were somewhat more sensitive to the second adapting value than to the first, and so their curves are translated leftward.

If the psychophysical tvi curve for a second test value were shown, the portion of it belonging to a particular analyzer would simply be a vertical translation of the portion in the curves illustrated (by the vertical displacement rule of Assumption 2).

3.3.2   The Stiles Model (Few Analyzers) and Chromatic Adaptation Results

Chromatic adaptation experiments, in which the adapting or background stimulus is a steady monochromatic field and the test is a superimposed monochromatic flash, lead to experimental results that look like the scalloped hypothetical curves in Fig. 3.8. Further, corresponding sections for different values seem to be vertical or horizontal translations of the same curve, as they should be on this model. Stiles used the vertical and/or horizontal displacements between the curves for many closely spaced test and adapting wavelengths to derive the sensitivities of individual analyzers (which are now known as Stiles's π mechanisms) as a function of wavelength. For pairs of wavelengths where relative sensitivities could be derived both from vertical and from horizontal displacements, there was excellent agreement, providing a check on many of the assumptions. Stiles's work is classic, and although the underlying substrates of the analyzers that his methods revealed (receptors?, higher order cells?) are just beginning to be understood, his work has had great effect. (See Boynton, 1979, Chap. 6, for a description.)

3.4 EMPIRICAL DISCREPANCIES IN SPATIAL-FREQUENCY ADAPTATION

3.4.1 Kinds of Discrepancies

As mentioned earlier, psychophysical tvi curves from spatial-frequency adaptation experiments do not always look like the horizontally translatable ones of the Swift and Smith (1982) study shown in Fig. 3.7. Consider, for example, the results from Georgeson and Harris (1984) shown in Fig. 3.9 for one test spatial frequency (4 c/deg) and many adapting spatial frequencies. The results of this second study differ from those of the first study in several ways: (a) For the same test frequency and different adapting frequencies, functions in the first study were horizontal translations of one another but functions in the second study were more like vertically scaled versions of one another (as was also found by

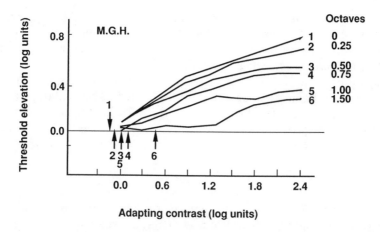

FIG. 3.9 Psychophysical threshold-versus-intensity (tvi) curves for spatial-frequency adaptation. Observer MGH. (From Fig. 2 of Georgeson & Harris, 1984; used by permission.)

Graham 1970, 1972; and Stromeyer, Klein, & Sternheim, 1977). (b) In the first set, individual curves are positively accelerating throughout the range of adapting contrasts (as is also true in Blakemore & Campbell, 1969; Blakemore & Nachmias, 1971; Graham, 1970; and for the most part in Movshon & Blakemore, 1973); but in the second set the curves turn downward for high adapting contrasts (as in Dealy & Tolhurst, 1974, and in some of the replotted results of Stecher, Sigel, & Lange, 1973a). (c) In the first set, the "adaptation threshold"—the adapting intensity at which the tvi curve starts to rise—seems to increase as the difference between the adapting and test frequencies increases; in the second the adaptation threshold changes little with frequency. Further, as we shall discuss later in this chapter, facilitation (threshold lowering) is sometimes reported when the adapting value is far from the test value (e.g., De Valois, 1977b), and at least one study has found oscillations in the tvi curves (little scallops) when the steps between adapting contrast values were only half as large as those for the studies shown here (Graham, 1970).

3.4.2   Effect of Time Course of Adaptation

The reason for the various discrepancies is far from clear. One candidate is the time course allowed for adaptation. In many studies (including the two illustrated), sessions are devoted to a single adapting frequency with adapting contrasts being run in increasing order. The time allowed for initial adaptation at any given adapting-contrast level was 60 to 75 seconds in the Swift and Smith study but 2 minutes in the Georgeson and Harris study, for example. Further, the Swift and Smith study—but not the second study—allowed a 2-minute "recovery period" between each adapting-contrast level and the next higher one. Georgeson and Harris speculated that this recovery period may account for the discrepancies between their results (Fig. 3.9) and those of Swift and Smith (Fig. 3.7). For recent evidence has shown that even a 2-minute adaptation period does not produce asymptotic elevation. Therefore, the 1-minute initial adaptation and 2-minute breaks between adapting-contrast levels in Swift and Smith's study may have prevented asymptotic adaptation from occurring in that study until quite late in the session (at the higher adapting contrasts), thereby underestimating the amount of threshold elevation at lower adapting contrasts.

3.4.3   Qualitative Criteria in Adaptation Experiments

Another likely cause of apparent discrepancies involves a feature of the experiment that is difficult to extract from the published literature. This is the criterion (quantitative but especially qualitative) used by an observer for deciding whether a stimulus was there. Even the use of forced-choice procedure cannot prevent an observer from ignoring some cues and, for example, basing a response only on the output of analyzers sensitive to certain spatial frequencies or to certain spatial positions rather than on all analyzers. Superficially, in all the spatial-frequency adaptation studies being discussed, the observers were supposed to be using the same criterion at all times—in particular, they were supposed to consider any perceptual effect different from that produced by the blank as indicating the presence of a grating. Different observers, however, may none-theless attend to (respond on the basis of) different aspects of their perceptions, and the same observer may attend to different aspects in different adaptation states. Some additional information makes this possibility seem particular likely.

Afterimages and Hallucinations. After adaptation to gratings, even blank fields do not look blank. There may be conventional negative afterimages; even if the observer is moving his or her eyes to try to avoid them and claims not to see them, weak ones or fragments thereof may exist. (From time to time these conventional afterimages have been suggested as the total explanation for spatial-frequency selective effects of adaptation. This possibility is considered and rejected in section 3.9.) These afterimages would presumably interfere: After adaptation to carefully fixated stationary gratings of low spatial frequencies, for example, conventional negative afterimages seem to actually increase the sensitivity of an observer to test stimuli in certain phases; when care is taken to eliminate the afterimages, sensitivity decreases (Bowker & Tulunay-Keesey, 1983; Smith, 1977).

Further, there may well be other kinds of leftover outputs from other levels of the visual system causing aftereffects on the blank field. "Hallucinations" that might result from higher level analyzers have sometimes been reported after adapting gratings are turned off (Georgeson, 1976, 1980).

Whatever their source, these nonblank perceptions on a nominally blank field are potentially confusing to observers instructed to consider any perceptual effect other than a blank field as indicating a grating. In fact, Georgeson and Harris (1984, p. 731) reported that data points for some stimuli (particularly lower spatial frequency, higher adapting contrasts) are omitted because the observers (who were the authors) were unable to "reliably distinguish the test grating from the 'hallucinations' or illusory gratings produced as an aftereffect of adaptation."

Differences in the degree to which apparently minor procedural details allow conventional afterimages and/or nonconventional hallucinations to form may explain some of the discrepancies among spatial-frequency selective adaptation results.

Further, even if conventional afterimages and hallucinations are constant across experiments, their effects on observers' thresholds might not be. For these nonblank perceptions on the nominally blank field turn the observer's task into something like a suprathreshold discrimination (a discrimination between two nonblank patterns). In fact, the task is very like that in a masking experiment: The observer must distinguish between a masker (the afterimage or hallucination) and the masker-plus-test. Such suprathreshold discriminations are known to exhibit individual differences and learning effects. (See section 1.5.2.) These differences may well be systematic across laboratories due to different instructions to and/or expectations of the observers (who are often also the investigators).

3.5 SOME STILES-TYPE MODELS ASSUMING MANY ANALYZERS

Scallops in psychophysical tvi curves, as predicted by the general Stiles model (like those shown in Fig. 3.8 bottom), are not clearly evident in any psychophysical tvi functions from pattern adaptation experiments. However, the scallops may be difficult to see if there are many of them (as there may be if there are many analyzers). And a small modification of the assumption about the observer's response will also tend to hide the scallops by smoothing over the transitions between them (see Assumption 7).

To try to account for their spatial-frequency adaptation results (some of which are in Fig. 3.9), Georgeson and Harris (1984) calculated the predictions from a number of versions of a general Stiles-type model. Figure 3.10 shows predictions from four versions. The main part of each panel shows predicted psychophysical tvi curves for a single test stimulus and for six adapting stimuli. The highest

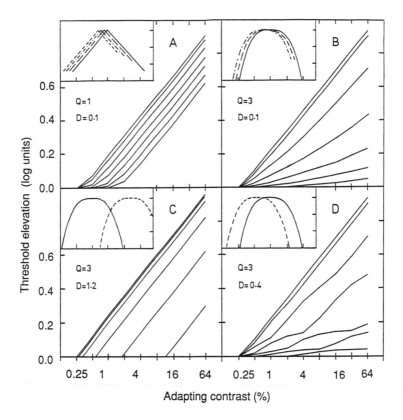

FIG. 3.10 Predicted threshold-versus-intensity (tvi) curves (main part of each panel) from several versions of Stiles-type models characterized by different assumptions about analyzer bandwidth and spacing (as shown in insets in each panel). (From Fig. 9 of Georgeson & Harris, 1984; used by permission.)

curve occurs when the adapting value equals the test value. Successively lower curves represent results for increases in adapting value of 0.25 octave apart on the dimension of interest (spatial frequency in these experimental results, but the particular dimension is irrelevant for the predictions). The inset in each panel shows the analyzers' sensitivity as a function of value on the dimension of interest.

3.5.1   General Assumptions

For all of Georgeson and Harris's predictions, Stiles's two displacement rules (Assumptions 1, 2, and 3) held, but the most sensitive analyzer was allowed to change after adaptation (Assumption 6). Also the most sensitive analyzer rule (Assumption 4) was replaced by a slight modification that smoothes over the sharp corners between scallops in tvi curves:

Assumption 7. Quick Pooling of Sensitivities.   *The observer's sensitivity to a stimulus is determined by the following nonlinear pooling of the sensitivities of all the analyzers:*

$$S_{\mathrm{obs}} = |\Sigma S_i^k|^{1/k}$$

where S_{obs} and S_i are the sensitivities of the ith analyzer and the observer, respectively, to the test stimulus in question after adaptation to whatever adapting stimulus is in question. The parameter k was taken to equal 3.5 in these calculations. This kind of pooling is discussed at length in Chapter 4. It implies that an observer's sensitivity is most heavily contributed to by the most sensitive analyzers but that the less sensitive analyzers contribute somewhat.

3.5.2   Assumptions About Specific Functions

In addition, Georgeson and Harris (1984) had to make assumptions about the specific functions involved in order to generate numerical predictions like those shown in Fig. 3.10.

For all four sets of predictions shown in Fig. 3.10, the following three assumptions were made:

Assumption 8. Uniform Peak Sensitivities.   *The peak sensitivities of all the analyzers are assumed to be equal.*

Assumption 9. Linear Transducer Function.   *The function f_i in Assumption 1 is the identity function, so that analyzer output is proportional to stimulus intensity (and the constant of proportionality is the analyzer sensitivity).*

Assumption 10. Power Adaptation Functions.   *The adaptation functions h_i are assumed to be flat until some adaptation threshold, above which they increase as a power function of input (alternately, log threshold elevation is linear with log input).*

Combining these last two assumptions, the function $g_i = h_i(f_i)$ that gives threshold elevation as a function of adapting contrast was assumed to equal

$$g_i(c_A) = 1 \qquad \text{for } c_A < c_0 \tag{3.1}$$

$$= \left[\frac{c_A \cdot S_i(V_A)}{c_0} \right]^m \qquad \text{for } c_A \geq c_0$$

where V_A and c_A are the values on the dimension of interest and contrast, respectively, of the adapting grating. The constant m was taken to be 0.4, leading to a slope of 0.4 on log-log coordinates. (In Fig. 3.10, the vertical and horizontal scales are different, so a line with a slope of 0.4 is at about 45 degrees.) The threshold for adaptation c_0 was set at 0.25.

What differentiates the four sets of predictions in Fig. 3.10 are the assumptions (described in assumptions 11–15) about the shape of analyzers' sensitivity functions (controlled by a parameter Georgeson and Harris [1984] called Q) and about the spacing of analyzers on the dimension of interest (controlled by a parameter they called D). Insets in each panel of Fig. 3.10 give these two parameter values as well as show sketches of the shape and spacing of analyzer sensitivity functions.

The two possible sensitivity function shapes could both be represented by the following equation:

$$S_i(V) = \exp\left[-\left(\frac{|V - V_i|}{K} \right)^Q \right] \tag{3.2}$$

where V_i is the best value of analyzer i and the parameter K determines the bandwidth and was held constant at 0.8 octave (corresponding to a half peak full bandwidth of 1.4 octave). The parameter Q (not to be mistaken with the Q in Chap. 2 used as the equivalent bandwidth) determines the shape as described further in the next two assumptions:

Assumption 11. Very Rounded. *The shape of each analyzer's sensitivity function is very rounded. $Q = 3$ in Eq. 3.2.*

Assumption 12. Very Peaked. *The shape of each analyzer's sensitivity function is very peaked when plotted as sensitivity versus value and is triangular when plotted as log sensitivity versus value. $Q = 1$ in Eq. 3.2.*

Georgeson and Harris considered three possible spacings of analyzers. Let the parameter D indicate the spacing in octaves along the dimension of interest, that is, the distance in octaves between the best values of two adjacent analyzers.

Assumption 13. Close Spacing. *The distance between two adjacent analyzers is small relative to the analyzers' bandwidth. In particular, $D = 0.1$ octave.*

(Remember the half peak full bandwidth was 1.4 octave.)

Assumption 14. Intermediate Spacing. *The distance $D = 0.4$ octave.*

Assumption 15. Sparse Spacing.   *The analyzers are very sparsely spaced relative to their bandwidths; D = 1.2 octave.*

3.5.3   Predictions of Stiles-Type Many-Analyzer Models

Although the most sensitive analyzer assumption (Assumption 4) has been replaced by the Quick-pooling assumption (Assumption 7), the following remains true: In conditions where a single analyzer is always the one most sensitive to a given test stimulus, the predicted psychophysical tvi curves will look like those of that single most sensitive analyzer and therefore will be horizontally translated versions of one another. As it turns out, when very peaked sensitivity functions are assumed whatever their spacing (panel a in Fig. 3.10 shows highly overlapping functions) or when sparsely spaced very-rounded functions are assumed (panel c), the predicted psychophysical tvi curves are horizontal translations of one another, as can be seen in Fig. 3.10.

When the very-rounded sensitivity functions are spaced every 0.4 octave (as in panel d) or even closer (0.1 octave in panel b), however, the predicted tvi functions are certainly not horizontal translations of one another. They are, in fact, very like vertically scaled versions of one another, just as were Georgeson and Harris's experimental results (Fig. 3.9).

To understand why this behavior is predicted, we will consider the tvi curves (on log-log plots) of all analyzers when the adapt value equals the test value. Call this value V^*. First consider the one analyzer that is most sensitive to the test value before adaptation (the analyzer having the lowest tvi curve when the adapting contrast is zero). Call this the * analyzer. Since we are considering the case where adapt and test values are equal, the tvi curve for any other analyzer is horizontally translated rightward from that of the * analyzer by the same amount it is vertically translated upward from it. (The actual amount of translation is the logarithm of the * analyzer's sensitivity to V^* divided by the other analyzer's sensitivity to V^*). But this leads to an overall slope (vertical translation divided by horizontal translation) of 1.0, which is steeper than the 0.4 slope postulated for an individual analyzer; see Eq. 3.1). Hence the tvi curve for the * analyzer remains lower than that for all other analyzers at all adapting contrasts. Although the observer's threshold is somewhat lower than that of the most sensitive analyzer (the * analyzer) by the Quick pooling assumption (Assumption 7), the psychophysical tvi curve for this case where adapt and test stimuli are equal—the top curve in Fig. 3.10 panel b or d—is still very similar to that individual analyzer's. In particular, it still has the same slope on log-log coordinates ($m = 0.4$).

When the adapt and test values are unequal, however, the tvi curves from different individual analyzers cross over, as in Fig. 3.8. Consider, for example, an analyzer that has a best value on the other side of the test value from the adapting value. Before adaptation, this side analyzer is less sensitive to the test value than is the analyzer centered at the test value. It will, however, also be less affected by the adapting stimulus than is the centered analyzer and may indeed cross over to become the more sensitive analyzer after adaptation (given the proper combination of analyzer shape, analyzer spacing, and slope *m*—see discussion in Georgeson and Harris, 1974). These crossovers make the slope of the psychophysical curve less than that for individual analyzers.

The slopes of the psychophysical tvi curves (normalized so the largest = 1.0) predicted from dome-shaped overlapping sensitivity functions are plotted as a function of the separation between adapting and test frequency in Fig. 3.11 (dotted line from predictions in panel b of Fig. 3.10, triangles from panel d). The solid points give the slopes from the experimental results. (Crosses and solid line are discussed in the following.) Notice that these predicted and measured slopes agree very well.

More Variants. None of the predicted tvi curves in Fig. 3.10, however, show the curvature that was apparent in Georgeson and Harris's 1984 results (Fig. 3.9) and also in Dealy and Tolhurst's 1974 results. A nonlinear compressive saturation can easily be introduced to account for this feature. The x's in Fig. 3.11 come from predictions including this feature.

Correcting these predictions for the fact that the actual contrast sensitivity function is not flat could be done in any of several ways. Georgeson and Harris (1984) showed an example of one way implemented by simply "correcting" the adapting contrast for relative psychophysical contrast sensitivity. When adapt-

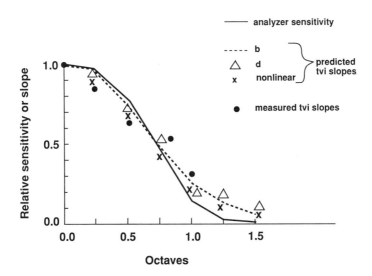

FIG. 3.11 Sensitivity function of a single analyzer (solid line) compared with slopes of psychophysical threshold-versus-intensity (tvi) curves predicted by general Stiles-type models. The dashed line and open triangles are computed from panels b and d of Fig. 3.10. The triangles are computed from predictions assuming an additional nonlinearity. The solid circles are experimentally measured slopes averaged over observers and frequencies. (From Fig. 10 of Georgeson & Harris, 1984; used by permission.)

ing frequencies are higher than the test frequency, this correction increases the distance between the adapting thresholds (the intercepts of the predicted psychophysical tvi curves with the horizontal axis) but otherwise affect the predictions little.

3.5.4   Estimating Bandwidth From the Many-Analyzer Stiles-Type Model

Another very convenient fact is shown in Fig. 3.11. The solid line there is the sensitivity function of the analyzers from which the predicted relative slopes of tvi curves (the dotted line, triangles, and x's) were calculated. Very conveniently, the predicted relative slopes of the tvi curves (from different adapting stimuli and the same test stimulus) turn out to be very similar to the relative sensitivity function of an individual analyzer.

This agreement suggests that plotting relative tvi slope versus adapting frequency may be a good way to estimate individual analyzer's sensitivity functions. Such plots are given in Georgeson and Harris (1984) for their two observers at test frequencies of 4 and 8 cpd and for a number of earlier studies. (Averaged across test frequencies and observers, such a plot is shown by the solid circles in Fig. 3.11.)

Alternatively, if all the tvi curves in a family intersect the zero threshold-elevation line at the same adapting contrast (see note 1), plotting a relative tvi slope is equivalent to plotting—for any single adapting contrast—the log threshold elevation for each adapting value divided by the maximal log threshold elevation (as is done in Graham, 1972).

3.5.5   A Word About the Numerical Modeling Approach

Sometimes you cannot derive analytically from a model the kind of qualitative relationships you wish to know, for example, the predicted relationship between some measure of psychophysical threshold elevation and the bandwidth of individual analyzers. In that situation it is often useful to do what Georgeson and Harris (1984) did. You choose some "representative" numerical values (e.g., the specific functions and the parameter values of Assumptions 8 through 15) and then calculate predictions. In those predictions you will sometimes find, approximately at least, that a qualitative relationship of the kind you want holds over some useful range of specific numerical values (e.g., the proportionality of tvi slope and analyzer sensitivity shown in Fig. 3.11).

3.6   EVEN MORE GENERAL FATIGUE MODELS

Loosening any of the first four assumptions discussed (Assumptions 1 through 4) may allow a fatigue model to predict very different results from those just described and may also allow very different versions of fatigue models to predict the same results. Several examples of such loosenings are given in this section. They may be skipped with little loss of continuity.

3.6.1 The Transducer-Function Assumption and a Physiological Aside

For example, suppose that the output of an analyzer does NOT depend on the product of sensitivity times intensity (contrary to Assumption 1) and that, therefore, the output-versus-log intensity curves for different stimuli are NOT horizontal translations like those in the bottom of Fig. 3.3. If the analyzer's output is not constrained in some way, any family at all of psychophysical tvi curves (for one test stimulus and different adapting stimuli) could be predicted by a fatigue model (Assumptions 2 through 5) by assuming that the family of tvi curves for the most sensitive analyzer was identical to the family of psychophysical curves one was trying to predict. Getting consistent predictions across different test stimuli by such a model might be harder. But it is clear that—without the intensity-sensitivity product assumption (Assumption 1)—it may be impossible to definitively rule out a fatigue model of selective adaptation.

Should the intensity-sensitivity product assumption (Assumption 1) be necessary for a model of analyzers? Not clearly. For example, the output of cortical neurons to gratings of different spatial frequency do NOT follow this assumption (Albrecht & Hamilton, 1982; Sclar & Freeman, 1982).

Cortical neurons, may, however, obey the following less restrictive assumption:

Assumption 16. Monotonic Transducer. *Analyzer output is a monotonic function of sensitivity (for different stimuli all at the same intensity) and also a monotonic function of intensity (for any given stimulus).*

Graphically, being a monotonic function of sensitivity means that the analyzer output-versus-contrast curves for different stimuli do not cross over. Much of the variation among cortical cells can be accounted for by multiplying a nonlinear saturating function of contrast (which does not depend on spatial frequency) by a factor that does depend on spatial frequency (Albrecht & Hamilton, 1982).

3.6.2 Adaptation's Effect on Different Test Values and Another Physiological Aside

Assumption 2 specifying uniform elevation for all test stimuli may not be a necessary property of the fatigue of a single analyzer. A less restrictive assumption would be:

Assumption 17. Not Selective for Value. *An analyzer's threshold elevation after adaptation is not selective for value.*

That is, if two adapting stimuli both elevate the analyzer's threshold for any one test stimulus by the same amount, they will elevate its threshold for any other test stimulus by the same amount (even though that amount might differ from that for the first test stimulus).

This assumption seems to be the crucial property for something to have been called an analyzer (or mechanism, etc.) in the context of selective-adaptation experiments. For, according to it, the analyzer must act as a unit and not itself show value-specific adaptation. In practice, however, what someone might willingly call an analyzer on other grounds might turn out to show value-specific adaptation. In fact, an individual cell in the visual cortex shows spatial-frequency selective adaptation (see end of this subsection). Does this mean that a single cell cannot be called a single analyzer?

In short, to know whether a single-analyzer model—a model in which only one analyzer is sensitive to values along the dimension of interest—can predict the results of selective-adaptation experiments, more must be known about the single analyzer. In the case of pattern vision, hovering behind the idea of a spatial-frequency analyzer was frequently a neuron with an excitatory-center/inhibitory-surround organization (or an array of neurons with receptive fields identical except for position). In this context, then, the question of whether a single-analyzer model could predict selective-adaptation effects reduced to the question of whether spatial-frequency selectivity could be explained without postulating different sizes of receptive fields.

In fact, a model was once constructed in which all neurons had one size of receptive field, and yet the model could predict spatial-frequency selective-adaptation results (Wilson, 1975). To do so, however, the model postulated selective fatigue of interconnections of different lengths AMONG neurons. The changes in these interconnections due to fatigue are something like changes in the shape of the receptive field. These different lengths of interconnections would be viewed by some people as multiple spatial-frequency analyzers in themselves. Formally, the changes in connections meant that individual neurons were showing spatial-frequency specific adaptation (a violation of Assumption 17). One unappealing feature about this model is that it ran into trouble explaining other psychophysical effects. A second was that it was very complicated to work with. Third, the adaptable interconnections are not very appealing on the basis of known neurophysiology. (This latter point is not, of course, devastating, since much remains unknown about neurophysiology.) Overall, it has not proved to be an attractive alternative to multiple spatial-frequency analyzers of the usual sort in models of pattern vision (that is, multiple sizes of receptive fields) and has been abandoned by its creator. It is at least, however, a very good lesson in the impossibility of ruling out everything that might reasonably be called a single-analyzer model in any context.

Pattern Adaptation of Cortical Cells. At least in the cat, adaptation to a high-contrast sinusoidal grating reduces the responsiveness of both simple and cortical cells (e.g., Maffei, Fiorentini, & Bisti, 1973; Vautin & Berkley, 1977). Whereas some cells' sensitivities for all spatial frequencies are depressed uniformly, other cells (both simple and complex) show spatial-frequency selective adaptation—a definitive violation of Assumption 17 (Movshon & Lennie, 1979).

In many cells, adaptation to a high-contrast pattern shifts the full response-versus-contrast curve to higher contrasts and may also lessen its slope when it is plotted as number of impulses versus log contrast (Albrecht, Farrar, & Hamilton, 1984; Dean, 1983; Ohzawa, Sclar, & Freeman, 1982).

3.7 INHIBITION PLUS FATIGUE

In addition to threshold elevation when adapting and test stimuli are close in value, two other effects have been reported in pattern adaptation experiments at threshold. These two effects—and the possibility that inhibition should be used to explain them—are discussed in this section.

3.7.1 *Facilitation at Far-Away Values*

Although the most typical effect of adaptation on thresholds is to elevate them, adaptation is sometimes reported to lower thresholds when the adapting and test values are far apart (e.g., De Valois, 1977b; see Fig. 3.2 right panel). Exactly how far apart the spatial frequencies need to be to produce lowered thresholds differs somewhat from report to report, but one to four octaves is the general range when adapting contrasts are high. Spatial frequencies closer together than that produce threshold elevation, and spatial frequencies further apart have no effect on each other. Low contrasts of adapting gratings seem to cause facilitation at some closer test frequencies when higher contrasts do not (Graham, 1970; Tolhurst & Barfield, 1978).

This facilitation has not always been found, and when it has been found, the method of adjustment was used. Thus changes in the qualitative criteria (i.e., some kind of response bias due to higher cognitive processing; see preceding discussion) may account for the result rather than properties of the analyzers of interest.

The commonly proposed explanation (e.g., De Valois, 1977b), however, postulates inhibition among analyzers as well as fatigue: The observer's sensitivity for certain test values (quite far from the adapting value) is actually greater after adaptation than it was before, because less inhibition is now being exerted on the TEST analyzers (the analyzers that are sensitive to those test stimuli) by the ADAPT analyzers (the analyzers that were desensitized by having responded to the adapting stimulus).

The brevity of this explanation hides the rather large number of analyzer properties that are assumed by it. Although not attempting to make a model of inhibition-plus-fatigue that is as well specified as the preceding models of fatigue, the following section indicates the kinds of assumptions that would be necessary to do so.

3.7.2   *Overview of Assumptions*

The pivotal assumption is that the total output of an analyzer R_i will be a function not only of its excitation $f_i(\text{stim})$—that depends only on the stimulus—but also of the inhibition exerted on this analyzer by each of the other analyzers.

Assumption 18. Output-dependent Inhibition.   *There is inhibition among analyzers (which has been called recurrent, or feedback, or response-dependent inhibition). The amount of inhibition exerted by analyzer j on analyzer i—denoted $K_{ij}(R_j)$—is an increasing monotonic function of the total output R_j of the inhibiting analyzer.*

One possible function (but far from the only one—e.g., Furman, 1965; Pinter, 1983; Sperling, 1970) for combining this excitation and inhibition is additive:

$$R_i(\text{stim}) = f_i(\text{stim}) - \sum_{j=1}^{N'} K_{ij}[R_j(\text{stim})]$$

If the functions K_{ij} are zero below some threshold value of R_j and then increase linearly for further increments of R_j, this equation describes well the eye of the horseshoe crab (where the individual analyzers in the model correspond to individual ommatidia in the eye). From this humble source came much of our initial knowledge of inhibition in the visual nervous system. (See Ratliff, 1965, for a delightful presentation.)

Although a complete quantitative specification of the inhibition (which would include specifications of the functions f_i and K_{ij} as well as their combination) is not necessary for our purposes, the following properties are definitely needed:

Assumption 19. Tonic Inhibition and Excitation.   *Even in the absence of stimulation, analyzers are excited to some extent (have a nonzero output) and also exert inhibition to some extent.*

Assumption 20. Inhibition Effective on Threshold and Below.   *Increasing the inhibition exerted on an analyzer will lower its tonic excitation (if it is unstimulated) or raise its threshold for all test stimuli.*

Also, something like the following must be specified to preclude the possibility that wild changes in inhibition due to the adapting stimulus might undermine the intended explanations of facilitation (or the compound-grating effect discussed later):

Assumption 21. Inhibitory Functions Not Affected by Adaptation.   *When a test stimulus is presented to an analyzer after an adapting stimulus, the function K_{ij} relating the amount of inhibition exerted by the analyzer to the magnitude of its output is unchanged.*

Note, however, that when an analyzer is unstimulated it exerts less inhibition when adapted than when not. (Adaptation leads to less tonic excitation which leads to less tonic inhibition.)

To prevent subsequent confusion, let me make the following implicit assumption explicit:

Assumption 22. Short-acting Inhibition. *The excitation and inhibition both have short enough time courses that the response to one stimulus (e.g., the adapting stimulus) is over by the time the next stimulus in the experiment (e.g., the test stimulus) arrives.*

Finally, assumptions about the fatigue (desensitization due to excitation) must be made also. The phrasings used in the transducer-function assumption (Assumption 1 or, alternately, 16) and the displacement rules (Assumptions 2 and 3) must be modified slightly to indicate whether the assumption applies only to the excitation of the analyzer (as it should in the case of the transducer-function assumption) or applies to the analyzer's total output (excitation and inhibition combined as in the displacement rules). And, of course, we still need an assumption specifying the transformation from analyzer outputs to the observer's response. Either the concept of most sensitive analyzer (Assumption 4) or of Quick pooling (Assumption 7) will do for this discussion.

3.7.3 Explanation of Facilitation Revisited

Let's consider separately two groups of analyzers. First, the ADAPT group contains the analyzers that are highly sensitive to the adapting stimulus. Second, the DISINHIBITED group contains the analyzers that are inhibited by analyzers in the adapt group although not themselves very sensitive to the adapting stimulus.

The analyzers in the ADAPT group will be affected in two ways by adaptation. First, they will all be less sensitive after adaptation than they were before (by fatigue assumptions). Therefore, for test values near the adapting value (near enough that analyzers in the adapt group are excited by the test stimulus), psychophysical thresholds will be elevated (just as in the fatigue models). Second, the analyzers in the adapt group will exert less tonic inhibition after adaptation than before (by Assumptions 20 and 21).

Consequently, the second group of analyzers will be less inhibited after adaptation than before; that is, they will be disinhibited. When a test stimulus affecting these disinhibited analyzers is presented, therefore, the observer's threshold for it will be lower than it was before adaptation. This lowering of threshold is the facilitation effect.

Note that the test stimulus values exciting the DISINHIBITED (showing facilitation) tend to be outside the range of values exciting the ADAPT (showing threshold elevation).

It will be useful to introduce the following terms. Let *inhibitory length* be some measure of the average distance between the best values of pairs of analyzers that inhibit one another. Let *excitatory length* be some measure of the average distance between a stimulus value and the best values of the analyzers excited by that stimulus. In these terms, the disinhibited group of analyzers have peak values that are roughly one inhibitory length plus one excitatory length away from the adapting stimulus value (since the disinhibited analyzers are simply the analyzers inhibited by the analyzers sensitive to the adapting stimulus). Hence, according to this inhibition-plus-fatigue model, facilitation should occur when test and adapting values are separated by about one inhibitory plus one excitatory length. (See De Valois, 1977b, p. 1063, for a related discussion in the particular case of spatial frequency.)

The effect of adapting contrast mentioned earlier—that facilitation may occur for much closer test and adapt frequencies when adapting contrast is low than when it is high—may be explainable by the increasing range of analyzers excited by and thereby desensitized by the adapting grating as its contrast is raised.

3.7.4   The Compound Adapting-Stimulus Effect

A second effect has been attributed to inhibition acting in concert with fatigue (starting with Tolhurst, 1972a): Adaptation to a compound stimulus sometimes produces less threshold elevation than adaptation to one of the components of the compound. This effect occurs with compounds containing component spatial frequencies that are quite close (Stecher, Sigel, & Lange, 1973b), that are in a ratio of 3 to 1 (Nachmias, Sansbury, Vassilev, & Weber, 1973; Tolhurst, 1972a) and that are in ratios spanning a range from very small to 4 to 1 (Georgeson, 1975, as described in Tolhurst & Barfield, 1978). The spatial frequency of the test grating has usually been the same as that of one component in the compound adapting grating. For all frequency ratios except some of the very smallest (in Georgeson's data), adaptation to the compound grating has led to less threshold elevation than adaptation to the component at (or near) the test frequency.

3.7.5   Explaining the Compound Effect With Inhibition-Plus-Fatigue

Briefly, a compound stimulus containing two rather far apart values (about one inhibitory length away from each other) would stimulate two sets of analyzers (one set responsive to each component); these two sets would inhibit each other. Any analyzer's output to the compound, therefore, is less than its output to the appropriate component (the component to which it is most sensitive). As a consequence, every analyzer will be desensitized less by adapting to the compound than by adapting to the appropriate component. For any test stimulus, therefore, the observer's threshold will be elevated less by adapting to the compound than by adapting to the appropriate component (the component closest in value to the test stimulus).

Notice that the diminished adapting effect of a compound relative to its components should occur maximally when the components are about one inhibitory length apart, since then the output to the compound will be minimal.

To explain this effect with fatigue only, one might just assume that "the output of an analyzer to a compound is less than its output to the appropriate component," but such an assumption seems to imply inhibition in some sense of the word, although the word is never used in stating the assumption.

3.7.6   Output-Dependent Versus Input-Dependent Inhibition

In the explanation of the compound-adapting-stimulus effect, inhibition is important only because it makes the output of each analyzer to the compound less than to the appropriate component. Another kind of inhibition can do this task just as well:

Assumption 23. Input-dependent Inhibition *(also called nonrecurrent, stimulus-dependent, feedforward inhibition). The amount of inhibition exerted on an analyzer can be expressed as a function only of the stimulus, with no explicit term for the outputs of other analyzers.*

When the term for excitation is also expressible as a function only of the stimulus (e.g., Assumption 1), the whole output of the analyzer will be expressible in the same way.

Such input-dependent inhibition can also explain the facilitation effect at faraway values if one assumes that an analyzer becomes MORE sensitive after being INHIBITED by an adapting stimulus (just as it become LESS sensitive after being EXCITED by an adapting stimulus).

Input-dependent inhibition cannot, however, predict true disinhibition of the sort predicted by output-dependent inhibition (e.g., see Ratliff, 1965).

Further discussion of conditions where it is or is not possible to tell output-dependent from input-dependent inhibition can be found in, for example, Edwards, 1983; Furman, 1965; Ratliff, 1965; and Varju, 1962.

3.7.7   Conclusions About Inhibition-Plus-Fatigue Models of Facilitation and of Compound-Grating Effects

The inhibition-plus-fatigue explanations of facilitation and of the compound-grating effect do not both require the same set of assumptions, but all the assumptions previously sketched appear to be consistent.

Whether this inhibition-plus-fatigue explanation will stand up under closer inspection remains to be seen, however. One way to further test this explanation is to consider the ranges of value separation for which the two effects occur. According to the inhibition-plus-fatigue explanation, facilitation should occur maximally when the adapt and test values are separated by about one inhibitory plus one excitatory length, and the compound-grating effect should occur maximally when the component values are separated by about one inhibitory length. Roughly (an excitatory length seems to be rather less than an inhibitory length), therefore, both effects should occur at the same value separation.

In the case of spatial frequency, both effects do seem to occur at roughly the same separation (as Tolhurst and Barfield [1978] concluded from the comparison of various investigators' results). Certainly this conclusion cannot be rejected. Unfortunately, no results, at least to my knowledge, compare the two effects in the same conditions—including the same contrast levels—on the same observers.

Certain results may provide some difficulty for the inhibition-plus-fatigue model, however. It is a bit tricky to explain why moving or jittering one of the components in the adapting grating reportedly abolishes the compound-adapting-stimulus effect (Klein & Stromeyer, 1980). The existence of tonic inhibition is potentially difficult to reconcile with the absence of the usual compound-grating effect when adapting to square-wave gratings of low contrast (Tolhurst, 1972a). It is not clear why the compound-grating effect occurs even when the frequencies are very close together (Stecher, Sigel, & Lange, 1973b).

3.7.8   *A Physiological Aside—Inhibition Among Cortical Cells*

A number of physiological and anatomical findings have suggested the presence of inhibition among cortical neurons (e.g., Bishop, Coombs, & Henry, 1973; Blakemore & Tobin, 1972; Maffei & Fiorentini, 1976; Movshon et al., 1978c; Petrov, Pigarev, & Zenkin, 1980). In neurons with maintained discharge, a spatial frequency differing from the cell's best frequency by more than an octave or an octave and a half (a factor of 2 or 3) may cause a decrease in the maintained discharge or a distinctive off response (De Valois & Tootell, 1983; Foster et al., 1985; Movshon et al., 1978c). Further, the responses of simple and complex cortical cells to suprathreshold compound gratings show inhibition (Bonds, 1983; De Valois & Tootell, 1983). When compounds contain the cell's best spatial frequency and a second harmonically related spatial frequency, for example, the response of 97% of all simple cells to the compound is less than to the best spatial frequency alone. Sometimes the response to the best frequency is even inhibited by frequencies that excite the cell when alone. This inhibition is much more common from higher spatial frequencies than from low, particularly from frequencies two to three times the best frequency. From lower frequencies, there is often facilitation instead of inhibition, in fact. In 40% of complex cells, the same result is obtained, again with inhibition being more common from high frequencies than from low. In simple but not complex cells, the extent of the inhibition is very dependent on the phase of the components in the compound; in fact, facilitation is sometimes observed at some phases where inhibition is observed at others. But the phase dependence is different from cell to cell, with maximum inhibition occurring throughout the whole phase range. The tight spatial-frequency tuning of the effect suggests that the inhibition arises from the cortex rather than from the lateral geniculate nucleus.

Orientation-dependent inhibition has also been demonstrated (Bonds, 1983; Burr et al., 1981; Morrone et al., 1982), as has temporal-frequency-dependent inhibition (Foster et al., 1985).

3.7.9   *An Aside About Some Suprathreshold Results*

Analogues to the opposite effect (facilitation) at far-apart values and to the compound-adapting-stimulus effect have both turned up in three kinds of suprathreshold experiments on one or both of the spatial-frequency and orientation dimensions (the only two dimensions for which I systematically examined the suprathreshold adaptation and masking literature).

Thresholds During Masking. When measuring thresholds in the presence of a mask stimulus (discrimination of test-plus-mask from mask alone), facilitation at far values has been reported on the spatial frequency dimension (Georgeson, 1975; Nachmias & Weber, 1975; Stromeyer & Klein; 1974, Tolhurst & Barfield, 1978) but may not exist on the orientation dimension. A compound effect has been reported on the orientation dimension (Lovegrove, 1976; Wenderoth & Tyler, 1979), but I know of no relevant information about the spatial-frequency dimension.

Perceived Suprathreshold Value After Adaptation. During measurement of the perceived orientation of suprathreshold stimuli after adaptation, both effects have been found. For the opposite effect at far values see Gibson and Radner, 1937; Logan, 1962 (replotted in O'Toole & Wenderoth, 1977); Morant and Harris, 1965; Muir and Over, 1970; and O'Toole and Wenderoth, 1977. For the compound-effect see Kurtenbach and Magnussen, 1979; and Magnussen and Kurtenbach, 1980. In this context also, these two effects have been taken as suggesting inhibition. (Also see Lennie 1971, 1972, and Tolhurst & Thompson, 1975, for related material.) Oddly, I know of no reports of such effects on perceived spatial frequency of suprathreshold stimuli after adaptation.

Perceived Suprathreshold Value During Masking. During measurement of the perceived value of suprathreshold stimuli in the presence of a mask stimulus, an opposite effect at far-apart values has been reported for orientation (Logan, 1962 [replotted in O'Toole & Wenderoth, 1977]; Over, Broerse, & Crassini, 1972; O'Toole & Wenderoth, 1977) but may not exist for spatial frequency (Klein, Stromeyer, & Ganz, 1974).

A compound-masking-stimulus effect has been reported for orientation (Blakemore, Carpenter, & Georgeson 1970, 1971; Carpenter & Blakemore, 1973; Kurtenbach & Magnussen, 1979; Magnussen & Kurtenbach, 1980; O'Toole, 1979). I know of no relevant information about spatial frequency.

Summary. Although the inconsistency between reports on the spatial-frequency and orientation dimensions is somewhat disturbing, overall the reports of compound-stimulus effects and opposite effects are rather impressive. Perhaps they should be taken as further evidence for inhibition among the low-level analyzers. But even if they are, there is a problem in interpretation. As Tolhurst and Barfield (1978) pointed out, although results are often taken individually to suggest inhibition among analyzers, it is difficult to reconcile—with any one model of inhibition—the ranges of values on the dimension of interest over which all the various masking and adaptation effects occur. Tolhurst and Barfield made this point in one context: measurement of thresholds after adaptation versus in the presence of a masking stimulus on the spatial-frequency dimension. To the extent that information is available about adapting and masking in three other contexts—perceived suprathreshold spatial frequency, thresholds on the orientation dimension, perceived suprathreshold orientation—the same kind of difficulty in interpretation seems to occur.

3.8   INHIBITION ONLY

3.8.1   *Explaining Threshold Elevations with Inhibition*

Another explanation of selective-adaptation effects at threshold postulates only inhibition, no fatigue (e.g., Blakemore et al., 1970; Kulikowski & King-Smith, 1973; Tolhurst, 1972a). To introduce this explanation, let's look briefly at the analogous explanation for masking experiments (although these masking experiments are outside the scope of this book; see section 1.11.1).

For masking experiments, the explanation can be stated simply: The threshold for a test stimulus is elevated by the simultaneous presence of a masking stimulus because the analyzers sensitive to the test stimulus are being inhibited by the analyzers sensitive to the masking stimulus. (Alternately, the analyzers sensitive to the test stimulus might be inhibited by the masking stimulus directly.)

The essence of this inhibition-only explanation applied to adaptation effects is thus: The threshold for the test stimulus is elevated after adaptation to the adapting stimulus because the analyzers sensitive to the test stimulus HAVE BEEN inhibited by the analyzers sensitive to the adapting stimulus or by the adapting stimulus directly. Except for the change in time—the masking effect is occurring simultaneously and the adapting effect successively—the inhibition-only explanations for the two effects are identical. (At this point, the explanation explains only threshold elevations. Discussion of facilitation and the compound-grating effect is postponed until section 3.8.3.) In the interest of brevity, we will not try to make explicit a set of assumptions corresponding to those implicit in the preceding verbal explanation, but one comment about possible alternative assumptions seems necessary for clarity.

Two Types of Prolonged Inhibition. At least two types of inhibitory process could have the necessary prolonged temporal properties: (a) The inhibition itself may be a much more sluggish process than excitation is, so that the adapting stimulus has to be on for some time before the inhibition builds up to its maximum, and the inhibition lasts some seconds after the adapting stimulus is turned off. (b) Although the inhibition itself ceases immediately when a stimulus goes off, the previously inhibited analyzer remains less sensitive for a while afterward. That is, the analyzer is fatigued by having been inhibited (instead of by having been excited, as in the conventional fatigue models).

Although these two possibilities might be distinguishable by some evidence (e.g., physiological recordings if the analyzers turn out to be single neurons), they cannot be distinguished by the kind of psychophysical results discussed here, unless further exact properties of both mechanisms are specified. At a qualitative level, either of them will serve our present purposes. They will be referred to interchangeably, therefore, as *prolonged inhibition.*

3.8.2 Predicted tvi Curves

According to the fatigue or fatigue-plus-inhibition models, no threshold elevation should occur until the adapting intensity is high enough that the adapting stimulus substantially excites the TEST analyzers (the analyzers sensitive to the test stimulus). In the inhibition-only model, however, the threshold elevation is controlled by how much the ADAPT analyzers respond to the adapting stimulus and by how much they inhibit the test analyzers. As adapting intensity is raised, therefore, threshold elevation should begin at the lowest intensity at which the ADAPT analyzers respond enough to inhibit the test analyzers. This intensity may be a good deal lower than the intensity at which the adapt stimulus excites the TEST analyzers. This intensity may even be less than the intensity at which the TEST stimulus excites the TEST analyzers (if the relative sensitivities of the analyzers, the dependence of magnitude of inhibition on adapting and test values, etc., are just right).

Dealy and Tolhurst (1974) reported one brief result of this kind and Stecher, Sigel, and Lange (1973a) showed another.

Less dramatically but still consistent with the inhibition-only explanations, the families of psychophysical tvi curves shown in Fig. 3.9 can be well described as vertically scaled functions that get shallower as adapt and test values get further apart, in exactly the way envisioned by Tolhurst (1972a) for an inhibition-only model.

Overall, however, this evidence for the inhibition-only model is not compelling. Determining the lowest adapting intensity at which one gets any adapting effect is quite tricky, since these threshold elevation effects are very small. Particularly with the method of adjustment, response biases or criterion shifts on the part of observers may dominate the results. And not everyone has found such an effect (Stromeyer, Klein, & Sternheim, 1977). Further, since Georgeson and Harris (1984; Fig. 3.10) have shown that vertically scaled psychophysical tvi curves are consistent with Stiles's-type fatigue models, the nature of these curves is little support for an inhibition-only model over a fatigue model.

3.8.3 Attempting Predictions of Facilitation and the Compound-Grating Effect

In the inhibition-plus-fatigue model, inhibition explained two effects—the facilitation at far-away values and the compound-stimulus effect—and fatigue explained a third—the threshold elevations at close values. In the inhibition-only model, this third effect—threshold elevations at close values—is explained by prolonged inhibition without any need to postulate fatigue. It would certainly be elegant if inhibition could be made to explain all three effects simultaneously without fatigue being assumed at all.

The most elegant of explanations would assume that there is only one distribution of inhibition across different values on the dimension of interest. More precisely, it would assume that, if any one of the three inhibitory properties that follow is true for a given pair of analyzers on the dimension of interest, then all three are true:

1. There is tonic inhibition to explain the facilitation.
2. Inhibition occurs when stimulation is present to explain the reduced effectiveness of a compound-adapting stimulus.
3. Inhibition has prolonged effects to explain the threshold elevations after adaptation.

Perhaps such an elegant inhibition-only explanation can be made to work, but not obviously. Facilitation can be predicted adequately; the argument is analogous to that used previously for predicting facilitation from the inhibition-plus-fatigue model. In particular, facilitation is predicted to occur for separations between test and adapt values that are larger than the separations for which threshold elevations occur. To account for the compound-grating effect, however, seems to require that the analyzers sensitive to one component of the compound inhibit the analyzers sensitive to the other component. Then the separation between the values of two components leading to a compound effect can be no greater than the separation over which inhibition acts. But then, by the second inhibition property, the compound-grating effect should occur only for components close enough together that use of one as an adapting stimulus would elevate the threshold of the other. The spatial-frequency compound-grating effect can occur, however, when the components are very far apart (Georgeson, 1975 [reported in Tolhurst & Barfield, 1978]). Thus, this kind of inhibition-only model does not seem consistent with spatial-frequency selective-adaptation results.

Perhaps there are two kinds of inhibition, one acting between analyzers having rather close peak values and having prolonged effects (leading to threshold elevations) and the other acting over wider value separations but having only short-term effects (leading to facilitation and compound-stimulus effects; Tolhurst, 1972a). Such a model cannot be ruled out by the present arguments, but is neither more parsimonious nor more elegant than the fatigue-plus-inhibition model.

3.8.4   Conclusions—Inhibition Versus Fatigue Explanations of Spatial-Frequency Selective Adaptation

Whether spatial-frequency-selective threshold elevations are due to fatigue or to prolonged inhibition is undecided; indeed, existing reports of the effect of varying contrast in the adapting gratings are quite discrepant. The fatigue explanation has the advantage at the moment, however, of being quantitatively consistent with at least some of the experimental data.

In any case, at least two processes seem necessary to explain all the effects of adaptation to gratings of different spatial frequencies: (a) something like fatigue or prolonged inhibition to explain the threshold elevations at close values, and (b) a second process to explain the facilitation and compound-grating effects. This second process might be a short-acting inhibition between far-apart values on the dimension of interest, a fancier form of the assumption linking analyzer outputs to observer responses (cognitive responses biases, qualitative criteria change, anchoring effects, etc.), or interaction/inhibition among analyzers responding to different values on dimensions (e.g., spatial position) other than the one being discussed.

3.9 POINT-BY-POINT FATIGUE (AFTERIMAGE) EXPLANATIONS

From time to time the possibility has been raised that these spatial-frequency-selective effects are the consequence of fatigue of individual receptors (cones and rods) or of other entities sensitive to a very small area (a point) of light, and not the consequence of spatial-frequency-selective analyzers at all. (The receptors or similar entities are spatial-position analyzers, since they are selectively sensitive to different ranges of spatial position. They are definitely not, however, spatial-frequency analyzers, since they are not sensitive to different ranges of spatial frequency.) This kind of explanation has been referred to by many names: *early local adaptation, point-by-point adaptation, receptor adaptation,* most often perhaps *afterimage* (although that may be a bit misleading). Here it will be called *point-by-point fatigue.* This explanation is an example of explanations that attribute selectivity in experimental results on one dimension to analyzers that are selective along some other dimension. The particular assumptions of such explanations vary a great deal with the context. The argument in this case runs as follows.

Both physiological and psychophysical results (e.g., conventional negative afterimages) strongly suggest that the receptors (or similar localized entities) are desensitized after having been excited. Although the observers in the spatial-frequency experiments are trying to move their eyes uniformly around on the adapting pattern to prevent the occurrence of conventional afterimages, they probably do not succeed completely. In fact, the typical kind of adaptation in this experiment—to a normally presented, unstabilized, high-contrast grating, with instructions to distribute fixation positions evenly across the light and dark bars—has been reported to be equivalent to looking at a stabilized grating of 12 to 25 times threshold contrast (Arend & Skavenski, 1979; although Tulunay-Keesey & Baker 1982 reported less dramatic effects). Afterimages of fixated gratings are even stronger, of course (see Georgeson & Turner, 1985, and references there). After the observer has adapted to a grating, therefore, receptor sensitivity may vary as an approximately sinusoidal function of position, where the sinusoidal function has the same spatial frequency and orientation as that of the adapting grating. Subsequently presented test gratings may then be differentially affected by this pattern of receptor sensitivity. If test gratings near the adapting spatial frequency and orientation are more affected than other gratings, this localized point-by-point fatigue may be the cause of the observed frequency-selective and orientation-selective effects.

Considerable conceptual difficulty arises in trying to make this argument rigorous, however. To do so, one must specify the transformation from analyzer outputs to observer responses. Suppose that the observer's threshold for a stimulus is the threshold of the most sensitive receptor. If the observer's eyes move over the test grating to some extent, every point on every test grating would have a chance to be detected by the maximally sensitive receptor. Thus no spatial-frequency selective adaptation could be predicted from this assumption. More complicated assumptions would have to be constructed to make the point-by-point fatigue explanation work.

In any case, there is quite good evidence against this point-by-point fatigue explanation. With specially designed equipment, a visual stimulus can be stabilized on the retina so that each point in the stimulus is always illuminating a particular receptor. If the stabilized stimulus itself is a moving or flickering grating rather than a stationary one, each receptor receives the same amount of illumination averaged across time. Even with such stimuli, spatial-frequency selective adaptation to gratings is obtained (Jones & Tulunay-Keesey, 1975; Kelly & Burbeck, 1980; middle of Fig. 3.2).

Of course, if recent illumination counts more in the desensitization than past illumination, as it must, there will still be some very slight differential point-by-point desensitization. Kelly and Burbeck (1980) tried to estimate this residual "sensitivity mask" by finding out the drift rates at which an observer could see a conventional afterimage. At the drift rate of a stabilized image that is most like unstabilized vision (0.15 degree/second, that used in Fig. 3.2 middle), some measurable sensitivity mask exists out to 5 or 10 c/deg. At a 10 times higher drift rate, however, no sensitivity mask exists (above 0.3 c/deg. in any case), and at this drift rate, exactly the same frequency-selective elevation is found (Kelly & Burbeck, 1980, Fig. 6). Thus, under conditions in which differential adaptation on the spatial-position dimension is eliminated, observers still show spatial-frequency selective adaptation.

This is a specific successful example of a general strategy: To reject the possibility that analyzers selective along a second dimension are the cause of experimental results selective on the first dimension, try to design stimuli that equate effects along the second dimension as much as possible.

Although we have just seen that point-by-point fatigue is not the explanation for the spatial-frequency selective effects, it does seem to elevate the thresholds in a nonselective manner, as demonstrated in the results with stabilized stationary gratings (Jones & Tulunay-Keesey, 1975, Fig. 4) or special fixation instructions in normal viewing (Smith, 1977). These point-by-point effects may well be the explanation for some discrepancies among the results of different experiments (see section 3.4.3).

3.10 WHAT IS THE FUNCTION OF PATTERN-SELECTIVE ADAPTATION?

In this book, selective adaptation is primarily a method for finding out about analyzers. The question of why there is selective adaptation at all is, however, a question of great intrinsic interest. At a general level, sensory or perceptual adaptation is often thought to allow observers to be particularly sensitive to novel stimuli, or alternatively, to adjust the operating range of the system so that the observer is now more sensitive to small changes that are likely to occur in the new environment (in the presence of the adapting stimulus).

The fact that there is facilitation at distant spatial frequencies after adaptation to gratings has been suggested as an example of an increased sensitivity to some novel stimuli (novel compared with the adapting spatial frequency). It is not too compelling an example, however. In any case, by far the most dramatic effect on threshold is the threshold elevations for the whole range of spatial frequencies around the adapting frequency. And these threshold elevations do mean that "novel" frequencies are going to be much more detectable than frequencies near the adapting frequency.

Discrimination among suprathreshold patterns is also affected by adaptation and is perhaps a better place to look for clues as to the function of adaptation (Barlow, Macleod, & van Meeteren, 1976; Greenlee & Heitger, 1988; Regan & Beverly, 1983b, 1985; Wilson & Regan, 1984). Spatial-frequency, orientation, and contrast discrimination may improve after adaptation, but the improvement is small and elusive. There are, however, substantial pattern-selective decreases in discriminability after adaptation (of rather interesting character; see foregoing references) that will tend to favor novel stimuli.

I think it unlikely that we yet understand the function (if any) of pattern-selective adaptation, although the results just discussed are suggestive.

3.11 SUMMARY

Selective adaptation occurs if, after adaptation, an observer's threshold is increased for test stimuli that are close in value to the adapting stimulus but is unchanged for other test stimuli.

One common explanation of selective adaptation is that multiple analyzers exist on the dimension of interest and that adaptation desensitizes (fatigues) the analyzers that are sensitive to the adapting stimulus.

Plots on logarithmic axes of threshold elevation due to adaptation versus intensity of the adapting stimulus are called threshold-versus-intensity (tvi) curves.

A typical fatigue model of selective adaptation (e.g., Stiles's model of color adaptation) assumes that (a) any single analyzer's tvi curves for one test stimulus and many adapting stimuli should be horizontal translations of one another, and

(b) any single analyzer's tvi curves for many test stimuli and one adapting stimulus should be vertical translations of one another. (Single cortical neurons, incidentally, do not follow these assumptions.)

If the most sensitive analyzer for a given test stimulus is always the same analyzer, no matter what the state of adaptation, then the observer's tvi curves for one test stimulus and many adapting stimuli should be horizontal translations of one another. This result is sometimes but not always reported for adaptation experiments on the spatial-frequency dimensions.

More often, however, which of the analyzers is most sensitive to the test stimulus will depend on the state of adaptation. In that case, an observer's tvi curves will contain sections controlled by different analyzers. Although each of the sections will follow the horizontal and vertical displacement assumptions just given, the whole tvi curves will not.

If there are many analyzers with appropriately shaped sensitivity functions, in fact, an observer's tvi curves may "fan out" and be approximately vertically scaled versions of one another. This result, also, is sometimes but not always reported for adaptation experiments on the spatial-frequency dimension.

Sometimes adaptation to a stimulus that is very far in value from the test stimulus will lead to threshold lowering (the opposite of the usual effect). Sometimes also, adaptation to a compound stimulus will cause less threshold elevation than adaptation to one of the components of the compound stimulus by itself. Inhibition among analyzers has been suggested as an explanation for these two effects.

Both of these effects have been reported on the spatial-frequency and orientation dimensions. Reports are also common of analogous effects for suprathreshold experiments on these dimensions.

Prolonged inhibition—rather than fatigue or desensitization—has sometimes been suggested as a cause for the threshold elevations typically found in adaptation experiments. It would be elegant if one kind of inhibition could be made to explain both these threshold elevations as well as opposite and compound effects, but that does not seem possible. Postulating two kinds of inhibition would work, but is no more appealing than postulating fatigue as well as inhibition.

Note

1. *Common intersections in families of tvi curves.* A common intersection might occur in a family of tvi curves for a single test frequency and many adapting frequencies (that is, the intersection might be determined by the test frequency) or in a family of tvi curves for many test frequencies and a single adapting frequency (that is, the intersection might be determined by the adapting frequency). The latter possibility is of great theoretical import and is discussed in section 3.8.2.

Strictly speaking, it is only the former possibility that would allow the simple division of log threshold elevation for each adapting value by maximal log threshold elevation (as done in Graham, 1972). Practically speaking, however, if either kind of common intersection exists, it will matter little to this calculation which kind of common intersection it is; the thresholds for adapt and test are only very different when they are far apart, in which case there is little adaptation anyway.

III

SUMMATION

4

Models for Far-Apart Values

4.1 A TYPICAL SUMMATION EXPERIMENT

In summation-at-threshold experiments, the observer's thresholds for a compound stimulus are compared with the thresholds for the components of the compound. (The observer is always in a neutral state of pattern adaptation.) The basic intuition behind these experiments is this: When two or more components of a compound stimulus both excite the same analyzer, that analyzer should respond much more to the compound than to either component alone. Hence, the observer should be much more sensitive to the compound than to either component. (Equivalently, a compound at fixed intensity should be substantially more detectable than its most detectable component. Or, as is often said, there should be substantial *summation*.) When components of a compound stimulus excite different analyzers, however, no analyzer will respond more to the compound than to some one of the components. Hence, the observer's sensitivity to the compound should about equal that to the most detectable component. (Equivalently, a compound of fixed intensity should be about as detectable as the most detectable component. That is, little or no summation is predicted. According to certain models discussed here, the compound may be slightly more detectable than the most detectable component due to *probability summation*—for now this is just a second-order detail, accounting for relatively little of the effect.)

Figure 4.1 shows possible results of a summation experiment that measures an observer's thresholds for a series of compound stimuli; each compound contains two components, one having a fixed value (V_0, marked by an arrow on the horizontal axis) and the other having a variable value plotted on the horizontal axis (V). On the vertical axis is plotted some measure of the amount of summation, that is, of how much more sensitive the observer is to the compound than to the most detectable component. (A number of different measures of summation will be discussed later.) Figure 4.1 shows value-selective behavior: As the two component values become further apart, less summation is found. The amount of summation found for very close-together values is that predicted when both components excite the same and only the same analyzers; the summation found for very far-apart values is that predicted when both components excite completely different analyzers. Ways to calculate these predicted amounts (which depend on many assumptions about the analyzers) are discussed at length in this chapter for experiments using far-apart values and in Chapter 6 for close values.

133

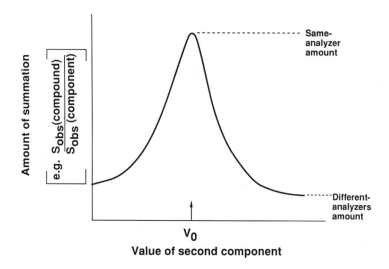

FIG. 4.1 Typical results of a summation-at-threshold experiment. Some measure of summation (how much an observer's sensitivity to a compound exceeds sensitivity to its components) is plotted on the vertical axis. The value of the second component is plotted on the horizontal axis. The value of the first component (V_0) is indicated by an arrow on the horizontal axis.

4.1.1   Introduction to Spatial-Frequency Summation Experiments

Typical stimuli for spatial-frequency summation experiments are shown in Fig. 2.1 as photographs and in the left column of Fig. 4.2 as luminance profiles: Two simple gratings having spatial frequencies differing by a factor of 3 (in the top two rows of the left column) and two compound gratings made up of those same frequencies but in different phases (in the bottom two rows of the left column). The contrasts of the two simple gratings are set so that each of them is just at its own threshold. The third row shows the component frequencies in "peaks-subtract phase": The peak (the brightest spot) of the higher frequency $3f$ is juxtaposed with the trough (the darkest spot) of the lower frequency f. The fourth row shows the "peaks-add phase": the peaks of the two frequencies juxtaposed. The middle and right columns show the predictions from models discussed below.

When the experiment in Fig. 4.2 was run, all four gratings turned out to be approximately equally detectable (Graham & Nachmias, 1971). In other words, there was no (or very little) summation, and the phase in the compound grating was irrelevant. This lack of summation is typically found for spatial frequencies a factor of 3 or more apart and sometimes at a factor of 2 apart (e.g., Campbell & Robson, 1964; Pantle, 1973; Quick & Reichert, 1975; Sachs, Nachmias, & Robson, 1971). For close-together spatial frequencies, the compound is much more detectable than the components, however (showing value-selective behavior like that in Fig. 4.1), and the phase matters.

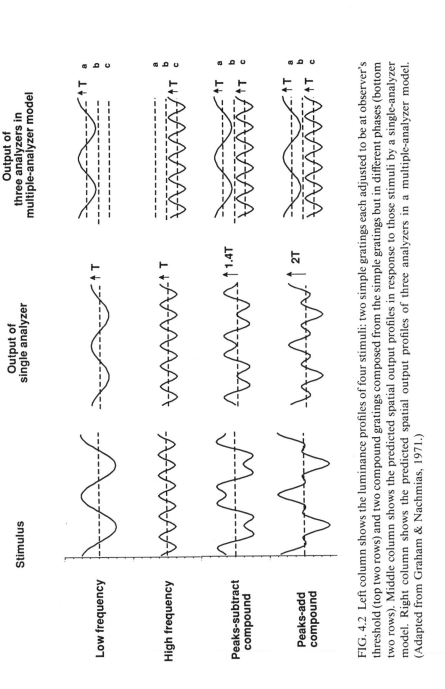

FIG. 4.2 Left column shows the luminance profiles of four stimuli: two simple gratings each adjusted to be at observer's threshold (top two rows) and two compound gratings composed from the simple gratings but in different phases (bottom two rows). Middle column shows the predicted spatial output profiles in response to those stimuli by a single-analyzer model. Right column shows the predicted spatial output profiles of three analyzers in a multiple-analyzer model. (Adapted from Graham & Nachmias, 1971.)

Historical Note. The earliest extensive experiments showing little summation among spatial frequencies a factor of 2 or 3 apart used compound stimuli that were complex gratings and thus contained many spatial frequencies (Campbell & Robson, 1964, 1968) or were aperiodic stimuli and thus even more complicated (reviewed in Thomas, 1970). These were very important and very influential experiments, but their complete interpretation is complicated by the presence of so many components.

4.1.2 Summation-Square Plots

When a compound stimulus contains only two components (as in Fig. 4.2), the measured thresholds and the thresholds predicted by models can be plotted on a *summation square* like that shown in Fig. 4.3. Relative intensity of one component—the actual intensity of the component in the compound divided by the threshold intensity for that component alone—is plotted on the horizontal axis. Relative intensity of the other component is plotted on the vertical axis.

To express this in symbols, let $c(V_j$ in cmpd) represent the intensity of the jth component in the compound stimulus. When the term $V_j in cmpd$ is used to name a stimulus in the argument of a symbol like c (as was just done), it can usually be safely translated (as it was) by the phrase "the jth component in the stimulus." Strictly speaking, however, as will be important in some other contexts, V_j *in cmpd* is a simple stimulus with a value V_j and the same intensity as

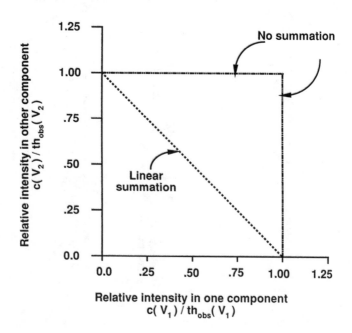

FIG. 4.3 A summation-square plot.

the component of value V_j in the compound. Let x and y be the horizontal and vertical coordinates of the summation square, respectively,

$$x = \frac{c(V_1 \text{ in cmpd})}{\text{th}_{\text{obs}}(V_1)} = c(V_1 \text{ in cmpd}) \cdot S_{\text{obs}}(V_1)$$

$$y = \frac{c(V_2 \text{ in cmpd})}{\text{th}_{\text{obs}}(V_2)} = c(V_2 \text{ in cmpd}) \cdot S_{\text{obs}}(V_2)$$

Each point on the summation-square plot, therefore, represents a compound stimulus containing two components having the intensities given by the horizontal and vertical coordinates. Points on the horizontal or vertical axis represent simple stimuli in which there is only one component (equivalently, the intensity of the other is zero). The points $(1, 0)$ and $(0, 1)$ represent the first and second component, respectively, when each is at its own threshold.

Points plotted on a particular ray through the origin represent compound stimuli containing some constant ratio of intensities in the two components. In summation experiments determining a compound's threshold, this ratio is usually kept constant while the absolute intensities are varied. In terms of the summation square, therefore, the stimulus is usually varied along some ray through the origin until the threshold is determined.

The upper and right lines of the summation square—the lines labeled "no summation" that connect the points $(1, 0)$ and $(0, 1)$ to the point $(1, 1)$—represent stimuli containing exactly the threshold intensity of one component and less than the threshold intensity of the other component. If there is no summation or any other kind of interaction between components, then the compound stimulus is exactly as detectable as its most detectable component, and the point for its threshold will fall on the upper or right edge of the summation square. To a first approximation, the results of summation experiments using spatial frequencies more than a factor of 2 or 3 apart do so. More exactly, however, they fall slightly inside at the corner. (Figure 4.11 shows an example of such results.)

The results of experiments on other dimensions to be considered later, for example, the temporal-frequency dimension, fall far inside the square, that is, the compound stimulus is at threshold even though each of its components is far below threshold. The negative diagonal in the summation square—labeled "linear summation" in Fig. 4.3—represents compound stimuli in which the sum of the relative intensities of the two components is constant and equal to 1.0.

If there is negative interaction between components so that any compound is actually less detectable than the most detectable component, the compound-stimuli thresholds will lie outside the square.

When some measure of the amount of summation is plotted against value on the dimension of interest (as in Fig. 4.1), the measure of summation indicates how close the compound's threshold is to the negative diagonal (or, equivalently, how far it is from the outside edges of the summation square). Different measures of summation have been used by different investigators; these will be presented later when they become relevant.

4.1.3   *Preview of the Rest of This Chapter*

This chapter presents five possible models of basic summation-at-threshold experiments.

The first two models each assume a single analyzer for the dimension of interest. They differ in whether that analyzer's output in response to a compound stimulus is completely additive (the first model) or not (the second). The second postulates a kind of nonadditivity that is particularly applicable to the spatial-frequency dimension, although it can be generalized to some other dimensions.

The third model is a basic, deterministic, multiple-analyzers model for far-apart values on a dimension of interest.

The fourth model—a nonuniform single-channel model—is specialized for spatial frequency and spatial position (or temporal position), but the general lesson generalizes to many pairs of sensory/perceptual dimensions.

The fifth model, which takes up the chapter's second half, is a multiple-analyzers model in which the analyzers are probabilistically independent. Like the first and third models, this fifth model is immediately generalizable to many sensory/perceptual dimensions.

In Chapters 5 and 6, where results from summation experiments along all spatial dimensions are discussed, this fifth model is gradually elaborated to cover all spatial dimensions simultaneously.

4.2   AN ADDITIVE SINGLE-ANALYZER MODEL

A rather common type of single-analyzer model on a sensory/perceptual dimension makes the following assumptions:

Assumption 24. One Analyzer.   *There is only a single analyzer on the dimension of interest.*

Assumption 25. Single-Number Output.   *To each presentation of a stimulus, the output of the analyzer can be represented as a single number.*

This output will be called R_0 (stim).

For the present discussion, it does not matter whether the output of the analyzer is deterministic (see Assumption 31) or varies over different presentations of the same stimulus. For generality's sake, we will assume:

Assumption 26. Variable Analyzer Output.   *The output of an analyzer to presentations of the same stimulus may change from trial to trial (is variable).*

The symbol $\overline{R}_0$(stim) represents the expected output (the average of the analyzer's output over all presentations of that stimulus).

Assumption 9. Linear Transducer.   *The expected output of an analyzer is proportional to the intensity of the stimulus.*

The constant of proportionality is the sensitivity of the analyzer to that stimulus $S_0(\text{stim})$. That is

$$\overline{R}_0(\text{stim}) = c(\text{stim}) \cdot S_0(\text{stim})$$

Assumption 27. Additivity (of Single-Number Outputs) to a Compound. *The expected output of an analyzer to a compound stimulus is the sum of its outputs to the components by themselves.*

Or, letting Cmpd be a compound stimulus composed of two components V_1 and V_2,

$$\overline{R}_0(\text{Cmpd}) = \overline{R}_0(V_1) + \overline{R}_0(V_2)$$

This assumption is a very important part of Assumption 47: Additive (Linear-System) Analyzers. The two have been separated only for ease of exposition.

Assumption 28. Only-Analyzer Rule. *The observer's sensitivity equals the sensitivity of the only analyzer. A stimulus is at (or above) the observer's threshold if and only if the analyzer's output is equal to (or greater than) 1.0.*

Since the only analyzer is of necessity the most sensitive analyzer as well, this assumption is equivalent to the most sensitive analyzer rule (Assumption 4) applied to this situation.

Predictions. These five assumptions predict that the thresholds of compound stimuli should fall on the negative diagonal in the summation square (Fig. 4.3). To see why, consider a compound stimulus containing two components each at a relative intensity of 1 (each at its own threshold). The analyzer's expected output to each of those components has magnitude 1.0, and therefore the analyzer's output to the compound has value 2.0. Hence the compound is way above the observer's threshold. To bring this compound down to threshold, the intensity of each component can be reduced by a factor of 2, since (by Assumption 9, linear transducer function) that will reduce the output to each component and hence to the compound by a factor of 2.

Additivity of Sensitivities. The linear transducer and additivity assumptions are sufficient to predict thresholds on the summation square's negative diagonal, but they are not necessary. Predictions on the negative diagonal simply mean that sensitivities add, that is

Assumption 29. Additivity of Sensitivities. *The sensitivity of an analyzer to a compound equals the sum of its sensitivities to the components.*

$$S_0(\text{Cmpd}) = S_0(V_1) + S_0(V_2)$$

Additivity of sensitivities may occur in the absence of additivity of outputs. Consider the following two-stage analyzer. The first stage obeys the linear transducer and additivity assumptions. The output of this first stage goes into a second stage, which nonlinearly transforms it (e.g., by taking the logarithm). The output of this second stage will not obey either the linear transducer or additivity of outputs assumptions, but will obey the additivity of sensitivity condition.

Comparison with Experimental Results. On the spatial-frequency dimension, the measured thresholds fall nowhere near the negative diagonal, but rather near the outside of the square. Hence this simple model is inadequate for these results. There are other dimensions where this simple model does much better (e.g., temporal frequency, direction of motion at low velocities). Even on these other dimensions, however, the simple model needs to be elaborated in ways explored further below.

4.3   A NONADDITIVE, UNIFORM, SINGLE-ANALYZER MODEL (A SINGLE-CHANNEL MODEL)

On many sensory/perceptual dimensions, the assumption of complete additivity of outputs (or even the weaker assumption of additivity of sensitivities) seems wrong. Other likely properties of the single analyzer prevent complete additivity. In this section we consider a single spatial-frequency analyzer to be a homogeneous array of a large number of mechanisms: Each mechanism is a linear system and the weighting functions of all are identical but are centered at different positions. Thus the analyzer is a two-dimensional translation-invariant linear system. A possible physiological substrate for such an analyzer is an array of neurons, which act linearly and have receptive fields identical in all characteristics except spatial position. We will sometimes call this a single-channel model. (See section 1.10 for definitions of mechanism and channel.)

4.3.1   Assumptions

In addition to assuming there is only a single analyzer for spatial frequency (Assumption 24), this model assumes:

Assumption 30. The Analyzer's Output is a Two-dimensional Function. *Not only is the stimulus (a visual spatial pattern) represented as a two-dimensional function of spatial coordinates x and y, but so is the analyzer's output.*

(The symbols x and y are being used here as the spatial coordinates for visual patterns, not for labeling the horizontal and vertical axes of summation squares as they were in the last section.)

Assumption 9. Linear Transducer. *The expected output of the analyzer (in this case, the value of the two-dimensional function at each point (x,y)) is proportional to the intensity of the stimulus.*

Assumption 27. Additivity (of Two-Dimensional Outputs) To a Compound. *The expected output to any compound stimulus is just the sum of the outputs to the two components.*

These last 2 assumptions are the same as the corresponding assumptions in the preceding subsection except that here the output is two-dimensional, a difference that is crucial in understanding the behavior of the analyzer.

Assumption 31. Translation-invariance. *If one stimulus is just a translation of another (a shifted version), the output to the first stimulus equals the output to the second version shifted by the same amount.*

Assumption 32. Deterministic Output (No Variability). *The output of the analyzer is the same to every presentation of a particular stimulus. Hence the expected or average output is the same as the output on a particular trial.*

Terminological Note. The channel being discussed here is supposed to be a single analyzer on the spatial-frequency dimension. What would happen if you considered each mechanism in the array to be a separate analyzer? Since the mechanisms' weighting functions are identical in everything except position, they all respond to the same range of spatial frequencies. Thus there would still be only a single analyzer on the spatial-frequency dimension. The individual mechanisms would be multiple analyzers on the spatial-position dimension, however.

The middle column of Fig. 4.2 shows one-dimensional cuts through the full two-dimensional output profiles described by Assumptions 9, 27, 30, 31, and 32. The predicted output to each simple sinusoidal grating is just a sinusoid (top two rows, middle column, Fig. 4.2); the output to the compound is just the sum of the outputs to the two sinusoidal components appropriately positioned to reflect their relative phase (bottom two rows, middle column, Fig. 4.2). For more explanation, see the brief introduction in Chapter 2 or any book on linear systems analysis.

To complete the predictions, we need as always to make an assumption about the transformation from the output of the analyzer to the observer's responses. We can continue to use the earlier assumption that the observer's sensitivity equals the analyzer's sensitivity (Assumption 4) if we define the analyzer's threshold with the following:

Assumption 33. Peak-in-Output-Profile Rule. *A pattern is at (or above) the analyzer's threshold if and only if the peak magnitude in the spatial output profile is at (or above) some criterion level T.*

According to this assumption, the threshold is determined entirely by the magnitude of the peak output, not by its spatial position. If you took the set of output magnitudes produced at different spatial positions and scrambled them into a new spatial order, you would still get the same predictions. In other words, *all* the spatial interactions (all the interactions that depend on the distances between points of light) are a result of the weighting function that characterizes the single analyzer.

4.3.2   Predicted Thresholds

As you can see in the second column of Fig. 4.2, the peaks in the single analyzer's output to the two simple gratings are the same and equal to the threshold criterion T (since we are assuming that the contrasts of these simple gratings have been set just at threshold). Now look at the peak outputs to the two compound gratings. They are both greater than T. In fact, the peak output to the peaks-subtract compound is $1.4T$ and to the peaks-add compound is $2T$. According to this single-analyzer model, therefore, these compound gratings are above threshold, and the peaks-add compound is further above threshold than the peaks-subtract compound.

If the contrast in each component of the peaks-add compound pattern were reduced by a factor of 2.0 and in each component of the peaks-subtract pattern by a factor of 1.4, then the peak output to each would have a value of T (since output magnitude is proportional to contrast by the linear-transducer assumption, Assumption 9). In other words, the two new compound patterns (with contrasts equal to ½ and 1/1.4 times the the contrasts shown in Fig. 4.2) would be just at the observer's threshold.

Where would these predicted compound gratings be plotted in the summation square of Fig. 4.3? For the peaks-add compound, the point is plotted at 0.5, 0.5, since the contrast of each component is at half its threshold when alone. That point is on the negative diagonal line labeled "linear summation." In general, in fact, this single-channel model predicts that the thresholds for peaks-add compound gratings (no matter what the ratio of frequencies or of contrasts) would fall on the negative diagonal.

The predictions for peaks-subtract compound gratings cannot be so simply summarized, however, except to say that values do not fall on the negative diagonal, although they usually fall nearer to it than to the outside edges of the square. For the case shown in Fig. 4.2—where the relative contrast in the two components a factor of 3 apart is the same—the point is at 1/1.4, 1/1.4. The predictions for all contrast ratios when frequencies differ by a factor of 3 are shown later as the line marked infinity in Fig. 5.2. They are always inside the summation square (and usually rather near the negative diagonal) except when the relative contrast of the f component is much larger than that of the $3f$ component; in this range the compound produces a smaller peak output than the f component by itself, and so the point falls outside the square. For other frequency ratios, further numerical calculations would need to be done.

Nonadditivity of Sensitivities.   In general, therefore, this single-channel model predicts thresholds that do not lie on the negative diagonal. That is, its predictions are inconsistent with additivity of sensitivities. This nonadditivity results because, although the full two-dimensional analyzer output has the additive property (Assumption 27), the relevant single number that determines the observer's threshold (the peak in the output, Assumption 33) does not.

Comparison with Experimental Results.   This model, like the last, is inadequate for spatial frequencies a factor of 2 or 3 or more apart (in the usual conditions) because it predicts too much summation. As will be discussed later, it does a better job on other dimensions, although even for these dimensions further modifications of it (in particular, the inclusion of independent variability at different positions, see next chapter) are necessary.

4.3.3 Relabeling the Entities in the Model

The single-channel model (the nonadditive uniform single-analyzer model) just discussed has been presented in alternate equivalent ways in the literature. Relabeling which entities in that model are to be included in the entity called an analyzer produces an entirely equivalent and useful description of the model. According to this relabeling, the analyzer is now a two-stage affair. The first stage is a two-dimensional translation-invariant linear system. This first stage was all there was to the analyzer in the original presentation. The analyzer of the relabeled model has a second stage: It calculates the peak in the spatial output profile from the first stage. This peak is now the output of the new two-stage analyzer. The observer's threshold is determined by this peak just as it was before. The predictions of the rephrased model will clearly be the same as those of the preceding model, as all that has occurred is a relabeling of entities.

With relabeling, however, all the assumptions change. To prevent confusion on reading the literature, let's go quickly through the changes:

1. This new two-stage analyzer's output is now a single number.
2. The analyzer does not generally display additivity of outputs, although it does for compound gratings in the peaks-add phase.
3. The analyzer's output obeys an even stronger kind of translation invariance than did the original analyzer, for now the single-number output remains exactly the same if the pattern is shifted.
4. The analyzer obeys the linear-transducer assumption.
5. There is still no variability.

With this relabeling, the relation of the second model (the nonadditive, uniform single-analyzer model or single-channel model) to the first model (the additive single analyzer) may seem clearer. The relabeled second model is the same as the first except that the analyzer's single-number output does not show additivity of outputs but rather a particular kind of nonadditivity; much of the structure of the second model goes to define this nonadditivity.

4.3.4 Alternative Assumptions

Time spent discussing alternative versions of assumptions seems worthwhile both for reading other authors' presentations and for increasing one's understanding of any model.

Assumption 33 uses the peak in the spatial output profile, but substituting peak-trough output (the difference between the maximum and the minimum output) would make no difference when the stimuli and the outputs are all symmetric above and below the mean output.

The property of translation invariance (weighting functions identical except for position) is certainly wrong for the spatial-position dimension, although perhaps correct for temporal position. Section 4.5 incorporates inhomogeneity (lack of translation-invariance) into a single-analyzer model.

Another assumption that might well be loosened is the assumption of no variability. Suppose there is "early" variability, in particular variability in the outputs of different mechanisms (variability in the magnitudes of the analyzer's output at different values of x and y). The case where the outputs at different positions are probabilistically independent of one another is considered in section 5.3.2, after the appropriate theoretical tools have been introduced.

The case where they are perfectly positively correlated, however, can be briefly summarized here, for the predictions remain the same as those from the non-additive single-analyzer (single-channel) model just discussed. To see why this is so, consider the following: Although the magnitude of the peak output will vary from trial to trial of a particular stimulus, the peak output will always occur at the same spatial position, for example, underneath where the peaks superimpose in the peaks-add compound grating. And the average at that spatial position will be what determines the observer's threshold; that average will act just like the deterministic model above.

Alternatively, if noise is assumed to be added after the peak of the output profile has been extracted ("late" variability), the predictions remain as from the single-channel model, since the peak output will always occur at the same spatial position.

Many assumptions other than Assumption 33—using more of the output than just the peak (or peak-trough) in the spatial profile, for example—have been considered over the years. To my knowledge, no reasonable one makes predictions very different from those of the single-analyzer models discussed here, that is, not different enough to make the model be consistent with summation of far-apart spatial frequencies. Predictions from what can be considered to be alternatives to Assumption 33 are shown in Fig. 5.2. (Remember the curve labeled "infinity" comes from this assumption.) Of course, if one makes a sufficiently complicated assumption—for example, postulating multiple analyzers coming after the single analyzer—one can dramatically change the predictions of the (nominal) single-analyzer model. But then the operative part of the model would be in the later stage, not in the single analyzer.

If a nonlinear stage comes after extraction of the peak output (e.g., a stage that changes the value of the peak output by squaring it), the predicted thresholds are unaffected. Because the value of the peak output is always the same at threshold, the subsequent nonlinearity is irrelevant.

An early nonlinearity (e.g., a nonlinear function transforming the value at each point of the luminance profile before it was input to the array of mechanisms) would, however, change the predictions. An early nonlinearity would, for example, effectively change a sinusoidal grating into a different kind of grating.

However, if the nonlinearity is slight, so will be the change in the predictions. And the most commonly assumed early nonlinearities (e.g., the light-adapting processes in the retina) are nonlinear only when very wide ranges of light intensity are involved. For the summation experiments here, where the contrasts are in general low (near threshold), all the intensities involved are close together, so these early nonlinearities may have little effect.

4.4 MULTIPLE-ANALYZERS MODEL

4.4.1 Assumptions

The right-hand column of Fig. 4.2 shows the predictions of a multiple-analyzers model for the summation of spatial frequencies a factor of 3 apart. The lines labeled "a," "b," and "c" represent the output profiles of three different analyzers, each of which is an array of mechanisms like that of the nonadditive single-analyzer model. Analyzer a is the analyzer that responds to the low-frequency sine wave f and does not respond to the high frequency at all; analyzer c responds to the high frequency $3f$ and does not respond to the low frequency at all. Analyzer b does not respond to either frequency and is a reminder that there are other analyzers besides a and c. In addition to a number of other analyzers that, like b, respond to neither of the frequencies, there may well be several other analyzers that respond at least somewhat to the low-frequency component (but not to the high) and still others that respond at least somewhat to the high-frequency component (but not to the low). What we will explicitly assume for this model is that no analyzer exists that responds to both spatial frequencies. Thus we replace the first assumption of the single-analyzer model with the following:

Assumption 34. Multiple Analyzers. *There are N' multiple analyzers having different sensitivity functions along the dimension of interest.*

Assumption 35. Nonoverlapping for Far-Apart Values. *For values far enough apart on the dimension of interest, no analyzer responds to both values.*

A factor of 3 will prove to be far enough apart on the spatial-frequency dimension in the typical experimental conditions. For the present we will also assume:

Assumption 32. Deterministic Analyzer Output. *The output of an analyzer in a given state of adaptation to a given stimulus is always the same.*

Assumption 25. Single-Number Analyzer Output. *The output of each analyzer to a given presentation of a stimulus is a single number.*

The output of the ith analyzer will be written R_i (stim).

In the right columns of Fig. 4.2, the output of each analyzer is drawn as a spatial output profile rather than as a single number, however. In drawing that figure, each of the multiple analyzers was taken to be a translation-invariant linear system with a two-dimensional function for an output (just as the single analyzer in the middle columns was assumed to be). One can easily turn the two-dimensional output profiles in Fig. 4.2 into single-number outputs by just taking the peak. Alternatively, one could consider each mechanism to be a separate analyzer and then it would have a single-number output. Either the two-stage analyzers (a linear translation-invariant system followed by a peak calculator) or individual mechanisms are sufficient as analyzers for our present purposes. But for our present purpose of dealing with far-apart components, we do not need to characterize the analyzers in anything like such great detail (although we will in Chap. 6 for close components). Further, such detail about the analyzers does not generalize to as many other sensory/perceptual dimensions. So in listing our assumptions we will use, instead of all these various detailed possibilities, the following weak property:

Assumption 36. The Ineffective-Stimulus Rule (Weak Additivity). *If a stimulus when presented alone has no effect on an analyzer, then that stimulus will have no effect when presented in a compound: The analyzer's expected output to the compound will be exactly like its output to the compound with that one stimulus removed.*

In short, ineffective stimuli are ineffective also in compounds. Or since we are assuming an analyzer's output is a single number, we can write
If

$$R_i(V_1) = 0$$

Then

$$R_i(V_1 + V_2) = R_i(V_2)$$

Thus, for example, in the right column of Fig. 4.2 the output of analyzer a to each compound stimulus containing f and $3f$ is just equal to its output to f alone (because $3f$ alone has no effect).

To avoid possible misunderstanding, one other assumption will be made explicit here:

Assumption 37. Noninteracting Analyzers. *The outputs of one analyzer have no effects (excitatory or inhibitory) on any other analyzer. The output of each analyzer can always be calculated directly from the stimulus regardless of what other analyzers may or may not be doing.*

The properties listed in Assumptions 35, 36, and 37 produce "perceptual separability," in the terminology of Ashby and Townsend (1986).

Now for the assumption about the transformation from the analyzer outputs to the observer's responses. We will use the assumption we used in Chapter 3, namely:

Assumption 4. Most Sensitive Analyzer Rule. *The observer's threshold (equivalently, sensitivity) for a stimulus equals the threshold (equivalently, sensitivity) of the one analyzer most sensitive to that stimulus.*

4.4.2 Predicted Thresholds

According to this set of assumptions, the output of analyzer a to either compound in Fig. 4.2 is identical to its output to the lower frequency component, and that output has magnitude equal to the threshold criterion T (since the component was assumed to be at threshold). Similarly the output of analyzer c to either compound is identical to its output to the higher frequency component, which equals the threshold criterion T. Consequently, if the contrast of either compound grating is reduced, the output of both analyzers a and c to the compound grating would be below threshold, and thus the compound grating would be below the observer's threshold. Hence the compound gratings shown in the figure are predicted to be just at threshold. More generally, this multiple-analyzers model predicts that any compound grating is below threshold unless at least one of its components is at threshold. Thus, its predictions fall on the outside edges of the summation square in Fig. 4.3. This prediction is quite unlike the predictions of the single-analyzer model and is in much better accord with the results of summation experiments using far-apart spatial frequencies (a factor of 2 or 3 or more apart).

As mentioned previously, however, the compound stimuli containing far-apart values are, in fact, slightly more detectable than their simple components (although still very near the outside edges of the summation square). In sections 4.6 through 4.9 we will see that a more sophisticated version of a multiple-analyzers model (incorporating independent variability in the outputs of analyzers) predicts exactly that.

4.5 A SINGLE NONUNIFORM CHANNEL (EXAMPLE OF INTERACTION BETWEEN TWO DIMENSIONS)

The nonadditive single analyzer presented earlier was spatially uniform in the sense shown in the top sketch of Fig. 4.4: The weighting functions (or, speaking in terms of the possible physiological substrate, the receptive fields) are identical at all positions in the visual field and thus sensitive to the same range of spatial frequencies. The analyzer was thus translation invariant.

The multiple spatial-frequency analyzers we used in drawing the predicted response profiles shown in Fig. 4.2 were also spatially uniform—see third row of Fig. 4.4. For the multiple-analyzers model, spatial nonuniformity (fourth row of Fig. 4.4) does not affect predictions of the type we have been discussing. (See section 4.5.5 for further clarification.)

The assumption of uniformity (translation invariance) is potentially critical in determining single-analyzer model predictions, however. Further, the uniformity we assumed previously is quite inconsistent with previously known experimental results. The thresholds for small patches of sinusoidal grating, for example, vary with spatial position (more precisely, with position on the retina). Some typical results are shown later in Fig. 5.6. The next several subsections consider the effect of allowing spatial nonuniformity in a single-analyzer model.

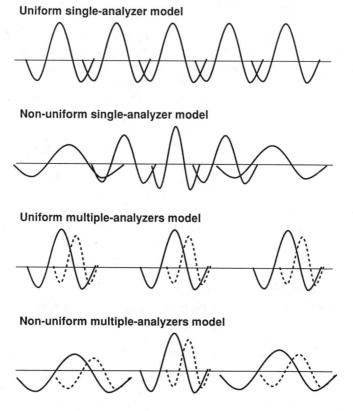

Uniform single-analyzer model

Non-uniform single-analyzer model

Uniform multiple-analyzers model

Non-uniform multiple-analyzers model

FIG. 4.4 A sample of individual mechanisms' weighting functions in four models.

4.5.1   *Modifying the Nonadditive Single-Analyzer Model*

To allow spatial nonuniformity, the single-analyzer model can be modified as shown in the second row of Fig. 4.4 to allow the weighting-function size and peak sensitivity to vary as a function of spatial position.

This modified model has been previously referred to as assuming a single analyzer for spatial frequency (e.g., Graham et al., 1978; Limb & Rubinstein, 1977). It might, however, be said to contain both multiple spatial-frequency analyzers (because it contains weighting functions of different sizes) and multiple spatial-position analyzers (because it contains weighting functions at different positions). The different sizes are at different positions in the visual field, rather than existing at the same position. This is exactly like the interactive joint selectivity illustrated in the upper right diagram of Fig. 11.3 (where dimensions A and B are replaced by spatial position and spatial frequency). As will be discussed in Chapter 11 for the general case, use of stimuli that are broad band on the nonexperimental dimension (in this case wide gratings, which are broad band on the spatial-position dimension) makes it very difficult to decide whether there are really multiple analyzers on the experimental dimension (e.g., spatial frequency) at each value on the nonexperimental dimension (e.g., spatial position) or whether there is interaction as in the upper right of Fig. 11.3. In the specific case we are discussing here (the single nonuniform analyzer model, second row of Fig. 4.4), the interpretational difficulties can be more fully described as in the next subsection (or see, e.g., van Doorn, Koenderink, & Bouman, 1972; Limb & Rubinstein, 1977).

4.5.2 Predictions for Large-Grating Spatial-Frequency Summation Experiments

When large gratings are used, the single nonuniform analyzer model (second row of Fig. 4.4) may behave like the multiple-analyzers model (third or fourth row of Fig. 4.4) and unlike the previous nonadditive uniform single-analyzer model (top row of Fig. 4.4): It may predict little summation between components of far-apart spatial frequencies. For the higher spatial-frequency component of the compound grating will be detected by mechanisms located nearer the fovea (having smaller receptive fields), and the lower frequency component will be detected by the mechanisms located more peripherally (having larger receptive fields). At each spatial position, therefore, the output to the compound might be no greater than the output to a single component. Consequently, the observer would be no more sensitive to the compound than to its most detectable component.

Quantitative consideration of exactly how the weighting functions must vary as a function of position to account for other results (e.g., measured sensitivity to small patches of sinusoidal grating or other localized stimuli) is probably sufficient to show that a realistic nonuniform single-analyzer model will not make the prediction suggested by the qualitative argument just given. Rather it will continue to predict that compound gratings are a good deal more detectable than their most detectable component (Graham et al., 1978). Such quantitative calculations, however, are always less convincing than they might be because they are difficult to follow and do depend on a number of assumptions. It seemed worthwhile, therefore, to do the following experiment.

4.5.3 Predictions for Small-Patch Spatial-Frequency Summation Experiments

Let's consider patches of grating that are quite small (narrow band on the spatial-position dimension as well as on the spatial-frequency dimension), like the Gabor patches shown in Fig. 4.5. Suppose that these stimuli are all shown at the same position in the visual field on different trials. According to the nonuniform single-channel model, only one size of weighting function is at a given position, even though the sizes change across the visual field. Therefore, according to that model, all the mechanisms stimulated by the patches will have almost exactly the same size weighting function. Consequently, the peak in the output profile

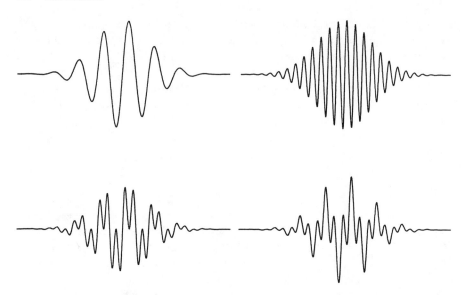

FIG. 4.5 Luminance profiles of four patches of sinusoidal grating (Gabor patches). Upper row shows simple stimuli, where the frequency on the right is three times that on the left. Lower row shows compounds made from the components above where the lower left is in peaks-subtract and lower right in peaks-add phase. In this figure, the amplitude of each component in the compound gratings (bottom row) is half that when it is alone (top row). (Figure 1 of Graham et al., 1978; reprinted by permission.)

to the compound-grating patch will be a good deal greater than the peak to either component, and phase will matter (just as was true for the uniform single-analyzer model). Calculations show that the sinusoidal patches in Fig. 4.5 are sufficiently localized in spatial position as well as in spatial frequency to be quite satisfactory for this experiment.

Comparison with Results. The results when small patches were used looked just like the results with full-field gratings. (The results with patches are shown in Fig. 4.11.) Thus, the results of a compound-grating experiment done with small patches of grating is strong evidence against the single nonuniform analyzer model for spatial-frequency summation (Graham et al., 1978). (Section 5.3 will elaborate the multiple-analyzers and the single-analyzer models to include independent variability at different spatial positions. But such independent variability does not change this conclusion.)

4.5.4   Including Both Spatial and Temporal Inhomogeneity

Just as different spatial frequencies might be detected at different spatial positions (suggesting the nonuniform single-analyzer model just discussed, different spatial frequencies might be detected at different temporal positions (at different times after the beginning of the stimulus). For there is abundant evidence that the responses to high and low spatial frequencies are of substantially different time course (see Chaps. 12 and 13). This produces an interpretational difficulty for temporal position and spatial frequency that is exactly analogous to the difficulty just discussed for spatial position and spatial frequency.

However, one does not postulate literally different mechanisms or neurons sensitive to different temporal positions and also sensitive to different spatial frequencies; rather one thinks of the output of the mechanisms at different points in time as having different spatial characteristics. Or to put it the other way around, one thinks of the output of a single mechanism or neuron as having different time courses to different spatial frequencies. How could this kind of spatiotemporal interaction occur in a mechanism or neuron? One likely way is for the time course of the output of the excitatory sections of the neuron's weighting function to be different from the time course of the output of the inhibitory sections.

Again, I suspect that careful quantitative considerations would show that a single-analyzer model with this kind of spatiotemporal interaction could not, in fact, account for the results of experiments using compound gratings of two different spatial frequencies. But such arguments are always difficult to see through intuitively, and they rest on a number of assumptions.

Thus another kind of compound-grating experiment to test this idea directly seems a good idea. If the different spatial-frequency components in a compound do not ordinarily summate because they elicit peak outputs at different times, they should summate if one is presented before the other by just the right amount of time to make the peak outputs juxtapose. In fact, however, the thresholds for compound gratings (either extended or small patches) containing far-apart frequencies (an octave or more apart) are not affected by temporal asynchrony between their components where the asynchronies are varied over a range of 400 milliseconds in either direction (Watson & Nachmias, 1980). Even including probability summation across time and accounting for the fact that not all asynchronies were tested (Limb, 1981), a single-analyzer model with spatiotemporal interaction cannot account for this result (Watson, 1981).

Thus, even allowing both temporal and spatial nonuniformity into a single-analyzer model does not make it consistent with available summation results using far-apart spatial frequencies.

4.5.5 *The Multiple-Analyzers Model Could Be Spatially Nonuniform or Uniform*

In the nonuniform version of the multiple-analyzer model (bottom row of Fig. 4.4), although there are multiple weighting functions at each point in the visual field (only two are shown in Fig. 4.4), the weighting functions at different positions range over a different set of sizes, being generally smaller near the fovea than in the periphery. This means, for example, that the analyzer having peak sensitivity to 3 cpd would not contain receptive fields at all spatial positions but only at those within some distance of the fovea. Notice that all the assumptions used in section 4.4 to describe a multiple-analyzer model (in particular, the assumption that ineffective stimuli are ineffective in compounds as well) are as true of the nonuniform version as of the uniform version. Thus both predict no summation between far apart spatial frequencies.

4.5.6   A Single Analyzer Followed by Multiple Analyzers

Although a single nonuniform analyzer model will not by itself account for pattern thresholds, it may be a reasonable model of a stage coming before the multiple-analyzer stage. Further, it may account for the "envelope" or overall contrast sensitivity as a function of spatial postion, spatial frequency, and so on (see, e.g., Kretz, Scarabin, & Bourguignat, 1979, p. 1644). It is the envelope that is discussed at length in Chapter 13 on parametric contrast sensitivity. If this early nonuniform single-analyzer stage and the subsequent multiple analyzers are linear systems, however, one will not be able to tell (from knowledge of stimuli and observer's responses) whether there are two such stages or only one. (See section 2.6.4.)

4.6   MULTIPLE-ANALYZERS MODELS INCORPORATING VARIABILITY

Once over their surprise that compound gratings were only slightly more detectable than their components (in contrast to single-analyzer models), the fact that they were slightly more detectable (in contradiction to the deterministic multiple-analyzer model) came as no surprise to those used to thinking about the consequences of variability, in particular, about the possibility of probability summation (Sachs, Nachmias, & Robson, 1971).

Observers' Variability. There is always a great deal of variability in the observer's responses over trials of the same stimulus. Over a large range of intensities of the stimulus, the observer's response is sometimes one thing (yes in a yes/no experiment, for example, or being correct in a forced-choice experiment) and sometimes another (no, or incorrect). The proportion only gradually increases from chance at low intensities to perfect behavior at high intensities. Operationally, the psychophysical threshold of a stimulus is not unambiguously defined but must be taken to equal the intensity producing a criterion performance level.

To explain this psychophysical variability, variability could be introduced into a model at any of a number of stages. Variability in the outputs of the analyzers is one candidate, and when that variability is probabilistically independent, it is the candidate that predicts probability summation.

Probability Summation. To understand probability summation, first consider what happens if you throw two coins rather than one in an attempt to get at least one head. (The outcomes of the two coin tosses are each variable—either head or tail—and probabilistically independent.) You are more likely to succeed if you throw two coins. In fact, given fair coins, the probability of getting at least one head with two coins is .75 (one minus the probability of getting two tails) while the probability of getting a head with one coin is only 0.5. This is an example of probability summation. Notice that the phrase *probability summation* does not mean the literal addition of probabilities.

How does this reasoning apply to multiple analyzers? Suppose there is variability in the output of each analyzer so that its output to any particular pattern varies from trial to trial. Suppose also the outputs of different analyzers are probabilistically independent. Let us suppose that a pattern is above the observer's threshold if and only if at least one analyzer's output is greater than criterion (the maximum-output detection rule, formally presented below as Assumption 40). Thus, an observer's trying to detect a compound grating containing two far-apart components is something like throwing two coins to get at least one head (to get at least one above-criterion output from two analyzers, e.g., analyzers a and c in Fig. 4.2); an observer's detecting a simple grating is like throwing one coin (only one of the two analyzers can detect the simple grating).

Exactly how much more detectable a compound is predicted to be due to this probability summation depends on a number of details of the multiple-analyzers model: on whether the variability is completely independent, on exactly what its probability distribution is, and on exactly what further elaboration of the decision rule is used to account for observer's "false alarms." In Chapter 7 we will discuss these issues at some length. In this chapter and the next two we will use a particularly simple model—one very close to the coin analogy, in fact. We will use it not because it is absolutely right but because it is exceedingly convenient, it has proved very useful to investigators of pattern vision, and it is a good introduction to the more complicated models. Before describing this model in detail, let's look at several issues relating to probability summation.

Appearance of Compound Stimuli. If on some trials the observer is detecting the compound stimulus because one analyzer (e.g., analyzer a in Fig. 4.2) detects it, sometimes because another analyzer (e.g., analyzer c) detects it, and sometimes because both analyzers detect it, you may wonder whether the appearance of the compound grating varies from trial to trial depending on which analyzer(s) detects it. See sections 10.4 through 10.6 for an answer.

Probability Summation Versus Summation Within an Analyzer. To clear up one possible confusion, let's explicitly distinguish between the two kinds of summation that we have met so far. First (although we met it second) there is probability summation. Even though components excite completely separate analyzers and no analyzer responds more to the compound than to one of the components, the detectability of the compound to the *observer* may be greater than the detectability of either component if there is independent variability in the outputs of these separate analyzers.

Second, there is summation within an analyzer. As in the single analyzer of Fig. 4.2 middle column, a particular analyzer may respond more to the compound than to either component. This can happen within a multiple-analyzers model if the two components get close enough together to both excite the same analyzers. The only multiple-analyzer model that would exclude this kind of summation is one in which the analyzers are extremely narrow-band and respond only to a single value along the dimension of interest. Such an analyzer is physiologically unreasonable in most cases (certainly in the cases of spatial frequency, orientation, etc.). Experiments in which the two components in compound stimuli are close enough together to give more summation than probability summation are discussed in Chap. 6. This extra summation is attributed to summation within an analyzer.

Three Possible Sources of Variability in a Spatial-Frequency Analyzer. If each spatial-frequency analyzer is taken to be an array of mechanisms at different positions in the visual field followed by something that calculates the peak output, there are at least three distinct sources for the variability in the analyzer's output: (a) The outputs at different spatial positions in the array may vary and vary independently. (b) The outputs at different spatial positions in the array vary but all are positively correlated. (c) The outputs from the array may not vary, but the calculation of the peak output may be noisy (variable).

These three sources of variability make identical predictions for compounds containing far-apart spatial frequencies, the topic of the present chapter. For compounds containing closer components that excite the same analyzer, however, the first leads to predictions for the amount of summation within an analyzer that are quite different from those of the second and third. (See Chap. 6.)

4.7 HIGH-THRESHOLD MULTIPLE-ANALYZERS MODEL

To discuss high-threshold models, the following terminology is conventional and useful. When an analyzer's output exceeds its threshold criterion, the analyzer is said to *detect the stimulus* or to *be in the detect state.* Since the threshold criterion is a fixed number, and the only important aspect of an analyzer's output will be whether it exceeds this criterion, there are essentially only two possible analyzer outputs of interest—being in the detect state (which is often called *1* when a number would be convenient) and being in the not-detect state (which can be called *0* when a number would be convenient).

Introductions to signal-detection theories (including high-threshold models) can be found in a number of sources, including Coombs et al. (1970), Egan (1975), Falmagne (1986), Gescheider (1976), Green and Swets (1966, 1974), Macmillan and Creelman (in press), MacNichol (1972), Nachmias (1972), and Sperling and Dosher (1986).

4.7.1 *Assumptions of High-Threshold Multiple-Analyzers Model*

These assumptions will be the same as for the multiple-analyzers model of section 4.4 with two important exceptions: the assumption of no-variability

(Assumption 32) and the most sensitive analyzer rule (Assumption 4) will be replaced.

First, a brief reminder of the unchanged assumptions: Assumption 34, multiple analyzers; Assumption 35, Nonoverlapping for far-apart values; Assumption 25, single-number analyzer outputs; Assumption 36, ineffective stimulus rule; and Assumption 37, noninteracting analyzers.

The no-variability assumption (Assumption 32) will be replaced by two assumptions:

Assumption 38. Probabilistically Independent Analyzers. *The output of each analyzer is variable, and the outputs of different analyzers are probabilistically independent of one another.*

Thus the probability that both analyzer A and analyzer B are in the detect state (both their outputs exceed criterion) is the product of the probabilities that each is in the detect state.

Assumption 39. High-Threshold Analyzers. *The probability of an analyzer being in the detect state is zero on every trial of the blank stimulus and also on every trial of any stimulus to which the analyzer is not sensitive.*

This last assumption is what leads to the name *high threshold,* suggesting that some internal threshold criterion has been set so high that it is never exceeded on trials of the blank stimulus.

Since the analyzers' outputs are not the same on each trial of a stimulus, we now need assumptions describing how the observer's response on each trial is determined by the outputs of the analyzers on each trial. (This replaces the most sensitive analyzer rule, Assumption 4.) The first assumption specifies a decision variable and the next two specify how the observer's response is based on that decision variable.

Assumption 40. Maximum-Output Detection Rule. *In all conditions, the observer's response is based on the maximum of the outputs from the monitored analyzers.*

In the high-threshold model, this maximum can have only two values—it equals a detect state if at least one of the analyzers is in a detect state (in which case we will say the observer is in a detect state), or it equals a not-detect state if all the analyzers are in a not-detect state (in which case we will say the observer is in a not-detect state).

We will make the conventional assumptions linking this decision variable to an observer's overt responses. In yes-no experiments, each single-alternative trial presents either a stimulus or a blank; the observer is to say "yes" to indicate the presence of a stimulus or "no" to indicate the presence of a blank.

Assumption 41. Yes-No Rule (Applied to High Threshold). *When the observer is in the detect state, the observer always says "yes." When the observer is in the not-detect state, the observer sometimes says "no" and sometimes guesses "yes."*

In a two-alternative forced-choice experiment, each trial contains two temporal intervals (or occasionally two spatial positions). In one of these intervals (randomly chosen) a blank stimulus is presented and in the other a nonblank stimulus is presented. The observer indicates which interval presented the nonblank stimulus.

Assumption 42. Forced-Choice Rule (Applied to High Threshold). *If the observer was in a detect state during one interval, the observer chooses that interval. If the observer was not in a detect state during either interval, the observer guesses.*

Note that a detect state will never occur in both intervals because the blank stimulus cannot produce a detect state in any of the analyzers and so can never produce a detect state in the observer. Or, as is sometimes said, there are no true false alarms according to this model.

An Aside About the Relationship of Maximum-Output and Most Sensitive Analyzer Rules. If multiple analyzers' outputs are either not variable (as in the deterministic multiple-analyzers model of section 4.4) or else perfectly positively correlated, the maximum output to a particular stimulus will always be the same and will always come from the same analyzer (or analyzers). In this case, therefore, application of the maximum-output rule (with the other assumptions linking the maximum-output decision variable to the observer's responses in the experiment) will lead to the same predictions as the most sensitive analyzer rule. I might have introduced the maximum-output rule in section 4.4 instead of the most sensitive analyzer rule, but did not do so for simplicity of exposition. (See Chap. 7 for further discussion of the maximum-output rule.)

4.7.2 Predicted Probability of Observer's Being in the Detect State

According to the independent-variability, high-threshold, and maximum-output rule assumptions, the only way that an observer *cannot* detect a stimulus is if *all* the analyzers fail to detect the stimulus. But, since the variability in the outputs of different analyzers is independent, the probability that all the analyzers fail to detect the stimulus is simply the product of the probabilities that each analyzer fails to detect. Thus, letting the symbol $P_j(\text{stim})$ denote the probability that analyzer j detects the stimulus, the symbol $P_{obs}(\text{stim})$ denote the probability that the observer detects the stimulus, and N' be the total number of analyzers, then:

$$1 - P_{obs}(\text{stim}) = \prod_{j=1}^{N'} [1 - P_j(\text{stim})] \qquad (4.1)$$

4.7.3 Predicted Observable Probabilities

We need to derive the relationship between $P_{obs}(\text{stim})$—the observer's probability of "detecting" a stimulus—and the probabilities of the responses given in an psychophysical experiment.

For Yes-No Experiments. Let g represent the probability that the observer guesses yes from a not-detect state (see Assumption 41). Let the "hit rate" be the probability of the observer's saying yes when a nonblank stimulus was presented and the "false-alarm rate" be the probability of the observer's saying "yes" when a blank was presented. Then, according to the high-threshold model

$$\text{Hit rate} = \Pr(\text{yes}\,|\,\text{stim})$$

$$= P_{\text{obs}}(\text{stim}) + g[1 - P_{\text{obs}}(\text{stim})] \tag{4.2}$$

$$\text{False-alarm rate} = \Pr(\text{yes}\,|\,\text{blank}) = g$$

An aside about conditional probabilities. The symbol $\Pr(A\,|\,B)$ can be read as "the probability that A occurs given that (conditional upon, assuming that) B occurs" or "the probability of A given B." The conditional probability $\Pr(\text{yes}\,|\,\text{blank})$, for example, can be read "the probability that the observer says 'yes' given that the blank is presented" or "the probability of 'yes' given blank." Letting "blank trials" be short for all the trials on which the blank is presented, $\Pr(\text{yes}\,|\,\text{blank})$ represents the proportion of blank trials on which the observer says "yes."

For Forced-Choice Experiments. On the standard forced-choice rule (Assumption 42), the observer will always be correct whenever one interval produces a detect state, because a blank stimulus never produces a detect state. However, if neither interval produces a detect state, the observer can be correct only half the time. (No residual information is available to the observer about the analyzer outputs beyond the fact that all were below threshold criterion, that is, in the non-detect state.) Thus

$$\Pr(\text{correct}) = P_{\text{obs}}(\text{stim}) + .5[1 - P_{\text{obs}}(\text{stim})] \tag{4.3}$$

In forced-choice experiments with more alternatives than two, the same equation holds except that the guessing probability is not .5 but rather the reciprocal of the number of alternatives.

Estimating the Observer's Probability of Detection. The preceding equations for observable probabilities (hit rate in yes-no and probability of correct in forced-choice) both have the same form except that the first equation has g [which can be estimated from data as $\Pr(\text{yes}\,|\,\text{blank})$] in the place where the second has .5 (more generally, 1/number of alternatives). Letting g serve for both these quantities now and abbreviating $P_{\text{obs}}(\text{stim})$—the probability that the observer detects the stimulus—to P, we find

$$\text{Observed probability} = P + (1 - P) \cdot g \tag{4.4}$$

$$= P \cdot (1 - g) + g$$

Consider what happens, according to this equation, as increases in stimulus intensity cause P to go from 0 to 1. Then the observed probability will trace out the same function of intensity that P does except that the observed probability function will be compressed vertically into the space between g and 1. This vertical compression is illustrated in Fig. 4.6 for yes-no (left panel) and two-alternative forced-choice (right panel) experiments.

The stimulus intensity (indicated in Fig 4.6 by a vertical dashed line) producing P equal to .5 is conventionally taken to define the stimulus threshold. (Notice that the concept of threshold as an intensity of a stimulus is quite distinct from the concept of an internal threshold or threshold criterion that an internal output can exceed.) At this stimulus intensity, the probability of being correct in a two-alternative forced-choice experiment is equal to 0.75, and the probability of saying yes in a yes-no experiment is equal to the value halfway between the false-alarm rate (the guessing rate—the probability of saying yes to a blank) and 1.0.

Correction for Guessing. More generally, it is easy to compute an estimate for $P = P_{obs}$(stim)—the probability of an observer's detecting the stimulus—from either value of observed probability by the following formula rearranged from Eq. 4.4:

$$P_{obs}(\text{stim}) = \frac{\text{observed probability} - g}{1 - g} \qquad (4.5)$$

This calculation is sometimes called *correcting the observed probability for guessing.*

4.7.4   A Failure of High-Threshold Models

This section can be skimmed or omitted with little loss of continuity.

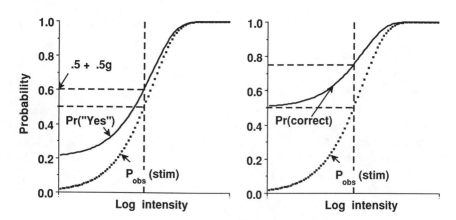

FIG. 4.6 Diagram of the predictions of a high-threshold model for psychometric functions from yes-no (left) and two-alternative forced-choice (right) procedures. In each procedure, the observed function [Pr(yes) or Pr(correct)] is a vertically compressed version of the function, giving the observer's probability of detecting a stimulus [P_{obs} (stim)].

Yes/No and Forced-Choice Experiments Results. Suppose the detectability of a certain stimulus is measured in several different experiments: a forced-choice experiment and several yes-no experiments using different instructions or pay-offs so that the false-alarm rate will be different in each. If the high-threshold model is correct, the probability of being correct in the forced-choice experiment and the probabilities of saying yes in the various yes-no experiments run at different false-alarm rates should yield consistent estimates of the observer's probability of detecting the stimulus when "corrected for guessing" as in Eq. 4.5.

Further, if several different intensities of the stimulus are used in each of the experiments to produce full psychometric functions, the psychometric functions should be the same except for different vertical compressions (as in Fig. 4.6).

In fact, however, for sinusoidal gratings (Nachmias, 1981) as well as for most other sensory/perceptual stimuli (Green & Swets, 1974), this prediction of the high-threshold model is wrong. A typical observer's performance in forced-choice experiments is better than it ought to be relative to performance in yes-no experiments; put another way, the probability of detecting a given stimulus $[P_{obs}(\text{stim})]$ is usually greater when estimated from forced-choice than from the yes-no experiment. Further, this probability is usually greater when estimated from yes-no experiments with high false-alarm rates than from those with low. See note 2 of Chapter 8 for further discussion.

ROC Curves. Another way of describing this failure is in terms of the high-threshold model's predicted ROC curve. An ROC curve is a plot of hit rate versus false-alarm rate for a particular stimulus (at a given intensity) in a yes-no experiment. (ROC curves can also be derived from rating-scale experiments.) Some ROC curves are shown in Fig. 7.5. According to a high-threshold model, variations in false-alarm rate are produced by variations in the guessing parameter g; thus the predicted ROC curve (when hit and false-alarm rates are plotted on linear coordinates) is simply a straight line derived from Eq. 4.2 where $P = P_{obs}(\text{stim})$:

$$\Pr(\text{yes}|\text{stim}) = P + \Pr(\text{yes}|\text{blank}) \cdot (1 - P)$$

ROC curves measured in psychophysical experiments, however, are typically not straight on linear coordinates but are bowed outward. This bowing means that estimates of $P_{obs}(\text{stim})$ obtained by running a high-threshold ROC curve through an experimental point at a high false-alarm rate would be greater than that obtained from an ROC curve through a point at a low false-alarm rate. The actual shape of measured ROC curves will be discussed in some detail in Chapter 7; some examples (plotted on normal probability or z axes) are shown in Fig. 7.5.

This failure of the high-threshold model means it is certainly wrong in detail. The high-threshold multiple-analyzers model also has many successes, however, in particular in predicting the results of summation experiments. For the time being (until Chap. 7), therefore, we end our discussion of its failures and move on to its successes.

4.7.5   Composite Analyzers—Reducing the General Case to the One-Analyzer-per-Component Case

In a number of places below, proofs become very easy to write symbolically if only one analyzer is sensitive to each component. But the theorems hold, in fact, no matter how many analyzers are sensitive to each component as long as no analyzer is sensitive to more than one component (which is what we mean by far-apart components). Thus, it will be convenient to show here how a proof written down for the one-analyzer-per-component case immediately generalizes to the many-analyzers-per-component case if components are far apart. Or, as mathematicians like to say, we can assume that only one analyzer is sensitive to each far-apart component "without loss of generality."

Composite Analyzers. Suppose that more than one analyzer is sensitive to each component in a compound. (Keep remembering that no analyzer is sensitive to more than one component, however, since we are assuming far-apart components.) Now consider the group of analyzers sensitive to the jth component and call this group the jth *composite analyzer.* Define the output of this composite analyzer to be the maximum of the outputs of the analyzers it contains. Similarly define composite analyzers for each component of the compound. Of this set of composite analyzers, only one composite analyzer is sensitive to a component! Sections 7.3.6 and 9.6 describe the formation of composites in more general cases than the high-threshold model considered here.

Verifying Assumptions. Next you check that each assumption you are dealing with holds for the composite analyzers just as it did for the original analyzers. For the present model (the high-threshold multiple-analyzers model), let's first consider the observer's decision variable. It was assumed to be the maximum of the original analyzers' outputs and is also, of necessity, equal to the maximum of the composite analyzers' outputs. Thus, the maximum-output detection rule (Assumption 40) and consequently the yes-no and forced-choice rules (Assumptions 41 and 42) hold for the composite analyzers.

Similarly, since the outputs of the original analyzers were probabilistically independent and no two composite analyzers contain the same original analyzer, the outputs of the composite analyzers are probabilistically independent (Assumption 38). One can continue straightforwardly to show that these composite analyzers obey the other assumptions of the high-threshold multiple-analyzers model (32, 34, 35, 35, 37, and 39) as long as the original analyzers did.

Reduction. Suppose a theorem has been proved (e.g., Eq. 4.6) for the case where only one analyzer is sensitive to a given component, but now you are considering a case where many analyzers are sensitive to each component. To show that the theorem holds in the second case, you consider composite analyzers formed from the analyzers in the second case; since only one of these composite analyzers is sensitive to each component, you apply the theorem you have proved to these composite analyzers and thus you know it holds in this second case as well.

Mechanisms and Channels—An Example of Forming Composite Analyzers. Suppose we start out with analyzers that are individual mechanisms having weighting functions of many different sizes and orientations and located at many different spatial positions. A component in a spatial-frequency summation experiment—a sinusoidal grating patch—will stimulate more than one of these analyzers. Now, however, suppose we form a composite analyzer by taking all the mechanisms that respond to a given component. These will all have weighting functions of about the same size and orientation—those matched to the grating—but the weighting-function positions may be scattered over a rather wide area (e.g., analyzers a, b, and c in Fig. 4.2 right column). In the terminology of section 1.10, this composite analyzer can also be called a *channel*. The output of this channel (this composite analyzer) is taken to be the peak of the outputs of the mechanisms (analyzers) forming it. Now, as long as the components are far enough apart that each mechanism responds to one (or none) of the components, then only one channel will respond to each component.

Algebraic Bookkeeping. If this approach of reducing the many-analyzer to the one-analyzer case is unsatisfying, the reader may use the following bookkeeping trick to modify algebraic proofs for the one-analyzer-per-component case to explicitly show that they hold for the many-analyzers-per-component case: renumber the analyzers using double subscripts, where the first subscript tells which component the analyzer is sensitive to and therefore which composite analyzer it is a member of. Then rewrite the equations involving products (or sums) into equations involving double products (or double sums), where one first multiplies (sums) over all analyzers within each composite analyzer and then multiplies (sums) over composite analyzers.

4.7.6 High-Threshold Predictions for Summation of Far-Apart Components

For any stimulus, the high-threshold model makes the prediction given in Eq. 4.1. This prediction contains quantities related to the observer's behavior (on the left side) and quantities expressing the properties of individual analyzers (on the right side). For compound stimuli that contain far-apart components, a prediction closely related to this one can be derived that is expressed entirely in terms of probabilities of the observer's behavior.

Suppose a compound stimulus (called *cmpd*) contains M far-apart components of values V_j, where j goes from 1 to M. The prediction of the high-threshold multiple-analyzers model is

$$1 - P_{\text{obs}}(\text{cmpd}) = \prod_{j=1}^{M} [1 - P_{\text{obs}}(V_j \text{ in cmpd})] \qquad (4.6)$$

In words, the observer's probability of not detecting the compound is simply the product of the observer's probabilities of not detecting each of the components by itself. (Remember that V_j in cmpd is, loosely, the jth component in the compound; more strictly, it is a simple stimulus with value V_j and the same intensity as the component of value V_j in the compound stimulus.) The derivation of Eq. 4.6 is given immediately hereafter. Then follow examples of predictions using Eq. 4.6, as these aid intuition.

Derivation of Eq. 4.6. Assume without loss of generality (see section 4.7.5) that only one anlyzer is sensitive to each of the M components in a compound. Let these M analyzers be numbered to accord with the numbering of the components, so that analyzer 1 is the analyzer sensitive to component 1, and so on. Since the only one of the observer's analyzers that is sensitive to component V_j is analyzer j, the probability that the observer detects a simple stimulus consisting of component j is equal to the probability that analyzer j detects that stimulus. In symbols:

$$P_{obs}(V_j \text{ in cmpd}) = P_j(V_j \text{ in cmpd}) \qquad (4.6a)$$

Also, the probability that the jth analyzer detects the compound is equal to the probability that the jth analyzer detects the corresponding component (since that is the only component the analyzer is sensitive to). In symbols:

$$P_j(\text{cmpd}) = P_j(V_j \text{ in cmpd}) \qquad (4.6b)$$

Combining these last two equations allows one to substitute $P_{obs}(V_j \text{ in cmpd})$ for $P_j(\text{cmpd})$ in Eq. 4.1 where cmpd has been substituted for stim. This leads directly to the desired prediction in Eq. 4.6.

Numerical Example of Summation Predictions. As an example, let's apply Eq. 4.6 to a compound of two far-apart components ($M = 2$), each at its own threshold:

$$P_{obs}(V_1 \text{ in cmpd}) = P_{obs}(V_2 \text{ in cmpd}) = .5$$

Then by Eq. 4.6 slightly re-arranged:

$$P_{obs}(\text{cmpd}) = 1 - (1 - .5)^2 = .75$$

In words, the observer fails to detect the compound only on that quarter of the trials where he or she failed to detect both far-apart components. So the compound is somewhat above threshold, although both components are at threshold.

How detectable does each component have to be (assuming both are equally detectable) for the compound to be detectable on half the trials (to be just at threshold)? Solving

$$.5 = P_{obs}(\text{cmpd}) = 1 - [1 - P_{obs}(V_1 \text{ in cmpd})]^2$$

says that the probability of detecting V_1 (or V_2) must be 1 minus the square root of .5, that is, .293.

To predict results of yes-no or forced-choice experiments, calculations like the example just given that use an observer's probability of being in a detect state must be sandwiched between transformations from and to the observed probabilities—the hit and false-alarm rates in a yes-no experiment of the percentage correct in a forced-choice experiment. Specifically:

1. The observed probabilities for the simple stimuli (the components by themselves) are used to estimate the observer's probabilities of detecting the components using Eq. 4.5.
2. These probabilities of detecting the components are then used to predict the observer's probability of detecting the compound (as in the previous simple example).
3. The observer's probability of detecting the compound is then used to estimate the observer's hit and false-alarm rates to the compound or the probability of being correct in a forced-choice experiment.

4.7.7 Predicted Psychometric Functions

Forced-choice psychometric functions for five different visual patterns are shown in Fig. 4.7. Three patterns were simple sinusoidal gratings having spatial frequencies in the ratio 1:3:9. Two patterns were compounds of the three simple gratings; in one the components were positioned so that the peaks of all three juxtaposed (cosine phase) and in the other so that the peaks of f and $9f$ added but the peaks of $3f$ subtracted (square wave or sine phase). The relative contrasts in the three components of the compound grating were adjusted so that all three

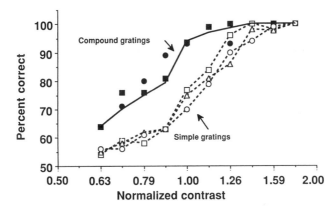

FIG. 4.7 Forced-choice psychometric functions for three simple gratings and two compounds made of those three. Contrast has been normalized so that the point giving percent correct for a compound grating (an open or closed circle) is directly above the three points giving percent correct for the three components of that grating by themselves. The solid lines connect the points for the simple gratings. The dotted line is the prediction of the high-threshold multiple-analyzers model for either compound grating's function. (Results from Robson and Graham in Graham, 1980.)

were (approximately) equally detectable when alone. To display this adjustment of relative contrasts, the horizontal axis in the figure gives "normalized" contrast (relative intensity), where the normalization was done by dividing the contrast of each component by (an estimate of) its threshold when alone. Once this normalization has been done, the compound grating represented by a particular circle in the figure is made up of the three components whose detectabilities are given by the three symbols directly below the circle. The predicted probability of correct for each compound grating (the dotted line) was calculated from the probabilities for its three components, using the high-threshold model as described above. As is typically found, the predictions are a good fit to the results. (Each point came from between 60 and 100 trials. In comparing the predictions with the results, remember that there is variability not only in the compound-grating thresholds but also in the predictions, since they are based on the simple-grating thresholds.)

In a study using unequally detectable components and a number of different spatial frequencies, Sachs et al. (1971) used a chi-square test to test directly a prediction that comes from Eq. 4.6: The probability that an observer says no to a compound is predicted to equal the product of the probabilities of saying no to each of the components (as long as the guessing rate g is the same for all of them, which it was in these experiments where compounds and components were intermixed within a block). The prediction fared well in their test.

Summation Square. The high-threshold model by itself makes no prediction for a summation-square plot. For to plot a point on the summation square one needs to know how much less contrast is required in each component of the compound for the compound to be at threshold than is required for the component by itself to be at threshold. In terms of the simple arithmetic example above, one needs to know the intensity at which an observer detects a component with probability .29 (and therefore the compound with probability .5) relative to the intensity at which the observer detects a component with probability .5. To know these intensities, the high-threshold model needs to be supplemented with a statement about how fast these probabilities grow with contrast. One way of supplementing the model is with empirical psychometric functions (e.g., those shown in Fig. 4.7). A second way is to choose an appropriate analytic form for the psychometric function. This is the way taken by the Quick pooling model described in the next subsection.

4.8 QUICK POOLING MODEL

4.8.1 *The Quick Psychometric Function*

To change the preceding high-threshold multiple-analyzers model into the form we will find most useful, we need to add one more assumption. This assumption specifies how the probability that an analyzer detects a stimulus depends on the intensity of the stimulus:

Assumption 43. Quick Psychometric Function. *The probability that the ith analyzer has an output that exceeds criterion equals*

$$P_i(\text{stim}) = 1 - 2^{-[c(\text{stim})S_i\ (\text{stim})]^k} \tag{4.7}$$

where k is a parameter determining the steepness of the psychometric function.

We could have had k depend on the analyzer i, but since we would almost immediately change and assume k to be the same for all i, we started out that way for notational ease.

Several examples of this function for different values of k are plotted in Fig. 4.8.

Historical Notes. The earliest attempts to deal with independent variability in the output of multiple spatial-frequency analyzers assumed that the variability in each analyzer's output had a normal (Gaussian) probability distribution (Sachs et al., 1971). Unfortunately, to make predictions from this assumption one has to use tables of the cumulative Gaussian distribution, which is time consuming (even on a computer) and does not permit simple analytic expressions. A few years later, Frank Quick pointed out the usefulness of Eq. 4.7, particularly when it is used in conjunction with the high-threshold model (Quick, 1974).

Since the function in Assmption 43 increases monotonically from 0.0 to 1.0, it can represent a cumulative probability distribution; as such it has been quite widely known as the *Weibull function* after one of its early users (see, e.g., Weibull, 1951). Indeed Weibull graph paper (analogous to normal or Gaussian graph paper) is commercially available. The Weibull cumulative probability distribution is a very good approximation to a cumulative Gaussian, which is, I think,

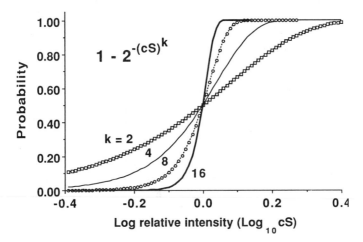

FIG. 4.8 Examples of Quick psychometric functions for several values of k (written next to each curve). The horizontal axis plots the logarithm (to the base 10) of the relative intensity (intensity divided by that intensity that produces a probability of .50.)

how Frank Quick came across it. In the Quick pooling model being presented in this chapter, however, an analyzer's psychometric function is not assumed to be a cumulative probability distribution of any sort; it is simply a function describing how the probability of detect changes with stimulus intensity. In Chapter 8, models will be presented in which an analyzer's psychometric function is closely related to a cumulative probability distribution describing the variability of the analyzer's output.

In vision, this function has also been previously discussed by Brindley (see, e.g., page 192 of his 1960 book and his short 1960 article) in a context similar to that discussed here, namely as a psychometric function for analyzers sensitive to different spatial (or temporal) positions.

Independence of Threshold Criterion. As the psychometric function is written in Eq. 4.7, S_i is easily seen to be the reciprocal of the contrast producing a probability of detection of .50. Thus the threshold intensity for a stimulus has been implicitly taken to be that producing a probability of detection of .50. Although this is conventional, it is essentially arbitrary. Changing the base from 2 to some other number will change the threshold criterion. A number of authors have used e as the base. None of the predictions derived below will depend on whether the performance level chosen is .50 or any other number (for the observer or the analyzer).

Changing the Intensity of a Compound Stimulus. To prevent possible confusion later when compound stimuli are discussed, let's clarify here what is meant by changing the intensity of a stimulus in the Quick psychometric function. In particular, consider a stimulus that is a compound containing several components. To change its intensity will mean to change the intensities of all the components by the same factor. It is that kind of change that is assumed to change the probability of an analyzer's detecting the stimulus in the way specified by the Quick function. If the intensity of components is changed by different factors, we will say a new stimulus has been formed rather than that the same stimulus has a new intensity.

4.8.2   Constraints on the Transducer Function

The following paragraphs clarifying the relationship between a psychometric function and a transducer function can be skipped without loss of continuity. Any psychometric function assumption (any assumption relating the probability of an analyzer's detecting the stimulus to the intensity of the stimulus) performs much the same role as an assumption about the form of the transducer function. In fact, a psychometric function assumption can be seen as a consequence of two other assumptions—one about the transducer function and one about the probability distribution (noise) in an analyzer's output. (See Chap. 8.)

It is interesting to note the following consequence of the Quick psychometric function assumption (Assumption 42) coupled with a second assumption that the probability that an analyzer detects a stimulus is a monotonic function of the analyzer's output. These two assumptions together imply that: An analyzer's output depends only on the product of sensitivity times intensity [c(stim) · S_i(stim)], that is, it obeys the intensity-sensitivity product assumption (Assumption 1). To see this, note that, according to the Quick function, the probability of detection is determined by the product of sensitivity times intensity [c(stim) · S_i(stim)]. Thus, if that product is the same for two different stimuli, the probability that the analyzer will detect the stimuli will be the same, and on the assumption that probability of detection is a monotonic function of output magnitude, the output magnitudes for the two stimuli must also be the same.

The Quick psychometric function (even with the additional assumption that detection probability is monotonically related to output magnitude) certainly does not imply that the transducer function is linear, however. Let's look at two alternatives. First, suppose the transducer function is linear (as in Assumption 9), that is, R_i(stim) = c(stim) · S_i(stim). Then the Quick psychometric function assumption is equivalent to the assumption that probability of detect is related to analyzer output by

$$P_i(\text{stim}) = 1 - 2^{-[R_i(\text{stim})]^k}$$

On the other hand, if the transducer function is a power function (with power k) of the product of sensitivity times intensity (as in assumption 92), that is, if

$$R_i(\text{stim}) = [c(\text{stim}) \cdot S_i(\text{stim})]^k$$

then the Quick psychometric function assumption is equivalent to the assumption that probability detect is related to analyzer output by

$$P_i(\text{stim}) = 1 - 2^{-R_i(\text{stim})}$$

4.8.3 Deriving the Observer's Psychometric Function and the Quick Pooling Formula

The convenient and aesthetically pleasing properties of the Quick psychometric function (Assumption 43) become apparent when it is substituted into the high-threshold model's expression for an observer's probability of nondetection as a function of the various analyzers' probabilities of nondetection (Eq. 4.1). By Assumption 42 the analyzers' probabilities of *not* detecting will all have the form: the number 2 raised to an exponent. Thus, when they are multiplied together in Eq. 4.1, the exponents simply add, giving

$$P_{\text{obs}} = 1 - 2^{-\sum_{i=1}^{N}(c \cdot S_i)^k} \tag{4.8}$$

Since all the contrasts, sensitivities, and probabilities in the derivations in this section involve the same arbitrary stimulus, the argument (stim) will be omitted everywhere to make the equations easier to read.

Now let S_{obs} be the following nonlinear summation of the individual analyzers' sensitivities:

$$S_{obs} = \left| \sum_{i=1}^{N'} S_i^k \right|^{1/k} \tag{4.9}$$

Then Eq. (4.8) can be rewritten as

$$P_{obs} = 1 - 2^{-(c \cdot S_{obs})^k} \tag{4.10}$$

(Eq. 4.10 is obtained by raising each side of Eq. 4.9 to the kth power, then multiplying each side of the result by c raised to the kth power, then using the result to substitute for the summation in Eq. 4.8.)

As the notation implies, S_{obs}—which was defined as the sum in Eq. 4.9—is equal to the observer's sensitivity to the stimulus; that is, as you can see in Eq. 4.10, it is the reciprocal of the stimulus intensity at which the observer detects the stimulus 50% of the time.

We will call Eq. 4.9 the Quick pooling formula. It and the predicted observer's psychometric function (Eq. 4.10) together express all the basic properties of the Quick pooling model.

4.8.4   *Properties of the Predicted Observer's Psychometric Function*

First notice that the observer's psychometric function in Eq. 4.10 has exactly the same form as the analyzers' psychometric function (Assumption 42). The predicted psychometric function observed in an experiment will have that same shape although it will be vertically compressed to begin at the guessing parameter (as in Fig. 4.6) Thus, one test of the Quick pooling model is its ability to predict the shape of the observed psychometric function. As one would expect from the long history of use of the cumulative Gaussian and the fact that the Quick function is a good approximation to the cumulative Gaussian, observed psychometric functions turn out to be well described by the Quick function. Examples of its success for visual patterns are shown and discussed later (Fig. 4.10).

Second, notice that the observer's psychometric function has exactly the same form for every stimulus. The stimulus intensity is simply multiplied by a different sensitivity value S_{obs}(stim) depending on the stimulus. Consequently, for all stimuli (equivalently, all values of S_{obs}), the plot of P_{obs} versus log stimulus intensity should have exactly the same shape; functions for different stimuli are simply horizontal translations of one another on a logarithmic intensity axis.

Or, in terms of observable quantities, the measured psychometric functions from forced-choice experiments (plots of percent correct vs. logarithmic intensity) should have the same shape on the log intensity axis for all stimuli; the measured psychometric functions from yes-no experiments at the same false-alarm rate (hit rate vs. logarithmic intensity) should also be the same for all stimuli.

4.8.5   *Properties of the Quick Pooling Formula*

Advantage. According to the Quick pooling model, the sensitivity of an observer to an arbitrary stimulus can easily be calculated by the Quick pooling formula of Eq. 4.9 whenever the sensitivities of all the individual analyzers to that stimulus are known. As will be seen in Chapter 7, this is in great contrast to the laborious calculations required from most other models of independent multiple analyzers. In them, no analytic expression for the observer's sensitivity in terms of individual analyzers' sensitivities is ever possible. And without such an expression there is no possibility of analytically working backward from observer's sensitivities to put constraints on analyzer sensitivities, as is necessary to solve a number of theoretical problems.

Alternative Interpretations. The derivation of the Quick pooling formula just shown—from a multiple-analyzers high-threshold model with each analyzer characterized by a Quick psychometric function—is not the only interpretation of that pooling formula. An alternative probabilistic interpretation of it for yes-no experiments will be discussed in section 8.5.

Alternative interpretations of the nonlinear pooling specified in the Quick pooling formula that do not involve assuming variability in the outputs of multiple analyzers at all also exist (Quick, 1974). We will look at two sets of assumptions that lead to the Quick pooling formula from deterministic analyzers.

The first set assumes a linear transducer function (as in Assumption 9), that is, the deterministic output of an analyzer is $R_i(\text{stim}) = c(\text{stim}) \cdot S_i(\text{stim})$. The deterministic outputs from different analyzers are assumed to pool nonlinearly as follows:

$$R_{\text{pool}}(\text{stim}) = \left| \sum_{i=1}^{N'} R_i(\text{stim})^k \right|^{1/k}$$

A stimulus is assumed to be at threshold for the observer if and only if $R_{\text{pool}} = 1.0$. To derive the Quick pooling formula in Eq. 4.9 from this first alternative set of assumptions, just substitute $c(\text{stim}) \cdot S_i(\text{stim})$ for $R_i(\text{stim})$ in the above equation and set contrast equal to the threshold contrast $c_{\text{obs}}(\text{stim})$. The left side now equals 1.0, for which $c_{\text{obs}}(\text{stim}) \cdot S_{\text{obs}}(\text{stim})$ should be substituted. Dividing all terms by $c_{\text{obs}}(\text{stim})$ turns this equation directly into the Quick pooling formula of Eq. 4.9.

The second set assumes a power transducer function (as in Assumption 92) so that the deterministic output of an analyzer is

$$R_i(\text{stim}) = [c(\text{stim}) \cdot S_i(\text{stim})]^k$$

The deterministic outputs from different analyzers are then assumed to pool linearly, that is

$$R_{\text{pool}}(\text{stim}) = \sum_{i=1}^{N'} R_i(\text{stim})$$

One can show that this set also leads to the Quick pooling formula of Eq. 4.9.

To account for variability in the observer's psychophysical responses under either of these two alternative interpretations, the outputs of the analyzers cannot be allowed to vary independently. Psychophysical variability must be assumed to arise in some other way, perhaps due to noisy transmission at some later stage than the nonlinear pooling. The precise detection rule for the observer's responses in a yes-no experiment might then be: An observer says yes if and only if $R_{pool}(stim)$ plus the error due to the noisy stage exceeds 1.0.

The relative merits as a description of pattern thresholds of this deterministic alternative interpretation of the Quick pooling formula and the full Quick pooling model will be discussed further in section 4.9.6.

Minkowski Metric. The Quick pooling formula in Eq. 4.9 can be viewed as a metric in the N'-dimensional space where each dimension represents S_i, the sensitivity of one of N' analyzers. Hence the title of Quick's 1974 paper, "A vector-magnitude model of contrast detection." These metrics are sometimes known as Minkowski metrics (see, e.g., appendix in Coombs et al., 1970). The origin in the space represents the blank stimulus, the stimulus for which all analyzers have sensitivity zero. The observer's sensitivity to a stimulus, $S_{obs}(stim)$, is the distance between the origin and the point representing the stimulus in question. (This approach can be extended to let the distance between any two points in the space represent the discriminability of any two stimuli. See Chap. 9.)

When k is 1 in Eq. 4.9—known as the *city-block metric*—the sensitivities of different analyzers are linearly summed or, to put it another way, the distance between the blank and the stimulus equals the sum of the two coordinates. When k is 2, the metric is the familiar Euclidian one. A value of k in the range somewhere from 3 to 5 will be suggested by visual pattern thresholds. When k is infinity, the observer's sensitivity equals the sensitivity of the most sensitive analyzer (the distance between the origin and a point is equal to the largest coordinate of the point). This is Assumption 4 of the deterministic multiple-analyzers model.

4.9   QUICK POOLING MODEL PREDICTIONS FOR SUMMATION OF FAR-APART COMPONENTS

The Quick pooling formula of Eq. 4.9 is written in terms of all the analyzers' sensitivities to the stimulus, quantities that are not directly observable. This indirectness is necessary in the case of an arbitrary stimulus. In the case of compound stimuli containing far-apart components, however, the Quick pooling formula can be rewritten in two different ways to include only observable quantities. The proofs are sketched in the appendix to this chapter, section 4.11; although the bookkeeping is more complicated, the proofs are similar to the proof that Eq. 4.1 for the high-threshold model implies Eq. 4.6 (see section 4.7.6).

4.9.1   First Form of Quick Pooling Formula for Far-Apart Components

This form is very close to the original Quick pooling formula given in Eq. 4.9. If a compound stimulus cmpd contains M far-apart components having values V_j ($j = 1, M$), then

$$S_{obs}(cmpd) = \left| \sum_{j=1}^{M} [S_{obs}(V_j) \cdot a_j(cmpd)]^k \right|^{1/k} \tag{4.11}$$

where

$$a_j(cmpd) = \frac{c(V_j \text{ in cmpd})}{c(cmpd)} \tag{4.12}$$

The quantities a_j do the bookkeeping necessary to keep track of the intensity in each component relative to the intensity in the compound no matter what convention is used in describing the contrast of the compound (e.g., whether it is set equal to peak-trough divided by mean luminance, or equal to the contrast in one component). See note 1 for an example. This kind of bookkeeping was not necessary in the original version of the Quick pooling formula (Eq. 4.9) because the same stimulus was involved in every term.

4.9.2 *Example with All Components Equally Detectable*

Some insight into Eq. 4.11 may be gained from considering the case where all the $S_{obs}(V_j)$'s and all the a_j's are equal to 1.0. This case applied to compound stimuli made up of equally detectable far-apart components when normalized contrast is used: (a) Contrast of the components is measured as relative intensity (defined in section 4.1.2, also used in Fig. 4.7), or in other words, the unit of contrast for each component is chosen so that $S_{obs}(V_j) = 1.0$ for all j; and (b) the unit of contrast for the compound is chosen to make its value equal to 1.0 when all of its components are just at their own thresholds (that is, when all have relative contrast 1.0). These choices of contrast units make all the a_j's equal to 1.0.

Now the (normalized) sensitivity of the observer will be the reciprocal of the compound's normalized contrast when the compound is at threshold, or equivalently, it will be the factor by which the contrast in each component of the compound would have to be reduced below that component's threshold for the compound to be at threshold (e.g., for the three-component compounds of Fig. 4.7 a factor of approximately $1/0.75 = 1.33$).

More generally, according to Eq. 4.11 with $S_{obs}(V_j)$ and a_j set equal to 1.0 for all j's, this factor will be

$$S_{obs}(cmpd) = M^{(1/k)} \tag{4.13a}$$

or

$$\log S_{obs}(cmpd) = (1/k) \log M \tag{4.13b}$$

Notice that this normalized sensitivity of the observer to a compound increases with the number of equally detectable far-apart components; in fact, the logarithm of the normalized sensitivity increases linearly with the logarithm of the number of far-apart components, and the slope of the relationships is the reciprocal of k (the steepness parameter from the Quick psychometric function).

Thus, the steeper the psychometric function, the slower the increase in sensitivity to the compound as the number of components is increased.

4.9.3   Second Form of Quick Pooling Formula for Far-Apart Components

For the second way of rewriting the Quick pooling formula in terms of observable quantities, we need another symbol—we will use *th.cmpd*—to mean the compound stimulus when it is just at the observer's threshold. Note, therefore, that $c(V_j$ in th.cmpd) is the contrast in the *j*th component when the compound is at the observer's threshold. Using these symbols, the second form of the Quick pooling formula can be written as

$$1.0 = \sum_{j=1}^{M} \left| \frac{c(V_j \text{ in th.cmpd})}{\text{th}_{obs}(V_j)} \right|^k \tag{4.14}$$

Remember that $\text{th}_{obs}(V_j)$ is the intensity in a simple stimulus of value V_j when that simple stimulus is at the observer's threshold (in other words, it is the observer's threshold for the *j*th component by itself).

Two Far-Apart Components. In particular, when compounds containing two far-apart components ($M = 2$) are at threshold, Eq. 4.14 says that the thresholds plotted on the summation square obey the following relationship, where x and y are the coordinates on the summation square (as in section 4.1.2) and can be substituted for the much more complicated but equivalent expression of Eq. 4.14:

$$1 = x^k + y^k \tag{4.15}$$

Contours obeying Eq. 4.15 for various values of k are shown in Fig. 4.9. (As an aside, these contours are the upper right quadrant of unit circles for Minkowski metrics. When the exponent k is 2, this is an ordinary circle.) Thus, according to the Quick pooling formula, the thresholds for all compounds containing two far-apart components should fall on the contours in Fig. 4.9 with the appropriate value of k.

4.9.4   Comparison of Predicted with Measured Psychometric Functions

Examples of psychometric functions for patches of sinusoidal gratings and their fit by Quick functions are shown in Fig. 4.10 using the empirical functions from Fig 4.7, and others can be found in Robson and Graham (1981) and Watson (1979). Deciding which exponent produces the best fit to a psychometric function is difficult. The possible precision of the answer is limited by the intrinsic binomial variability of proportions estimated from relatively small numbers of trials (say 100 at each stimulus intensity). Collecting more trials is not the answer to the problem, however, since drifts in sensitivity across time seem to exist and cause functions collected over a long time to be shallower than the true

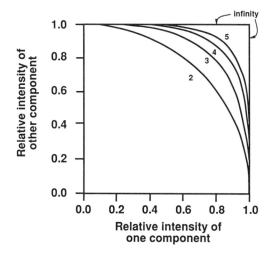

FIG. 4.9 Predictions of the Quick pooling model using each of several values of the exponent k for the thresholds of compound stimuli composed of two far-apart components. (Figure 4 relabelled from Graham et al., 1978; reprinted by permission.)

instantaneous function (e.g., Hallett, 1969). In any case, the Quick function does describe psychometric functions for visual patterns like sinusoidal gratings, at least to a very good approximation. The values of exponent in the range from 3 to 6 are typically found. (See Watson, 1979, for more details and a method of fitting to a maximum-likelihood criterion.)

There are, however, at least two ways in which the predictions of the Quick pooling model for psychometric functions are inaccurate for visual patterns. The first is common to all high-threshold models and was discussed in section 4.7.4.

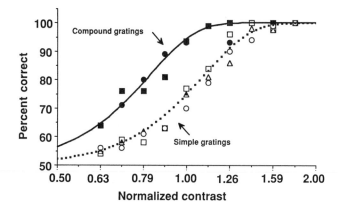

FIG. 4.10 Results from Fig. 4.7 replotted with Quick psychometric functions having an exponent k of 4.

A second failure is the existence of some differences among the steepnesses of functions for different visual patterns. The best documented difference is slight (Nachmias, 1981), with the functions for an edge stimulus being somewhat shallower (estimates of k being 20 to 60% lower) than those for a 12-cpd grating. It is possible that allowing the steepness parameter to be different for different analyzers would easily correct this deficiency. To do so would complicate the model quite drastically, however, and since the model works reasonably well without this complication we will continue to avoid it. In any case, the steepnesses of the psychometric functions for all stimuli are approximately the same, which has been one of the interesting facts of psychophysics for many years.

4.9.5　Comparison of Predicted with Measured Summation

A prediction based on the first observable form of the Quick pooling formula (Eq. 4.11) is illustrated in Fig. 4.10. The experimental results are those from Fig. 4.7, but here they are fit by Quick psychometric functions. The predicted horizontal distance between the function for the three simple sinusoidal gratings and that for the compound gratings can be easily calculated from Eq. 4.11 or, since the contrast is appropriately normalized, from Eq. 4.13. Since there are three components and $k = 4$, the compound's threshold should be $1/1.32 = 0.76$ of the components' threshold in these normalized coordinates. This is the factor separating the curves drawn in Fig. 4.10.

A prediction based on the second observable form of the Quick pooling formula (Eq. 4.14) is shown in Fig. 4.11. These summation-square plots compare the predictions of the Quick pooling model with results from spatial-frequency summation experiments using small patches of grating either in the fovea or in the periphery. The curves shown are the predictions from the Quick pooling model with $k = 3$ or 4. The results for both observers and for both periphery and fovea are consistent with these predictions. It would be very difficult to say, however, that one value of k was better than the other or to rule out slightly higher or slightly lower values of k (Graham et al., 1978).

A number of other studies have investigated the summation of far-apart spatial frequencies and found results similar to those shown here (e.g., Mostafavi & Sakrison, 1976; Quick, Mullins, & Reichert, 1978; Sachs et al., 1971; see Chap. 12 for further references).

More precision in the estimate of k from summation experiments could be obtained if compounds contained a large number of far-apart components. On the spatial-frequency dimension, more than three or four are not possible. On the spatial-position dimension, however, more are. As will be discussed later, summation experiments on the spatial-position dimension suggest a value of 3.5, values of 3 and 4 being somewhat too small and too large, respectively (Robson & Graham, 1981). This value is consistent with those from spatial-frequency summation experiments.

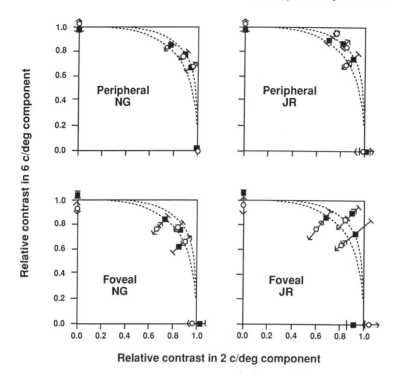

FIG. 4.11 Obtained thresholds for patches of compound gratings containing 2 and/or 6 cpd shown in summation-square plots. Thresholds for peaks-subtract and peaks-add phases are given by solid squares and open circles, respectively. Results are shown for two observers and for two positions (foveal and 7.5 degrees peripheral; more data were collected in the periphery than in the fovea). Bars through the symbols represent ± 1 standard error of the mean. The curves are the predictions of the Quick pooling model with exponents of 3 and 4. (Figure 3 from Graham et al., 1978; reprinted by permission.)

4.9.6 Agreement Between Exponents Estimated From Psychometric Function Steepness and From Summation

If the Quick pooling model in its entirety were absolutely correct, then the value of k estimated from the steepness of individual psychometric functions should exactly equal the value estimated from the amount of summation. If, however, the alternative interpretation of the Quick pooling formula as deterministic nonlinear pooling were correct, the steepness of the psychometric function would bear no necessary relationship to the amount of summation.

Several studies have examined the question of whether the two estimates of k are equal (Robson & Graham, 1981; Watson, 1979). They have found equality (e.g., Fig. 4.10 compared with Fig. 4.11), or rather differences that are indistinguishable from equality. (Given the difficulties in either estimation of k, such differences may be rather large.)

It would be somewhat surprising to find perfect agreement between the two estimates in any case. For one thing, as mentioned previously, psychometric functions collected over longer periods of time seem to be shallower than those collected over short periods (Hallett, 1969). And thus the slope of any empirically collected psychometric function may well be shallower than that of the true instantaneous one (the one describing the system's behavior at any one moment in time and determining the amount of summation). This may be due to drifts over time in the observer's sensitivity (perhaps due to something as peripheral as changes in accommodation) which change the horizontal position of the instantaneous underlying psychometric function while leaving the slope constant. Second, the high-threshold model is admittedly wrong, as was discussed in section 4.7.4 and at greater length in Chapter 7. Third, the form of the Quick psychometric function, while a good fit to observed results, may not be perfect. It is particularly difficult to know about the shape of psychometric functions near the bottom (at low values). Unfortunately, predictions in summation experiments depend on the bottom.

4.9.7   Some Discrepant Findings

Uncertainty Effects. Occasional experiments have seemed to find *no* summation between far-apart spatial frequencies, that is, have seemed to support a deterministic multiple-analyzers model without probability summation. Sometimes this is because investigators have been interested in larger questions and simply have not determined whether the compound grating was a little more detectable than its most detectable component. In some experiments, however (e.g., Graham & Nachmias, 1971), the thresholds for compound gratings most certainly do not lie as far inside the sides of the summation square as in other experiments or as one might expect from probability summation. Sometimes at least, this smaller amount of summation is a result of the particular experimental procedure used—the smaller amount of summation is found when the observer knows on each trial which stimulus will be presented, while the larger amount is found when the observer does not know. Chapter 7 discusses this effect at length and provides an explanation for it. Although the high-threshold multiple-analyzers model (and therefore the Quick pooling model as presented here) cannot predict this effect, other models with probabilistically independent multiple-analyzers can.

Inhibition? The results of one other experiment showed less summation between far-apart spatial frequencies than expected from the independently variable multiple-analyzers model. Olzak and Thomas (1981) measured the thresholds for various compounds containing far-apart frequencies. They found less summation between 3 and 18 cpd than between 3 and 9 or 3 and 12 cpd. The results for these latter compounds were those expected from independent multiple analyzers. Yet, although 3 and 18 cpd are even further apart and therefore should certainly stimulate separate analyzers if the closer pairs did, there was less summation between 3 and 18 than between the closer pairs of frequencies. Although this effect has not been replicated, some discussion seems worthwhile, because it provides an occasion to discuss the effect of modifying assumptions of the multiple-anlyzers model. Several modifications could account for the finding:

1. The variability in the outputs of the 3 and 18 cpd analyzers might be positively correlated even though the variability in the outputs of 3 and 9 or 3 and 12 cpd analyzers was independent. In the extreme, if two analyzers are perfectly positively correlated, there is no probability summation, no advantage to having two analyzers rather than one. But positive correlation is unappealing here, since there seems no good reason why the further apart analyzers should be more highly correlated than the closer ones.
2. Inhibition may exist between very far-apart analyzers (e.g., 3 and 18 cpd) but not between closer ones (e.g., 3 and 9 or 3 and 12 cpd).
3. Higher stages of the visual system may be unable always to simultaneously monitor the outputs of two very-far-apart analyzers (so that on some trials of compounds containing far-apart components the observer's response would be based on something less than the maximum output). The question of whether an observer can always monitor the outputs of multiple channels is taken up in Chapter 7.

Too Much Summation. A third complication, of a quite different kind, is a finding of *much more* summation than expected from multiple analyzers (Wilson, 1980a). Here the results for compound gratings containing frequencies a factor of 3 apart were consistent with the single-analyzer model predictions. In this study, however, very low spatial frequencies and a time course of presentation emphasizing very high temporal frequencies were used, which, as the author intended, presumably isolated a single extreme one of the multiple analyzers. (See Chap. 12 for more discussion of spatiotemporal interactions.)

4.10 SUMMARY

If a compound stimulus is more detectable than either component, *summation* is said to have occurred.

An additive single-analyzer model predicts a great deal of summation between components even if they are very far apart on the dimension of interest. In particular, it predicts that the intensities of each of two components could be half their individual thresholds and the compound would still be detectable. This is much more summation than typically found between far-apart spatial frequencies.

A nonadditive single-analyzer model (a single-channel model) is more appropriate for the spatial-frequency dimension. In this model the analyzer is a set of mechanisms (hence called a *channel*) with weighting functions at many different places in the visual field but identical in other respects. It predicts more summation than is usually found between far-apart spatial frequencies; it also predicts a dependence on the phase between the two components of different spatial frequency, and such a dependence is not generally found.

This model can be modified to allow nonuniformity of weighting functions at different spatial positions (but still only one mechanism centered at each position). Then it predicts less (but still too much for the spatial-frequency dimension) summation and phase dependence. This nonuniform single-channel model is an example of interaction between two dimensions (in this case spatial frequency and spatial position).

Multiple-analyzers models predict much less summation. Indeed, a simple deterministic form predicts no summation. Empirically, however, some summation is usually found between far-apart spatial frequencies, an amount consistent with the existence of variable analyzers that have probabilistically independent outputs.

A particular model of the variability in the analyzers—the high-threshold model—is convenient to work with, especially when coupled with an assumption that an analyzer's psychometric function is described by a Quick (Weibull) function. This combination of assumptions (called the *Quick pooling model* here) leads to two important, convenient, and useful analytical results.

First, the observer's psychometric function for any stimulus is also of the Quick (Weibull) form. Hence the psychometric functions for all stimuli should have the same shape when plotted against logarithmic intensity.

Second, the observer's sensitivity to any stimulus can be easily calculated as a power sum of the sensitivities of the individual analyzers. This calculation of the observer's sensitivity is here called the *Quick pooling formula.*

Another way to describe the Quick pooling formula is that it says that the detectability of a stimulus is given by the distance between the origin and the stimulus in a space where each dimension gives the output of an individual analyzer. The measure of distance is a Minkowski metric. (Empirically an exponent of 3 or 4 seems about right where an exponent of 2 is ordinary Euclidian distance.)

For far-apart components (so far apart that no analyzer responds to both), these two analytic results (originally written in terms of the observer's sensitivity and various analyzers' sensitivities to the compound) can be rewritten in terms of the observer's sensitivity to the compound versus the observer's sensitivities to the components. This provides easy tests of the model.

4.11   APPENDIX. DERIVATION OF OBSERVABLE QUICK POOLING FORMULAS

We will assume here without loss of generality that only one analyzer is sensitive to each of the far-apart components. (All the assumptions of the Quick pooling model are the same as those of the high-threshold model except for the addition of the Quick psychometric function. We have already verified that only one analyzer can be assumed without loss of generality for the high-threshold model— see section 4.7.5. If the Quick psychometric function holds for an analyzer, it can easily be shown to hold for a composite analyzer.)

4.11.1 Derivation of Intermediate Results

To derive an intermediate result from which both observable forms of the Quick pooling formula follow, start with the Quick pooling formula in Eq. 4.9 applied to the compound stimulus. Multiply both sides by the contrast in the compound stimulus:

$$[c(\text{cmpd}) \cdot S_{\text{obs}}(\text{cmpd})]^k = \sum_{i=1}^{N'} [c(\text{cmpd}) \cdot S_i(\text{cmpd})]^k \qquad (4.16)$$

Next we need two equations analogous to Eq. 4.6a and 4.6b used earlier in deriving the prediction of the general high-threshold model. The equation analogous to Eq. 4.6a is easy to find: If there is only one analyzer sensitive to each component, then the sensitivity of the observer to that component must equal the sensitivity of the one analyzer to that component, that is,

$$S_{\text{obs}}(V_j) = S_j(V_j) \qquad \text{for all } j \qquad (4.17)$$

We now need an equation analogous to Eq. 4.6b, but here the problem of keeping track of the intensity of the compound relative to that of the component arises (as in Eq. 4.12). We will deal with this problem here by keeping track of intensities as well as sensitivities. Since each analyzer responds to only one component of the compound, the relative intensity of the compound can be expressed conveniently either in terms of the compound itself (Eq. 4.18 left) or equivalently in terms of the one component the analyzer is sensitive to (Eq. 4.18 right):

$$\frac{c(\text{cmpd})}{\text{th}_j(\text{cmpd})} = \frac{c(V_j \text{ in cmpd})}{\text{th}_j(V_j)} \qquad (4.18)$$

Substituting sensitivities for thresholds in this last equation gives

$$c(\text{cmpd}) \cdot S_j(\text{cmpd}) = c(V_j \text{ in cmpd}) \cdot S_j(V_j) \qquad (4.19)$$

Now, substituting $S_{\text{obs}}(V_j)$ for $S_j(V_j)$ in Eq. 4.19, as allowed by Eq. 4.17, gives

$$c(\text{cmpd}) \cdot S_j(\text{cmpd}) = c(V_j \text{ in cmpd}) \cdot S_{\text{obs}}(V_j) \qquad (4.20)$$

Combining Eqs. 4.16 and 4.20 and remembering that, of the N' original analyzers, only the first M (by our numbering scheme) have nonzero sensitivity for this compound, gives the desired intermediate result:

$$[c(\text{cmpd}) \cdot S_{\text{obs}}(\text{cmpd})]^k = \sum_{j=1}^{M} [c(V_j \text{ in cmpd}) \cdot S_{\text{obs}}(V_j)]^k \qquad (4.21)$$

4.11.2   *Derivation of Observable Pooling Formulas From Intermediate Result*

To derive the first observable form of the Quick pooling formula (Eq. 4.11) requires two simple steps:

1. Divide both sides of the intermediate result (Eq. 4.21) by c(cmpd).
2. Substitute a_j for $c(V_j$ in cmpd)$/c$(cmpd) on the right.

The result is the first observable form (Eq. 4.11).

To derive the second observable form of the Quick pooling formula (Eq. 4.14) also requires two simple steps:

1. Apply the intermediate result (Eq. 4.21) to the case of a compound stimulus that is exactly at the observer's threshold. That is, make the following two replacements: The left side of the intermediate result is now equal to 1.0. And in the right side, the contrast in the jth component—$c(V_j$ in cmpd)—is now equal to the contrast in the jth component at the compound threshold—$c(V_j$ in th.cmpd).
2. Replace $S_{obs}(V_j)$ on the right by the reciprocal of $th_{obs}(V_j)$, which it equals by definition.

You now should have the second observable form (Eq. 4.14).

Note

1. To see how the use of the a_j's corrects appropriately no matter what convention is used for the contrast of the compound, let's work through an example. Consider a particular compound grating, one in peaks-add phase containing frequencies in a ratio of 1:3 (like that at bottom left of Fig. 4.2). We will suppose the contrast in the first lower frequency component is 2.5 times that in the second higher frequency component. (The absolute level of contrast clearly does not affect the a_j's.) First, see what happens to the a_j's if we let contrast of the compound be the difference between the peak and trough luminance divided by the mean luminance (our usual definition of contrast). Since this is a peaks-add compound stimulus, the contrast in the compound (by this definition) is simply the sum of the contrasts in the two components: a_1 will be 2.5/3.5 and a_2 will be 1/3.5.

Now consider the case where the contrast of the compound is taken to equal the contrast in the first component (as a number of authors have done on a number of sensory/perceptual dimensions). Then a_1 would be 1.0 and a_2 would be 1/2.5; each is 3.5 times greater than by the first definition of compound contrast. And, by Eq. 4.11, the sensitivity of the observer to the compound (the reciprocal of the compound's intensity at threshold) would also be 3.5 times greater than by the first definition (as it should).

5
Far-Apart Values on Spatial Dimensions

5.1 OVERVIEW

To illustrate the explanations of summation experiments using far-apart values along any dimension, the previous chapter presented experimental results on the spatial-frequency dimension. Those results can be summarized by the answers to two questions: (a) Are there multiple analyzers along the dimension? (b) If so, is there probability summation among the analyzers? For spatial frequency, the answers are both yes.

In this chapter we discuss results at far-apart values on the remaining spatial dimensions discussed in section 2.3.4 and illustrated in Fig. 2.7: orientation, spatial position (two dimensions), spatial extent (two dimensions), and spatial phase. To the extent allowed by the existing evidence, the two questions just presented will be answered on each dimension. Interpretation of the results on any one spatial dimension is substantially affected by one's assumptions about multiple analyzers and probability summation on the other dimensions. Results for the temporal dimensions (Fig. 2.8) and other dimensions (Fig. 2.9) are reviewed in Chapter 12.

5.2 FAR-APART ORIENTATIONS

Figure 5.1 illustrates the predictions of models assuming single- or multiple-orientation analyzers. Three patterns are represented in the left column: simple sinusoidal gratings of very different orientations but the same spatial frequency and a compound grating composed of the two simple ones. Since this set of patterns varies in two dimensions, one-dimensional luminance profiles cannot be used to represent them. Instead, square-wave gratings are shown for ease of illustration (although sinusoidal gratings are being discussed). The numbers indicate the luminances at the central point of each region (the points of greatest and least luminance when the gratings are sinusoidal). The numbers written into the sketches give the luminance in arbitrary units relative to mean luminance. For example, $+1$ marks an area of peak luminance in a simple grating and indicates that it is 1 arbitrary unit of luminance brighter than the mean. Similarly -1 indicates the area of trough luminance in a simple grating. The two simple gratings are assumed to be at threshold. They are shown as containing identical contrast, since the human visual system's sensitivity for all orientations is quite similar (except for a small "oblique effect"—see Chap. 13) but they could be shown at different contrasts (as was done for different spatial frequencies in Fig. 4.2)

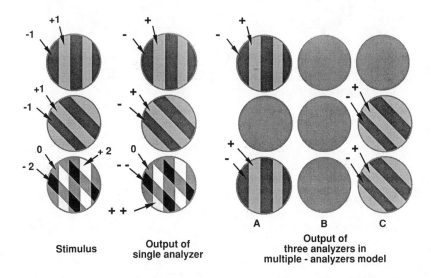

Stimulus	Output of single analyzer	Output of three analyzers in multiple - analyzers model

FIG. 5.1 Left column illustrates three stimuli: two simple gratings of different orientations and a compound grating composed of the two simple ones. The next column shows the predicted outputs of a single-orientation-analyzer model. The group of three columns on the right shows the predicted outputs of three analyzers in a multiple-orientation-analyzer model. Numbers or symbols indicate the luminance at the midpoint of each region (stimulus sketches in left column) or the output from the maximally-responding mechanism in that region (analyzer output sketches in right four columns).

without affecting the following argument. Since the compound is the sum of the components' excursions from the mean luminance, the numbers in each position in the sketch of the compound grating are the sums of the numbers for that position in the simple gratings.

5.2.1 A Nonadditive, Uniform, Single-Orientation-Analyzer Model

The second column of Fig. 5.1 shows the predictions of a particular model assuming a single-orientation analyzer. This single analyzer is a single channel; it is an array of mechanisms (each a linear system) having weighting functions at different positions but all responsive to the same range of orientations. Thus it is just like the nonadditive, uniform, single-analyzer model of section 4.3. Since this single-orientation analyzer must be assumed to respond to all orientations to which the human visual system is sensitive, and since humans are approximately equally sensitive to all orientations, these mechanisms' weighting functions must be concentric or nearly so. (The oblique effect could be taken care of by making the receptive fields not quite concentric.) Whether there are multiple spatial-frequency analyzers—several different sizes of weighting function centered at each position—or only a single one is irrelevant here, because only those responsive to the spatial frequency of the stimuli used need be considered.

In the second column of Fig. 5.1, the symbol next to an arrow pointing to any region of the sketch represents the output from the one mechanism that has a weighting function centered at that midpoint. (We assume for simplicity that the weighting functions of the mechanisms are even-symmetric so that the maxmium output of the single-orientation analyzer always occurs in the middle of a stripe in the grating. The argument holds for any symmetry however.) The maximal output of the analyzer when a pattern is just at threshold (as the two simple gratings of Fig. 5.1 are presumed to be) will occur in the middle of the bright bar and is designated by a single + symbol. The output at each position to the compound grating is just the sum of the outputs to the components. (The sketches in the first and second column are identical—except that each 1 in the first column is replaced by a + and each 2 is replaced by + +—because the two simple gratings were assumed to be equally detectable.) According to this model, therefore, the contrast in each of the components of the compound could be turned down by a factor of 2 and the compound would just be at threshold. That is, the compound should be much more detectable than either component.

5.2.2 Multiple-Orientation-Analyzers Models

The third, fourth, and fifth columns show the outputs of a multiple orientation-analyzers model to these patterns (analogous to the right column of Fig. 4.2; see section 4.4). Three of the analyzers are represented. A responds to vertical but not oblique, C responds to oblique but not vertical, and B responds to neither. Thus the outputs of analyzers A and B to the compound grating are exactly like their outputs to the vertical and oblique components, respectively (assuming only the weak form of additivity that ineffective stimuli are ineffective in compounds). For the moment let's assume that an observer's sensitivity equals that of the most sensitive analyzer (Assumption 4). The multiple-orientation-analyzers model then predicts that the compound in Fig. 5.1 should be just at threshold (bottom right three sketches).

If one assumes instead that there is independent variability in the output of the multiple-orientation analyzers (Assumption 38) and that the observer's decision variable is, for example, the maximum of the outputs from the analyzers (Assumption 40), then the compound should be slightly more detectable than its components; that is, probability summation across orientations is predicted.

5.2.3 Experimental Results

Gratings. In experimental results collected with sinusoidal gratings over a wide range of spatial frequencies and luminances, the compound gratings containing two or three very different orientations were not (much) more detectable than their components, contrary to the prediction of a single-analyzer model and in better accord with those of a multiple-analyzers model (Carlson, Cohen, & Gorog, 1977; Kelly, 1982a; Kulikowski, Abadi, & King-Smith, 1973; Wilson, McFarlane, & Phillips, 1983) except at high velocities (Kelly & Burbeck, 1987). Noise gratings produce the same results (Mayhew & Frisby, 1978).

Aperiodic Stimuli. An experiment with lines rather than gratings produced quite similar results, although compounds containing lines an intermediate distance apart in orientation (15–25 angular degrees) were somewhat less detectable than either component. This may be the result of inhibition between analyzers tuned to orientations this far apart (Thomas & Shimamura 1975), although it is not clear whether a more up-to-date analysis considering, for example, probability summation, would support this possibility.

Circularly Symmetric Gratings. Rather than superimposing ordinary sinusoidal gratings (called rectilinear gratings here) of different orientations (as in Fig. 5.1), consider arranging many small patches of gratings of different orientations around a circle, with the bars in neighboring patches touching end to end (that is, the orientation of the bars in each patch is perpendicular to the radius at that point). In the limit as the bars of each patch were made infinitely short, a perfect circle would be made from such patches. Further rings of patches all at the same spatial frequency could be added inside and/or outside the first ring of patches. Thus a circularly symmetric pattern that is a compound of many different orientations (all at the same spatial frequency) would be made. The results of comparing the thresholds for these circularly symmetric compounds with the thresholds for rectilinear gratings (Kelly, 1982a; Kelly & Magnuski, 1975) are inconsistent with a single-analyzer model and at least qualitatively consistent with a multiple-analyzers model.

Probability Summation. If mechanisms sensitive to different spatial frequencies have independent variability, it seems reasonable that those sensitive to different orientations should. On the other hand, they might not. As it turns out, compounds containing two sinusoidal gratings or narrow-band noise patterns of very different orientations are indeed slightly more detectable than their components by an amount appropriate for probability summation (Carlson et al., 1977; Mayhew & Frisby, 1978; Phillips & Wilson, 1984).

5.2.4   *Singly Selective Versus Doubly Selective Analyzers, and an Extension of the Quick Pooling Model to Cover Spatial Frequency and Orientation*

When selectivity has been shown on two dimensions, there remains the question of whether each putative analyzer is selective along both dimensions (is doubly selective) or is broadly tuned on one dimension and narrowly tuned on the other (singly selective). How to answer this question is discussed at length in section 11.2. When summation experiments show no more summation than probability summation for far-apart values on two dimensions (as with spatial frequency and orientation), the answer is rather clear: The analyzers (at least the most sensitive analyzers, all those involved in determining the thresholds for the patterns in the summation experiments) must be doubly selective.

The Quick pooling model of section 4.8 can be taken to apply directly to these analyzers that are doubly selective for spatial frequency and orientation. Simply let N' be the total number of such analyzers in, for example, Eqs. 4.8 and 4.9 of section 4.8.3.

5.3 THE EFFECT OF PROBABILITY SUMMATION ACROSS SPACE ON SPATIAL-FREQUENCY AND ORIENTATION MODELS

5.3.1 A Preview of Spatial-Position Summation Results

In exact analogy to the spatial-frequency dimension, the question of whether there is more than one analyzer on the spatial-position dimension can be answered by summation-at-threshold experiments. The threshold for a compound stimulus containing several patches of sinusoidal grating at widely spaced spatial positions (but all of the same spatial frequency and orientation), for example, could be compared with the thresholds for the component patches alone. If there were only a single spatial-position analyzer sensitive to that spatial frequency and orientation (e.g., a single mechanism having a weighting function of many lobes stretching across the whole visual field or at least as much of the visual field as occupied by the compound stimulus), the threshold for the compound would be much lower than that for the component patches. If there are multiple analyzers, however, the threshold for the compound might be little different from that for the most detectable component; it should be slightly lower if there is independent variability in the outputs of those analyzers producing probability summation across spatial positions, as suggested by a number of investigators (e.g., Graham & Rogowitz, 1976; Granger, 1973; Howell & Hess, 1978; King-Smith & Kulikowski, 1975a; Legge, 1978b; Mostafavi & Sakrison, 1976; Stromeyer & Klein, 1975; Wilson, 1978a; the idea has a long history, however, and some of the older history is reviewed in Blackwell, 1972, p. 94). This experiment has not been published in this form to my knowledge (but see Cannon & Fullencamp, 1987), but the results can be confidently predicted from other results described later. The compound should turn out to be slightly more detectable than the most detectable component; the results should turn out to be consistent with multiple analyzers along the spatial-position dimension where the outputs of the multiple analyzers sensitive to different spatial positions are probabilistically independent. Or, as is often said, the results should show "probability summation across spatial position," or more briefly, "across space."

Having opened up the possibility of probability summation across space (see note 1) we need to reexamine the spatial-frequency and orientation models of the last chapter and this chapter to make sure that the multiple-analyzers models are still consistent with the results and that the single-analyzer models are still unable to account for them. For, as is explained in the next subsection, adding spatial probability summation to the single spatial-frequency or orientation channel models changes their predictions for the summation of far-apart spatial frequencies and orientations; and the new predictions are more like the experimental results than are the old (e.g., Granger, personal communication, 1973; Limb & Rubinstein, 1977; Stromeyer & Klein, 1975).

5.3.2   Inclusion of Probability Summation Across Space in a Single Spatial-Frequency or -Orientation Channel Model

If there is independent variability in the outputs of mechanisms sensitive to different positions, the derivation we used for the predictions of a single-channel model for spatial frequency (Fig. 4.2) and for orientation (Fig. 5.1) is unsatisfactory. The output profiles drawn in Fig. 4.2, for example, must now be considered average-output profiles—profiles of the outputs at each position averaged over repeated presentations of the same stimulus. They can no longer represent the output on each and every trial. In fact, on any one trial, the output profile will look very ragged, since some mechanisms will be responding more than their average and some less. We still assume that a pattern is at threshold whenever the peak in the output profile reaches a criterion (Assumption 33), but the particular location (or occasionally locations) that produces the peak output will vary from time to time. Hence, the more spatial positions there are at which the *average* outputs are very large, the more chances there are on any particular *trial* to get a large enough peak output to exceed the threshold criterion. And the more likely, therefore, that the single channel and hence the observer will detect the pattern. For example, as the number of cycles in a grating is increased, the single analyzer's sensitivity to the grating will increase because the number of locations at which the analyzer has a chance to detect the grating will increase.

Now let's get back to the question of summation of far-apart spatial frequencies. (An exactly analogous argument applies for summation of far-apart orientations, so it will be omitted.) Consider the average-output profiles in the middle column of Fig. 4.2. Note that there are fewer locations at which peak or near-peak outputs occur in the average-output profile for either compound than there are for the simple gratings. Consider what happens, therefore, if you attenuate the contrast in the peaks-add compound by a factor of 2. Although the peaks in the average-output profiles to the attenuated compound and to each simple component will all now be equally high, the channel will not detect the compound grating on as many trials as it detects either simple component because there are fewer locations at which peaks and near-peaks occur for the compound. Thus, according to this model, the peaks-add compound with its contrast turned down by a factor of 2 will be *less* detectable than the original simple gratings, while in the original deterministic model of section 4.3 it was just as detectable. To put it another way, the compound in its original state (without the contrast turned down) is not, according to this model, as much more detectable than its components as predicted by the original deterministic single-analyzer (single-channel) model. In still other words, there is not as much summation between components in this version of the single-analyzer model as in the original deterministic version. Furthermore, although it may not be immediately obvious, the predicted difference between the peaks-add and peaks-subtract compounds is also reduced.

Therefore, the predictions of the single-channel model including probability summation across space differ from the predictions of the original single-channel model in just the direction necessary to better fit the data (e.g., Fig. 4.11). The next subsection derives quantitative predictions (see note 2).

5.3.3   Using the Quick Pooling Model to Derive Quantitative Predictions From a Single Spatial-Frequency Channel Model With Probability Summation Across Space

To find out whether a single spatial-frequency channel model including probability summation across space can actually account for observers' thresholds, you need to make quantitative predictions. Although these predictions can be made assuming the variability at each position is normally distributed, that is, using the cumulative Gaussian function for the psychometric function (Granger, 1973; Limb & Rubinstein, 1977), using the Quick psychometric function produces very similar results but is much simpler. Thus, all assumptions of the single spatial-frequency channel model in section 4.3 will remain the same except that the following will be substituted for the deterministic output assumption (Assumption 32):

Assumption 44. Independent Variability at Different Positions. *The probability that the output at one position exceeds any level is independent of the probability that the output at any other position does.*

Since each mechanism in the spatial-frequency/orientation channel is itself a spatial-position analyzer (sensitive only to a range of spatial positions), Assumption 44 can be rephrased to say that there is independent variability in the outputs of the multiple spatial-positions analyzers comprising one spatial-frequency/orientation analyzer (channel). The probability that the output at any one spatial position i in the single spatial-frequency/orientation channel exceeds criterion will be assumed to be given by the Quick psychometric function, Eq. 4.7, where S_i(stim) in the equation is the sensitivity at that position i. That is, it equals the reciprocal of the average output of the mechanism (the spatial-position analyzer) at that spatial position to that stimulus. (This is Assumption 43 applied to spatial-position analyzers.)

To derive quantitative predictions one just applies the Quick pooling model (Eq. 4.9 of section 4.8.3) to the multiple probabilistically independent spatial-position analyzers within the single spatial-frequency/orientation analyzer (channel). Predictions were calculated both for simple gratings and for many ratios of contrasts in compound gratings (where the frequency ratio is 1:3 in both peaks-add and peaks-subtract phases) as well as for several values of the exponent k (Graham et al., 1978). These predictions are shown in Fig. 5.2.

The predictions when k equals infinity are the same as those of the deterministic single-channel model of section 4.3. For when k equals infinity, the psycho-

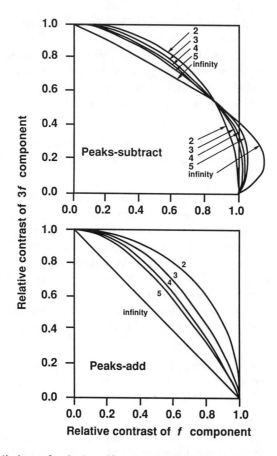

FIG. 5.2 Predictions of a single uniform spatial-frequency analyzer model incorporating probability summation across space for the thresholds of gratings containing two components a factor of 3 apart in spatial frequency and in either of two phases (two panels). Relative contrast in the lower and higher frequency components is shown on the horizontal and vertical axes, respectively. The number labeling each curve gives the exponent used in the Quick pooling formula to generate that curve. (From Fig. 5 of Graham et al., 1978; reprinted by permission.)

metric function goes from chance performance to perfect performance instantaneously, which is equivalent to postulating that there is no range over which the performance varies, that is, that there is no variability in the outputs of the individual mechanisms.

The curves when $k = 2$ are the same for compounds of both phases and can be derived analytically (see Graham et al., 1978). In fact, they each turn out to be a quadrant of a circle. This is the same as the prediction of a multiple spatial-frequency analyzer model including probability summation across analyzers with a k of 2 (Fig. 4.9). As you can also see from Figs. 5.2 and 4.9, however, for all higher values of k the single spatial-frequency analyzer (channel) model including probability summation across space predicts more summation across spatial frequencies than does the multiple spatial-frequency analyzer model (i.e., predicts that the compounds should be much more detectable relative to their spatial-frequency components). And the single spatial-frequency analyzer model but not the multiple spatial-frequency analyzer model also predicts that phase should make a difference (compare the two panels of Fig. 5.2).

The predictions shown in Fig. 5.2 were calculated for wide-field gratings. It is quite easy to modify the calculations to apply to smaller gratings and to take nonuniformity across spatial position into account. The predictions for small patches of grating like those used to collect the experimental results shown in Fig. 4.11 are indistinguishable from the predictions shown in Fig. 5.2, however (Graham, et al., 1978). Further, even when the spatial nonuniformity is slightly overemphasized, the predictions for compound gratings remain extremely close to those shown in Fig. 5.2 (both for full-field gratings and for the small patches). Thus, a single spatial-frequency analyzer model cannot account for the thresholds of simple and compound sinusoidal gratings (the results shown in Fig. 4.11) even if spatial nonuniformity and probability summation across space are allowed.

Nonliner Spatial Pooling. We originally derived the Quick pooling formula from the assumption of independent variability in different analyzers' outputs where the Quick psychometric function described that variability. But, as mentioned before, there are other interpretations of that formula. In particular, the equation might just be an expression of nonlinear pooling of deterministic outputs from different locations, where changing the exponent changes the degree of nonlinearity in the pooling.

Why Spatial Position But Not Orientation? Why is it that conclusions about spatial-frequency summation experiments cannot be made without consideration of probability summation across spatial position, but we do not have to consider orientation similarly? Simply because the stimuli used in the spatial-frequency summation experiments are rectilinear sinusoidal gratings; these are broad-band on the spatial position dimension but not on the orientation dimension. In general, whenever a summation (or other kind of analyzer-revealing experiment) on one dimension (e.g., spatial frequency) is done with stimuli that are broad-band on another (e.g., spatial position), that second dimension can introduce a variety of complications. These include the contaminating effects of independent variability among analyzers on that second dimension (just discussed here) and nonuniformity on that second dimension (discussed in section 4.5). These complications do not arise for dimensions on which the stimuli are narrow-band. Chapter 11 discusses this problem in a general context.

5.3.4   Spatial Probability Summation and Nonuniformity in the Multiple Spatial-Frequency/Orientation Analyzers Model

If the multiple spatial-frequency and/or orientation analyzer model is revised to include spatial probability summation (or nonlinear spatial pooling), will the model still predict accurately the summation of far-apart spatial frequencies (e.g., as in Fig. 4.11) and far-apart orientations? To do this revision we take each spatial-frequency/orientation analyzer to be a collection of mechanisms having identical weighting functions except at different positions. The answer then is a clear yes. In fact, the predictions of the revised model for summation of far-apart spatial frequencies and orientations are exactly like the predictions of the original model. Each spatial-frequency/orientation analyzer's output to the compound is exactly the same at its output to one of the components; hence, spatial probability summation and spatial nonuniformity affect both the same way; therefore the predicted detectability of the compound relative to its components is unaltered.

To see this argument in more detail, consider the following: According to the revised model, the little drawings in the right-hand column of Fig. 4.2 represent average-output profiles of individual spatial-frequency channels. The average-output profile to the compound stimulus is identical to the average-output profile to one of the components. And therefore, according to this revised model (as well as the original model), each compound stimulus in Fig. 4.2 is just at channel A's and at channel C's threshold. If the two channels are probabilistically independent, the compound is slightly above the observer's threshold (just as before). A formal presentation of this argument could be derived from the equations presented below if one desired.

5.3.5   Quick Pooling Model for Spatial Frequency, Orientation, and Spatial Position

To extend the independent-analyzers models of Chapter 4—in particular, the Quick pooling model—to this case is analogous to the extension to orientation (section 5.2.4) and again very simple. All the previous equations hold, but each analyzer (indexed by i) is now taken to be analogous to a single mechanism, that is, to be an analyzer triply selective for spatial position, spatial frequency, and orientation. Accordingly, the multiplication (as in Eq. 4.1 in section 4.7.2) or the summation (as in Eq. 4.9 of section 4.8.3) is now calculated over all such triply selective analyzers. The notation can be left as is with a single product or summation sign (where N' is now the total number of triply selective analyzers). More revealing for some purposes, double product and summation signs can be used to indicate multiplication or summation over spatial positions *within* a single spatial-frequency/orientation channel (that is, over mechanisms having weighting functions identical except at different spatial positions) separately from the multiplication or summation over the different spatial-frequency/orientation channels (where each channel is characterized by a different center size and different orientation of weighting function). Let's look at several of the important equations from the Quick pooling model, using the double product and summation signs for clarity of several points.

Let j be the index for the spatial-frequency/orientation channels (analyzers), and let M equal the total number of spatial-frequency/orientation analyzers. Let i be the index for the mechanisms within a particular spatial-frequency/orientation analyzer, and let n_j be the total number of mechanisms in analyzer j. (Then the sum of the n_j from $j = 1$ to $j = M$ is equal to N', the total number of mechanisms.) Let $P_{j,i}$ be the probability that the ith mechanism in the jth spatial-frequency/orientation analyzer detects the stimulus. Then Eq. 4.1 becomes

$$1 - P_{\text{obs}}(\text{stim}) = \prod_{j=1}^{M} \prod_{i=1}^{nj} [1 - P_{j,i}(\text{stim})] \qquad (5.1)$$

Equation 4.10 for the observer's psychometric function remains as is. Equation 4.9 giving the observer's sensitivity is now a double summation, where $S_{j,i}$ indicates the sensitivity of the ith receptive field in the jth channel:

$$S_{\text{obs}}(\text{stim}) = \left| \sum_{j=1}^{M} \sum_{i=1}^{nj} S_{j,i}(\text{stim})^k \right|^{(1/k)} \qquad (5.2)$$

Two Equivalent Assumptions. One way of viewing Eqs. 5.1 and 5.2 is as an embodiment of the assumption: An observer detects a stimulus if and only if one of the individual mechanisms does. An equivalent assumption, however, is: An observer detects a stimulus if and only if one of the spatial-frequency/orientation channels does, and a spatial-frequency channel detects a stimulus if and only if one of the mechanisms in it does.

Nonuniformity of the Visual Field. It is conceptually simple to include nonuniformity in this Quick pooling model. The sensitivities of the individual mechanisms $S_{j,i}$ are simply adjusted to account for the sensitivity to small patches of sinusoidal grating of different spatial frequencies and orientations (indexed by j) at different positions (indexed by i) in the visual field. In practice, since any small patch may be responded to by a number of mechanisms of slightly different best spatial frequency, orientation, and spatial position, choosing an appropriate set of $S_{j,i}$ can be a bit tricky. (The parametric variation of sensitivity with spatial position is summarized in Chap. 13.) For components that are far apart in spatial frequency, orientation, or spatial position, however, the problem is simplified, since sensitivity to the compound can be computed directly from sensitivity to the components, using the formulas given earlier (section 4.9).

5.3.6 Summation Index

For many purposes it is desirable to have a summary measure of amount of summation rather than working with the full contrast interrelationship functions plotted on summation squares like those in Fig. 4.11. One common measure for replotting results from compounds near the diagonal has been called by a number of names, for example, relative sensitivity (e.g., Quick et al., 1978), threshold ratio (e.g., Watson, 1982a), or sensitivity ratio (e.g., Arditi, Anderson, & Movshon, 1981), but no name has become standard. It will be called the *summation index* here.

Consider a compound stimulus that is at the observer's threshold and also is on the positive diagonal of the summation square, that is, a threshold compound in which both of its components have the same relative intensity. The summation index is defined to be the reciprocal of this contrast.

To put it another way, if you start with two components each of which is just at the observer's threshold and then put the two together into a compound, the summation index is the factor by which you turn both components' contrasts down to make the compound be just at the observer's threshold.

In symbols, when the compound is on the positive diagonal of the summation square the summation index is

$$\text{Summation index} = \frac{th_{\text{obs}}(V_1)}{c(V_1 \text{ in th.cmpd})} = \frac{S_{\text{obs}}(V_1 \text{ in cmpd})}{S_{\text{obs}}(V_1)}$$

or the same equations with V_2 instead.

This summation index goes from 1.0 in the case of no summation to 2.0 in the case of complete summation.

Even in cases where the threshold compound is not on the positive diagonal, results have often been (and will be below) summarized using this summation index by extrapolating or interpolating to determine the point on the positive diagonal and then using that to compute the summation index.

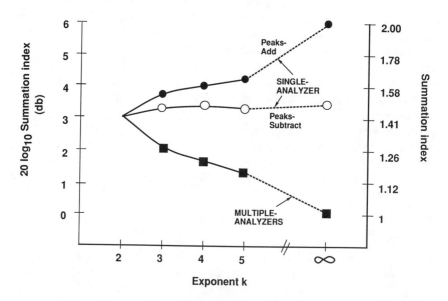

FIG. 5.3 Value of the summation index (right vertical axis) or its decibel form (left vertical axis) as predicted by two models for the thresholds of compound gratings containing two components a factor of 3 apart in spatial frequency. Circles show the predictions of the single-analyzer model for peaks-add (closed circles) and peaks-subtract (open circles) compounds. Squares show the prediction of a multiple-analyzers model.

Summation Index in Logarithmic and Decibel Forms. For some purposes, as in Fig. 5.3—taking the logarithm of the summation index emphasizes the comparisons of interest. Partly for historical reasons but also because it simplifies one interesting prediction, this logarithm (to the base 10) of the summation index is often multiplied by 20 (see note 3). This gives the summation index in decibels, or in other words, the number of decibels by which you turn down the contrast in each component to make the compound be just at threshold (Arditi et al., 1981; Watson, Thompson, Murphy, & Nachmias, 1980). Decibels is often abbreviated db.

5.3.7 Comparison of Multiple- Versus Single-Analyzer Predictions for the Summation Index

An analytic expression for the summation index predicted by the multiple-analyzers model for far-apart components is easily available. When there are M equally detectable far-apart components, the multiple-analyzers model predicts that the summation index is M raised to the $1/k$th power (Eq. 4.13 in section 4.9.2). When the number of components M is just 2, therefore, the model predicts that:

$$\text{Summation index} = 2^{1/k}$$

$$\text{Db summation index} = 20 \cdot \log_{10} 2^{1/k} = \frac{6}{k}$$

Figure 5.3 compares predicted summation-index values from the multiple spatial-frequency-analyzer models in which there is probability summation across spatial frequencies and may or may not be probability summation across space (as in the equation just given and Fig. 4.9) and from the single spatial-frequency-analyzer models in which there is probability summation across space (Fig. 5.2). These are the predictions for summation of spatial frequencies a factor of 3 apart in either of two phases. The predicted summation index is plotted against the exponent in the Quick pooling formula. The three curves in Fig. 5.3 give the values predicted by the multiple-analyzers model for either phase (bottom curve) and by the single-analyzer model for peaks-subtract (middle curve) and peaks-add (top curve) phases. The predicted values can be verified by finding the intersections of the positive diagonal with the predicted curves in Figs. 4.9 and 5.2 and taking their reciprocals. For the multiple-analyzers model, they can also be calculated simply as 6/k (see above).

As just mentioned, all three predicted summation indices for an exponent of 2 in Fig. 5.3 have the same value—1.4, or in decibels, 3. The differences between curves increase as the exponent increases, reaching a maximum for an exponent of infinity (that is, for deterministic models). A similar figure for summation of opposite directions of motion (where temporal as well as spatial probability summation is a consideration) is shown in Watson et al. (1980).

5.4   SUMMATION OF FAR-APART SPATIAL POSITIONS

5.4.1   *Difficulties in Interpreting the Results of Varying the Spatial Extent of a Grating*

A very common summation experiment on the spatial-position dimension measures the sensitivity to sinusoidal gratings of varying numbers of cycles (see Howell and Hess, 1978; Legge, 1978b, Chap. 12). The individual components are single cycles and the compound is the many-cycle grating. In general, these experiments have found that sensitivity first increases as the number of cycles increases and then levels off, showing little if any further increase in sensitivity.

Several factors make the results of this summation experiment difficult to interpret, particularly so once the existence of multiple spatial-frequency analyzers is allowed for. Difficulties arise in trying to decide whether multiple spatial-position analyzers exist; and, more seriously, in trying to decide whether the multiple spatial-position analyzers are probabilistically independent (whether there is probability summation across space). Three distinct factors cause these difficulties.

Factor One: Summation Within Individual Spatial-Position Analyzers (Within Individual Weighting Functions). The first problem arises because the components (single cycles) are not all very far apart from one another on the spatial-position dimension, and thus two or more components will certainly stimulate the same spatial-position analyzer (mechanism) even if there are multiple spatial-position analyzers. As the number of cycles in a grating is increased from a very small to a somewhat larger number, an increase in sensitivity is sure to occur as a result of the increased stimulation of an individual analyzer (two or more cycles will fall within the same mechanism's weighting function). Compare the second and third sketches from the top in Fig. 5.4, for example. The second one shows a stimulus containing ½ cycle of a grating (a bright bar) centered on a weighting function of a mechanism that is sensitive to the appropriate spatial frequency and orientation. Only one excitatory lobe is stimulated, and that by a bright bar, causing a net excitatory output from the mechanism. If the extent of the grating is increased to 1½ cycles (third sketch), one excitatory lobe will be stimulated by a bright bar (as in the second sketch) but the two inhibitory lobes will be stimulated by dark bars, thus adding to the net excitatory output of the mechanism. If the grating is extended to 3½ cycles (bottom sketch Fig. 5.4), the individual mechanism responds just as if there were still only 1½ cycles.

Now consider a different weighting function having three excitatory lobes and four inhibitory lobes (Fig. 5.5; the sensitivity profile is in the top row and the weighting function map in the middle row). Consider gratings positioned so that bright bars stimulate the excitatory lobes and dark bars the inhibitory ones (bottom row). Although the side lobes are not as sensitive as the center lobe, they are somewhat sensitive, and the total output of the mechanism will be substantially larger to a grating containing 3½ cycles than to one containing 1½ cycles.

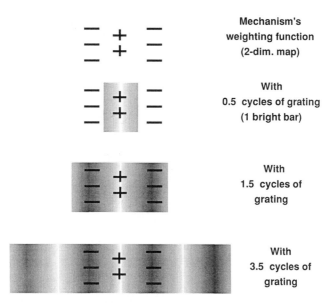

FIG. 5.4 Sketches of gratings patches containing varying numbers of cycles (0.5 cycle in second row, 1.5 cycles in third row, and 3.5 cycles in fourth row) juxtaposed on weighting function (shown alone in top row) of mechanism centered under the grating patch.

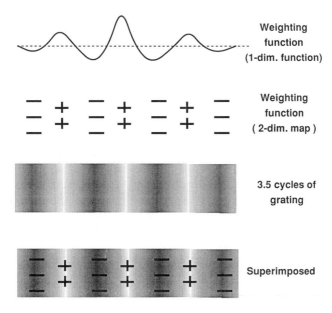

FIG. 5.5 A weighting function containing more lobes than that in the previous figure. It is illustrated both as a sensitivity profile (top row) and as a two-dimensional excitation/inhibition map (second row), and is then juxtaposed with a 3.5-cycle grating patch (bottom row).

Thus, the number of inhibitory and excitatory lobes in the field (see comparison in Figs. 5.4 and 5.5) determines the number of cycles over which sensitivity will continue to increase as a result of summation within individual spatial-position analyzers (individual mechanisms). The narrowest estimates of spatial-frequency bandwidth suggest weighting functions with eight or nine lobes (e.g., Kulikowski & King-Smith, 1973; Sachs et al., 1971; see note 4). Thus, increases in sensitivity with increases in number of cycles up to four or five might still be considered a possible result of summation within a single analyzer and cannot be attributed to probability summation across space (to probabilistically independent multiple spatial-position analyzers).

Note that using component sinusoidal patches at widely separated spatial positions (rather than increasing the number of cycles within a single grating) would completely avoid this problem of within-analyzer summation, just as using gratings of widely different spatial frequency avoids the analogous problem on the spatial-frequency dimension. No such experiment has been publsihed to my knowledge, however (but see Cannon & Fullencamp 1987).

Factor Two: Frequency Spread. A second difficulty in interpretation of experiments varying the number of cycles arises because, as the number of cycles is increased, the spatial-frequency content of the patch is changed, thereby changing which subset of mechanisms responds most to the pattern. Any patch of grating contains a range of spatial frequencies around its nominal spatial frequency (see section 2.4.2). The smaller the patch, the wider this range of spatial frequencies. To show this frequency spread in Fig. 5.4 would require drawing a number of weighting functions having slightly different sizes of excitatory and inhibitory lobes (slightly different best spatial frequencies) all centered at the same location, and showing that more of these different sizes were effectively stimulated by the ½-cycle stimulus in the second row than by the 1½-cycle stimulus in the third row.

For relatively high spatial frequencies, the effect of this spread of frequencies around the nominal frequency is the opposite of summation; it causes sensitivity to decrease as the number of cycles increases. This decrease happens because the observer is substantially more sensitive to the frequencies spread on the low side of a relatively high nominal frequency than to the nominal frequency itself. As the number of cycles in the patch of grating is increased and the spread of frequencies is decreased, these lower frequencies to which the observer is most sensitive disappear from the patch. This decrease in sensitivity with increasing number of cycles due to frequency spread (at high spatial frequencies) could mask any summation effect (either summation within single analyzers or probability summation across analyzers).

The problem of frequency spread is negligible once there are a large number of cycles in a grating; how large is large enough can be calculated from the spatial-frequency content of the patches and consideration of spatial-frequency bandwidth estimates.

Factor Three: Spatial Nonuniformity. To avoid the contaminating effects of both summation within individual weighting functions and of frequency spread, you want to be able to increase the number of cycles in a patch of grating to quite large numbers, certainly more than 4 or 5. This brings us to our third difficulty. In the typical experiment in which the number of cycles in a grating has been increased, the observer has looked directly at the grating so that the grating has extended across the foveal region. Unfortunately, sensitivity is not uniform across this region of the visual field. On the contrary, sensitivity to most kinds of stimuli is much greater at the fovea and drops off rapidly as you move away. (See Chap. 13.) Thus as the number of cycles in a grating patch centered on the fovea is increased, the observer is less and less sensitive to each added cycle. The further cycles are, in effect, hardly there at all.

Figure 5.6 shows the sensitivity measured for small patches of grating at var-

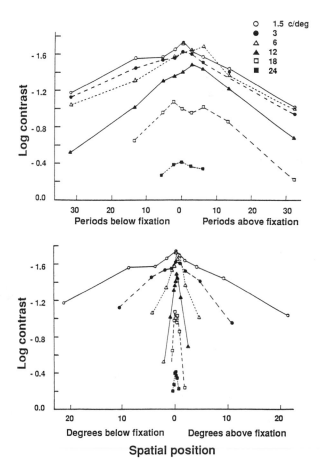

FIG. 5.6 Log threshold contrast for 4-cycle patches of grating as a function of distance above and below the fixation point. Thresholds are plotted as a function of eccentricity measuring distance either in periods of the relevant spatial frequency (top panel) or in degrees of visual angle (bottom panel). The grating patches contained horizontal bars. [Figure 4 from Robson and Graham, (1981); used by permission.]

ious distances from foveal center (at intermediate temporal frequencies, Robson & Graham, 1981). When distance is given in terms of periods, as in the top panel, the functions for different spatial frequencies are quite similar. As you can see there, once a grating has the 4 or 5 cycles necessary to avoid the first two difficulties, the addition of further cycles will have hardly any effect, simply because the observer is much less sensitive to these extra cycles (as will be shown in Fig. 5.7).

This last difficulty could be avoided if the contrast in the portions of the grating (or better, in separated patches of grating) was nonuniform in just the manner to offset the decrease in sensitivity with distance from the fovea. This has not been done extensively, however.

5.4.2   Varying the Number of Cycles in a Horizontal Strip Above the Fovea

Another way around this difficulty is to find a place in the visual field where sensitivity is more uniform than across the fovea. This has been done and is summarized in Fig. 5.7 (Robson & Graham, 1981; also see Jamar, Kwakman, & Koenderink, 1984, and the results of Mayer & Tyler, 1986, at large number of periods—their results with small numbers of cycles are difficult to interpret due to the presence of sharp edges). Without doing precise measurements at all distances, we settled on using, for a given spatial frequency of grating patch, the strip that was 42 periods of that spatial frequency above the fovea. The sensitivity was, in general, very uniform (see original paper).

Figure 5.7 shows the sensitivity (vertical axis) to gratings of different numbers of cycles (horizontal axis) for several different spatial frequencies and two observers; the gratings were presented either in a vertical strip through the fovea (left panel), where the sensitivity as a function of spatial position was very nonuniform as shown in Fig. 5.6, or in the horizontal strip 42 periods above the fovea (right panel), where the sensitivity was almost uniform. (The onsets and offsets were gradual; the spatial edges were gradual; the length of all bars in all gratings was approximately 4 cycles of the grating.)

As you can see, in the strip above the fovea where sensitivity is practically uniform, the observer's sensitivity to the grating continues to grow as the number of cycles is increased to 32 or 64, although in the strip through the fovea sensitivity grows substantially only for the first 8 or 16 cycles.

The summation in the peripheral strip, although continuing over many cycles, is too little to be consistent with a single spatial-position analyzer model. Doubling the number of cycles (which is equivalent to forming a compound made of two equally detectable components) only increases the sensitivity by a factor of about 1.2 (one 10th of a log unit). This is much less than the factor of 2 predicted by a reasonable single spatial-position-analyzer model—the model in which there is only a single mechanism (sensitive to the given spatial frequency and orientation) and in which, therefore, the weighting function of the single mechanism covers the visual field.

The summation over number of cycles in both the peripheral and the foveal

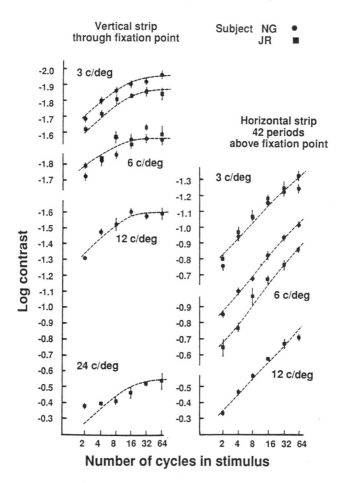

FIG. 5.7 Log threshold contrast as a function of number of cycles contained in the grating patch (on a logarithmic axis). The left half shows results for grating patches located within a thin vertical strip centered on the fixation point (the strip for which sensitivity measurements are shown in Fig. 5.6). The right shows results for grating patches located within a horizontal strip whose center was 42 periods vertically above the fixation point. (In this strip sensitivity is very close to uniform). All grating patches were centered in the strip within which they would appear. The orientation of the bars in each grating patch was perpendicular to the orientation of the strip. The dashed curves show the predictions of a model incorporation probability across space as described in text. (Figure 3 from Robson & Graham, 1981; used by permission.)

regions is, however, of just the right magnitude to be consistent with probabilistically independent multiple spatial-position analyzers (probability summation over space) or equivalent nonlinear pooling. [An interesting candidate for a nonprobabilistic pooling process across cycles of a grating has been qualitatively described by Grossberg (1983).] The predictions from a Quick pooling model are shown by the dotted lines in Fig. 5.7. The fit of the predictions to the data is very good. The only discrepancies, in fact, are due to certain approximations in the predictions—in particular the neglecting of the first two factors mentioned above (summation within individual analyzers and frequency spread), which affect the calculations at small numbers of cycles. (See details in Robson and Graham, 1981, and see note 5 for further discussion.) The implications of these results for spatial-frequency bandwidths is mentioned in section 6.6.1.

That these predictions for the horizontal strip 42 periods above the fovea are nearly straight lines on a logarithmic axis is not a coincidence but a direct consequence within the Quick pooling formula of the fact that sensitivity is nearly uniform there. If sensitivity were perfectly uniform, the lines would be perfectly straight with a slope equal to the reciprocal of the exponent (see Eq. 4.13). The exponent used here was 3.5. (Exponents of 3 and 4 predicted too much and too little summation, respectively.)

5.4.3   More Spatial-Position Summation Experiments—Evidence Consistent with Probability Summation Across Space

The results of the experiments briefly described in this subsection increase one's confidence in the existence of probabilistically independent multiple spatial-position analyzers (or equivalent nonlinear spatial pooling), although none of the results alone is compelling evidence. Many of the experiments are quite clever; the collection of more experimental results (including information on the sensitivity of the observer at different positions) and/or more extensive quantitative modeling could turn them into compelling evidence.

With a Masking Grating. Legge (1978b) measured threshold as a function of the number of cycles in a 3 c/deg test grating when a low-contrast mask grating of the same spatial frequency was always present. The masking grating was hoped to isolate only those mechanisms sensitive to 3 c/deg (avoiding frequency spread). Summation with a single weighting function was estimated from the data by the use of a quantitative model.

Far-Apart Aperiodic Stimuli. The use of lines at different spatial positions rather than cycles of grating (King-Smith & Kulikowski, 1975a) produced results at least qualitatively consistent with nonlinear spatial pooling. (Although there are small deviations between the data and the predictions of a high-threshold model of spatial probability summation, the total amount of data is small and the possibility of frequency spread and summation within single analyzers was not considered.)

Similarly, the detectability of three spots at far-apart spatial positions compared with that of each spot alone is consistent with probabilistically independent multiple spatial-position analyzers (Wickelgren, 1967).

Very Close Spatial Frequencies. If there is spatial probability summation, the summation of very close spatial frequencies will be strongly affected. The results of such summation experiments (further described in Chap. 6) are consistent with spatial probability summation and the known spatial nonuniformity. Such results are very difficult to explain without spatial probability summation, and thus seem further evidence for its existence.

Frequency-Modulated Gratings. Another potential way to investigate the existence of spatial probability summation and other forms of spatial pooling is to use compound gratings that contain the same spatial frequencies but in different phases. Along this line, a compound grating in which all the local peaks are of much the same height (an analogue to frequency-modulated—FM—radio signals) can be compared with compounds more like the peaks-add one shown in Fig. 4.2, where the peaks are of different heights (Stromeyer & Klein, 1975). A model assuming *no* spatial probability summation but very narrow spatial-frequency bandwidths is probably consistent with the experimental results; however, a model assuming spatial probability summation and medium spatial-frequency bandwidths seems to provide the best fit to the data (Graham & Rogowitz, 1976).

Summation of Close Lines. Wilson (1978a) argued that the results for compounds containing two lines separated by various amounts (further discussed in Chap. 6) cannot be accounted for by narrow spatial-frequency bandwidth analyzers without spatial probability summation. The results can be accounted for by medium spatial-frequency bandwidth analyzers with spatial probability summation. (The implications of multiple spatial-frequency bandwidths may not have been thought out for these cases).

Coherence Length of Rectangular Gratings. By using components that are light and dark lines (all of the same width) but varying the rules by which the light and dark bars are positioned, a wide variety of patterns can be composed ranging from homogeneous fields (only light lines allowed) to rectangular gratings (alternation of light and dark lines). If the coherence length (the average distance over which light and dark bars alternate regularly) is just one line, the placement of light and dark bars is totally random, producing a totally incoherent pattern. If the coherence length is as large as the total pattern width, the pattern is totally coherent (a rectangular grating). As it turns out, observers' sensitivities to these patterns continue to grow as the number of cycles increases, no matter whether the pattern is coherent or incoherent or in between (Koenderink & van Doorn, 1980). This result is again consistent with spatial probability summation or equivalent nonlinear spatial pooling. (Although the authors tentatively concluded in favor of "physiological" rather than "probability" summation, apparently on the basis of presumed disagreements between the amount of summation measured with number of bars and the steepness of the psychometric function, this conclusion is premature. The effects of summation within individual weighting functions, frequency spread, retinal inhomogeneity, and use of a dark surround immediately contiguous to their patterns would need to be further and quantitatively investigated.)

Coherent Grating Patches. A somewhat similar experiment used separated patches of grating in which the phases were either coherent across the patches (as if they were cut from one full grating) or incoherent (Halter, as reported by Mostafavi & Sakrison, 1976). As in the preceding, the results suggest spatial probability summation or equivalent nonlinear spatial pooling, since there was as much summation for the incoherent case as for the coherent case. Again, however, the contamination of possible within-receptive-field summation by the opposite effect of frequency spread prevents this from being telling evidence for spatial probability summation.

Peaked Narrow-Band Noise Patterns. Mostafavi and Sakrison (1976) used a series of stimuli that were variations on a narrow-band noise stimulus. Each member of this series was generated by starting with a particular narrow-band noise stimulus (a noisy sinusoidal grating) and (a) raising the difference between the luminance at each point in the original pattern and the mean luminance to a power q although retaining the sign of the difference, and (b) then keeping the spatial-frequency content the same by some slight spatial-frequency filtering. As the power q increases from 1, intensities far from the mean are made still further away relative to intensities near the mean. That is, the peaks in the luminance profile become more peaked as q gets higher. The exponent in the Quick pooling model that best fit Mostafavi and Sakrison's data was near 6. They suggested that the discrepancy between this value of 6 and the value of 3.5 necessary to fit the results for sinusoidal gratings is due to the existence of a slightly more complicated nonlinearity than that represented by the Quick psychometric function. Before we accept the necessity of this more complicated nonlinear operation, however, further results with their patterns should probably be carefully collected and analyzed (and the analysis should not neglect the existence of multiple spatial-frequency analyzers as the original analysis did).

Varying Length. A grating containing long lines or bars can be thought of as composed of short-bar gratings stimuli lined up end to end. Thus experiments varying the lengths of bars are spatial-position summation experiments analogous to those varying the numbers of cycles, and they run into precisely the same difficulties of interpretation: (a) summation within an analyzer (along the length of an individual mechanism's oriented weighting function); (b) orientation spread (as the bars get longer, the range of orientations contained in the pattern is less; see Wright, 1982, for some examples), and (c) spatial nonuniformity (the observer's sensitivity at different locations along the longer length bars must be known).

Some experiments varying the length of the bars have been done (e.g., Bacon & King-Smith, 1977; Howell & Hess, 1978; Kulikowski, 1969; Wright, 1982; see these and Chap. 13 for other references), although to my knowledge no experiment concomitantly measuring the sensitivity at different locations along the length of the bars has been published. The results all seem consistent with the conclusions drawn earlier from the experiments varying the number of cycles. In particular, as the length of the bars in a grating is increased, the observer's sensitivity tends to increase rather noticeably until a "critical length" is reached. There is some agreement that the value of this critical length decreases in inverse proportion to the spatial frequency of the grating, or to put it another way, the value of this critical length is approximately the same when expressed in periods of the spatial frequency of the grating.

In the absence of information about sensitivity along the length of the bars (and without calculations for the effect of orientation/frequency spread), it is not possible to interpret definitively the critical length arrived at by existing studies. The length is probably some conglomerate of the effect of summation within single analyzers coupled with spatial probability summation attenuated by the nonuniformity of the visual field in the direction parallel to the bars. That the critical length seems to be the same when length is measured in periods of the nominal spatial frequency probably reflects the following: (a) The length-to-width ratio of every weighting function's excitatory and inhibitory sections is the same, and/or (b) sensitivity as a function of spatial position in the direction parallel to the bars is the same for different spatial frequencies when spatial position is measured in number of periods.

5.4.4 A Physiological Aside: Independent or Correlated Variability in Neurons' Outputs?

On the basis of known neurophysiology and anatomy, strict probabilistic independence would not be expected; the outputs of at least some neurons at any one level in the visual pathways (e.g., the retina, or V1) would be expected to be positively or negatively correlated (across presentations to the same stimulus) either because they share inputs or because they directly interact with one another. Correlation seems particularly likely for neurons sensitive to the same or nearby spatial locations, because they tend both to share inputs and to directly interact. This observation might lead one to doubt the probabilistic independence of analyzer outputs that we assumed when discussing probability summation. And, indeed, strict probabilistic independence is almost certainly an oversimplification for neurons and for the analyzers needed to explain psychophysical results. Although more theoretical work ought to be done to determine the effect of assuming some correlation among analyzers, I suspect the following is true: If the correlations are not too strong and if their direct effects are limited to near neighbors on some or all dimensions, their existence will have negligible effect on the predictions for experiments using far-apart values. Their existence may, however, have some decided effect on the results using close-together values (results from which bandwidth estimates are typically made, as in the next chapter).

Recently, neurophysiologists have begun to study the actual pattern of correlations among neurons, both in their spontaneous activity and in their responses to stimuli. [Some relatively recent articles that contain references to older articles are Mastronarde, (1983a, 1983b, 1983c), Tanaka (1983), and Toyama, Kimura, & Tanaka (1981a, 1981b).] At least for the spontaneous activity of cat retinal ganglion cells, correlations appeared only if the receptive-field centers of the neurons overlap, and the strength of the correlation depended on the degree of overlap (Mastronarde, 1983).

5.5   SUMMATION EXPERIMENTS ON THE SPATIAL-EXTENT DIMENSION

In spatial-extent summation experiments with sinusoidal patches, the observer's sensitivity to a compound stimulus containing component patches of two different spatial extents must be compared with the sensitivity for the components by themselves. (The extents might differ either perpendicular or parallel to the bars, or both, that is, either in spatial-frequency or orientation bandwidth, or both.) As far as I know, no experiment of this type has been done using sinusoidal patches. However, some elegant experiments adding an aperiodic stimulus (an aperiodic stimulus is like a sinusoidal patch containing a very small number of cycles) to a wide sinusoid (a sinusoidal patch of many cycles) have been done (Hauske, Wolf, & Lupp, 1976; Kulikowski & King-Smith, 1973; Shapley & Tolhurst, 1973) and their results will be briefly considered here and more extensively in Chapter 6.

5.5.1   *Components That Are Grating Patches of Differing Numbers of Cycles*

An example of a summation experiment using sinusoidal components of differing numbers of cycles is illustrated in Fig. 5.8. The left column shows the luminance profiles and the right column the Fourier amplitude spectra of each of two component stimuli (two top rows) and a compound stimulus (bottom row). In terms of spatial frequency, the difference between the two component stimuli—which have the same nominal spatial frequency—is in the bandwidth of spatial frequencies each contains. The bandwidth of the 2-cycle component is much broader than that of the 5-cycle component.

What If Such an Experiment Showed Very Little Summation? Suppose the results of such a summation experiment showed very little summation, as little as would be expected from probability summation between two independent analyzers. How would we interpret them? As with any dimension, a reasonable interpretation would postulate (at least) two analyzers with nonoverlapping sensitivities on the dimension of interest—in this case, one analyzer sensitive to the 2-cycle component but not to the 5-cycle component in Fig. 5.8 and a second analyzer sensitive to the 5-cycle but not to the 2-cycle component.

Although this is a reasonable explanation, the kind of mechanism we have considered so far cannot serve as such an analyzer. For a mechanism having a weighting function of two excitatory and two inhibitory lobes (ideally suited for

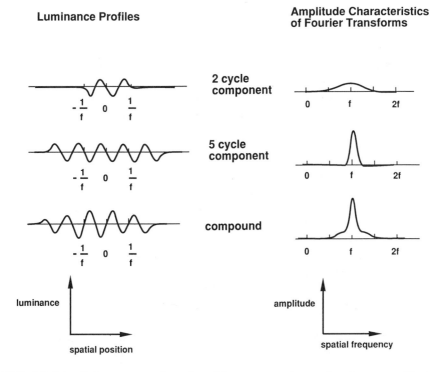

FIG. 5.8 Stimuli for a summation-of-spatial-extent experiment. Luminance profiles in the left column illustrate the two simple stimuli (top rows) and the compound stimulus (bottom row). The amplitude parts of the Fourier transform are crudely sketched in the right column. (The abrupt edges on the stimuli in the left column mean that the full Fourier amplitude plots should contain secondary negative and positive lobes; these have been omitted to make the important details more visible.)

detection of the 2-cycle component) will respond just as much to the 5-cycle component as to the 2. A mechanism having a weighting function of five excitatory and five inhibitory lobes (ideally suited for detection of the 5-cycle component) will respond to some extent to the 2-cycle component. Thus, even if there are mechanisms having weighting functions of different numbers of lobes (but the same size of lobe, at the same spatial position, orientation, etc.), they will have heavily overlapping sensitivities on the spatial-extent (spatial-frequency bandwidth) dimension and one would expect to find a good deal of summation between components having different spatial extents (different numbers of cycles). If the results of a spatial-extent summation experiment like that in Fig. 5.8 actually came out showing as little summation as would be expected from nonoverlapping analyzers on the spatial-extent dimension, one would have to consider mechanisms very different from those we have considered here.

In fact, however, the results of the aperiodic-stimulus-plus-sine experiments (see section 6.7) all show a good deal of summation, so we do not need to consider this possibility further.

Can Such an Experiment Distinguish Between Multiple Versus Single Analyzers on the Spatial-Extent Dimension? Since, as we have just argued, a good deal of summation between stimuli of different spatial extents may be shown even if there are multiple analyzers on the spatial-extent dimension (multiple spatial-frequency bandwidths at a given spatial frequency, orientation, position, etc.), the question arises whether this kind of experiment can possibly distinguish between the existence of multiple analyzers and the existence of only a single analyzer on the spatial-extent dimension. I am not sure, but my experience analyzing the aperiodic-test-plus-sine experiments (see section 6.7) convinces me that such a distinction is very tricky to make for reasons outlined here.

If there were only a single analyzer on the spatial-extent dimension (at each spatial frequency, orientation, spatial position, etc.), one might hope to get the completely linear summation typical of a single analyzer. Judging from the aperiodic-plus-sine results, however, one would not get this much summation. Does this rule out a single analyzer on the spatial-extent dimension (a single spatial-frequency bandwidth)? No, for the actual prediction assuming a single analyzer on the spatial-extent dimension is complicated by spatial-frequency spread: The smaller and larger stimulus components will maximally stimulate somewhat different subsets of analyzers on the spatial-frequency dimension. In particular, the smaller stimulus component (e.g., the 2-cycle component in Fig. 5.8) will stimulate more different spatial-frequency analyzers, for example, mechanisms having more different sizes of weighting-function lobes, than the larger stimulus component does. And thus, even if there is only a single analyzer on the spatial-extent dimension, one would not get the completely linear summation typical of a single analyzer. Calculations showing much less than complete summation between spatial extents—even if only a single analyzer exists on the spatial-extent dimension—will be presented in section 6.7.

Another factor that may slightly complicate the calculation for spatial-extent summation experiments is the fact that the larger component occupies more spatial positions than does the smaller, and thus existence of multiple spatial-position analyzers with probability summation among them must enter into any complete calculation.

Throughout this section, we have discussed stimuli of differing spatial extent that are all centered at the same spatial position. Offsetting one complicates the calculations greatly, by introducing phase differences that may make the compound quite unlike the components.

5.5.2   *Components That Are Grating Patches of Different Bar Lengths*

Arguments exactly analogous to those of the last section apply to the summation of gratings having different spatial extents in the direction parallel to the bars (but all centered at the same position). Here analyzers of different orientations play the role played above by analyzers of different spatial frequencies.

5.5.3 Components That Are Aperiodic Stimuli of Different Extents

Summation experiments using compounds of homogeneous stimuli of two different spatial extents (e.g., disks of different diameters, bars of different widths) have been done by Thomas and his colleagues (Bagrash, Kerr, & Thomas, 1971; Thomas, 1970; Thomas, Bagrash, & Kerr, 1969; Thomas & Kerr, 1971; Thomas, Padilla, & Rourke, 1969). In these experiments the two components differed markedly both in spatial-frequency content (the wider disk or bar had lower spatial frequencies) and in spatial-frequency bandwidth (the wider disk or bar had a smaller spatial-frequency bandwidth) and also, when bars were used, in orientation bandwidth (the wider bar had a larger orientation bandwidth). Thus the experiment is a combination of a spatial-frequency and spatial-extent summation experiment. The small amount of summation found when the two components differed greatly in size might be consistent with multiple analyzers on either the spatial-frequency or spatial-extent dimensions. The interpretation in the original paper (backed up by quantitative predictions) postulates multiple analyzers on the spatial-frequency dimension only (that is, postulates that weighting functions differ in the sizes of their lobes but not in the number of their lobes).

5.6 SUMMATION EXPERIMENTS ON THE SPATIAL-PHASE DIMENSION

5.6.1 Symmetries Versus Positions of Mechanisms

Consider what a summation experiment on the spatial phase dimension is. The compound is formed from two sinusoidal components both identical except in spatial phase (that is, both of the same spatial frequency and orientation and temporal frequency and phase with the same spatial and temporal extents and positions). Although no one has explicitly done such an experiment, its results are easy to predict from known results. For the compound is just another sinusoidal grating of the same frequency as the original two components but, in general, of different phase and amplitude. That is, the compound is just a simple stimulus having another value on the phase dimension. Let us assume that the thresholds for slightly different spatial phases (spatial positions within one period) of a sinusoidal grating are identical. (In fact, they might not quite be, but visual field nonuniformity is rather slight within one period.) On this assumption, we can easily predict the result of the phase summation experiment. When the two components are of the same phase (zero phase difference), there will be complete summation, because the compound has twice the amplitude of either component but is otherwise identical. As the components are made to differ in phase, the summation will decrease as the amplitude of the compound decreases (to 1.41 at a phase difference of 90 degrees and to zero at a phase difference of 180 degrees, where the two components just cancel each other out). Thus there is very strongly value-selective summation on the spatial-phase dimension.

By analogy with conclusions drawn on other dimensions, one might suggest multiple analyzers on the phase dimension. Is there anything wrong with this conclusion? No, except if "phase analyzer" is overinterpreted—a problem that arises from the intimate relationship between spatial position and phase.

There are at least two quite distinct ways—within the multiple-mechanism framework we have been discussing—of having analyzers selectively different to different phases. First, some mechanisms might have even-symmetric weighting functions, some odd-symmetric, and some in between (although all are centered at the same spatial position, sensitive to the same spatial frequency, orientation, etc.). To many people, this is the most interesting way to have phase analyzers. Unfortunately, mechanisms with weighting functions all of the same symmetry but centered at slightly different positions also serve quite well as phase analyzers in the present situation. Assuming, for example, that all weighting functions are even symmetric, the mechanisms centered under the peaks of a grating will respond most, and thus different mechanisms will respond most to different phases.

Within the multiple-mechanism framework, therefore, the results of the spatial-phase summation experiment described above may be telling us either that (a) there are weighting functions of the same symmetry at many different positions so that no matter what the spatial phase of the sinusoidal grating, its brightest point is superimposed on the very center of some weighting function, or (b) that there are weighting functions of different symmetries.

5.6.2   On the Interaction of Spatial Phase with Other Dimensions in Summation Experiments

Experiments on one of the other pattern dimensions (e.g., spatial frequency) sometimes also manipulate the relative spatial phase between the two components. Experiments that manipulated the relative spatial phase between components as well as changing value on another dimension (e.g., spatial frequency) probably fit best into the classification framework as an interaction experiment between the other dimension and phase (e.g., spatial frequency and spatial phase). For the effect of differences between the two components on both dimensions are simultaneously investigated. Here these experiments are briefly listed with some discussion of the ones that speak to the question of whether different symmetries of weighting function exist.

With Far-Apart Spatial Frequencies. As discussed in Chapter 4, the phase between two sinusoidal gratings of different spatial frequency has been varied in several summation experiments using far-apart spatial frequencies. In the usual conditions, no difference between the phases is found, as one would expect if the components activate separate analyzers (e.g., Graham et al., 1978).

At very low spatial frequencies, however, where there is substantial summation among far-apart spatial frequencies, one finds the differences due to spatial phase expected from summation within an individual analyzer that is characterized by an even-symmetric weighting function—that is, peaks-add compounds are considerably more detectable than peaks-subtract (Wilson, 1980a).

Spatial frequencies within about a two-octave band centered around 7 cpd were added together so that their relative amplitudes were always the same but their relative spatial phases were different (Henning, Derrington, & Madden, 1983). Two of the relative-phase conditions were (a) an even-symmetric stimulus that looked like one tall excitatory peak, with two much smaller inhibitory troughs and then just a hint of further rippling, and (b) an odd-symmetric stimulus that had one large excitatory and one large inhibitory peak with subsequent smaller secondary lobes and a hint of further rippling. (The temporal onsets and offsets were gradual.) The even-and odd-symmetric stimuli (of same amplitude spectra) were equally detectable. As the authors pointed out, this is consistent with there being two different symmetries (even and odd) of weighting function having approximately equal sensitivity. They also considered the possibility that there is only one symmetry of weighting function (even) and that the odd-symmetric stimulus is detected by that kind of weighting function centered on the bright peak. They argued against this possibility on the grounds that then the observer should be 1.5 times less sensitive to the odd-symmetric stimulus than to the even-symmetric stimulus. This calculated factor is apparently based, however, on a model neglecting spatial probability summation. A full model with probability summation across spatial frequencies and spatial position might predict greater similarity in the three patterns' thresholds, if only because the odd-symmetric stimulus gains by having both a substantial peak and a trough whereas the symmetric one has only a substantial peak. Therefore, although the authors' conclusion that there are different symmetries of weighting functions is intriguing, more calculations would need to be done to make the conclusion from this experiment compelling.

With Spatial Position. One experiment, briefly described in section 5.4.3, varied the relative spatial phases of three small patches of grating at different spatial positions (Halter, described by Mostafavi & Sakrison, 1976); but these results have no implication for the possible symmetries of receptive fields.

With Spatial Extent. In the experiments adding sinusoidal gratings to aperiodic stimuli, the phase of the grating with respect to the aperiodic stimulus was sometimes varied (e.g., Kulikowski & King-Smith, 1973; Shapley & Tolhurst, 1973). When the added sinusoid is in phase with the aperiodic stimulus' component of the same spatial frequency, there is summation. When the added sinusoid is out of phase, there is inhibition. In-between phases yield in-between results. Qualitatively at least, the effect is as expected on almost any model, including probability summation among multiple spatial-frequency analyzers, even if all weighting functions have the same symmetry [as in the Graham (1977) reinterpretation of these studies].

5.7 SUMMARY

Summation experiments using far-apart values on the spatial dimensions have produced evidence for multiple analyzers with probability summation among them on several dimensions: spatial frequency, orientation, and both spatial position dimensions. (A possible physiological substrate for such analyzers are neurons having elongated excitatory-inhibitory receptive fields with varying orientations, widths of excitatory/inhibitory lobes, and positions.) Each such mechanism is simultaneously sensitive to narrow ranges of spatial frequencies, or orientations, and of spatial positions. Such joint selectivity on all dimensions is necessitated by the finding of almost no summation at far values.

There is no evidence for multiple analyzers on either of the two spatial-extent dimensions or on the spatial-phase dimension. In terms of the multiple-mechanism model, there is no evidence for weighting functions having different numbers of lobes, different lengths of lobes, or different symmetries (while having the same width of lobe, the same orientation, and the same spatial position). In most of the following discussion we will assume, therefore, that multiple analyzers on these latter dimensions do not exist (at least none that are active at threshold; some less sensitive analyzers may well exist). It is worth remembering, however, that there is also no completely compelling evidence against the existence of multiple spatial-extent analyzers (see further discussion in the next chapter) and almost no evidence one way or the other about spatial-phase analyzers, so some future puzzle at threshold may be solved by postulating multiple analyzers on one of these dimensions.

Notes

1. *The logical possibility of probability summation across spatial frequency and orientation but not across spatial position.* Logically, probability summation across spatial frequencies could exist without probability summation across spatial positions (and vice versa). In terms of possible physiological substrate, for example, there could be independent variability in the outputs of neurons in different spatial-frequency analyzers (neurons with receptive fields of different sizes or orientations) and yet completely correlated variability in all neurons of a given spatial-frequency analyzer (neurons with the same shape of receptive field but in different positions). Alternatively, the source of variability in a spatial-frequency analyzer's output might be variability in the threshold criterion for that analyzer (the size of the peak output necessary for an analyzer to detect a grating). This kind of variability, although undoubtedly neural also, may be at some level in the nervous system higher than that of the array. Then, if this higher level variability is the only source of variability, one would not predict probability summation across space.

2. *Appropriate form of Quick pooling formula.* The forms of the Quick pooling formula for far-apart components derived in section 4.9 cannot be used in deriving the predictions of the single-channel model with spatial probability summation for far-apart spatial frequencies. For the stimuli of concern are various simple and compound sinusoidal gratings that, although they contain far-apart spatial frequencies, contain very-close-together spatial positions. Instead, the sensitivity of each spatial-position analyzer to each stimulus must be computed, as indicated in Fig. 4.2, from the output of the single translation-invariant system, and the summation in Eq. 4.9 must be done. See Graham, Robson, and Nachmias (1978) for more details.

The question of how many such spatial-position analyzers there should be (of how closely packed the positions of weighting functions should be) was answered—as is frequently done—by assuming an effective continuum, that is, by assuming they are so close together that making them closer together, say by a factor of 2, does not affect the predictions.

3. *Decibels.* It may seem strange that there are 20 decibels in each logarithmic unit of contrast in spite of the "deci" in the name, which means 10, and in spite of the "bel," which originally referred to units of auditory intensity. This is a historical accident; many early experiments generated sinusoidal gratings using waveform generators and attenuators that had originally been designed for use in auditory experiments. A decibel was a 10th of a logarithmic unit of power. But power is the square of intensity, so you only raise intensity by half a log unit to raise power by a whole log unit. And contrast is the analogue of auditory intensity. Hence there are 10 decibels in half a logarithmic unit of contrast.

4. *Interaction between spatial frequencies and spatial positions.* Spatial-frequency bandwidth can be estimated from the results of experiments in which compound gratings containing close frequencies are used (as will be done in Chap. 6). Unfortunately for our present purposes, however, the bandwidth estimated from these experiments depends a good deal on whether there is probability summation across space, one of the questions we are trying to answer at present. Thus, to be conservative in the present argument, one must take the estimates using the largest number of lobes (the estimates assuming there is no probability summation across space).

5. *Multiple spatial-frequency-bandwidth model and varying number of cycles.* One more possible model is worth considering. Perhaps the increase in sensitivity as number of cycles increases—although so little as to rule out the existence of only a single spatial-position analyzer—is the result of summation within individual spatial-position analyzers (factor one) rather than spatial probability summation or equivalent nonlinear pooling across the outputs of different analyzers. If so, the weighting function of at least some individual spatial-position analyzers must have at least 32 or 64 pairs of excitatory and inhibitory regions (although the far-out ones may be relatively insensitive). This is many more than has even been suggested by any other kind of psychophysical evidence, in particular by the summation of close spatial frequencies discussed in Chapter 6. Therefore, to account for the summation of far-apart spatial frequencies, there would need to be, in addition to the weighting functions with 32 or more pairs of lobes necessary to account for the number-of-cycles data, weighting functions with smaller numbers of excitatory and inhibitory lobes (larger spatial-frequency bandwidths). These smaller ones would have to be of exactly the right sensitivity to camouflage the effects of the weighting functions with 32 pairs of lobes in the spatial-frequency summation experiments. I do not think this model postulating multiple spatial-frequency bandwidths (in addition to multiple spatial-position, spatial-frequency, and orientation analyzers) can be conclusively rejected, but its complexity and coincidental nature (how do the sensitivities manage to exactly balance out?) are unappealing, and it will generally be ignored in the following.

6

Close Values on Spatial Dimensions

6.1 OVERVIEW

Summation experiments using close values are usually done to estimate analyzers' "bandwidth," or more formally, to estimate an individual analyzer's sensitivity as a function of value on a particular dimension. The logic of bandwidth estimation is much like that used to distinguish single-analyzer from multiple-analyzers models. (The analyzer in a single-analyzer model is a very broad-band analyzer indeed.)

Let's consider a dimension on which multiple analyzers are indicated by summation experiments using far-apart values. A compound formed from two far-apart components on such a dimension is only a little more detectable than the most detectable component. That little bit of extra detectability is attributed to probability summation among analyzers—no individual analyzer is thought to be sensitive to both values. When, however, the two components are brought closer together, one typically finds that the compound becomes more detectable (relative to its components). This further increment in detectability is attributed to summation within analyzers; at least one analyzer's output to the compound is thought to be greater than its output to either component. The greater this extra detectability, the more sensitive some individual analyzer is thought to be to both components. By varying the difference between the two values in the compound, therefore, the sensitivity of an individual analyzer to values various distances apart can be found.

The exact estimation of the sensitivity depends on the assumptions one is willing to make about the analyzers, however. Further, the existence of analyzers on several dimensions (e.g., spatial frequency, orientation, spatial position—even perhaps spatial-extent or spatial-frequency bandwidth) complicates bandwidth estimation on any one dimension (e.g., spatial frequency; see below).

This chapter starts with the estimation of bandwidth in the case of very simple assumptions—two linear, deterministic analyzers. Not only is this simple model useful as an introduction to the later more complex ones, but this reasoning is the prototypical reasoning found for summation experiments in many sensory/perceptual domains. The effects on bandwidth estimates of loosening these assumptions will then be considered. The second part of the chapter reviews the current bandwidth estimates from summation experiments on the spatial dimensions. (See Chap. 12 for references to bandwidth estimates from other kinds of experiments and on other dimensions.)

6.2 TWO ADDITIVE, DETERMINISTIC ANALYZERS (THE NAIVE MODEL)

6.2.1 Assumptions

This simple calculation of analyzer sensitivity from summation experiments can be defined by four assumptions:

Assumption 45. Two Relevant Analyzers. *There are only two relevant analyzers—one analyzer most sensitive to the value of one component in the compound and the other analyzer most sensitive to the value of the other component.*

Assumption 27. Additivity to a Compound. *Each analyzer's output to the compound is the sum of its outputs to the two components.*

(In the case of spatial-frequency summation experiments, this assumption is reasonable only in the peaks-add phase. Thus, most spatial-frequency summation experiments at close values have used peaks-add phase.)

Assumption 32. Deterministic Output (No Variability). *The output of an analyzer in a given state of adaptation to a given stimulus is always the same.*

Assumption 40. Maximum-Output Detection Rule. *In all conditions, the observer's response is based on the maxmium of the outputs from the monitored analyzers.*

These last two assumptions imply the following (which is a version of Assumption 4):

Assumption 46. Most Sensitive Analyzer Detection Rule. *An observer's threshold for the compound equals the threshold of the most sensitive of the two analyzers.*

6.2.2 Predictions of the Naive (Two Deterministic Analyzers) Model

Summation Squares and Intensity Interrelationship Functions. Figure 6.1 shows summation squares for four different hypothetical pairs of components. Component A is assumed to be the same in all four pairs, but component B varies from having the same value as A (upper left summation square) to having a very different value (lower right). The absolute intensities of component A and of component B are plotted on the right vertical axis and the top horizontal axis. The relative intensities of A and B are plotted on the left vertical and bottom horizontal axes.

The heavy solid line in each of the four drawings shows the thresholds of "analyzer A," the analyzer that is most sensitive to component A. Notice that in all four drawings the heavy solid line for analyzer A intersects the vertical relative-intensity axis at point 1.0, since, by the foregoing assumptions, the psychophysical threshold for component A must equal the threshold of this one

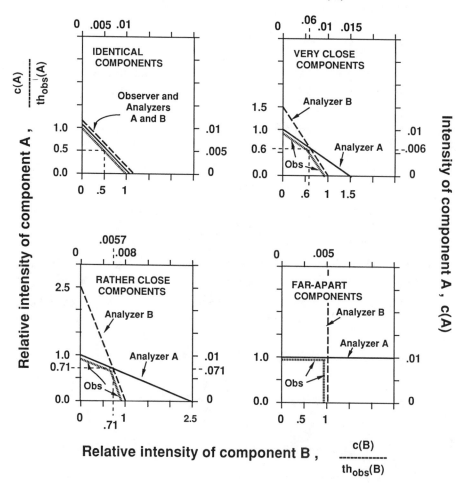

FIG. 6.1 Hypothetical summation-square plots from the naive model (two additive, deterministic analyzers) for four cases: components that are identical, very close, rather close, and far-apart in value on the relevant dimension. Curves that would lie on top of one another have been offset in the drawing for visual clarity. See text for more details.

analyzer. The absolute intensity at the observer's threshold for component A is assumed to be 0.01 in this example, as is indicated on the right vertical axis.

Similarly, the heavy dashed line shows the thresholds of analyzer B, the analyzer most sensitive to component B. The heavy dashed line intersects the horizontal axis at a relative intensity of 1.0. Since the value of B varies, so does the absolute intensity at the observer's threshold for component B; it is indicated on the top horizontal axis. The observer's thresholds for component B are replotted in Fig. 6.2 in the curve marked "observer." The left vertical axis in Fig. 6.2 is labeled with the threshold intensities and the right by their reciprocals.

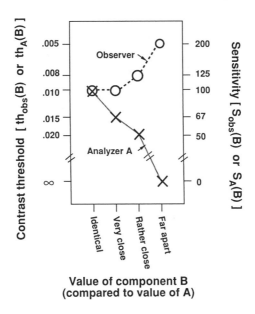

FIG. 6.2 Observer's (open circles) and analyzer A's (X's) thresholds for component B from the four cases of Fig. 6.1.

In the drawings of Fig. 6.1, the following symmetry assumption has been made: The intersection of analyzer B's curve with the relative-intensity-of-component-A axis is shown as identical to the intersection of analyzer A's curve with the relative-intensity-of-component-B axis. This assumption is probably not strictly justified in most cases but is sometimes used as a simplifying assumption. (In the upper left drawing, the heavy dashed line and solid lines, although drawn slightly offset from one another for clarity, are supposed to be identical because the two stimulus components are identical.)

The heavy dotted lines in Fig. 6.1 show the observer's thresholds as predicted by this model. They always are identical to those of the most sensitive analyzer by Assumption 46, although offset somewhat in the figure for visual clarity.

The light dashed lines in Fig. 6.1 indicate the coordinates of the intersections of the observer's threshold curve with the positive diagonal.

Notice that in the lower right drawing where the two components are assumed to be so far apart that no analyzer is sensitive to both components, the predicted observer's thresholds lie on the upper and right edges of the summation square. This is the same prediction illustrated in Fig. 4.9 for a multiple-analyzers model for the case of no probability summation among analyzers (the exponent of infinity).

Terminological Note. Intensity Interrelationship Functions. In the following, curves showing thresholds on summation squares will sometimes be called *intensity interrelationship functions* for the sake of (relative) brevity. Thus, in Fig. 6.1, for example, the heavy solid lines, heavy dashed lines, and dotted lines might be called intensity interrelationship functions for analyzer A, for analyzer B, and for the observer, respectively. The latter will sometimes be called *psychophysical intensity interrelationship functions* (and have sometimes been called *psychophysical contrast interrelationship functions* in the pattern-vision literature).

Analyzer A's Sensitivity for Component B. The intersections of the heavy solid lines in Fig. 6.1 with the bottom horizontal axis show analyzer A's thresholds for component B by itself (for component B when the intensity in component A is zero). The top axis gives these thresholds in absolute intensity as 0.01, 0.015, 0.02, and infinity, respectively. These thresholds are plotted in the lower curve of Fig. 6.2.

6.2.3   *Naive Estimates—Linear Extrapolation from Low Intensities*

According to this simple model of section 6.2.1, the sensitivity of analyzer A to component B—$S_A(B)$—can easily be measured without measuring the whole function giving the observer's thresholds. All that is needed is the observer's thresholds for 2 compounds in the left of the summation square (compounds in which component B's relative intensity is so low that analyzer A determines the observer's threshold). These 2 thresholds determine analyzer A's threshold line from which one can then extrapolate, as illustrated in Fig. 6.3, to the intersection of analyzer A's line with the horizontal axis. Called y in Fig. 4.3, this intersection

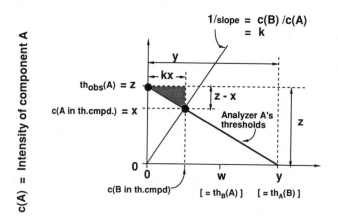

c(B) = Intensity of component B

FIG. 6.3 Illustration of the extrapolation from the observer's thresholds for two stimuli (solid circles) to the naive estimate of analyzer A's threshold for component B (the intersection of the line through the solid points with the horizontal axis). One of the two stimuli is component A by itself and the other is a compound containing so little of component B that the observer's threshold is completely determined by analyzer A. See text for further details.

is equal to th$_A$(B)—the threshold of analyzer A for component B—and its reciprocal is S_A(B). (Even if the whole psychophysical contrast interrelationship curve has been measured, it is necessary to extrapolate if an estimate of analyzer A's sensitivity is desired.)

Rather than doing the extrapolation graphically, there are many different but equivalent algebraic representations of this extrapolation, one of which is illustrated in Fig. 6.3. and described in the following. (A reader can skip to Eq. 6.1— if willing to believe that equation—without loss of continuity.) For clarity in this discussion, the single-letter symbols w, x, y, z, and k will be used to represent various quantities—as shown on Fig. 6.3—usually represented by longer-symbols. Note that the symbols c(A in th.cmpd) and c(B in th.cmpd) mean the contrasts in components A and B, respectively, when the compound is just at the observer's threshold. Consider the small shaded right triangle in Fig. 6.3 with base of length kx and height of length $(z - x)$ and the larger right triangle containing it—the triangle having analyzer A's line for a hypotenuse—that has a base of length y and height of length z. These two triangles are similar (in the technical geometrical sense) because both triangles are right triangles and share the same angle on the upper left. Hence the lengths of corresponding sides are proportional. Thus

$$\frac{z}{y} = \frac{z - x}{k \cdot x}$$

Simple algebraic manipulation gives

$$\frac{1}{y} = \frac{1}{k} \cdot \left| \frac{1}{x} - \frac{1}{z} \right|$$

which is written out as

$$\frac{1}{\text{th}_A(B)} = \frac{1}{k} \left| \frac{1}{c(A \text{ in th cmpd})} - \frac{1}{\text{th}_{\text{obs}}(A)} \right|$$

Let S_{obs}(A in cmpd) be the sensitivity of the observer for component A when it is in the compound, or equivalently, the reciprocal of c(A in th cmpd), which is the intensity in component A when the compound is at the observer's threshold. Then the above equation can be rewritten

$$S_A(B) = \frac{1}{k} [S_{\text{obs}}(A \text{ in cmpd}) - S_{\text{obs}}(A)] \qquad (6.1)$$

The quantity on the right side of Eq. 6.1 is thus equal to S_A(B) according to this model and can be used to estimate S_A(B) from experimental results. This estimate of S_A(B) in Eq. (6.1) has been used many times in the visual literature. In order to have a short name for it in the following, it will be referred to as the *naive* estimate, although the negative connotations of naive are not entirely appropriate here.

If naive estimates of S_A(B) are plotted against different values of component

B, the bandwidth of the resulting sensitivity function will be called the *naive estimate of bandwidth.*

This procedure always has the virtues of simplicity and some descriptive power; in some situations, the procedure may even turn out to be essentially correct. In any case, this procedure of estimating sensitivity or bandwidth from summation experiments is the one typically used in the initial stages of investigating analyzers on some dimension (sometimes without consideration of all the assumptions entailed, however). What is sufficient and necessary for this naive procedure to be valid is that the two (or more) observer's thresholds from which one is extrapolating are equal to analyzer A's thresholds and that the locus of all of analyzer A's thresholds is a straight line.

6.2.4   Relation of Naive Estimate to Summation Index

In Fig. 6.1, light dashed lines are drawn horizontally and vertically from the observer's threshold on the positive diagonal to the axes (except that the lines were not drawn in the lower right—they are the same as the heavy dotted lines). As these lines show, the relative intensity in each component is 0.5, 0.6, 0.714, and 1.0 for the four cases from upper left to lower right. It is the reciprocal of this intensity that is the summation index (that is, 2.0, 1.67, 1.4, and 1.0 for the four cases of Fig. 6.1) and is plotted (on the left vertical axis) in Fig. 6.4 for the four cases of Fig. 61.

This summation index bears a close relationship to the naive estimate of $S_A(B)$ in Eq. 6.1. In fact (the derivation is outlined below)

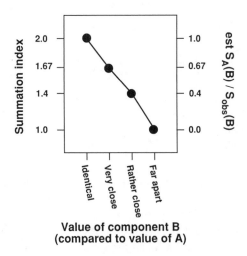

FIG. 6.4 Summation indices (left axis) for the four hypothetical cases of Fig. 6.1 (indicated by value of component B on the horizontal axis). The labels on the right axis give the naive estimate of analyzer A's sensitivity to B relative to the observer's sensitivity to B. This naive estimate equals the summation index minus 1.0.

$$\frac{\text{est } S_A(B)}{S_{obs}(B)} = \text{summation index} - 1.0 \qquad (6.2)$$

Notice now that the quantity on the left side of this expression is the reciprocal of the intersection of analyzer A's line with the relative-intensity horizontal axis on summation squares like those in Fig. 6.1. (For the four cases in Fig. 6.1 starting from the upper left, the intersections were 1.0, 1.5, 2.5, and infinity, respectively, and thus the reciprocals were 1, 0.67, 0.4, and 0, as plotted on the right axis of Fig. 6.4.)

The naive estimate of the half-amplitude full-bandwidth can be obtained directly from the summation index by doubling the difference in values that gives a summation index of 1.5.

Outline of Derivation of Eq. 6.2.

1. Compute the naive estimate for a compound located on the positive diagonal by substituting $S_{obs}(B)/S_{obs}(A)$ for $1/k$ (since these quantities are equal on the positive diagonal) in Eq. 6.1.
2. Into the result substitute "summation index" for its definition $S_{obs}(A$ in cmpd$)/S_{obs}(A)$.
3. Divide both sides by $S_{obs}(B)$.

Interpreting the Summation Index. The relationship in Eq. 6.2 between the summation index and the naive estimate means that the summation index is straightforward to interpret in one case, the case where (a) the intersection of the observer's thresholds with the positive diagonal is always a point on analyzer A's curve (there is no probability summation, no other analyzer interferes, etc.); (b) analyzer A is additive so its thresholds fall on a straight line; (c) the observer's thresholds for all values on the dimension of interest are identical (as may be at least approximately true on the orientation dimension, for example, and may also be true within restricted portions of most dimensions) so the distinction between relative intensity and absolute intensity can be ignored. In this one case, the value of the summation index minus 1.0 is simply proportional to the sensitivity of analyzer A to B.

If the analyzers are not additive, if the observer's threshold is determined by more than one analyzer, or if the psychophysical thresholds for all values are not equal, there will be no simple relationship between the summation index and underlying analyzer sensitivity. The next few sections illustrate qualitatively the ways in which these complications affect the summation index.

6.3 MORE SOPHISTICATED MULTIPLE-ANALYZERS MODELS

6.3.1 *Allowing for Probability Summation Among Analyzers*

As we have seen (Chaps. 4 and 5), evidence exists for probability summation (or equivalent nonlinear pooling) among analyzers sensitive to far-apart values on several pattern dimensions. Thus, there is reason to suppose that probability summation may exist among all analyzers on those dimensions, including between those sensitive to close values. Formally, the outputs of all analyzers on that dimension may be probabilistically independent, and Assumption 32 and its implication (Assumption 46) of the naive model should be replaced by Assumption 38:

Assumption 38. Probabilistically Independent Variability. *The output of each analyzer is variable and the outputs of different analyzers are probabilistically independent of one another.*

As earlier, the effect of assuming probability summation among analyzers is to make a compound stimulus more detectable than it would be in the case of deterministic analyzers, or, in other words, to increase the amount of summation measured psychophysically between the components. To illustrate this effect, the drawing from Fig. 6.1 for very close components is shown again in the left side of Fig. 6.5 but this time with the observer's intensity interrelationship function (dotted curve) bowed somewhat inside the corner where the two analyzer's intensity interrelationship functions intersect. The measured summation index (the reciprocal of the coordinates of the intersection of the observer's function with the positive diagonal) will now be somewhat larger than in the original deterministic model, as indicated on the right side of Fig. 6.5.

6.3.2   Allowing for More Than Two Analyzers

Suppose that, in addition to the two analyzers most sensitive to the two components (those shown in Fig. 6.1), there is a third analyzer quite sensitive to both components although less sensitive than analyzer A to component A and less sensitive than analyzer B to component B. (This third analyzer might be most sensitive to a value intermediate between those of A and B, for example.) As illustrated in the left panel of Fig. 6.6, it may be this third analyzer that will determine the psychophysical threshold for compound stimuli near the positive diagonal. In this case the summation index (right panel of Fig. 6.6) will be somewhat larger than in the original two-analyzer model. (The observer's intensity interrelationship function in Fig. 6.6 is drawn on the assumption of deterministic analyzers; the same kind of effect of a third analyzer will hold in the case where analyzers' outputs vary independently.)

6.3.3   Allowing for Nonadditive Summation Within an Analyzer

Suppose the thresholds for a single analyzer cannot be represented by a straight line on summation-square diagrams like those in Fig. 6.1. For example, in the case of spatial-frequency analyzers conceived of as arrays of mechanisms, probability summation across space or equivalent nonlinear spatial pooling means that an individual analyzer's intensity interrelationship function will not be a straight line but a curve, even if the phase between the components is peaks-add

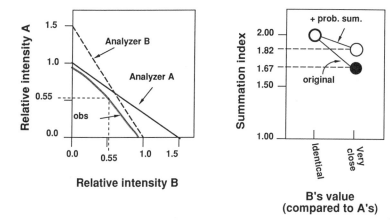

FIG. 6.5 Effect of probability summation across analyzers. The left panel shows the very-close summation square from Fig. 6.1 except that—as expected if there is independent variability in the output of the two analyzers (probability summation across analyzers)—the observer's threshold curve is now bowed somewhat inside that in the original figure. The observer's threshold curve now intersects the positive diagonal at (0.55, 0.55) rather than at (0.6, 0.6) as it did originally. Thus the summation index (right panel) is now 1.82 (open circles) rather than 1.67 (closed circles).

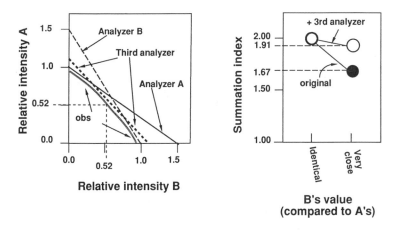

FIG. 6.6 Effect of intrusion of third analyzer. The left panel shows the very-close summation square from Fig. 6.1 except that it shows a threshold curve for a third analyzer that, for each component, has a threshold contrast 1.1 times that of the observer. The observer's threshold for compounds near the positive diagonal is now determined by that third analyzer, so the observer's curve now intersects the positive diagonal at (0.52, 0.52) rather than at (0.6, 0.6) as it did originally. Thus the summation index (right panel) is now 1.91 (open circles) rather than 1.67 (closed circles).

(e.g., Fig. 5.2 bottom). Figure 6.7 shows once again the summation square from Fig. 6.1 for the case of components very close together. Two different lines are shown for each analyzer, however, representing two different assumptions—straight lines for the additive assumption (exactly as in Fig. 6.1) and bowed-out curves for the nonadditive assumption. We will call analyzers with this kind of bowed-out intensity interrelationship function convexly nonadditive. (See note 1.) The case of nonadditive analyzers where the curvature is in the opposite direction has not yet arisen in the pattern-vision literature but could be dealt with in the analogous fashion and would produce the opposite effect.

As can be seen by examining Fig. 6.7, the observer's intensity interrelationship function determined by the curved analyzer functions is further from the origin than the observer's function (also not shown) determined by the straight lines. This is true whether the analyzers are assumed to be deterministic—as assumed in computing the summation index in the right panel of Fig. 6.7—or independently variable. Thus, the sensitivity of an observer with convexly nonadditive analyzers to compounds (e.g., the summation index in the right panel of Fig. 6.7) is less than that of an observer with additive analyzers when both observers have the same sensitivities to the components alone (the same intersections with the horizontal and vertical axes on summation squares).

6.3.4 Effects on Naive Bandwidth Estimates

Probability Summation Among Analyzers or Among More Than Two Analyzers. Compared with the case where there are two additive, deterministic

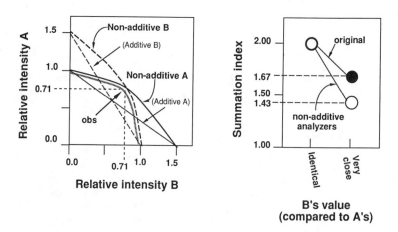

FIG. 6.7 Effect of nonadditive (nonlinear) analyzers. The left panel shows the very-close summation square from Fig. 6.1 except that the thresholds for each of the two analyzers now fall on a bowed-out curve rather than on a straight line. (The original straight lines are shown for comparison.) The observer's threshold curve is consequently also bowed out relative to that in the original case; it intersects the positive diagonal at (0.7, 0.7) rather than at (0.6, 0.6) as it did originally. Thus the summation index (right panel) is now 1.43 (open circles) rather than 1.67 (closed circles).

analyzers (Fig. 6.1), the effect either of assuming independent variability in the outputs of analyzers or of including more than two analyzers (Figs. 6.5 and 6.6) is to increase the amount of summation measured psychophysically, that is, to increase the observer's sensitivity to a compound stimulus relative to the components. Thus, although the bandwidth of analyzer A is the same in the naive and the more sophisticated models, the function giving summation index versus component B's value is wider—and the naive estimate of bandwidth consequently greater—than if there were only two deterministic analyzers. In short, if there is probability summation among analyzers or more than two analyzers, the naive estimate of bandwidth is an overestimate of the analyzer's bandwidth.

Convexly Nonlinear Analyzers. If analyzers are convexly nonadditive, however, less summation is measured than with additive analyzers. That is, a compound is less detectable relative to its components (Fig. 6.7). Thus, by the same logic as the preceding, the naive estimate of bandwidth will be an underestimate.

If we were lucky, the overestimates and underestimates would balance one another out, and the naive estimate of bandwith would be a good one. Such is not usually the case, however, as the more quantitative discussions that follow will show.

6.3.5 Procedures: Unbalanced Versus Balanced Intensities

Two procedures have commonly been used in summation experiments. In one, the thresholds are measured for three stimuli: the two components alone and a compound as close as possible to the positive diagonal.

In the other common experimental procedure, thresholds are measured for compounds in the very left of the summation square, compounds containing much more (at least a factor of 2 more) relative intensity in component A (the fixed component) than in the other varying component.

The second procedure has two disadvantages relative to the first (see note 2): (a) It is not measuring thresholds in the region most sensitive to the differences between models one is trying to investigate (near the diagonal; see Figs. 5.2, and 4.11 for examples); (b) It is trying to extrapolate from very small differences (between the threshold for component A by itself and the threshold for a compound containing mostly component A).

The second procedure does have some potential advantages, however. By staying away from the diagonal, it may also avoid some of the contaminating effects of probability summation among analyzers and of intermediate analyzers, since these effects are greatest near the diagonal. It seems unlikely, however, that this advantage outweighs the disadvantages.

6.3.6 Models and the Shape of Intensity Interrelationship Functions

If psychophysical data were good enough, the precise shape of the measured observer's intensity interrelationship would yield information about the correct model. For example, if there were only two additive, deterministic analyzers, there would be two linear segments to the curve. In fact, as the experimental results in Fig. 4.11 (which come from a very extended summation experiment) demonstrate, such details of shape would be difficult or impossible to find in measured functions.

Even the question of whether the function is linear at low intensities is less revealing than has sometimes been hoped. King-Smith and Kulikowski (1975b) compared the shapes of the psychophysical intensity interrelationship functions at low contrasts for pattern and flicker detection. Their functions for pattern were more linear than for flicker at low contrasts. This was consistent with the analyzers operative in pattern detection being additive and those in flicker being convexly nonadditive.

Unfortunately for this distinction, however, once the model is more complicated than two additive, deterministric analyzers, even additive analyzers can produce psychophysical functions at low intensities due to probability summation across analyzers and intrusion of intermediate analyzers (as in Figs. 6.5 and 6.6). Conversely, even if there are intermediate analyzers and probability summation among analyzers, you may get psychophysical intensity interrelationship functions that are very linear over a large range of low intensities (certainly for relative intensities in component B of up to 0.5), as example calculations show (e.g., Graham, 1977).

6.4   SUMMATION OF CLOSE SPATIAL FREQUENCIES

6.4.1   *Naive Estimates of Spatial-Frequency Analyzer Bandwidths*

Figure 6.8 shows typical results from experiments using close spatial frequencies. The summation index (called relative sensitivity by these authors) is plotted on the vertical scale and the difference between the two spatial frequencies on the horizontal scale. (These results are from Quick & Reichert (1975); the first such results were published by Sachs et al. (1971) and have been replicated many times since—e.g., Arend & Lange, 1980; Bergen, Wilson, & Cowan, 1979; Blake & Levinson, 1977; Kulikowski & King-Smith, 1973; Lange, Sigel, & Stecher, 1973; Watson, 1982a.)

Remember that if there were only two linear, deterministic analyzers, subtracting 1.0 from the quantity plotted on the vertical axis would give the sensitivity of an analyzer (except for the correction necessary for differences between the psychophysical thresholds of the first and second components, a relatively minor problem for spatial frequencies close together). The naive estimate of half-amplitude full-bandwidth—obtained by doubling the Δf at the point giving a summation index of 1.5—is definitely narrow, although a bit difficult to specify exactly from these results, since there is a plateau in the function at just about that height. (This plateau is of considerable theoretical significance as it turns out; see section 6.4.5.) Roughly, this bandwidth would be about 2 c/deg no matter what the spatial frequency, or equivalently, decreasing from about 0.5 to 0.16 octave with increasing spatial frequency over the range studied.

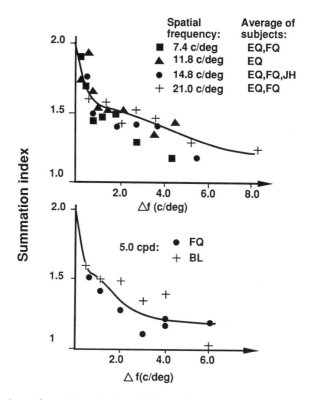

FIG. 6.8 Comparison of model predictions with experimental results from summation of close spatial frequencies. Compounds contained two frequencies spaced a distance Δ-*f* apart (plotted on the horizontal axis) centered at the frequency indicated by the symbol (see inset). The solid lines are the predictions of a multiple-analyzers model with probability summation across spatial frequencies and spatial positions. See text for further details. (Relabelled from Fig. 4 of Mullins, and Reichert, 1978; used by permission.)

Discussion of These Naive Estimates. To the extent that these naive bandwidth estimates were wrong in assuming the action of only two analyzers and the nonexistence of probability summation among analyzers, these estimates were too broad. Since, however, the original estimates were already very narrow (much narrower than those from adaptation and masking experiments, for example) and since Sachs et al. (1971) had carefully considered probability summation among analyzers, worry about the possible errors introduced in this direction were minimal.

To the extent that these original estimates were wrong in assuming additive (linearly acting) analyzers, however, the error was in the opposite direction, making the original spatial-frequency bandwidth estimates much too narrow. Further, as calculations show, the error can be quite large if the spatial-frequency analyzers are nonadditive in the manner expected from probability summation across space or equivalent nonlinear spatial pooling (Bergen et al., 1979; Graham & Rogowitz, 1976; King-Smith & Kulikowski, 1975a; Mostafavi & Sakrison, 1976; Quick et al., 1978; Stromeyer & Klein, 1975). The analogous problem in estimating the bandwidth of analyzers' sensitivity to auditory frequency was noted at approximately the same time (Hall & Sondhi, 1977).

6.4.2 Assumptions of Multiple-Mechanism Models Used to Estimate Bandwidth

Later estimates of the spatial-frequency bandwidth of analyzers are based on models allowing for probability summation (or some equivalent form of nonlinear pooling) across spatial frequency and spatial position and incorporating the effect of many analyzers. Subsection 6.4.3 will present three of these estimates by (a) Quick, Mullins, and Reichert, (b) Wilson and his colleagues, and (c) Watson. This section describes the multiple-mechanisms models used for these three estimates. Further details can be found in the original papers and in the appendix to this chapter.

Each analyzer in these models is a single mechanism that is selective for spatial frequency and (in principle) for both dimensions of spatial position. That is

Assumption 33. Multiple Analyzers. *There are N' multiple analyzers having different sensitivity functions along the dimensions of interest.*

Assumption 25. Single-Number Output. *To each presentation of a stimulus, the output of the analyzer can be represented as a single number.*

Assumption 26. Variable Output. *The output of an analyzer to presentations of the same stimulus is variable.*

Assumption 47. Additive (Linear-System) Analyzers. *The expected output of each mechanism in the model can be calculated as the product of a weighting function and the luminance profile of the stimulus.*

Assumption 37. Noninteracting Analyzers. *The outputs of one analyzer have no effects (excitatory or inhibitory) on any other analyzer. The output of each analyzer can always be calculated directly from the stimulus regardless of what other analyzers may or may not be doing.*

Assumption 7. Quick Pooling. *As observer's sensitivity to a stimulus is determined by probability summation across all analyzers or by equivalent nonlinear pooling.*

Exponents in the Quick pooling formula within the range from 3 to 5 are used below.

Assumption 48. Only One Spatial-Frequency Bandwidth of Analyzer. *Only one spatial-extent analyzer (only one spatial-frequency bandwidth of analyzer at each spatial frequency and spatial position) is assumed in any of these models.*

Selectivity Along Some Other Dimensions Ignored. Possible selective tuning along other dimensions—in particular, temporal frequency and orientation (except orientation in the model of Watson, 1983; see section 6.9.2)—and its possible interaction with spatial-frequency selectivity are also ignored in these calculations. Ignoring these factors may lead to an underestimate of spatial-frequency bandwidth, just as ignoring tuning on the spatial-position dimension does. The effect of this simplification is not too great, however, when the stimuli in any one experiment are constant along the other ignored dimensions, particularly not when the stimulus is narrow-band on these other dimensions, that is, contains only a small range of value (as has always been true for the orientation dimension and sometimes for the temporal-frequency dimension). The spatial-frequency bandwidth estimates derived, of course, can only apply to the orientation, temporal parameters, and so on, that were used in the particular experiment. Possible variations in spatial-frequency bandwidth as a function of these other dimensions is taken up in Chapter 12.

Phase Selectivity Irrelevant. Including weighting functions of odd symmetry as well as of even symmetry has been tried and apparently does not affect the calculations.

Other Details. Exact details of the calculations (for example, the exponent in the pooling formula, the shape of the analyzers' weighting function, the spacing of analyzers on the spatial-frequency dimension, the spacing of analyzers in the visual field, and the variation in sensitivity with spatial frequency and with eccentricity in the visual field) had, in fact, to be specified in the model in order to make the predictions. In general, the predictions seem not to be particularly sensitive to many of these factors.

6.4.3 *Spatial-Frequency Bandwidth Estimates From Multiple-Mechanisms Models*

Extended-Grating Summation. The solid curves in Fig. 6.8 are the predictions calculated by Quick et al. (1978) from a multiple-mechanisms model like that just described to compare with the data from Quick and Reichert (1975). The sharp drop or "needle" in the predicted curves at small frequency separations is due almost entirely to probability summation (or equivalent nonlinear pooling) across spatial position (futher discussed in section 6.4.5). At larger frequency separations there is a more gradual decrease in sensitivity—the *skirt*. This skirt is a fairly accurate although scaled-down version of the function giving a single analyzer's relative sensitivity at each frequency separation. For the results at 5 c/deg in the bottom panel of Fig. 6.8, the curve shown is the prediction assuming a half-amplitude full-bandwidth of about 3.5 c/deg in a Gaussian-shaped analyzer-sensitivity function. The curve in the top panel for the higher spatial frequencies assumes a bandwidth twice as large (about 7 c/deg). In octaves, these assumed bandwidths vary from about one octave at 5 c/deg to slightly less than that at 12 c/deg, decreasing to about half an octave at 21 c/deg.

How stable these bandwidth estimates are is not clear. The major problem is the intrinsic variability in experimental estimates of the summation index coupled with the limited possible height of the skirt of the function. When there is probability summation across spatial position, the maximal amount of summation possible between any two nonidentical spatial frequencies (using extended gratings on a uniform retina) corresponds to a summation index of about 1.6 for exponents near 4. (See, e.g., the full summation-square plots in Fig. 5.2 for the case of a single spatial-frequency analyzer.) The minimal amount of summation possible between any two spatial frequencies when there is probability summation across spatial frequencies (even if no analyzer responds to both frequencies) corresponds to a summation index of about 1.2 for exponents near 4. Thus there is only the range between summation indices of about 1.2 and 1.6 in which to measure the spatial-frequency bandwidth of an analyzer accurately.

Not only does a good deal of variability necessarily exist in the summation index computed from experimental results, but the variability is hard to estimate. (For one thing, in the experiment of Fig. 6.8 the thresholds of some of the simple gratings were determined at times quite removed from the thresholds for the compound. The commonly found existence of shifts in sensitivity between sessions makes this procedure less than optimal.) And the predictions from different bandwidths do not differ all that greatly.

Wilson's Estimates. In fact, Bergen, Wilson, and Cowan (1979, Fig. 13) claimed that much larger spatial-frequency bandwidths of the sort incorporated in their models (see section 6.9.1 for more details) can account satisfactorily for the Quick and Reichert (1975) data, although their prediction, as they pointed out, is slightly too broad.

They also measured (a) the thresholds for single sinusoidal gratings (Wilson & Bergen, 1979) and (b) thresholds for compound gratings containing two frequencies (Bergen et al., 1979) and compared the data with predictions from their model. Their fits were good. But in predictions for single gratings, several factors—bandwidth, number of analyzers, and peak sensitivities of analyzers—will trade off: If you assume smaller bandwidths, you will need more analyzers to predict the thresholds of single gratings, that is all. And the compound gratings used by Wilson and his colleagues were rather far from the diagonal of the summation square—the relative contrast of one component in the compound gratings was twice that of the other component—which reduces the differences between predictions of different models (in particular between models assuming different bandwidths).

Summation of Grating Patches and Watson's Estimates. The limitations placed on full-grating summation experiments by spatial probability summation suggest using small patches of grating. Two close spatial frequencies will sum more completely in patches than in full gratings if the patches are small enough. Watson (1982a) measured thresholds near the diagonal of the summation square for compounds containing patches of two spatial frequencies, either 1 or 16 c/deg paired with some higher frequency. He compared these results with predictions from the four-mechanisms model of Wilson and his colleagues and from models postulating narrower spatial-frequency bandwidths (e.g., half-amplitude full-bandwidths of 0.25, 0.75, and one octave). As it turned out, a bandwidth of 0.25 octave is probably too small and a bandwidth of 0.75 or one octave is probably too large both at 1 and 16 c/deg. The overall best estimate of analyzer bandwidth is about 0.50 octave. A later model of Watson's incorporating mechanisms of different orientations as well as spatial position (1983; see section 6.9.2) uses a one-octave half-amplitude full-bandwidth and leads to predicted summation results that are slightly too wide. A 0.8 octave bandwidth seems about right in that model.

The model of Wilson and his colleagues (because of its greater than one-octave bandwidths) clearly predicts too much summation for these grating-patch results. I tend to think that Wilson's experiments were too insensitive to bandwidth, and that the narrower bandwidths are closer to correct for typical experimental conditions and subject. See further discussion in notes 3 and 4.

Number of Different Spatial-Frequency Mechanisms Estimated From Summation Results. Watson (1982a) argued that his results imply the existence of a minimum of seven mechanisms in the fovea serving the frequency range between 1 and 32 c/deg and probably (accepting 0.50 octave as the analyzer bandwidth) at least 20 mechanisms.

The models of Wilson and his colleagues can include fewer different spatial-frequency mechanisms at any one location because the bandwidths are broader. Only four mechanisms were included at the fovea (covering the range from 1 to 16 c/deg) in the models they compared with spatial-frequency summation results, although later models have included more.

6.4.4 Spatial Weighting Functions Corresponding to the Spatial-Frequency Bandwidth Estimates

Taking the inverse Fourier transform of an analyzer's sensitivity as a function of spatial frequency can give a plot of the mechanism's sensitivity as a function of spatial position (i.e., the spatial weighting function) as long as some assumption about spatial phase is made. An assumption either of perfect even symmetry or perfect odd symmetry is quite sufficient (and plausible in the spatial case) and is often made.

The top panel of Fig. 6.9 shows an odd-symmetric weighting function corresponding to the spatial-frequency sensitivity function shown in the bottom panel—a 0.78-octave half-amplitude full-bandwidth Gaussian function. The Gabor function has 1.67 cycles at half-amplitude (or, equivalently, 2.8 cycles within plus and minus 2 standard deviations of the center). Were the bandwidth (in octave or logarithmic terms, or equivalently, linear bandwidth divided by peak frequency) narrower, as suggested for high spatial frequencies by Watson (1982a) and by Quick et al. (1978), there would be even more excitatory-inhibitory cycles. Were the bandwidth broader, as in the four-mechanisms model of Bergen, Wilson, and Cowan (1979), there would be fewer (see section 6.9.1).

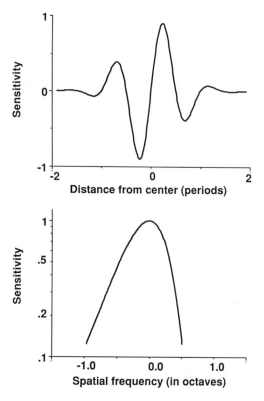

FIG. 6.9 A weighting function (top) and the amplitude of its Fourier transform normalized to be 1.0 at the peak frequency (bottom). (From Figure 7 in Watson in 1982a; used by permission.)

6.4.5   Summation of Very-Close Spatial Frequencies Is Predicted by Spatial Probability Summation and Spatial Nonuniformity

According to the multiple-mechanisms models, the sharp drop in sensitivity found as the frequency difference increases from zero—the needle in Fig. 6.8— is primarily a result of spatial probability summation (or equivalent nonlinear spatial pooling) across the beat pattern present in the compound (e.g., Hall & Sondhi, 1977; Quick et al., 1978). The width of the needle does not depend, therefore, on the spatial-frequency bandwidth of the analyzers. It does depend strongly on the function relating sensitivity to position in the visual field, because that function determines how much of the beat pattern in the compound is effectively seen by the eye. This dependence is described at some length in Graham and Robson (1987), who attempt to provide intuitions behind it.

To briefly describe this dependence: According to these multiple-mechanisms models, the more uniform the sensitivity, the narrower the needle should be. In the extreme case, where sensitivity is uniform over an infinite visual field, the needle would have zero width, and as soon as the components were not of absolutely identical spatial frequency (as soon as the spatial-frequency difference was greater than zero, no matter how small the nonzero difference), the summation index would fall from its value of 2.0 (for identical components) to a much smaller value (about 1.6 depending on the exponent in the model).

Two consequences of this general prediction were tested. (a) The needle measured in the very nonuniform foveal region should be wider than the needle measured in a nearly uniform peripheral region. (b) Since sensitivity falls off faster with distance from the fovea for higher spatial frequencies than for low (when distance is measured in degrees of visual angle; e.g., Fig. 5.6), the needle should be narrower (plotted against frequency difference as in Fig. 6.8) for summation experiments done in a high spatial frequency range than in a low range. (The needle should be about the same width when plotted against frequency ratio, however; cf. top of Fig. 5.6.)

Both predictions were quantitatively consistent with the results (Graham & Robson, 1987). The summation of very-close spatial frequencies—at least under these experimental conditions—is quite well predicted by multiple-mechanisms models incorporating probability summation across space and the measured fall-off in sensitivity with eccentricity.

Interestingly, a similar needle occurs in the summation of auditory frequencies. From the form of this needle, Hall and Sondhi (1977) deduced the properties of the nonlinear temporal integration mechanism (the analogue in their case to spatial probability summation coupled with sensitivity as a function of spatial position in this case).

6.5   SUMMATION OF CLOSE ORIENTATIONS

Grating Stimuli. Naive estimates of orientation bandwidth are very narrow. For example, in the earliest study, sensitivity dropped to a half when the angle between the two gratings was only 3 angular degrees yielding a half-peak-amplitude bandwidth of 6 angular degrees (Kulikowski et al., 1973). The results shown in the left panel of Fig. 6.10 (using 13.5 cpd and a "sustained" time course containing predominantly low temporal frequencies) lead to a similarly narrow naive estimate of orientation bandwidth, whereas the results in the right panel (using 3.4 cpd and a transient time course containing no low temporal frequencies) lead to a somewhat larger naive estimate.

Spatial probability summation affects orientation bandwidth estimates in the same way it affects spatial-frequency bandwidth estimates. If there is spatial probability summation, an analyzer's sensitivity to a stimulus is determined not only by the peak in the average output profile but by the number of locations at which that peak occurs. When the stimulus is a compound grating containing two orientations, there are fewer locations in the average output profile at which peak or near-peak responses occur than when the stimulus is a simple grating (cf. Fig. 5.1, although the orientations would have to be somewhat closer

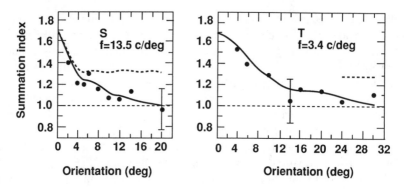

FIG. 6.10 Summation of orientations. The two components were sinusoidal gratings that differed in orientation (horizontal axis) but both had the same spatial frequency and time course (13.5 cpd and a sustained time course in left panel; 3.4 cpd and a transient time course in right panel). See text for more details. (From Figures 7 and 8 in Phillips & Wilson, 1984; used by permission.)

together than those in Fig. 5.1 to make it reasonable that an individual analyzer of a multiple-analyzers model would respond to both orientations). Thus, there is less summation between components of different orientation when probability summation across space exists than when it does not, and the orientation bandwidth derived assuming no probability summation across space is too narrow if, in fact, there is probability summation across space.

Spatial probability summation was explicitly considered by Phillips and Wilson (1984) in the analysis of their orientation-summation results. They used the Quick pooling formula. On the basis of other (masking) studies, they had estimated half-amplitude full-bandwidth for orientation to range from 60 angular degrees at a very low spatial frequency (½ c/deg) to about 30 angular degrees at a medium spatial frequency (8 c/deg). They then used these values to predict the results of the orientation-summation experiments shown in Fig. 6.10. The fit of these predictions, shown as solid lines, is quite satisfactory. But it is also apparent from the scatter of the data points and the indicated error bars that equally satisfactory fits could be obtained with a good deal broader or narrower bandwidths.

Some predictions of a single-orientation-analyzer model (e.g., one in which all weighting functions were circularly symmetric) are shown by the dashed curves. Notice the needle in the predicted curve at very close orientations (in the left panel); it is exactly analogous to the needle for very-close spatial frequencies. Another orientation bandwidth estimate is briefly described in note 4.

Line Stimuli. When thin lines differing in orientation by 5 angular degrees were used, the compound was more detectable than either component; at 15 degrees difference in orientation, however—the next smallest difference used— there was not summation, but inhibition (Thomas & Shimamura, 1975). This suggests a crude upper limit to orientation bandwidth of something less than 15 degrees, which is not out of line with the estimates previously given. (The region at the intersection of the lines, however, was the same contrast as the rest of the line, so the compound was not quite a true sum. The "inhibition" is also a complication.)

To date, there are few estimates of orientation bandwidth from summation studies, and the range of uncertainty left by the existing estimates is large. Possible changes of orientation bandwidth with other parameters—in particular, spatial frequency—are considered in Chapter 12.

6.6 SUMMATION OF CLOSE SPATIAL POSITIONS

In the framework of multiple-mechanisms models, compound stimuli containing components close together on the spatial-position dimension (e.g., adjacent lines or small bits of sinusoidal grating) should be more detectable than the individual components as a result of summation within a single mechanism (a single spatial-position analyzer). In fact, a number of such summation experiments have been done in an attempt to derive the spatial weighting functions of individual mechanisms. As we will see, however, the interpretation of these spatial-position summation experiments is just as dependent on assumptions about spatial-frequency and orientation analyzers as the interpretation of spatial-frequency and orientation summation experiments was dependent on assumptions about multiple spatial-position analyzers.

6.6.1 *Increasing the Spatial Extent of a Stimulus*

Varying the Number of Cycles in a Grating. Any estimate of a spatial weighting function from increasing the number of cycles in a grating will be very tricky, because frequency spread will disguise the summation within individual analyzers. (See section 5.4.1.) It is unlikely, therefore, that such experiments could distinguish between subtle differences in spatial weighting functions. On the other hand, the fact that all the summation as the number of cycles is increased from 2—and certainly as it is increased from 4 (in Fig. 5.7)—can be accounted for by spatial probability summation is completely consistent with a weighting function containing very few cycles (e.g., those in Fig. 6.9). See note 5 for a (suprathreshold) variant.

Varying the Length of Bars in a Grating. In using the effects of increasing length to estimate orientation bandwidth, the same problems arise as in using the effects of increasing number of cycles to estimate spatial-frequency bandwidth. (See section 5.4.3.) One must consider orientation spread (the fact that gratings contain a wider and wider range of orientations as the bars get shorter) as well as spatial probability summation and spatial nonuniformity. To date, in any case, no satisfactory estimate of orientation bandwidth has been calculated from such studies.

6.6.2   *Summation of Parallel Lines at Different Separations*

A large number of studies have varied the distance between two lines or between a center line and two flanking lines and measured the sensitivity for the compound as a function of separation (e.g., Blommaert & Roufs, 1981; Hines, 1976; King-Smith & Kulikowski, 1975a, 1975b; Kulikowski & King-Smith, 1973; Limb & Rubenstein, 1977; Wilson, 1978a; Wilson & Bergen, 1979; Wilson et al., 1979). Some typical results (from Wilson and Bergen, 1978) are shown as the data points in Fig. 6.11 where the compound contained a center line (component A) and two flanking lines (component B) where each flanking line contained three eighths the contrast of the center line. The separation between each flanking line and the center line is given on the horizontal axis. The sensitivity measure plotted on the vertical axis is the reciprocal of the contrast of the center line when the compound is at the observer's threshold—that is, S_{obs}(A in cmpd). This (by Eq. 6.1) is simply a scaled (by three fourths) and translated upward [by S_{obs}(A)] version of the naive estimate of the S_A(B)—the sensitivity of the center line's mechanism to the flanking lines. If the naive estimate were justified, the sensitivity function it generated would be equivalent to the one-dimensional spatial weighting function of an individual mechanism.

In Fig. 6.11, the sensitivity to the compound declines as separation is increased, reaching a minimum (typically at 0.1 degree or less) and then, at least

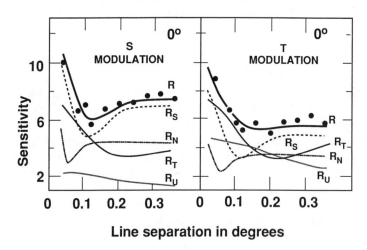

Line separation in degrees

FIG. 6.11 Summation of close spatial positions. The sensitivity to a compound stimulus is plotted as a function of difference between its components' spatial positions (the distance between a central line and each of two flanking lines). The flanking lines had three eighths the contrast of the central line. Both panels show results when the central line is at the fixation point; the left panel shows results for a sustained time course and the right panel for a transient time course. R_N, R_S, R_T, and R_U are the sensitivities to the compound of the individual mechanisms in the four-mechanisms model; R is the sensitivity of the observer predicted by that model. [From Figure 8 in Wilson & Bergen (1979); used by permission.]

for the sustained time courses that are typically used (e.g., left panel) climbs again at far separations, although never reaching a level as high as for very-close separations. Usually, as in these results, there is no overshoot or secondary excitatory lobe in the function. That is, after having reached a minimum, sensitivity climbs steadily toward an asymptote equal to the observer's sensitivity for the center line by itself (or perhaps slightly higher due to spatial probability summation if the other lines are of contrast comparable to the center line). There has been one report of a secondary excitatory lobe, by Rentschler and Hilz (1976), but it seems to occur only in what is basically a masking paradigm (see note 2), and may reflect discrimination strategies quite different from the detection rules in the models here.

In interpreting these line-plus-line experiments, the problems of spatial probability summation and, more subtly but even more importantly, of spatial-frequency spread reappear. As the separation between two lines increases from zero, the spatial-frequency content changes dramatically from very wide band (at separation zero) to a spectrum that is still wide band but is dominated by the frequency equal to the reciprocal of the interline separation. Thus, at different separations between the lines, different populations of spatial-frequency analyzers (different sizes of weighting-function centers) may be detecting the lines.

Figure 6.11 shows an example of this. Here the four-mechanism model of Wilson and his colleagues (see section 6.9.1) is used to predict the results given by the data points. The four lower lines give the sensitivity of each of the four mechanisms. The upper solid line is the model's prediction of the observer's sensitivity, which results from probability summation among the four separate mechanisms and is, thus, roughly the envelope of the four. It is clear in Fig. 6.11 that the four-mechanisms model does quite a good job at predicting this experiment and that—according to this model—different mechanisms are primarily responsible for detecting the compound at different separations.

Spatial-Frequency Bandwidth Estimates. Such line-plus-line experiments are probably not a particularly sensitive way to deduce the details of the spatial weighting functions (e.g., the exact spatial-frequency bandwidth), however. Even with only four mechanisms postulated, as in this figure, the characteristics of any one may be disguised. Note in particular, in the case of T modulation, that the observer's threshold at very small separations is determined by the S and T mechanisms, which are equally sensitive. Then at low to medium separations, the T mechanism is most sensitive. At medium to large separations, the S mechanism is most sensitive. At very large separations both S and T are almost equally sensitive again. If the true spatial-frequency bandwidth of individual mechanisms were narrower there would be even more mechanisms and more shifting among them.

In particular, weighting functions with secondary excitatory lobes outside the inhibitory lobes (corresponding to narrower bandwidth analyzers than those used by Wilson) could predict psychophysical results like these in which there is no secondary excitatory lobe. Any one such weighting function would predict a second rise in sensitivity (sometimes called disinhibition) at medium line separations. But overall, no such rise would be seen in the psychophysical results if the effects of the secondary excitatory lobes in weighting functions having smaller width lobes were outweighed by the effects of the inhibitory lobes in weighting functions having larger width lobes. Since probability summation among different analyzers emphasizes the ones with larger outputs; however, the secondary excitatory lobes would need to be fairly small to be so outweighed. Thus, the fact that most investigators doing line-plus-line experiments have found no secondary excitatory lobe may well put some limits on how narrow the spatial-frequency bandwidth of the analyzers involved in detecting these lines could be. (See Wilson, 1978a, for some calculations.) For example, these results may rule out analyzers that have spatial-frequency bandwidths as narrow as 0.5 octave at all spatial frequencies. On the other hand, spatial-frequency bandwidths as narrow as 0.5 octave at the higher spatial frequencies (e.g., a half-amplitude full-bandwidth of 4 c/deg at 20 c/deg) and wider at the lower ones are clearly consistent with these results.

6.6.3 Increasing the Width of Aperiodic Stimuli (Areal Summation Experiments)

Many experiments increasing the width of aperiodic stimuli have been done, for example, classic areal summation experiments. Within the framework of multiple-mechanisms models, the results of any such experiment depend on the precise balance of sensitivities and other characteristics of many types of mechanisms. As the width of an aperiodic stimulus is changed, the spatial-frequency content changes dramatically, thus changing which populations of mechanisms (which sizes of weighting-function centers) are maximally stimulated.

Thomas (1970) presented the earliest interpretation of the results of this kind of experiment within the theoretical framework of mechanisms having different sizes of weighting-function centers. The smallest aperiodic stimuli are detected by mechanisms having the smallest weighting-function centers. As stimulus width is increased, if there were only a single size of weighting-function center, sensitivity would stop increasing once the stimulus was bigger than this center. Further, sensitivity would actually decrease as the disk encroached on the one weighting functions' inhibitory surround. With multiple mechanisms, however, as stimulus width is increased, mechanisms having larger and larger weighting-function centers take turns becoming the most sensitive mechanism and determining the observer's threshold for the disk. Thus, an inhibitory segment is never seen in the psychophysical function. Probability summation between mechanisms of different sizes will smooth out any local dips in the curve.

Wilson (1978b) and Wilson and Bergen (1979) presented their four-mechanisms model's predictions for variations in width of two kinds of aperiodic stimuli: half cycles of cosine gratings and stimuli having a difference-of-Gaussians luminance profile. It is these analyses in fact that drove these investigators to postulate at least four mechanisms (four sizes of receptive field at a single position).

Blommaert and Roufs (1981) started out trying to explain the results of a classic areal summation experiment (increasing the radius of a disk) with only a single size of weighting function. That weighting function was specified by the naive estimate from varying the separation between two localized stimuli (a point and an annulus) plus some considerations of inhomogeneity. The single-weighting-function predictions do not fit the experimental results for large disk sizes. These investigators ended up using a model with four sizes of weighting function; it predicts the results quite well. (Any number of sizes between three and infinity would probably have done as well.)

6.7 SUMMATION OF CLOSE SPATIAL FREQUENCIES— INTERACTION WITH SPATIAL EXTENT

6.7.1 *Aperiodic Test Stimuli Added to Sinusoidal Gratings*

Figure 6.12 shows results of "test-plus-sine" summation experiments in which one component was an aperiodic "test" stimulus and the second component was a sinusoidal grating (Kulikowski & King-Smith, 1973; Shapley & Tolhurst, 1973). The luminance profile of the aperiodic test stimulus is shown as an inset. A number of different spatial frequencies of sinusoidal grating were used, and spatial frequency is plotted on the horizontal axis.

Although the two components in this experiment differed both in spatial extent (i.e., spatial-frequency bandwidth, with the aperiodic stimulus having much wider spatial-frequency bandwidth than the sine) and in central spatial frequency, it is on the spatial-frequency dimension that the two stimuli are sometimes close.

The solid points give the "naive" estimates of the sensitivity of one analyzer (the analyzer most responsive to the aperiodic test stimulus—it would be called analyzer A in section 6.2) to the component of spatial-frequency f (component B in section 6.2). This estimate will be called $S_{\text{test}}(f)$ here. The curves through the points are predictions discussed shortly. (The top curves in each panel show $S_{\text{obs}}(f)$—the observer's sensitivity to a sinusoidal grating of frequency f.)

6.7.2 *Interpretation in Terms of Multiple Analyzers on the Spatial-Extent Dimension*

These test-plus-sine results were originally interpreted as evidence for the existence of multiple analyzers on the spatial-extent dimension. In favor of this interpretation is the fact that there is incomplete (less than linear or additive) summation between test and sine; this shows up in Fig. 6.12 as the fact that $S_{\text{test}}(f)$ is always less than $S_{\text{obs}}(f)$.

On this interpretation the data points plotted in any panel of Fig. 6.12 were taken as the sensitivities of a particular analyzer to different spatial frequencies; that is, they were taken to be the amplitude characteristic of the Fourier transform of a particular weighting function. Note that these sensitivity functions are

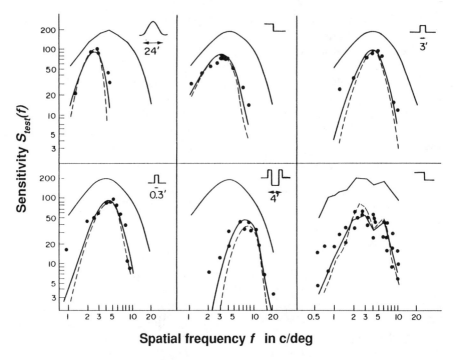

Spatial frequency f in c/deg

FIG. 6.12 Summation of stimuli differing in spatial extent and spatial frequency. Each compound stimulus contained a many-cycle sinusoidal grating of spatial frequency f (on the horizontal axis) and a localized aperiodic test stimulus (the luminance profile inset in the upper right of each panel). The vertical axis gives S_{test} (f)—the naive estimate of the test-stimulus's analyzer's sensitivity to a sinusoidal grating of frequency f. The solid circles show experimental results. Those in the lower right panel are from Shapley and Tolhurst (1973) plotted at one third their actual value. Those in the other panels are from Kulikowski and King-Smith (1973). The lower two curves in each panel are predictions from two slightly different versions of a model assuming only one spatial-frequency bandwidth of analyzer with probability summation among analyzers. The upper curve in each panel is the observer's sensitivity to sinusoidal gratings (the psychophysical contrast sensitivity function). (From Figure 3 in Graham, 1977; used by permission.)

quite wide, much wider than the width obtained when using a sinusoidal grating as a test stimulus (e.g., Fig. 6.8). Hence if these estimates are accepted, the analyzer detecting an aperiodic stimulus has broader spatial-frequency bandwidth than that detecting a sinusoidal grating. In other words, multiple spatial-frequency bandwidths of analyzer exist, or equivalently, multiple analyzers exist on the spatial-extent dimension (at a given spatial frequency, orientation, and spatial position).

   In still further support of their interpretation, the original investigators made quantitative predictions from these broad-band analyzers for various other compounds—like edges and lines added together—and for the edges or lines by themselves and checked them against results. The predictions worked quite well.

6.7.3 Interpretation in Terms of Pooling Across Different Spatial-Frequency Analyzers With Only a Single Analyzer on the Spatial-Extent Dimension

The bothersome thing about the original interpretation is that probability summation among analyzers sensitive to different spatial frequencies and spatial positions has been overlooked. The assumption of the naive model that there is no probability summation was a reasonable one to begin with—particularly since it is much easier to work with in this very complicated situation and did lead to nice predictions. But, as Jack Nachmias pointed out to me, the known probability summation should not be completely ignored. As briefly described in the next paragraph, qualitative considerations suggested that a model involving probability summation across spatial frequencies might explain the results very well even if there were only a single analyzer on the spatial-extent dimension (only a single spatial-frequency bandwidth of analyzer).

Consider the following argument: An aperiodic test stimulus contains a broad range of spatial frequencies activating a range of analyzers sensitive to different spatial frequencies. All of the analyzers sensitive to any spatial frequency contained in the aperiodic test stimulus will play some role, even if minor, in determining the threshold for the test stimulus. Therefore, if a sinusoid anywhere in that range of spatial frequencies is added to the test stimulus, the activity in some analyzer responsive to the test stimulus is increased. Consequently, the contrast in the test stimulus necessary for the test-plus-sine compound to be at psychophysical threshold is less than that for the test stimulus alone. On this argument, the amount by which the added sine wave reduces the necessary test contrast [this amount is the operational definition of the quantity $S_{test}(f)$] should depend on how much of the frequency is contained in the test stimulus to begin with. Notice in Fig. 6.12 that, indeed, when a blurry bar—which contains only low spatial frequencies—was used (upper left), $S_{test}(f)$ was nonzero only at low spatial frequencies. When a triphasic light-dark-light pattern—which contains only high spatial frequencies—was used (lower middle Fig. 6.12), $S_{test}(f)$ was nonzero only at high spatial frequencies. (A fuller description of these intuitions can be found in Graham, 1980.)

The two lower curves in each panel of Fig. 6.12 are predictions from slightly different versions of a model in which (a) only a single spatial-frequency bandwidth of analyzer exists at each spatial frequency and this bandwidth is consistent with estimates from the summation of close spatial frequencies (section 6.4), and (b) probability summation among spatial frequencies is allowed. These predictions fit the data very well indeed. (Including probability summation across space, although it can be done, is relatively unimportant, because with or without it the results can be predicted. It does, of course, affect the spatial-frequency bandwidth estimates in the usual way.)

Although details of the procedures necessary to generate these calculations are not general enough to be worth going into here (see Graham 1977, 1980), it might be worth pointing out that considerably fewer parameters are involved in these predictions than in the original interpretation.

Although not conveniently shown on Fig. 6.12, another prediction of the models was successful (Graham, 1977): The threshold for each test stimulus alone is successfully accounted for by the model at the same time it accounts for $S_{test}(f)$. Thus, for these experimental results in any case, the thresholds for thin lines are consistent with the existence of only one spatial-frequency bandwidth of analyzer where that bandwidth is narrow enough to be consistent with sine-plus-sine results (but see appendix A, part 2 of Klein and Levi, 1985).

Subsequent test-plus-sine experiments of King-Smith and Kulikowski (1975b) have also been predicted with the same success. Still a further test-plus-sine experiment by Hauske, Wolf, and Lupp (1976) has not been similarly modeled, but the results are very much like those of the earlier experiments. The investigators quantitatively described their results, in fact, by almost exactly the same function used in Graham (1980).

Conclusion. Summation-at-threshold results from experiments using compounds of aperiodic test stimuli and sinusoidal gratings provide no compelling evidence for more than a single analyzer on the spatial-extent dimension (at a given spatial frequency, orientation, spatial position, etc.). The original interpretation of these experiments in terms of multiple analyzers on the spatial-extent dimension might still be correct, but then the question of what happened in this situation to the probability summation among spatial-frequency analyzers has to be dealt with. Notice that, even if only a single analyzer on the spatial-extent dimension is important in determining the thresholds for all these patterns, there may be some less sensitive analyzers (too insensitive to detect these compounds at threshold) which are of smaller spatial extent (i.e., of broader spatial-frequency bandwidth) and operate above threshold. Indeed, much suprathreshold evidence is consistenct with the existence of broader spatial-frequency bandwidth analyzers (e.g., Klein & Levi, 1985; Nachmias & Weber, 1975), as is the known neurophysiology (see section 12.7.1).

6.7.4   *Matched Filters*

Hauske et al. (1976) had a rather different explanation of their test-plus-sine results than the models here. Their explanation is an interesting idea in its own right, and also points to an interesting attribute of models involving probability summation or similar nonlinear pooling. They interpreted $S_{test}(f)$ as the result of the processing of the aperiodic test stimulus by a "matched filter"—a filter designed to optimally detect that one particular aperiodic test stimulus in white noise (filtered through the contrast sensitivity function of the human). Thus it is as if the visual system were constructing a filter matched to the particular requirements of the task.

On the multiple-analyzers models here, the visual system does not literally change its wiring at some lower level to produce a matched filter. However, the existence of multiple analyzers on various dimensions (spatial frequency, spatial position) with some nonlinear pooling (e.g., probability summation) among them means that the subset of analyzers responsible for detection does change from stimulus to stimulus. Thus the model acts much as if a new matched filter were being constructed for each stimulus being detected.

6.8 SUMMARY

One common and simple way of estimating analyzer bandwidth from a summation experiment on any dimension assumes that analyzers are additive and deterministic and that the observer's thresholds for all the compounds in the experiment are determined by the same analyzer or by two symmetric analyzers. These "naive" bandwidth estimates are too broad if there is probability summation among analyzers or if there are other analyzers sensitive to the compound. These naive estimates are too narrow to the extent that individual analyzers are nonadditive rather than additive.

For spatial-frequency and orientation summation experiments, the last-mentioned factor (the nonadditivity) turns out to be much more important than the first two. Thus recent estimates from multiple-mechanisms models of spatial-frequency and orientation bandwidths are a good deal broader than the early naive estimates based on the simpler assumptions. Current estimates suggest half-amplitude full-bandwidths of something like one octave on the spatial frequency dimension (increasing somewhat on a logarithmic scale as spatial frequency gets lower) and perhaps 30 degrees of orientation. (These estimates are not yet very precise and should be taken cautiously. For those interested in modeling, the appendix to this chapter gives the spatial parameters of two current multiple-mechanisms models. Notice that the bulk of the estimates come from conditions involving low to medium temporal frequencies. Possible changes in bandwidth with other conditions are reviewed in Chapter 12.)

Results from spatial-position summation experiments also seem consistent with current multiple-mechanisms models, but they may be consistent with any of a wide range of spatial-frequency and/or orientation bandwidths. The absence of a secondary excitatory lobe in the line-plus-line results may rule out half-amplitude full-bandwidths as narrow as 0.5 octave at all spatial frequencies (although it is consistent with that narrow a bandwidth at high spatial frequencies if there is a larger bandwidth at low). The results from increasing the width of periodic stimuli (gratings) or aperiodic stimuli (classic areal summation experiments) are certainly consistent with these models, although they probably put few constraints on exact parameters of the model. When these results are coupled with line-plus-line results, the absence of an inhibitory lobe and the range of widths over which increased sensitivity occurs may be sufficient to rule out the notion of only one or two sizes of weighting-function centers at a single location.

The results of aperiodic-test-plus-sine summation experiments (where the components differ in both spatial extent and spatial frequency) were originally interpreted in terms of multiple analyzers on the spatial-extent dimension (multiple spatial-frequency bandwidths of analyzers), but they can be interpreted at least as well in terms of probability summation among analyzers on the spatial-frequency dimension with only a single analyzer on the spatial-extent dimension (only a single spatial-frequency bandwidth of analyzer).

6.9 APPENDIX. DETAILS OF TWO MULTIPLE-MECHANISMS MODELS

6.9.1 *The Four-Mechanisms Model of Wilson and His Colleagues*

The 1979 model of Wilson and his colleagues (Bergen et al., 1979; Wilson & Bergen, 1979) is illustrated in Fig. 6.13. It contains only four sizes of weighting-function centers at each location in the visual field, but contains many more sizes altogether, since these sizes vary with eccentricity. The temporal characteristics of the outputs of these four mechanisms differ, the mechanisms having larger weighting-function centers (sensitive to lower spatial frequencies) also having faster, more transient outputs than the mechanisms with smaller weighting-function centers (see bar graphs on right of Fig. 6.13). In the fovea, the half-amplitude bandwidths of the two smaller mechanisms (whose peak sensitivities are centered at 4.4 and 8.8 c/deg and whose temporal responses are sustained) are about 1.5 octave. (Bandwidth at 71% peak is one octave; Wilson & Bergen, 1979, p. 28. Half-amplitude full-bandwidth is about 1.5 times as big.) The two weighting functions in the fovea having the larger excitatory centers have no inhibitory surround at all, so their sensitivity as a function of spatial frequency extends unattenuated down to zero spatial frequency, making their bandwidth in octaves infinite.

The increase in size with eccentricty is illustrated in Fig. 6.13.

The parameters for this four-mechanism model were derived from the results of experiments using aperiodic stimuli, primarily line-plus-line experiments at a number of different eccentricities. Initially, in fact, the two line-sensitivity functions collected under sustained and transient time courses (e.g., Fig. 6.11) were simply corrected for probability summation across space and taken to represent two different sizes of weighting functions at a given spatial location [with the nonuniformity of the visual field taken into account by measuring these two line-sensitivity functions at many positions (Wilson, 1978b)]. This assumption of only two weighting functions per location proved inadequate to explain thresholds for stimuli other than line-plus-line compounds [e.g., the thresholds for different widths of DOG stimuli (differences of Gaussian functions and much like 1.5 cycles of a grating) and also the thresholds for sinusoidal gratings of relatively low and high spatial frequency]. The model was expanded to include the minimum number of extra weighting functions at each position to account for the stimuli's thresholds to the investigator's satisfaction. This number was two, so the expanded model contained four (Bergen et al., 1979; Wilson

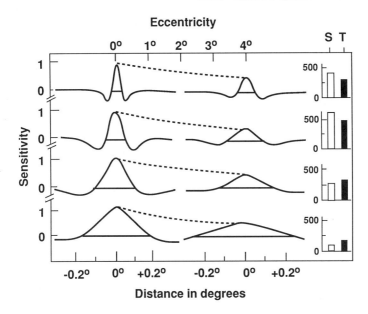

FIG. 6.13 Summary diagram of Wilson and Bergen's (1979) four-mechanisms model. The line-spread function (the spatial weighting function integrated along one dimension) is plotted for each of the four mechanisms centered at the fixation point (left) and for each of the four mechanisms centered at an eccentricity of 4 degrees (right). Distance relative to the midpoint of the weighting functions appears on the lower horizontal axis; the horizontal line within each weighting function shows the extent of its excitatory center. Each of the spatial weighting functions on the left has been normalized to have the same height. The spatial weighting functions at 4 degrees are shown with the correct heights relative to those at the fixation point. The top horizontal axis gives eccentricity of the weighting function's center. The dashed lines indicate the variation in relative sensitivity as a function of eccentricity of the weighting function's center. The bar graphs to the right of the figure plot the absolute sensitivity of each mechanism at foveal center to a line presented with either of two temporal envelopes: a Gaussian with a full width at half amplitide of about 400 milliseconds (indicated by *S* for sustained—empty bars) or a single cycle of an 8-Hz square wave (transient, indicated by *T*—solid bars). (From Figure 9 in Wilson & Bergen, 1979; used by permission.)

& Bergen, 1979). Then probability summation among these different sizes of weighting function was included as well as probability summation over space.

The ability of their four-mechanisms model to predict the results using aperiodic stimuli is impressive and important. The predictions for these stimuli, however, are probably relatively insensitive to spatial-frequency bandwidth, since the stimuli themselves contain such a broad range of spatial frequencies.

Wilson and his colleagues have tested the predictions of their model against (a) the thresholds for single sinusoidal gratings (Wilson & Bergen, 1979) and (b) the results of summation experiments measuring the thresholds for compound gratings containing two frequencies (Bergen et al., 1979). The fit of the predictions to the results were very good. These tests also, however, are relatively insensitive to spatial-frequency bandwidth and probably could not distinguish between the bandwidths of Fig. 6.9 and the somewhat larger bandwidths of the four-mechanisms model (as Bergen, Wilson, and Cowan pointed out).

Later versions of Wilson and his colleagues' model are largely based on suprathreshold results and thus are beyond the scope of this book. But it is interesting to note that these later versions have increased slightly the number of different sizes of weighting-function centers at each location (partly due to increasing the range of spatial frequencies considered, but I think also partly due to having used stimuli containing narrower bands of spatial frequency). These later versions have also added specification of the orientation selectivity of the mechanisms as described in section 6.5 (e.g., Wilson et al., 1983; Phillips & Wilson, 1984).

6.9.2   The Multiple-Mechanisms Model of Watson (1983)

The original article—Watson (1983)—should be consulted for justifications and cautions. Watson used "sensor" for what I call "mechanism" here.

Properties of the Mechanisms. The spatial weighting functions are two-dimensional Gabor functions with a half-amplitude full-bandwidth of one octave on the spatial-frequency dimension and 38 degrees on the orientation dimension.

At each position in space, there are eight different sizes of weighting function; the sizes increase with distance from foveal center. You can group the mechanisms into eight families (one of which is illustrated in Fig. 13.4). In any one family the weighting-function size increases with eccentricity e according to the function $s = 1 + ke$, where the value of k may differ from observer to observer; it is 0.4 for Watson's own eyes. For the eight mechanisms at foveal center, the peak spatial frequencies range from 0.25 to 32 c/deg in octave steps. Some further details are given in section 13.4.2.

The peak sensitivities of the eight mechanisms at the fovea were chosen so that the overall response of the model to sine waves of different spatial frequencies was like that of the human observer for grating patches at the fovea. The peak sensitivities of mechanisms inside the same family but outside the fovea are inversely proportional to their excitatory-center area to make spatial processing homogeneous irrespective of eccentricity.

See section 13.4.2 for more information.

Decision Rule. The general model in Watson (1983) incorporates an ideal observer—an "optimal Bayesian classifier"—as will be discussed in Chapters 9 and 10 for identification experiments. When predicting results of summation experiments, however, Watson (1983) used a Quick pooling formula with an exponent of 3.5 as a good-enough approximation to the ideal observer in this case.

Notes

1. *Convexity and nonlinear pooling.* Mullins (1978) has proved that whenever detection by some entity is the result of nonlinear pooling described by the Quick pooling formula across many linearly acting subentities, the resulting threshold curve on a summation square will always be convexly curved (if not straight) as are the curves in Fig. 6.7. In particular, this theorem applies to what we are calling a *channel* here. Since each mechanism contained in the channel is a linear system, the overall threshold curve for that channel will be convexly rather than concavely nonadditive. Similarly, the threshold curve for an observer will be convexly curved (if not straight) as long as it is occurring by probability summation or equivalent nonlinear pooling among many linearly acting mechanisms. A concavity, for example a cusp at a particular potent stimulus, would be evidence against Quick pooling among linearly acting mechanisms. To my knowledge, all reported psychophysical contrast interrelationship functions are either straight or convex within the precision of experimental error.

2. *Masking versus summation experimental paradigms.* The second procedure mentioned in section 6.3.5 has often been done with the low-contrast component B on continuously and the observer adjusting component A. Potentially this changes this experiment from a true summation experiment (the discrimination of a compound from a blank) into a masking experiment (the discrimination of component B from the compound), although of course component B is far below threshold. This fact seems to have had little effect on the results, since in those cases (e.g., compounds involving gratings of two different spatial frequencies) where experiments have been done both ways, very similar results have been obtained. If the contrast of component B is made high enough, this procedural difference will certainly have an effect. See Wilson, Phillips, Rentschler, and Hilz (1979) for an example.

3. *Further comments on the spatial-frequency bandwidths in the four-mechanism model.* Wilson's and his colleagues' experimental results leading to the parameters of the four-mechanism model cover only the frequency range up to 16 c/deg and thus have always allowed for the possibility of another mechanism serving higher frequencies. The discrepancy, therefore, described in section 6.4.3 between the model's predictions and the 16 c/deg summation results is less suprising than that for the 1 c/deg summation results. It is possible, furthermore, that under Wilson's experimental conditions (e.g., lower mean luminance, different subjects), the spatial-frequency bandwidths are broader than under Watson's conditions. (However, Quick and Reichert's mean luminance was also lower and their bandwidths are less like Wilson's than Watson's.)

4. *Spatial-frequency and orientation bandwidth estimates from noise gratings.* Another estimate of spatial-frequency and orientation bandwidths (Mostafavi & Sakrison, 1976) used results from noise stimuli containing different ranges of spatial frequency of orientation (around a center frequency of 4.5 c/deg with a center orientation of vertical, using any of a range of exponents and Gaussian-shaped filters). Although the calculation carefully took into account nonlinear pooling across spatial position, it did not allow for nonlinear pooling (e.g., probability summation) across spatial frequencies and orientations, which may be why it led to such a large spatial-frequency bandwidth estimate—roughly 6 c/deg at 4.5 c/deg half-amplitude full-bandwidth, that is, more than two octaves and broader than the others described in section 6.4.3. Their orientation estimate was somewhat narrower than others mentioned in section 6.5, however (a half-amplitude full-bandwidth of 23.6 angular degrees ± 4.8 degrees), which is somewhat puzzling. Relatively few data went into these estimates, however.

5. *Legge's number-of-cycles experiment.* An interesting variant of the number-of-cyles experiments mentioned in section 6.6.1 is the previously mentioned experiment of Legge (1978b) that attempted to isolate one spatial-frequency analyzer by choosing the spatial frequency (3.0 c/deg) at the peak of the contrast sensitivity function and superimposing all the test stimuli on top of it. On the assumption that this did isolate the 3.0 c/deg analyzer (which allowed him to ignore the problems of frequency spread), Legge computed backward from the sensitivity increase as a function of number of cycles to a presumed spatial weighting profile (properly taking spatial probability summation into account). This profile shows an inhibitory surround reaching maximum depth at about 6 minutes from the center and then a second excitatory flank, weak but extending from 10 minutes to 20 minutes. If future understanding of masking experiments should confirm the assumption that Legge's procedure isolated the 3.0 c/deg analyzer, this calculated sensitivity function would lend some supporting evidence to the claim that bandwidths are as narrow as those in Fig. 6.9. Until masking experiments are better understood, however, the evidence from this experiment about the spatial weighting function should be considered very tentative indeed.

IV

UNCERTAINTY

7

Extrinsic Uncertainty
and Summation Revisited

7.1 INTRODUCTION

7.1.1 Typical Uncertainty Experiment

In uncertainty experiments, the detectability of a stimulus when it is the only stimulus presented in a block of trials (the *alone condition*) is compared with its detectability when trials of it are randomly intermixed with trials of other stimuli (the *intermixed condition*). Frequently, the detectability of each stimulus is greater in the alone condition, when the observer can be certain about which stimulus will be presented, than in the intermixed condition, when the observer is necessarily uncertain about which stimulus will be presented. The decrement in performance going from the alone to the intermixed condition is said to be an *uncertainty effect* (or, sometimes, a *set-size* effect).

Figure 7.1 shows results from a hypothetical uncertainty experiment measuring the detectability of each of a number of simple stimuli of different values V (plotted on the horizontal axis) in two conditions: an alone condition (top curve) and an intermixed condition (bottom curve) containing equal numbers of trials of the stimulus of value V and of a fixed stimulus of value V_0. (V_0 is marked by an arrow on the horizontal axis.) When V equals V_0, two identical stimuli are intermixed together so that the intermixed condition is exactly the same as the alone condition. When, however, two stimuli of far-apart values are intermixed, there is frequently a substantial uncertainty effect. This value-selective behavior is clearly shown in the bottom of the figure, where the difference between performance in the alone condition and performance in the intermixed condition is plotted so that no effect (a zero difference) is at the top of the scale.

Extrinsic Uncertainty. Uncertainty experiments and effects like those just described will sometimes be called *extrinsic-uncertainty experiments* and *effects,* because the uncertainty is extrinsic to the observer. Intrinsic uncertainty is discussed in the next chapter.

7.1.2 Effects of Uncertainty About Spatial Frequency

A number of uncertainty experiments have been done on the spatial-frequency dimension studying combinations of far-apart values, however. (Early references include Cormack & Blake, 1980; Davis & Graham, 1981; Davis, Kramer,

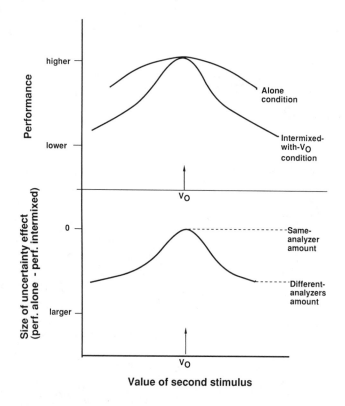

FIG. 7.1 Results from a hypothetical uncertainty experiment.

& Graham, 1983; Graham et al., 1978.) When measured in terms of performance at a constant contrast, the uncertainty effect at far-apart spatial frequencies can seem rather large (e.g., 10 to 15 percentage points when measuring percent correct in two-alternative forced-choice detection). However, the amount
by which the contrast in the alone condition would have to exceed contrast in
the intermixed condition to make performance in both conditions equivalent is
less than one fourth log unit (less than a factor of 1.8), perhaps only one tenth
of a log unit (a factor of about 1.2).

Cormack and Blake (1980) reported that the magnitude of the spatial-frequency uncertainty effect is inversely proportional to the difference between two
intermixed spatial frequencies, but they gave no further information. (Also see
section 7.2.3 for a different paradigm using closer spatial frequencies.)

7.1.3 Overview of Explanations

Although the common explanations of uncertainty effects differ in detail, they
all assume the existence of analyzers that are differentially sensitive to the different stimuli used in the intermixed condition. These analyzers need not, of
course, be the same as the ones revealed in adaptation-at-threshold or summa-

tion-at-threshold experiments. They might, for example, occur at much higher levels in the visual system. Available evidence suggests the analyzers may well be the same, however.

In this chapter we will look at several classes of explanation for these effects.

Limited-Attention-Capacity-Models (Single-Band Models). In previous chapters, the observer's response has been assumed to be based on the outputs from the full set of all analyzers. To explain uncertainty effects, however, the observer's capacity to "monitor" different analyzers is sometimes assumed to be limited. In the first model discussed here, capacity is assumed to be so limited that on any trial the observer can monitor only one analyzer. Thus, in the intermixed condition, he or she will often be monitoring the wrong analyzer—an analyzer that is not at all sensitive to the stimulus actually presented on the trial (although in the alone condition the correct analyzer can always be monitored). This kind of model has sometimes been called a *singleband* model (especially in the auditory literature), but to more explicitly distinguish it from the single-analyzer models of Chapters 3 and 4, we will sometimes call this kind a *single-attention-band* model.

Noise-Limited (Independent-Analyzers) Models. In these models, there is no limit to how many analyzers the observer can monitor. But because the observer is uncertain which stimulus will be presented on the next trial in an intermixed condition, he or she monitors more analyzers in the intermixed condition than in the alone condition. Thus there are more sources of noise in the intermixed than in the alone condition (noise from which the response to the signal must be discriminated).

Revisiting Models for Summation Experiments. Each version of this noise-limited independent-analyzers class of models will be discussed as applied not only to uncertainty experiments but also to summation experiments, since one is interested in finding a model adequate for both. In general, the noise-limited independent-analyzers models all tend to predict "probability summation," as did the independent-analyzers models of Chapters 4 through 6. (Once the class of models has been expanded, some care is necessary to use the term *probability summation* without misleading the reader. Note 1 discusses various usages of this term.)

About Monitoring and Labeled Lines. All the models in this chapter assume that the observer's response can be based on a particular subset of analyzers rather than on all analyzers. This implicitly includes an assumption that the higher processes can keep track of which output comes from which analyzer, at least to some extent, as if the output were "labeled" with the name of the analyzer or subset of analyzers it comes from. Such an assumption is sometimes called a *labeled-lines* or *labeled-outputs* assumption in the pattern vision literature; it is related to Muller and Helmholtz's idea of specific nerve energies (e.g., Watson & Robson, 1981).

7.2   SINGLE-ATTENTION-BAND MODELS

7.2.1   *Switching Single-Band Models*

We will talk here, for ease of expression as if there were only one analyzer sensitive to each of the far-apart stimuli. But, as in sections 4.7.5 and 7.3.6, the argument applies as well to the case where there are many analyzers sensitive to each of the far-apart stimuli, for example, many mechanisms in the multiple-mechanisms model. One simply forms appropriate composite analyzers, only one of which is sensitive to each of the far-apart stimuli.

The crucial assumption of a switching single-band model is

Assumption 49. Switching Single-Band Model.   *The observer monitors only one analyzer on a given trial, but which analyzer it is will switch from trial to trial if more than one stimulus is possible on a trial.*

This switching is often thought to be the result of limited capacity, that is, the observer is thought to be unable to monitor more than one analyzer at a time. It may be, however, that the observer just chooses to monitor only one at a time in certain experimental conditions but could monitor more in others.

It is easy to see why a switching single-band model predicts an uncertainty effect for far-apart stimuli. On many trials in an intermixed condition, the observer will monitor the "wrong" analyzer (that is, an analyzer insensitive to the stimulus presented) and will thus be correct only by chance. On every trial in the alone condition, however, the observer monitors the correct analyzer and thus has a higher probability of being correct.

To calculate predictions from a switching single-band model for uncertainty experiments using far-apart values requires an assumption about the proportion of trials in which the observer attends to each analyzer. Let a be the proportion of time the observer spends monitoring the analyzer for a given stimulus in the intermixed block. Then

$$\text{Pr}_{obs}(\text{correct}\,|\,\text{stim,intermixed}) = a \cdot \text{Pr}_{obs}(\text{correct}\,|\,\text{stim,alone}) + 0.5(1 - a)$$

where Pr_{obs} (correct | stim,condition) is the probability that the observer is correct on a given stimulus in the given condition. These equations say that the predicted probability of being correct on a particular stimulus in an intermixed block will be a (the proportion of time spent monitoring the correct analyzer for that stimulus) times the probability of being correct in the alone block (in which the correct analyzer is monitored all the time) plus $(1 - a)$ times the probability of being correct by chance (which is .5 in two interval forced choice).

As it turns out, these predicted probabilities are much too low (the predicted uncertainty effect is much too big) to explain results for far-apart spatial frequencies in uncertainty experiments like those described above (e.g., Davis et al., 1983). However, a condition that has evoked behavior consistent with some switching between analyzers is described in section 7.2.3.

7.2.2 Stationary Single-Band Models

The crucial assumption of a stationary single-band model is:

Assumption 50. Stationary Single-Band Model. *The observer monitors the same single analyzer on every trial of an intermixed block.*

Like the switching single-band model of which it is an extreme form, this stationary single-band model predicts uncertainty effects much larger than those found on the spatial-frequency dimension when intermixed and alone are compared conditions, as described above (e.g., Davis et al., 1983), but see the next subsection for a condition in which it may work. Also this model may be appropriate for direction-of-motion uncertainty effects, at least under some conditions (see section 12.3.5).

7.2.3 Primary-Plus-Probe Uncertainty Experiments

Another kind of uncertainty experiment uses an unbalanced intermixed condition containing a preponderance of trials of one "primary" value randomly intermixed with trials of many other "probe" values (e.g., Davis & Graham, 1981; Greenberg & Larkin, 1968; Macmillan & Schwartz, 1975; Scharf, Quigley, Peachey, & Reeves, 1987). These unbalanced intermixed blocks are used in an effort to get the observer to attend only to the single analyzer sensitive to the primary value; in other words, to get the observer to obey the stationary single-band model. (Here also the single attended analyzer may actually be a composite analyzer composed of all analyzers—e.g., mechanisms—sensitive to the value of interest and perhaps to nearby values on the dimension of interest.)

If this effort succeeds, there should be little uncertainty effect for the primary value and for values close to it (all those values detected by the single analyzer being monitored), but there should be a substantial uncertainty effect at values far from the primary. The results should look like the hypothetical results sketched in Fig. 7.1, in fact, where the primary has value V_0 (although that figure was originally described as illustrating results from uncertainty experiments in which the intermixed conditions contained equal amounts of two stimuli of value V_0 and V). For spatial frequencies, the predicted tuning of the uncertainty effect was found (Davis & Graham, 1981). The lack of consistent sequential dependencies in this condition was also consistent with the assumption that the same (composite) analyzer was being monitored from trial to trial.

When the proportion of trials on which the primary spatial frequency was presented decreased from 95 to 80%, the tuning became broader, suggesting that the composite analyzer monitored in the 95% condition contained fewer mechanisms (only those with preferred values very close to the primary value) than the composite analyzer monitored in the 80% condition. [Compare Johnson and Hafter's (1980) suggestion that bandwidth of monitoring of auditory frequencies influences detection.]

Information About Bandwidth. Given the intrinsic variability of these measurements and the small size of uncertainty effects, it is difficult to specify precisely a bandwidth of these effects at all, but the following can be said about the spatial-frequency results: The obtained bandwidth of the uncertainty effect measured as difference between performance in the alone and unbalanced-intermixed conditions (when the primary was presented on 95% of the trials) was at least as broad as spatial-frequency bandwidths of individual analyzers estimated from adaptation or summation at threshold experiments (Davis & Graham, 1981).

Monitoring Two Far-Apart Values—An Intermediate Strategy. In another kind of intermixed condition, two primary spatial frequencies were spaced very far apart (Davis, 1981). The results showed large uncertainty effects at probe frequencies in the middle between the primary spatial frequencies and almost no uncertainty effect at one of the primaries (1 c/deg) with intermediate-sized effects both at the other primary (16 c/deg) and at a frequency close to the first primary (2.5 c/deg). This pattern is consistent with a model in which the observer monitors only the 1-c/deg analyzer on some trials and both the 1- and 16-c/deg analyzers on other trials, while never monitoring analyzers tuned to a range of frequencies intermediate between the two (Davis, 1981).

7.3   INDEPENDENT-ANALYZERS (ATTENTION-SHARING, NOISE-LIMITED, MULTIPLE-BAND) MODELS

7.3.1   Perfect Monitoring (Selective and Unlimited)

This class of models assumes that there is either no limit to an observer's attention capacity or that the limit is so high that it is not reached in the situations under consideration. More formally, it assumes

Assumption 51. Perfect Monitoring (Selective and Unlimited). *On each trial the observer monitors all the relevant analyzers and only the relevant analyzers, where the relevant analyzers are those sensitive to any stimulus the observer thinks might be presented on that trial. The probability distribution of the random variable representing the analyzer output is not affected by whether the analyzer is being monitored.*

These models have sometimes been called *attention sharing* (because the observer can share his or her attention over all relevant analyzers) or *noise limited* (because it is the variability or noise in analyzer outputs that leads to the effect); a subclass of them have been called *multiple band* or *multiband* (because the observer is simultaneously monitoring multiple bands or analyzers). Here they will usually be referred to as *independent-analyzers* models of uncertainty effects.

7.3.2   *Insight Into Prediction of Uncertainty Effects*

To understand why most versions (but not all—see end of this subsection) of independent-analyzers models predict uncertainty effects, consider an experiment where simple stimuli of four far-apart values (V_1, V_2, V_3, and V_4) are used; their detectabilities are measured in both alone and intermixed conditions; the psychophysical procedure is two alternative, forced choice. The possible output magnitudes from four analyzers are shown in Fig. 7.2, where each analyzer is sensitive to exactly one of V_1, V_2, V_3, or V_4, as indicated on the figure. Two probability density functions are shown for each analyzer: The "noise" density function on the left gives the probability density when the stimulus is either a blank or a stimulus to which the analyzer is not sensitive; the "signal" density function on the right gives the probability density when the stimulus is the simple stimulus (of the four used) to which the analyzer is sensitive. (The density functions are drawn as identical for all analyzers, which is appropriate when the four far-apart stimuli are equally detectable.)

In an alone-condition for a stimulus of value V_1, the observer monitors only the V_1 analyzer. Figure 7.3 illustrates the output of that analyzer during the stimulus interval (top left) and the blank interval (top right) of a two-alternative forced-choice trial by shading in the appropriate density function. The observer will be correct on a trial as long as this one analyzer's output during the stimulus interval (characterized by the right-hand density function) is bigger than its output during the blank interval (characterized by the left-hand density function). The only time the observer is incorrect is when the output during the blank interval happens by chance to be unusually large and bigger than the output during the stimulus interval.

In the intermixed condition the observer monitors all four analyzers on each

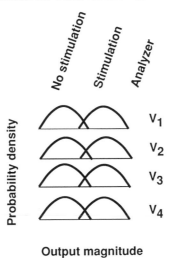

Output magnitude

FIG. 7.2 Schematic probability density functions for the outputs of each of four far-apart analyzers to no stimulation (left) and to stimulation (right).

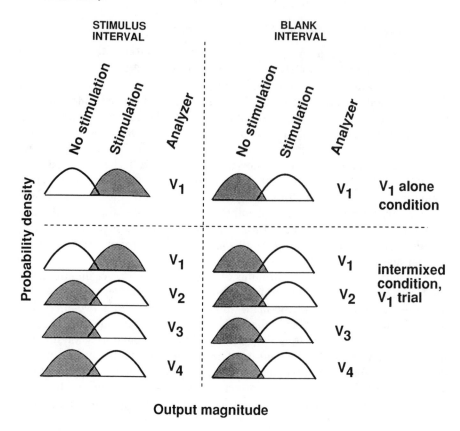

Output magnitude

FIG. 7.3 Illustration of independent-analyzers models' predictions for uncertainty experiments in which the detectability of four far-apart stimuli is measured in alone (certain)
and intermixed (uncertain) conditions.

trial. The appropriate density functions for the stimulus and blank interval of a
trial when V_1 is presented are shaded in the bottom part of Fig. 7.3. For this
example, let us assume the maximum-output detection rule (Assumption 40).
In a stimulus interval in the intermixed condition (bottom left of figure), the
maximum output will almost always come from the V_1 analyzer although, very
occasionally, it may come from one of the other three analyzers. Thus the maximum output on a stimulus interval in the intermixed condition will tend to be
only a little bigger than that during a stimulus interval in the alone condition
(upper left). During the blank interval of a trial in the intermixed condition
(lower right), however, any one of four analyzers is equally likely to produce the
maximum output. And thus the maximum output during a blank interval in the
intermixed condition (lower right) will tend to be a good deal greater than that
during a blank interval in the alone condition (upper right).

To put it another way: In the intermixed condition there are four opportuni-
ties to get an output on the blank interval that is greater by chance than the

"correct output" (the output from the V_1 analyzer during the stimulus interval—which output is usually the maximum output during the stimulus interval even in the intermixed condition). In the alone condition, however, there is only one opportunity. Hence the observer will say the wrong interval (the blank interval) more often in the intermixed condition than in the alone condition. Thus there will be a decrement in performance due to uncertainty.

The High-Threshold Model. The model of this class that was described earlier (section 4.7)—the high-threshold version—predicts no uncertainty effect, however. The analyzer outputs for the high-threshold version do not take on any of a range of values, as in the drawings of Fig. 7.2 and 7.3, but rather take on only two values; the detect state and the not-detect state. Further, a blank stimulus never causes a detect state. Therefore, the extra analyzers monitored on any trial in the intermixed condition (those that are not sensitive to the stimulus on that trial) never mislead the observer by giving an output that is actually greater than the output of the "correct" analyzer.

7.3.3 Basic Assumptions of Independent-Analyzers Models

The assumptions will be the same as those in section 4.7 for a high-threshold multiple-analyzers model incorporating variability except (a) the perfect selective and unlimited monitoring assumption (Assumption 51) replaces a previously implicit assumption that all analyzers were always monitored, (b) alternative probability distributions in addition to the high-threshold distribution will be considered, as listed in section 7.3.4, and (c) several alternative decision variables in addition to the maximum-output decision variable will be considered, as listed in section 7.3.5. The assumptions repeated from section 4.7 without modification or alternatives are the following: 25, Single Number Output; 34, Multiple Analyzers; 35, Non-overlapping for Far-Apart Values; 36, Ineffective Stimulus Rule; 37, Non-interacting Analyzers; and 38, Probabilistically Independent Analyzers. The last three assumptions need hold here only for far-apart stimuli, although stated more generally previously.

We will make explicit here the following:

Assumption 52. Probabilistically Independent Trials. *The outputs of an analyzer on different trials (or different intervals of a two-alternative forced-choice trial) are probabilistically independent of each other.*

We also make explicit an assumption that exactly one analyzer is sensitive to each of the far-apart stimuli, although as was true earlier, this assumption is made without loss of generality if the proper interpretations are applied (see section 7.3.6):

Assumption 53. One Analyzer per Stimulus. *For a set of far-apart simple stimuli, there is exactly one (and only one) analyzer that is sensitive to each simple stimulus in the set.*

In Chapter 4 the following was implied by the high-threshold assumption, but it is worthwhile making it explicit now to avoid confusion as we generalize to alternative probability distributions.

Assumption 54. Identical Probability Distribution Families. *All analyzers' noise density functions are identical. Further, if any two far-apart simple stimuli are equally detectable when measured in alone conditions, the signal density functions of the relevant two analyzers' outputs (to those two stimuli) are identical.*

This last assumption does reduce the generality of the independent-analyzers model. It has testable consequences, however, and for a number of dimensions (e.g., spatial frequency and spatial position of visual stimuli) it is supported by the strong similarities among the ROC functions or psychometric functions measured for different stimuli (e.g., sinusoidal gratings of different spatial frequencies or spatial positions).

7.3.4   Alternative Probability Distribution Families

Why These Six? We will explicitly consider six alternative families here. Each of these six is a one-parameter family, and we will call that parameter the *signal-strength parameter*. We originally looked at these and other distributions because they were used in the visual and auditory psychophysical literature. We choose to present these six here for two reasons. First, as a group, their predictions span the interesting range and thus demonstrate the possible behaviors of a much larger class of distributions. Thus, for many purposes a reader could skip the following description of the particular distributions. Second, however, individual ones of these six hold special interest. The high-threshold distribution has already been much discussed (Chaps. 4, 5, and 6); the constant-variance Gaussian function is often used because of its convenience; and three others (the exponential and the increasing-variance Gaussians) are the best predictors of ROC slopes, as discussed below. The sixth one—the double-exponential—while it has several intriguing properties (Graham, Kramer, & Yager, 1987; Yellott, 1977), is here primarily to be the end of the range. For each of the six families, Fig. 7.4 sketches the noise density function and one signal density function (for a signal at a moderate level of detectability).

Assumption 55. High-Threshold Family. *The density function describing an analyzer's output to a particular stimulus is a discrete two-state (the detect and not-detect states) function. The signal-strength parameter p is the probability of being in the detect state. Its value is 0.0 for the blank stimulus (noise).*

Letting the detect state be indicated by an output of 1.0 and the not-detect state by 0.0 (as in Fig. 7.4), the density function can be written using delta functions (see section 2.2.1) as

$$f_i(z) = p_i \cdot \delta(z - 1.0) + (1 - p_i)\delta(z)$$

In row a of Fig. 7.4 the signal and noise functions at 0 have been offset horizontally from one another for clarity.

Assumption 56. Spread-Exponentials Family. *The density function describing an analyzer's output to a particular stimulus has the form:*

$$f_i(z) = 0 \qquad\qquad \text{for } z < 0$$

$$= k_i \cdot \exp(-k_i \cdot z) \qquad \text{for } z \geq 0$$

where $0 \leq k \leq 1$ and k equals 1 for the noise stimulus. The signal strength parameter is

$$k' = 2 \cdot \log_{10}(1/k)$$

It is zero for the noise stimulus and increases from zero with stimulus strength.

We find k' convenient because its magnitude is very similar to that of the d' in Gaussian models (see below) that predicts similar levels of detectability. These exponential densities all start at the same output magnitude but have different variance.

Three one-parameter Gaussian families are shown in rows c, d, and e of Fig. 7.4. If μ_S and μ_N are the means of the signal and noise density functions, respectively, and σ_S and σ_N are the standard deviations, the signal strength parameter is taken to be:

$$d' = \frac{\mu_S - \mu_N}{\sigma_N}$$

The value of d' is zero for the noise stimulus.

The parameter r distinguishing the three Gaussian families from one another describes the rate at which the variance of the signal distribution increases as the mean increases:

$$\frac{\sigma_S}{\sigma_N} = 1 + r \cdot d'$$

Assumption 57. Increasing-Variance Gaussians ($r = \frac{1}{3}$). *The density function describing an analyzer's output is Gaussian. The signal strength parameter d' is the difference between the means in response to signal and to the blank (noise) divided by the standard deviation in response to the blank. The ratio of the standard deviations in response to a signal and in response to noise is $1 + \frac{1}{3} d'$.*

Assumption 58. Increasing-Variance Gaussians ($r = \frac{1}{4}$). *Like Assumption 57 but the ratio of the signal to the noise standard deviations is $1 + \frac{1}{4} d'$.*

Assumption 59. Constant-Variance Gaussians ($r = 0$). *Like Assumption 57 but the ratio of the signal to the noise standard deviations is 1.0.*

Row f of Fig. 7.4 shows the sixth family:

Assumption 60. Shifted Double-Exponentials Family. *The density function describing an analyzer's output has the form*

$$f_i(z) = \exp(z - U_i) \cdot \exp\{-\exp[-(z + U_i)]\}$$

The signal-strength parameter is U. Its value is 0.0 for the noise distribution.

The double-exponential density functions used here all have the same variance but are horizontally shifted from one another.

7.3.5   *Alternative Decision Variables*

Decision Variables. The decision variable R used by the observer is assumed to be a combination of the outputs from the monitored analyzers. The symbol M' denotes the number of monitored analyzers. The random variables R_i representing analyzer outputs have been numbered so that the first M' of them are the outputs of the M'-monitored analyzers.

We will start by considering two potential decision rules, one already given and one new one. After examining the predictions from them, we will enlarge our focus to include two more (see section 7.4.7).

Assumption 40. Maximum-Output Detection Rule. *In all conditions, the observer's response is based on the maximum of the outputs from the monitored analyzers:*

$$R = \overset{M'}{\underset{i=1}{\mathrm{MAX}}}\, R_i$$

Assumption 61. Sum-of-Outputs Detection Rule. *In all conditions, the observer's response is based on the sum of the outputs from the monitored analyzers:*

$$R = \sum_{i=1}^{M'} R_i$$

The decision variable R is assumed to determine the observer's response in psychophysical experiments according to the assumptions of standard signal detection theory.

Assumption 41. Yes-No Rule. *For continuous probability distribution families, the observer says yes on a trial if and only if the decision variable R on that trial is greater than some criterion level λ. In the high-threshold case, the observer says yes if R is the detect state; otherwise the observer says no or guesses yes.*

Assumption 42. Forced-Choice Rule. *In two-interval forced-choice, the observer is assumed to say whichever interval yielded the larger value of the decision variable R. (If both intervals yield the same value, as they will with the high-threshold family, the observer guesses with no bias toward either interval.)*

When we compare experimental with theoretically predicted quantities, we will make the following conventional assumption:

Assumption 62. No Criterion Variance. *The criterion λ (or, in the case of the high-threshold model, the guessing paramater g) is assumed to be constant throughout the block of trials from which results are pooled to get an empirical measurement.*

This last assumption is made for tractability. Potential implications of criterion variance across trials (random and systematic) are discussed occasionally here, but have been considered more deeply by, for example, Johnson (1980a), Nachmias (1981), Nachmias and Kocher (1970), Treisman and Williams (1984), and Wickelgren (1968).

Why These Two Decision Variables? An infinite number of decision variables could be considered. These two were used for several reasons. (a) They are mathematically tractable—see section 7.6. (b) They have been used by a number of others—see note 2 of this chapter. (c) They are closely related to the ends of a continuum of useful decision variables, where each is some measure of distance between the blank stimulus and the stimulus in question—see section 9.8.1. (d) The optimal decision variable, which is not so tractable in the general case, is known to be well described by the sum or the maximum in certain situations.

Because of this last reason, in fact, we will later consider the two more decision variables (described in more detail in section 7.4.7). The first is a hybrid of the two above:

Assumption 63. Hybrid Decision Rule. *In different conditions, the observer uses whichever of the maximum-output or sum-of-outputs decision rule is better.*

The second new decision variable is sometimes (in circumstances described in more detail later and in other sources) the optimal decision variable, that is, it leads the observer to produce the best possible performance where *best* is appropriately defined. Let $R_i, i = 1, M'$ be the outputs of the analyzers observed on a particular trial. The "likelihood given the signal" is defined to equal the probability of producing exactly those outputs ($R_i, i = 1, M'$) given that a signal (a nonblank stimulus the observer is supposed to be detecting) was presented. In other words, the likelihood given the signal (of a particular set of outputs) is the proportion of all signal trials on which exactly those outputs occur. Similarly, the likelihood given the blank (of a particular set of outputs) is the probability of producing exactly those outputs given that a blank was presented. Then the decision variable of interest here is:

Assumption 64. Likelihood-Ratio Decision Rule. *The observer's decision variable is the likelihood given the signal divided by the likelihood given the blank:*

$$\frac{\Pr(R_1, R_2, \ldots, R_{M'} | \text{signal})}{\Pr(R_1, R_2, \ldots, R_{M'} | \text{blank})}$$

Ten Distinct Models. Of the 12 possible combinations of the six probability distribution families (section 7.3.4) paired with each of the basic two decision variables (maximum and sum-of-outputs detection rules, Assumptions 40 and 61), predictions were calculated from 11 (Graham et al., 1987) and will be summarized here. For all 11, all the other assumptions just listed were assumed to hold. The 12th—the sum-of-outputs rule with the shifted double-exponentials probability-distribution family—required more work than was merited by what seemed likely to be learned from it.

For the high-threshold distribution, the sum-of-outputs rule makes exactly the same predictions as the maximum-output rule. Therefore, only 10 of the 11 sets of predictions are distinct from one another.

Each of these models will be referred to by a short name reflecting both the decision rule and the probability distribution family, e.g., "sum-of-constant-variance-Gaussians model" for the independent-analyzers model including the sum-of-outputs decision rule and the constant-variance Gaussian family. (The words *spread* and *shifted* will generally be omitted. Since either decision rule coupled with the high-threshold distribution makes the same predictions we will often refer simply to the high-threshold model.)

7.3.6   When More Than One Analyzer Is Sensitive to a Simple Stimulus

Although we assume for the calculations that follow that only one analyzer is sensitive to each of a set of far-apart stimuli, this assumption is not restrictive as long as the proper interpretations are made.

Just as was done in section 4.7.5, we form composite analyzers by grouping together all the original analyzers that are sensitive to a particular simple stimulus. (In fact, as will become important in the next chapter, one can group into the analyzers some entities that are not sensitive to any stimulus under consideration as long as each entity is grouped into at most one analyzer. See note 3 for discussion of composite analyzers within the framework of the multiple-mechanism model.)

The output of each of the new composite analyzers is taken to be a combination of the outputs from all the original entities—the combination that is consistent with the decision variable used by the observer. Thus, if the observer's decision variable is to be the sum (respectively, maximum) of the outputs of the composite analyzers, then the output of the composite analyzer is taken to be the sum (respectively, maximum) of the outputs of the original entities.

Now suppose the original analyzers satisfied all the basic assumptions of independent-analyzers models (section 7.3.3) except for the one-analyzer-per-stimulus assumption. Then so will the new composite analyzers, with the clarifications discussed in the next paragraphs.

Given stimuli that are far enough apart that none of the original entities was sensitive to more than one, then none of the new analyzers will be sensitive to more than one. When the original entities are noninteracting and probabilistically independent, so are the new analyzers. If ineffective stimuli are ineffective in compounds for the original entities, so are they for the new analyzers.

However, the exact signal and noise densities (which are specified in section 7.3.4) will not be the same for the new random variables (the composite analyzer outputs) as they were for the original ones (the original entities' outputs). In fact, whether these new random variables even have the same kind of probability distribution as did the original ones depends on both the probability distributions and the combination rule. (They will have, incidentally, for the high-threshold model, the sum-of-constant-variance-Gaussians model, and the maximum-of-double-exponentials models. For the sum-of-increasing-variance-Gaussians model, the new random variable will again be Gaussian but the variance will not depend on signal strength in the same way as did the originals.) If, however, the behavior of a model with the restriction that only one analyzer is sensitive to each far-apart simple stimulus were known for *all* possible families of probability distributions, then the behavior of the model without that restriction would also be known. We will not, of course, calculate the predictions for *all* possible families but we will compute them for a large enough variety to give a good idea of the behavior for all of them.

For the perfect monitoring assumption to apply to the composite analyzers it is not necessary (although it is sufficient) that it apply to the original entities. The following weaker assumption can apply to the original entities instead. The set of entities monitored when the observer is uncertain as to which of several stimuli will occur (an intermixed condition) must be the union of the sets monitored in the alone conditions for each of those stimuli, and also these two added restrictions must hold: (a) The set of entities monitored in the alone condition for any one of the far-apart simple stimuli must be the set that was combined to form the composite analyzer for that stimulus. (b) None of the entities monitored in the alone condition for one of the far-apart simple stimuli can also be monitored in the alone condition for another. Notice that this weaker assumption does not require "perfect" monitoring of the original entities; for, in an alone condition, the observer may monitor some entities that are not actually sensitive to the stimulus (as in the intrinsic-uncertainty version considered later).

Since the observer's decision variable computed over the original entities is either the maximum output or the sum of the outputs, and since that same combination rule has been used to form the new analyzers' outputs from the original entities' outputs, then the observer's decision variable computed over the new analyzers (either maximum or sum appropriately) will exactly equal the observer's decision variable computed over the original entities.

A specific example of composite analyzers is explored in the next chapter (section 8.1).

7.4 PREDICTIONS OF INDEPENDENT-ANALYZERS MODELS

7.4.1 *Three Predictions Independent of Probability Distribution and of Combination Rule*

Table 7.1. The stimulus conditions of each of the kinds of experiments considered in this chapter are shown in Table 7.1. For each kind, we will consider in this chapter only the case where the M simple stimuli are equally detectable and far apart.

In simple-uncertainty experiments, the detectability of simple stimuli in an alone condition is compared with detectability measured when trials of M simple stimuli are intermixed.

Two types of summation experiments are considered. In blocked-summation experiments, the detectability of each of M components is measured in a simple-alone condition and the detectability of the compound is measured in a compound-alone condition. (In a compound-alone condition, a compound is the only stimulus presented).

In intermixed-summation experiments, the detectability of each component and of the compound are measured simultaneously in a simple-and-compound-intermixed condition.

The column second from the right in Table 7.1 shows M'—the number of analyzers monitored according to Assumption 51. The right column shows P'—the number of analyzers characterized by a signal probability distribution according to assumptions 35, 36, 37, and 53.

Let's use the symbol Dn to denote predicted detectability for the nth row of Table 7.1. Then $(D5 - D4)$ is the amount of summation in an intermixed-summation experiment (as indicated by the solid bracket connecting rows 4 and 5 in the table). We will call this the *intermixed-summation effect* for short. Also $(D1 - D2)$ is the amount of summation in a blocked-summation experiment (see corresponding solid bracket) or the *blocked-summation effect*. And $(D2 - D3)$ is the amount of loss due to uncertainty in a simple-uncertainty experiment (see corresponding solid bracket) or the *simple-uncertainty effect*.

The dotted-line brackets in the left part of the table connect pairs of rows having the same values of both M' and P'.

Three Predictions. If the observer uses the same combination rule to form his or her decision variable in all conditions (as is, for example, assumed by the maximum-output and sum-of-outputs rules given in Assumptions 40 and 61), then three predictions follow immediately and do not depend either on the probability distribution family or on the exact form of the decision variable (e.g., on whether it is the sum of the outputs or the maximum output).

Since two rows connected by a dotted-line bracket in the left column of Table 7.1 have the same values of M' and P', those conditions are predicted to lead to equal detectability as long as the same decision variable is used in both conditions. Hence, two immediate predictions are:

1. $D1 = D5$, the detectability of a compound stimulus should be the same whether measured in an alone condition (row 1) or a compound-and-simple intermixed condition (row 5). In other words, there should not be an uncertainty effect for the compound.
2. $D3 = D4$, the detectability of a simple stimulus should be the same whether it is measured in a simple intermixed condition (row 3) or in a compound-and-simple intermixed condition (row 4).

By the equalities in these predictions, it is easy to show that $(D5 - D4) = (D1 - D3)$. Simple algebra (or a glance at the top three rows in Table 7.1) also shows that $(D1 - D3) = (D1 - D2) + (D2 - D3)$. Therefore, the third prediction follows:

3. $D5 - D4 = (D1 - D2) + (D2 - D3)$, or, in words,

TABLE 7.1.

Row	Stimulus Conditions	Kinds of Experiments	Number of Analyzers Monitored M'	Number of Analyzers with Signal Distributions P'
1	Compound Alone (M components)		M	M
		Blocked-summation experiment		
2	Simple Alone		1	1
		Simple-uncertainty experiment		
3	Simple Intermixed (M simple stimuli)		M	1
	Compound and Simple Intermixed (M simple stimuli)			
4	Simple Stimulus		M	1
		Intermixed-summation experiment		
5	Compound Stimulus		M	M

$$\begin{array}{ccc} \text{The} & \text{the} & \text{the} \\ \text{intermixed-} & \text{blocked-} & \text{simple-} \\ \text{summation} = \text{summation} + \text{uncertainty} \\ \text{effect} & \text{effect} & \text{effect} \end{array}$$

7.4.2 *Numerical Predictions From Specific Probability Distributions*

ROC Curves. As it turned out, the effects of probability distribution family depend primarily on the slopes of the ROC curves predicted by each family, so let's look at these slopes first. Figure 7.5 shows two sets of ROC curves predicted for the simple-alone condition. It is useful to plot these curves on z-score axes. (A z score is a value that corresponds to a given probability from the Gaussian distribution having mean 0,0 and standard deviation 1.0. Z scores are also called *standard normal deviates,* because that Gaussian distribution is also called the *standard normal distribution*). In Fig. 7.5, the z score corresponding to the probability of saying yes given a nonblank stimulus (a hit) is shown on the vertical axis or given a blank stimulus (a false alarm) is shown on the horizontal axis. The curves are labeled as were the probability distribution families in Fig. 7.4. The signal strength parameter for each family was chosen to make the predicted ROC curve intersect the negative diagonal at a vertical coordinate of +1.0 (left panel) or +0.5 (right panel). The curves in the left panel come from the signal-strength parameters of the distributions illustrated in Fig. 7.4.

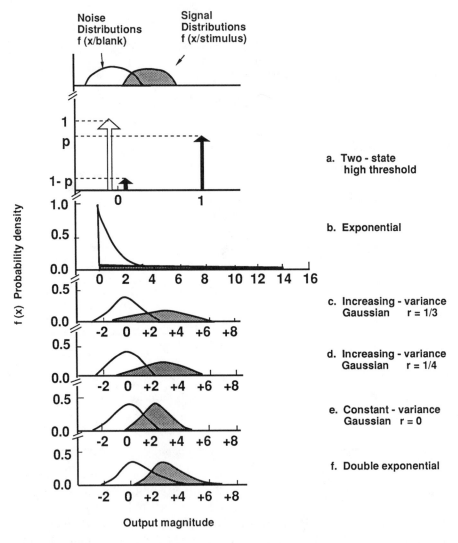

FIG. 7.4 Six families of probability density functions. For the high-threshold family, the noise and signal functions near zero should be exactly overlapping but have been offset horizontally from each other for clarity. (Adapted from Kramer et al., 1985.)

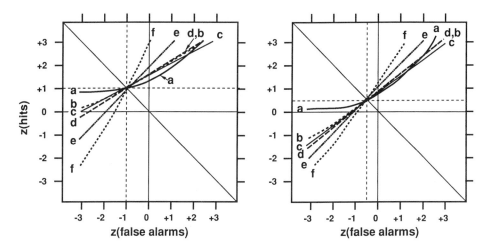

FIG. 7.5 ROC curves for the simple-alone condition predicted by the independent-ana-lyzers model, assuming each of six different families of probability density function (labeled as they were in the previous figure). (Adapted from Graham et al., 1987.)

As is well known, the Gaussian simple-alone ROC curves are straight lines on *z*-score coordinates where the lines have a slope equal to σ_N/σ_S and an intersection with the horizontal axis at the negative of the value of d'. Thus, for the constant-variance Gaussian family (the curves marked e), the slope stays constant at 1.0. And for the increasing-variance Gaussian families (curves c and d), the slope gets shallower with increased detectability, with the reciprocal of the slope always equaling 1.0 plus *r* times the absolute value of the horizontal intercept. (Remember that *r* is ¼ and ⅓ for families d and c, respectively).

The ROC curves predicted by the exponential family (curves b) are also well known to be very close to straight lines on normal-normal coordinates (examples can be found in Egan, 1975, or Green & Swets, 1974). Further, their slopes change with detectability in much the same way that the two unequal-variance families' slopes do. (At low false-alarm rates, the exponential is more like family c; at high more like d.)

The ROC curves from the high-threshold family are very shallow and also concave upward (curves a), whereas those for the double-exponential family (curves f) are very steep.

We computed ROC curves at several levels of detectability for all the conditions of Table 7.1. Always, the slopes of the ROC curves were ordered as were the six probability distribution families in Fig. 7.4 except for some minor reversals among the ones with very similar slopes (families b, c, and d).

Uncertainty and Summation Experiments. Figures 7.6, 7.7, and 7.8 show some predicted results for simple-uncertainty, blocked-summation, and inter-mixed-summation experiments, respectively, using two or four simple stimuli (all run as two-alternative forced-choice experiments). The *z* score correspond-

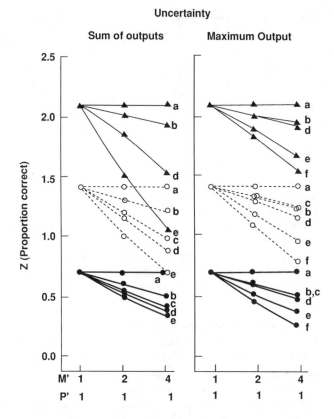

Uncertainty

FIG. 7.6 Predictions of the independent-analyzers model for a simple-uncertainty experiment where *M* (the number of far-apart simple stimuli) could be 1, 2, or 4. The horizontal
axis shows the number of analyzers monitored (*M'*, which equals *M* in this case) and the
number of monitored analyzers characterized by signal distributions on stimulus trials
(*P'*, which equals 1 in this case). The standard normal deviate (*z* score) corresponding to
predicted proportion correct in two alternative forced choice is shown on the vertical axis.
Predictions from each of the six different families of probability density functions are
labeled by the same letters used in the previous figures; the sum-of-outputs and maximum-output predictions are shown in the left and right panels, respectively. (Provided by
Patricia Kramer from calculations in Kramer, 1984.)

ing to the predicted percent correct is plotted on the vertical axis and the stimulus condition on the horizontal axis (indicated by *M'* and *P'* values). The sum
and the maximum decision variables were used for the left and right halves of
each figure, respectively. Each curve (lettered as usual) connects predicted points
for a particular stimulus strength parameter in a particular probability distribution family. Signal strength parameters were chosen to make the *z* score in
the one-stimulus condition equal to 0.707 (the bottom set of curves in each
panel), to 1.414 (the middle set of curves—dashed lines), or to 2.121 (the top set
of curves). The signal strength parameters predicting *z* scores of 1.414 in the one-

stimulus condition were very close to those generating the ROC curves in the left panel of Fig. 7.5 and the probability distributions in Fig. 7.4. In Fig. 7.8 for the intermixed-summation experiments, there are separate sets of curves for the two-component and the four-component experiments, because the signal strength parameters necessary to produce a given performance on the single-component stimulus are different for the two experiments, since performance is measured with trials of two simple stimuli intermixed in one case and four intermixed in the other.

Notice two features of these results. Except for sum-of-outputs and intermixed-summation (left panel of Fig. 7.8), the curves always tend to be ordered as were the probability distribution families in Fig. 7.4, with the curves from family a (high-threshold) on the top and the curves from family f (double-exponential) on the bottom. Second, the curves for the sum-of-outputs rule tend to be steeper than those for the maximum-output rule. The next subsections discuss the implications of the first of these features; section 7.4.6 discusses the second.

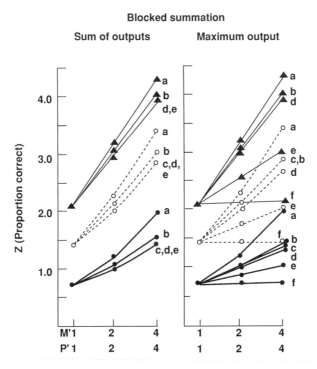

Blocked summation

Sum of outputs   **Maximum output**

FIG. 7.7 Predictions for a blocked-summation experiment. Same conventions as previous figure except that for these experiments M' will equal P', which will equal the number of far-apart components in a compound stimulus measured in a compound-alone block and can be 1, 2, or 4. (Provided by Patricia Kramer from calculations in Kramer, 1984.)

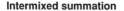

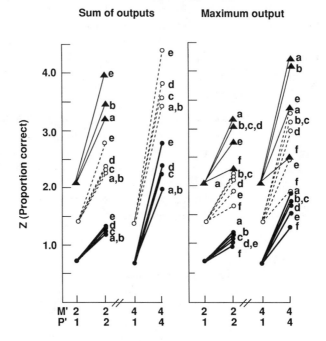

FIG. 7.8 Predictions for an intermixed-summation experiment. Same conventions as previous two figures except that (see text) the predictions for two-component (in which case $M' = 2$) and four-component (in which case $M' = 4$) experiments have been separated into separate subpanels. P' again equals the number of components in the stimulus. Provided by Patricia Kramer from calculations in Kramer (1984).

If the intersection of the ROC curve with the negative diagonal is plotted (as in Graham et al., 1987) instead of being given as proportion correct, the figures look very much like those here. (The predictions from these models are plotted in still other ways in Graham et al., 1987; Kramer, 1984; and Kramer et al., 1985.)

7.4.3   Shallower ROC Slopes, Smaller Simple-Uncertainty Effects, and Greater Blocked-Summation Effects

Another way of describing the ordering of the curves in Figs. 7.6 and 7.7 is to say the following. For either decision rule, distributions predicting ROC curves of shallower slope (letters closer to the beginning of the alphabet—Fig. 7.5) predict smaller decrements due to extrinsic uncertainty (shallower curves in Fig. 7.6) and larger increments due to summation in blocked-summation experiments (steeper curves in Fig. 7.7).

For intermixed-summation experiments (Fig. 7.8), these two trends counteract each other, since the intermixed-summation effect equals the blocked-summation effect plus the simple-uncertainty effect (see the end of section 7.4.1 and Table 7.1). Thus probability distribution should make less difference for inter-mixed-summation experiments; indeed it makes relatively little difference with the maximum-output rule (right panel Fig. 7.8); with the sum-of-outputs rule (left panel), the ordering actually reverses.

7.4.4 Some Insight Into the Effect of Probability Distribution

This section attempts to provide some understanding of why the slope of the ROC curve is related to the amount of uncertainty and summation effects. A somewhat more rigorous version of this argument plus a discussion of its gen-erality can be found in Graham et al. (1987).

When an observer monitors additional analyzers (while keeping his criterion λ constant), there are always two effects—extra hits (due to above-criterion val-ues of the decision variable on stimulus trials) and extra false alarms (due to above-criterion values of the decision variable on blank trials).

Loosely speaking, on a shallow ROC curve, each hit is worth several false alarms. (You add several extra false alarms for every extra hit to stay on the same ROC curve.) Conversely, on a steep ROC curve, each false alarm is worth several hits. (You add several extra hits for every false alarm to stay on the same ROC curve.)

Simple-Uncertainty Experiments. The decrement in simple-uncertainty experiments is the amount by which performance is worse in simple-intermixed than in simple-alone conditions. It will be determined by the balance between the extra hits and extra false alarms that come from the extra analyzers moni-tored in the intermixed condition. (See Fig. 7.3.) These extra hits are "spurious" hits—that is, hits produced by analyzers that are not sensitive to the stimulus in question.

The decrement due to uncertainty, therefore, is the effect of extra false alarms on blank trials in the simple-intermixed condition "minus" the effect of extra spurious hits on simple-stimulus trials in that same condition. So the more effec-tive a false alarm is relative to a hit (the steeper the slope of the ROC curve), the bigger the decrement due to uncertainty. If an ROC curve is shallow enough, however (e.g., the high-threshold model), the extra hits may completely coun-teract the extra false alarms and there will be no decrement due to uncertainty.

Blocked-Summation Experiments. Similarly but oppositely, the increment in blocked-summation experiments is the amount by which performance is better in compound-alone than in simple-alone conditions. It is the effect of extra hits on compound-stimulus trials in the compound-alone condition "minus" the effect of extra false alarms on blank trials in the compound-alone condition. So the more effective a hit is relative to a false alarm (the shallower the slope of the ROC), the bigger the increment due to summation. If an ROC curve is steep enough (the double-exponential), the extra false alarms may completely balance out the extra hits and there will be no increment due to summation. See Graham et al. (1987) for even steeper cases.

Intermixed-Summation Experiments—Maximum-Output Rule. As discussed earlier (see end of section 7.4.1 and Table 7.1), the intermixed-summation effect is the sum of the blocked-summation and simple-uncertainty effects. These latter two effects vary in opposite ways (one getting larger and one getting smaller) with changes in ROC slope. For the maximum-output rule, in fact, if hit rate at a fixed false-alarm rate is the measure of performance, the increment due to summation in intermixed-summation experiments is totally independent of ROC slope (of probability distribution). One manifestation of this independence is that probabilities of the observer's saying no, when corrected for guessing, multiply when the maximum-output rule is used. In symbols, Eq. 4.6 in section 4.7.6 holds for all maximum-output models—not just for the high-threshold model as originally introduced—if $P_{obs}(\text{stim})$ is interpreted simply as the observer's probability of saying yes manipulated as in the correction for guessing of Eq. 4.5 in section 4.7.3. (See section 7.6.6 for derivation.) When other measures of performance are used (proportion correct in forced choice—as in Fig. 7.8 here—or the intersection of the ROC curve with the negative diagonal—as in Graham et al., 1987), there is a small effect of probability distribution on intermixed-summation predictions even with the maximum-output rule. Notice that the effect is in the same direction as that on blocked summation (the shallower the ROC slope, the greater the summation).

Intermixed-Summation Experiments—Sum-of-Outputs Rule. With the sum-of-outputs rule, the effects of probability distribution on simple-uncertainty predictions seem generally to be greater than the effects on blocked summation (e.g., the vertical distance between any curve labeled a and the corresponding curve labeled e is greater in the left panel of Fig. 7.6 than in the left panel of Fig. 7.7). With the sum-of-outputs rule, therefore, there is always a small net effect of probability distribution on the intermixed-summation effect, where the effect is the opposite of that on blocked summation; here the shallower the ROC slope, the smaller the intermixed-summation effect (curve a is on the bottom of each panel of curves in the left panel of Fig. 7.8).

7.4.5   Implications for Use of the Quick Pooling Formula

For intermixed-summation experiments, as we just discussed, probability distribution has relatively little effect on predictions. Therefore, predictions assuming high-threshold distributions (e.g., as in the Quick pooling model used throughout Chaps. 4, 5, and 6) are not so very different from those assuming other probability distributions that do predict simple-uncertainty effects. The previous successes of the Quick pooling model may rest on this fact. The predictions of the Quick pooling model—most frequently in the form of the Quick pooling formula—have usually been compared with results of experiments where all the stimuli have been intermixed within blocks. These are essentially intermixed-summation experiments (although not using equally detectable far-apart stimuli), so the observer may well be monitoring all the relevant analyzers.

In the future, therefore, if one wishes to use the Quick pooling formula to calculate predictions from multiple-mechanisms models, it is probably safer to always compare its predictions with results from experiments where trials of the various stimuli have been intermixed.

7.4.6   Sum-of-Outputs Versus Maximum-Output Decision Variables

The sum-of-outputs detection rule tends to predict both bigger increments, due to summation, and greater decrements, due to uncertainty, than does the maximum-output detection rule. (For example, the curves in the left panels of Figs. 7.6, 7.7, and 7.8 are steeper than the corresponding curves in the right.) Loosely speaking, summing the outputs makes an observer more susceptible to both the effects of extra noisy analyzers (in simple-uncertainty experiments) and extra signal-carrying analyzers (in summation experiments) than does taking the maximum of the outputs. (Remember, however, that for the high-threshold family, both combination rules lead to exactly the same predictions.)

An alternative way of stating the effect of combination rule is in terms of what stimulus condition each rule does better on: (a) The sum-of-outputs rule usually predicts better performance on the compound stimulus than does the maximum-output rule. (Thus it usually predicts greater detectability of the compound in blocked-summation experiments and therefore a greater blocked-summation effect.) This is particularly true for the constant-variance Gaussian case (family e) and less true for the others. (b) The maximum-output rule usually predicts better performance on simple stimuli in intermixed conditions (thus leading to smaller uncertainty effects) than does the sum-of-outputs rule.

Some Insight.   With the sum-of-outputs rule, the additional random variables monitored as M' gets larger affect the decision variable (the sum) on every trial. With the maximum-output rule, however, the additional random variables affect the decision variable (the maximum) only on those trials on which one of them happens to produce the maximum output. Looked at this way, it seems reasonable that both the decrements due to uncertainty effects and the increments due to summation—both of which are effects of the monitoring of additional random variables—should tend to be greater with the sum-of-outputs than with the maximum-output rule.

That the effects of changing from the maximum-output to the sum-of-output rule are different for different probability distributions is straightforward to explain. The maximum-output predictions depend only on the ROC curve for the simple-alone condition, or to put it another way, depend only on the ratios of signal to noise probability densities at various criteria. Consider what happens if one takes a given pair of signal and noise density functions and nonuniformly stretches the axis underneath both: The maximum-output rule predictions stay the same because the ratios of signal to noise density stay the same. The sum-of-output predictions do not stay the same after nonuniform stretching, however, because the distribution of the sum depends on the actual magnitudes of all the numbers that went into it.

7.4.7   *Hybrid and Optimal Decision Rules*

For the probability distributions used here (see above), the sum is generally better in the compound-alone condition and the maximum is generally better in the simple-intermixed condition. If observers have control (conscious or unconscious) over which decision rule is used, therefore, they ought to exercise this control. Let's consider the predictions of the hybrid decision rule introduced earlier (section 7.3.5):

Assumption 63. Hybrid Decision Rule—Maximum Output or Sum of Outputs, Whichever Is Better.   *In different conditions, the observer uses whichever of the maximum output or sum of outputs decision rules is better.*

The question of which is better in the simple-and-compound-intermixed condition is more complicated. The maximum output is better for the simple stimuli but the sum of outputs is better for the compound stimulus, and yet the observer (not knowing which stimulus will be presented when) has to use the same decision rule on each trial. When simple stimuli occur on the majority of the trials of this condition (as they do in the spatial-frequency experiments considered later), an observer who is attempting to achieve the best performance possible might well use the maximum output rule in those experiments. So for our purposes here, we will assume the observer does use this rule. The hybrid decision rule can then be rephrased as the following table:

Condition	*Decision Variable*
Compound alone	Sum of outputs
Simple alone	Sum of outputs = Maximum output
Simple intermixed	Maximum output
Compound and simple intermixed	Maximum output

Predictions from Hybrid Decision Rule—Compound Uncertainty Effect. The predictions (a) for simple-uncertainty experiments are identical to those shown previously using the maximum-output decision rule (right Fig. 7.6), (b) for blocked-summation experiments are identical to those shown previously using the sum-of-outputs decision rule (left Fig. 7.7), and (c) for intermixed-summation experiments are identical to those shown previously for the maximum-output decision rule (right Fig. 7.8).

This new decision rule does make one completely new prediction, however. Remember that, whenever the same decision rule was used in a pair of conditions joined by dotted-line brackets in Table 7.1, performance was predicted to be the same in both (because M' and P' are the same—assuming the same stimuli are used in both, of course). Even with the new decision rule, the same performance is still predicted for rows 3 and 4 because the new decision rule equals the maximum output for both. However, this hybrid decision rule predicts, in general, better performance in the compound-alone condition (row 1) than on trials of the compound stimulus in the simple-and-compound-intermixed condition (row 5), because the hybrid is equivalent to the sum of outputs in the former and the maximum output in the latter. That is, the hybrid decision rule predicts a compound-uncertainty effect. The predicted difference is very small for four of the probability distribution families (a through d—in fact, is zero for high threshold) but is large enough to be of some practical significance for the constant-variance Gaussians (curve e).

If one considered an alternative hybrid decision rule, the same as this one except that the sum-of-outputs rule was used in the simple-and-compound-intermixed condition rather than the maximum-output rule, no compound uncertainty effect would be predicted. But then simple stimuli should be more detectable in the simple-intermixed condition than in the simple-and-compound-intermixed condition.

Optimal Behavior. We will consider one more decision rule (introduced in section 7.3.5) because of its relationship to optimal behavior.

Assumption 64. Likelihood-Ratio Decision Rule. *The observer uses the following likelihood ratio as the decision variable in a detection task:*

$$\frac{\Pr(R_1, R_2, \ldots, R_{M'} \mid \text{signal})}{\Pr(R_1, R_2, \ldots, R_{M'} \mid \text{blank})}$$

Proper use of the likelihood ratio as the decision rule can produce optimal behavior. Such use requires that the criterion used be appropriately based on the presentation probabilities of different stimuli and the payoffs (usually implicit, e.g., how bad or good each kind of correct or wrong answer seems to the observer). If the observer uses this appropriate criterion, the expected value of the observer's behavior (the average payoff over many trials) will be maximized. (See presentation in, for example, Chap. 6 of Coombs et al., 1970.)

If the payoffs are such that the two ways of being correct are equally valued and the two mistakes are equally abhorred, then maximizing the expected value is equivalent to maximizing the posterior probability—that is, to maximizing the probability that the observer's response is correct (yes when a signal or no when a blank).

If the presentation probabilities for a blank and a signal are equal, then the "appropriately calculated criterion" just equals 1.0. Thus the observer should say yes if the numerator of the ratio given above is greater than that in the denominator and should say no otherwise. Equivalently, the observer's response should correspond to the maximum of the two likelihoods. Frequently, therefore, a *maximum-likelihood assumption* (choosing the larger or largest of two or more likelihoods) is stated explicitly and used.

Other senses in which use of the likelihood decision variable is optimal are discussed in Chapter 1 of Green and Swets (1966 or 1974).

For Constant-Variance Gaussians. In general, the maximum-likelihood decision rule is much harder to work with than the sum-of-outputs or maximum-output rule. For the case of constant-variance Gaussian probability families and equally detectable far-apart components, however, two results are known: (a) For compound stimuli in any condition, the likelihood decision rule is equivalent to the sum-of-outputs decision rule (Green & Swets, 1974, appendix 9a) and (b) for simple stimuli in a simple-intermixed condition, the likelihood decision rule is approximately equivalent to the maximum-output decision rule [Nolte and Jaarsma, 1967; see also Cohn (1978), who includes the Poisson case, and Klein (1985)].

7.4.8 Uncertainty and Summation Results on the Spatial-Frequency Dimension

ROC Slope. The slope of the ROC curve turns out to be very important, and I could find very few published ROC curves using sinusoidal gratings. Thus Fig. 7.9 shows the most relevant evidence I could find even though the experiment from which these results were extracted was not quite one of those discussed in this chapter (see figure legend.). In Fig. 7.9 the slopes of ROC curves (on z axes)

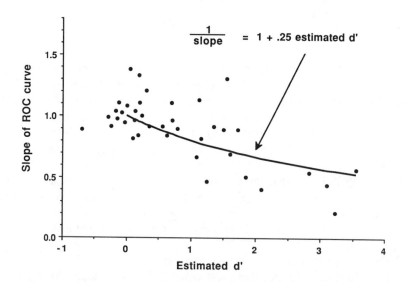

FIG. 7.9 Slope of ROC curve (on z-score axes) plotted against estimated d'. These ROC curves were extracted from the results of the concurrent identification study published in Hirsch, Hylton, and Graham (1982). Each point here represents an ROC curve from a single session plotted from the 50 to 100 trials on which the stimulus was a 3-c/deg grating; the response on which the ROC curve was based was the observer's confidence rating that 3 c/deg was present. (On each trial the observer also rated his or her confidence that 9 c/deg had been presented. See Chapter 10 for more details of this paradigm.) The relationship predicted by the increasing-variance Gaussian family with $r = 0.25$ (solid curve) has been previously reported for other stimuli.

are plotted as a function of estimated d' (-1 multiplied by the intersection of the ROC curve with the horizontal z axis). The solid line is the prediction of the increasing-variance Gaussian family with $r = \frac{1}{4}$ (family d). In spite of the considerable scatter, the ROC slopes for sinusoidal gratings clearly decrease with increasing detectability in the way previously reported for other stimuli (e.g., Green & Swets, 1974; Nachmias & Kocher, 1970). We have many such plots for different spatial frequencies and different observers, and we almost always have found this trend.

Uncertainty and Summation Effects. The size of the uncertainty effects predicted by independent-analyzers models depends on the details of the particular model. The uncertainty effects found on the spatial-frequency dimension are consistent with the predictions of models within this independent-analyzers class and are much too small to be consistent with limited-attention single-band models. At present, however, exactly which model of the independent-analyzers class does the best job at simultaneously predicting uncertainty and summation effects is still unclear. (See Davis et al., 1983; Kramer, Graham, & Yager, 1985; Yager, Kramer, Shaw, & Graham, 1984.)

The models that currently appeal to me most are ones that combine the maximum-output or hybrid decision rule (the latter as a stand-in for the optimal decision rule) with a probability distribution predicting slopes that get shallower with detectability in the way reported empirically (e.g., the exponential or increasing-variance Gaussians, or the intrinsic-uncertainty distribution in the next chapter). Choosing the probability distribution this way builds in the advantage of predicting ROC slope appropriately. The attractiveness of the hybrid decision variable is increased by the small compound-uncertainty effect found on the spatial-frequency dimension (Kramer et al., 1985).

Any of the models in this attractive group do quite a good job at simultaneously predicting uncertainty and summation effects, with one exception: On the basis of available experimental results (which are still somewhat too sparse), none of the models we are considering seem able to simultaneously account for the effect of uncertainty as M increases from 1 to something more and for the effect as M increases from 2 or more. The effect as M increases from 2 is smaller and is more consistent with the slope of the ROC curves (within the framework of this class of models) than is the effect as M increases from 1.

Imperfect Monitoring—Observer's Uncertainty Growing Faster than Experimental Uncertainty. To account for all the results, therefore, some assumption of the above models probably must be changed. One change that would certainly help is a change in the perfect-monitoring assumption. Perhaps an observer's uncertainty in simple-intermixed conditions (measured as M', the number of analyzers sensitive to different simple stimuli) increases faster than the number of stimulus alternatives (M) for low values of M. This might happen because an observer becomes "confused" about which analyzers to monitor as soon as he or she has to monitor more than one.

Formally, one might assume:

Assumption 65. Monitoring Too Many Analyzers in Intermixed Conditions.
When $M = 1$, $M' = 1$. As M increases from 1 to 2 or 3, M' increases faster (perhaps to 4 or 5) so the ratio M'/M becomes substantially greater than 1.0. For higher values of M, the increase in M' slows down so the ratio M'/M becomes approximately equal to 1.0 again.

Whether this kind of change in the perfect monitoring assumption would produce a model that predicts all the experimental results remains to be seen.

7.5 SUMMARY

Uncertainty effects on the spatial-frequency dimension exist but are not big enough to require assuming any limitation to the observer's ability to monitor all the relevant analyzers simultaneously.

Uncertainty effects on the spatial-frequency dimension are of a size explainable by the noise limitations inherent in independent-analyzers models even when the observer can simultaneously monitor all relevant analyzers.

A number of versions of independent-analyzers models are discussed in this chapter, and their predictions for both uncertainty experiments and summation experiments are calculated. The models differ in their assumption about the probability distribution characterizing each analyzer's output and in their assumption about how the multiple analyzer's outputs are combined to form the observer's decision rule (maximum output, sum of outputs, or a hybrid of the two that is closer to the optimal decision rule).

In general, probability distributions predicting shallower ROC slopes predict larger summation effects in blocked-summation experiments, but smaller uncertainty effects. (The ROC slope reflects the relative importance of extra hits and extra false alarms.)

The size of the summation effect predicted for intermixed-summation experiments by these models is approximately the sum of the predicted uncertainty effect's size plus the predicted blocked summation's effect size. Since these latter two sizes are related in opposite ways to ROC slope, the predictions of different models for intermixed-summation experiments are similar to one another.

This last point provides some insight into why the Quick pooling formula (developed in Chap. 4 from a high-threshold model) may work so well for intermixed-summation effects, although high-threshold independent-analyzers models do not predict empirical uncertainty effects nor empirical ROC curves correctly.

Thus, it is probably all right to use the very convenient Quick pooling formula to analyze the results of intermixed-summation experiments and to deduce the properties of individual analyzers from such experiments (as was done in Chaps. 4–6).

7.6 APPENDIX. CALCULATING THE INDEPENDENT-ANALYZERS PREDICTIONS

7.6.1 Basic Assumptions Restated in Combined Form

We calculated predictions for the following stimulus set presented in any of several conditions: (a) blank stimulus, (b) M far-apart but equally detectable simple stimuli denoted by their values on some dimension of interest ($V_j, j = 1, M$), and (c) a compound C containing all M of the simple stimuli. This stimulus set contains the ingredients for both summation and uncertainty experiments.

The basic assumptions 25, 33, 35, 36, 37, 52, and 53 can be restated for this set of stimuli as follows, where the number of analyzers is N' and the density function of the ith analyzer in response to a stimulus "stim" is denoted $f_i(z|\text{stim})$.

There are N' mutually probabilistically independent random variables. The whole set of N' random variables is numbered so that the ones sensitive to the M simple stimuli in the stimulus set ($V_j, j = 1, M$) come first and are numbered in the same order as the simple stimuli.

For the first M random variables ($j = 1, M$),

$$f_j(z|C) = f_j(z|V_j) = f_1(z|V_1)$$

When i is not equal to j,

$$f_j(z|V_i) = f_j(z|\text{blank}) = f_1(z|\text{blank})$$

For the last $N' - M$ random variables ($j = M + 1, N'$) and for any simple stimulus ($i = 1, M$),

$$f_j(z|C) = f_j(z|V_i)$$
$$= f_j(z|\text{blank}) = f_1(z|\text{blank})$$

7.6.2 General Methods for Calculating Predictions

ROC Curves. For each of the 10 models and for each of a large number of signal-strength parameters, predicted ROC curves were computed for each row of Table 7.1. In symbols, where $f(z|\text{stim})$ and $F(z|\text{stim})$ are the probability density and distribution functions, respectively, of the decision variable R:

$$\text{Hit rate} = \int_{\lambda}^{+\infty} f(z|\text{stim})\, dz$$
$$= 1 - F(\lambda|\text{stim})$$

And the false-alarm rate is just the hit rate when the stimulus is the blank stimulus.

Forced-Choice. For two-alternative forced-choice experiments, predicted percent correct is the area underneath the corresponding ROC curves for models assuming continuous random variables. For the high-threshold model, an expression for percent correct can be derived directly from the assumptions; as it happens, predicted percent correct is again equal to the area under the high-threshold ROC curve. For these forced-choice predictions, it should be noted, we are assuming that (as in Assumption 42) there is no response bias in favor of one interval or the other and that (Assumption 25) there is no correlation between the outputs in the two intervals.

7.6.3   Computations for the Maximum-Output Decision Rule

The probability that the maximum output is less than some value z just equals the probability that all of the monitored analyzers' outputs are less than z. Since the analyzers are probabilistically independent, this last probability is just the product of the probabilities that each analyzer's output is less than z. Hence

$$\Pr(R < z \,|\, \text{stim}) = \prod_{i=1}^{M'} \Pr(R_i < z \,|\, \text{stim})$$

or in terms of distribution functions

$$F(z \,|\, \text{stim}) = \prod_{i=1}^{M'} F_i(z \,|\, \text{stim})$$

Of the M' monitored analyzers, P' are characterized by the signal density (since we are considering equally detectable far-apart simple stimuli) and $M' - P'$ are characterized by the noise density. Therefore

$$F(z \,|\, \text{stim}) = |F_1(z \,|\, \text{signal})|^{P'} \, |F_1(z \,|\, \text{noise})|^{(M'-P')}$$

From here, it is easy to derive the following relationship between (a) the hit and false-alarm rates for the simple-alone condition, which we will call x_1 and y_1 (since in this condition, the decision variable R equals the output of the first analyzer) and (b) the hit and false-alarm rates for the condition where the number of analyzers monitored is M' and the number of analyzers sensitive to a signal is P' (call them x and y).

$$1 - y = (1 - y_1)^{P'}(1 - x_1)^{M'-P'}$$
$$1 - x = (1 - x_1)^{M'}$$

Thus, for the maximum-output rule with any probability distribution and for any condition of summation and uncertainty experiments (i.e., any values of M' and P'), the ROC curve that would be generated by varying λ can be generated from the ROC curve for the simple-stimulus alone condition using the above equation. (The segments of the high-threshold ROC curve generated by changing the guessing parameter also obey this relationship as it happens.)

Constant-Variance Gaussians. For computing predictions from the constant-variance Gaussian family for forced-choice performance in uncertainty experiments (or for identification performance—see Chap. 9), one can use Elliot's tables in Swets (1964), which have recently been improved by Hacker and Ratcliff (1979) and an algorithm for extending them suggested by J.E.K. Smith (1982).

7.6.4 Computations for the Sum-of-Outputs Decision Rule

When the decision rule is the sum of M' random variables, there is no solution for the general ROC curve (when either $M' > 1$ or $P' > 1$ or both) in terms of the ROC curve for the simple-alone condition ($M' = P' = 1$).

To calculate the general ROC, one needs to compute the distribution function of the decision variable R, that is, of the sum of the R_i (for i from 1 to M'). In general, the probability density and distribution functions for the sum of independent random variables can be calculated as the convolution (appropriately defined) of the individual random variables' density or distribution functions, respectively (e.g., see Feller, 1966).

For any kind of probability density functions one could compute these convolutions numerically. We did not use this approach, however, and thus were limited to cases where we could compute analytic results. For the case of Gaussians, the result is well known: The sum of random variables that have Gaussian distributions has a Gaussian distribution. For the high-threshold and exponential distributions, the required convolution is easily done analytically. The case of double exponentials was not done.

7.6.5 The Sum-of-Outputs Rule With Gaussian Families

To derive predictions for Gaussian models with the sum-of-outputs decision rule (and all the other assumptions of section 7.3), one simply considers the mean and standard deviation of the observer's decision variable R in each condition with the following facts in mind:

1. A sum of random variables that have Gaussian distributions has a Gaussian distribution. (Thus an ROC curve for any stimulus in any condition will be linear on z axes according to those models. Its horizontal intercept will be the d' value computed from the decision variable and its slope will be the reciprocal of the ratio of the signal-to-noise standard deviations for that decision variable.)
2. The mean of a sum of random variables is equal to the sum of the means of the individual random variables.
3. If the random variables are independent, the variance of the sum equals the sum of the individual variances.

Euclidian d' Summation Rule for Blocked Summation. The following is an oft-quoted rule for summation of d' values over, for example, the M components of a compound stimulus:

$$d' = \left| \sum_{i=1}^{M} d_i^2 \right|^{1/2}$$

or, in the case of equal d_i' values ($d_i' = d_1'$ for all i),

$$d' = M^{1/2} \, d_1'$$

As is fairly straightforward to show from these assumptions, this is the prediction of any of the Gaussian families (even unequal variance) sum-of-output models for blocked-summation experiments. (It is worth emphasizing that, for this prediction, the d_i' values from single analyzers must have been estimated in conditions where the observer was monitoring only that single analyzer, as in a simple-alone condition.)

This same relationship holds for negative diagonal d' values and for z scores corresponding to percent correct in forced-choice experiments (see Fig. 7.7).

Uncertainty Effect. The observer's d' for a simple stimulus in an intermixed condition is

$$d'(\text{simple, intermixed}) = \frac{d_1'}{M^{1/2}}$$

where d_1' is the value in the simple-alone condition. This is true for both constant-variance and increasing-variance Gaussians. If negative diagonal d' values or z scores corresponding to forced-choice proportions correct (Fig. 7.6) are considered, however, the uncertainty effect gets smaller as the variance of the signal increases relative to the variance of the noise.

Intermixed Summation. For an intermixed-summation experiment (again assuming equally detectable far-apart components), the d' value for a compound is compared with that for any one of the simple components in an intermixed condition. Doing so yields

$$d'(\text{compound}) = M \cdot d'(\text{simple, intermixed})$$

This is true for both constant-variance and increasing-variance Gaussians. If negative diagonal d' values or z scores corresponding to forced-choice percent correct (Fig. 7.7) are considered, however, the predicted amount of summation becomes smaller as the signal variance increases relative to the noise variance.

ROC Slopes. For the compound stimulus (in either an alone or intermixed condition), the slope of the ROC curve is the same as that for any of its equally detectable far-apart components. For the simple stimulus in an intermixed condition, the slope of the ROC curve is

$$\frac{M^{1/2}}{|\sigma_S^2 + M - 1|^{1/2}}$$

7.6.6 *Intermixed-Summation Experiments and the Maximum-Output Decision Rule*

Assuming the maximum-output rule, and no matter what the probability distribution, the following result can be derived for intermixed-summation experiments using a compound made of P' far-apart components:

$$\text{Pr}^*_{\text{obs}}(\text{no}\,|\,\text{cmpd},\lambda) = \prod_{i-1}^{P'} \text{Pr}^*_{\text{obs}}(\text{no}\,|\,\text{simple}_i,\lambda)$$

where

$$\text{Pr}^*_{\text{obs}}(\text{no}\,|\,\text{stim}) = \frac{\text{Pr}(\text{no}\,|\,\text{stim})}{\text{Pr}(\text{no}\,|\,\text{blank})}$$

is the probability of saying no corrected for guessing.

In words, no matter what the probability distribution, the corrected probability of saying no to the compound will be the product of the corrected probabilities of saying no to the components.

This is the same relationship derived for high-threshold models in Eq. 4.6, where the corrected probabilities of saying yes or no here correspond, respectively, to the probabilities of the observer being in the detect state [$\text{Pr}_{\text{obs}}(\text{stim})$] or the not-detect state.

This multiplication of probabilities lends itself nicely to chi-square statistical tests (Sachs et al. 1971; Shaw, 1982).

Sketch of Derivation. Given the maximum-output rule, the following equation gives the predicted probability that the observer will say no to a stimulus:

$$\text{Pr}_{\text{obs}}(\text{no}\,|\,\text{stim},\lambda) = \text{Pr}(R < \lambda\,|\,\text{stim}) = \prod_{i=1}^{M'} \text{Pr}(R_i < \lambda\,|\,\text{stim})$$

To derive the desired rule from this last formula, the same M' analyzers must be monitored for both the compound and its components, and the same criterion λ must be used for both (so there is the same false-alarm rate for both). A simple-and-compound-intermixed summation condition will have these properties according to our assumptions. Then (a) apply the immediately preceding equation to the compound, the simple stimuli, and the blank in turn, (b) convert the expressions for the compound and the simple stimuli into corrected probabilities by dividing them by the expressions for the blank, and (c) arrange terms into the desired result given at the beginning of this section 7.6.6.

Comments. Some readers may be interested in noting that the use of the same criterion λ for every analyzer's output—which follows from the maximum-output decision rule—is not actually essential in the above proof. If one instead had a decision rule according to which every analyzer's output was separately compared with its own criterion and the observer detected a stimulus if and only if at least one of the analyzer's outputs was larger than criterion, the same predictions would result. It is, in fact, this decision variable that Sachs, Nachmias, and Robson (1971) used in their study of spatial-frequency summation.

For results collected with a forced-choice procedure, however, observed probabilities corrected for guessing will not in general multiply in the above way, although they do in the high-threshold models (see Eq. 4.6 and following discussion). This is another reflection of the fact that the predicted intermixed-summation effect measured in forced-choice experiments does depend on probability distribution (even when the maximum-output rule is used throughout), as shown in Fig. 7.8, although the dependence is not as great as that in uncertainty and blocked-summation results.

Notes

1. *Terminology—probability summation.* The term *probability summation* has not been used consistently by all authors. The use of "probability summation" in Chapters 4 through 6 was, I hope, unambiguous; the term referred either to the empirical finding that a compound was slightly more detectable than its components (when those components were so far apart as presumably to affect completely separate analyzers) or to the major explanation offered for that empirical effect—namely, the high-threshold version of a multiple-analyzers model incorporating variability. However, another explanation— deterministic nonlinear pooling—was offered (section 4.8.5), and, in spite of editing efforts, I may have slipped and included that explanation under the term probability summation on occasion. For, in some contexts at least, a number of people, including me, have used the term rather loosely to mean any summation due to the presence of multiple analyzers, that is, any summation other than summation within an analyzer.

This terminological problem becomes more acute in the later parts of the current chapter where more different versions of multiple-analyzers models are considered. Many of them can predict probability summation in the sense of the empirical finding that a compound containing far-apart components is slightly more detectable than its components (due to something other than summation within an analyzer). Further, all these explanations do assume the "probabilistic independence" of the analyzers, and this probabilistic independence always contributes to the predicted summation. However, in some of these models that predicted summation is due not only to the probabilistic independence but also to the literal summing of outputs of different analyzers. In this latter case, probability summation does not seem a very good description of the theoretical mechanism. I have tried to avoid the term probability summation in ambiguous contexts, therefore.

Some others have used probability summation to refer only to the high-threshold multiple-analyzers model of the last chapter; still others have used it to refer only to the kind of calculation embodied in Eq. 4.6 and section 7.6.6 (the multiplication of probabilities of not detecting, that is, of observed probabilities corrected for guessing). Pelli (1985, 1987) used the word in an interesting fashion to name certain interesting properties of independent-analyzers models (some but not all of the properties of the high-threshold version).

2. *Alternate terminology for decision variables.* The maximum-output rule here (section 7.3.5) is sometimes referred to as a *decision-threshold model* or as a *combination of decisions* (one for each analyzer). Then the sum-of-outputs rule is referred to as an *integration*

model (where the multiple observations are "integrated" into a single observation) or as a *combination of observations* (e.g., Green & Swets, 1974; section 9.2). Wickelgren (1967) referred to them as a *multiplicative probability rule* (see section 7.6.6) versus an *additive strength rule*. In the terminology of Shaw (1982), the maximum-output models here are equivalent to second-order integration with either continuous or discrete distributions and fixed sharing. The sum-of-outputs models are equivalent to first-order integration with continuous distributions and fixed sharing.

3. *Composite-analyzers in the multiple-mechanisms model.* Within the framework of the multiple-mechanisms model for pattern vision, the analyzers referred to in this and subsequent chapters should certainly be taken to be composite analyzers (section 7.3.6). Indeed, each should presumably be a channel (a subset of mechanisms) and might well be called a *stimulus-defined channel* or a *channel for a particular stimulus*. Such a channel is whatever the observer monitors in the alone condition for that stimulus. Within the multiple-mechanisms model, it would be a subset of the full set of mechanisms or, more generally—when temporal dimensions are to be taken into consideration—a subset of the full set of elements.

It is interesting to consider the relationship of a stimulus-defined channel to what might be called a *dimensionally defined channel* or a *channel for particular values on particular dimensions* (e.g., for 3 cpd and vertical orientation). Such a channel is a subset of mechanisms that are homogeneous in the following sense: all the mechanisms in the subset are sensitive to the same values along the one or more dimensions of interest (e.g., sensitive to 3 cpd and to a vertical orientation) although sensitive to different values along other dimensions. To encompass temporal dimensions, we can easily generalize this definition to groups of elements at the same value along the temporal position dimension.

In general, a dimensionally defined channel need never contain exactly the same elements as any stimulus-defined channel, but it will often contain many of the same ones. Consider, for example, a channel defined by a stimulus that is narrow-band along one or more dimensions of interest but broad-band along others—a 3 c/deg vertical grating presented for a long time and containing many cycles. It seems plausible that the stimulus-defined channel for that stimulus (the elements monitored by the observer in an alone condition for that stimulus) will contain a great many elements, all of which are responsive to 3 c/deg and to vertical orientation, although sensitive to different spatial positions and temporal positions. All these elements are also in the corresponding dimensionally defined channel, the one sensitive to 3 c/deg and to vertical orientation. The dimensionally defined channel may contain still other elements, however, ones responsive to spatial and temporal positions beyond the boundaries of the stimulus.

8

Intrinsic Uncertainty
and Transducer Functions

8.1 INTRINSIC-UNCERTAINTY VERSION OF INDEPENDENT-ANALYZERS MODEL

The last chapter considered uncertainty arising from sources extrinsic to the observer, in particular, from the observer's ignorance on any given trial as to which of several alternative stimuli would be presented. The first part of the present chapter considers uncertainty arising from sources intrinsic to the observer—in particular, the observer's inability to remember exactly what the set of possible stimuli in the present condition is and/or inability to ignore all irrelevant information. This intrinsic uncertainty will be incorporated into the independent-analyzers models following a suggestion made by Tanner (1961) and since developed by a number of authors (e.g., Cohn, Thibos, & Kleinstein, 1974; Nachmias & Kocher, 1970; Pelli, 1985).

8.1.1 The Intrinsic-Uncertainty Probability Distribution Family

Let's start with the formal assumption that we will use to incorporate intrinsic uncertainty into the independent-analyzers models of the last chapter (section 7.3). This is an assumption describing a seventh alternative probability distribution (which does not have a conventional name to my knowledge). As first stated, it may seem opaque, but the ensuing discussion will, I hope, illuminate it.

Assumption 66. Intrinsic-Uncertainty Probability Distribution Family. *The distribution of the jth analyzer's output is the distribution of the random variable*

$$R_j(\text{stim}) = \overset{M_j'}{\underset{i=1}{\text{MAX}}} \; R_{ji}(\text{stim})$$

where the R_{ji} ($i = 1, M_j'$) are independent and have Gaussian distributions all of the same variance. The means of the first P_j' of the R_{ji} increase with detectability level, but the means of the other $M_j' - P_j'$ remain at zero.

We will consider this seventh probability distribution only in conjunction with the maximum-output detection rule (Assumption 40). Note that we are still assuming that exactly one of the analyzers is sensitive to each of a set of far-apart stimuli (Assumption 53). Thus, exactly one stimulus in the set of far-apart simple stimuli in an experiment corresponds to analyzer j.

Now let's consider the motivation for this probability distribution family.

The analyzer mentioned in assumption 66 is a composite analyzer (as discussed previously in sections 4.7.5 and 7.3.6). For clarity in the present discussion, we will call the smaller entities composing the composite analyzer *microanalyzers*. There are M'_j of the microanalyzers in analyzer j. The output of the ith microanalyzer in the jth analyzer in response to a stimulus is $R_{ji}(\text{stim})$.

The first P'_j of the microanalyzers in analyzer j are sensitive to the simple stimulus corresponding to analyzer j; accordingly, their mean outputs will increase with increasing signal strength. Exactly how the mean outputs increase is a topic for the second part of this chapter.

But the other $M'_j - P'_j$ microanalyzers are not sensitive to the stimulus; accordingly, their means are zero at all signal strength levels. It is the fact that the analyzer output (and therefore the observer's decision) depends on insensitive microanalyzers as well as on the sensitive microanalyzers that represents "intrinsic uncertainty." The underlying cause of this intrinsic uncertainty might be any of a number of things—the observer may not remember perfectly what each stimulus is and therefore higher level visual processes may not be able to "choose" correctly the microanalyzers that are sensitive to each stimulus to include in the appropriate analyzer. Or perhaps the microanalyzer outputs are not labeled perfectly but only approximately.

For assumption 66 each microanalyzer's output is assumed to have a constant-variance Gaussian family probability distribution. (See next subsection for motivation.)

For the other assumptions of the independent-analyzers models to hold (see section 7.3), certain further constraints must be put on the microanalyzers and their relationships to one another:

They must be independent and noninteracting (at least for far-apart simple stimuli) and any ineffective stimulus must also be ineffective in a compound.

Further, for far-apart stimuli, the sets of microanalyzers composing different analyzers must be disjoint (must not contain any of the same microanalyzers). The total number of microanalyzers (M'_j) and the number of microanalyzers sensitive to the stimulus corresponding to that analyzer (P'_j) must be the same for all analyzers j.

8.1.2 Each Microanalyzer Could Be a Mechanism With Photon Noise

For complete generality, one would wish to consider all possible probability distributions characterizing the microanalyzers. The constant-variance Gaussian is the only one considered by Pelli (1985), however, and it does have a particular appeal if one wishes to put an intrinsic-uncertainty model into the framework of earlier signal-detection work and into the framework of the multiple-mechanisms model earlier. Earlier signal-detection work had a particular interest in noise arising from the stimulus itself—in the case of visual patterns, photon noise. The mechanisms in the multiple-mechanisms model are linear systems.

If the noise or variability in the output of each mechanism originates entirely in the photon noise of the light stimulus itself, then two consequences follow:

1. For near-threshold visual patterns on a moderate background, photon noise is well modeled by the constant-variance Gaussian family.

Argument. Photon statistics are described by the Poisson distribution; the mean and variance of a Poisson are always equal to each other, and—in the limit for a large number of events per unit time or space—a Poisson is well approximated by a Gaussian. Thus, if the noise distribution of an analyzer is Poisson with a high mean and if the signal distribution is Poisson with a slightly higher mean, the pair of Poisson distributions will be well approximated by Gaussian distributions of constant variance. As an example, consider the case of noise and signal distributions having means of 100 and 110, respectively (corresponding to a contrast of 10%). The two means are separated by 1 standard deviation of the noise distribution—equivalent to a d' of 1.0—and the ratio of the standard deviations is little greater than 1 (1.05 to be exact, which is much less, for example, than the 1.25 ratio at $d' = 1$ in the increasing-variance Gaussian families used previously).

2. The outputs of many of these mechanisms will be probabilistically independent (or nearly so).

Argument. Technically, this second fact is only true for mechanisms having what are known as orthogonal weighting functions (functions that, when multiplied together and integrated over, give zero). But the majority of mechanisms postulated in a typical multiple-mechanisms model do have orthogonal or near-orthogonal weighting functions. Note that two functions that do not overlap in space or two functions that do not overlap in time are orthogonal. So are two sine waves of different frequencies, and consequently, two Gabor functions may be nearly orthogonal if each contains several cycles.

Given orthogonal weighting functions, the lack of correlation between outputs is a result of the fact that photon noise at different spatial and temporal positions is not correlated. And, since the probability distribution functions are Gaussians or approximately so, zero correlation implies probabilistic independence. A fuller proof can be found in Pelli (1985). (See note 1.)

8.1.3   *Properties of the Intrinsic-Uncertainty Probability Distribution Family*

The quantitative details of this family depend, of course, on the values chosen for M_j and P_j. Qualitative features of this probability distribution family are illustrated in Fig. 8.1. The left column shows the probability density functions for a set of three microanalyzers. The three functions are shown both in response to the blank or noise stimulus (at the top) and in response to increasingly higher intensity levels of the stimulus to which the analyzer is sensitive. Each density function in the left column is a Gaussian with the same variance. One of the

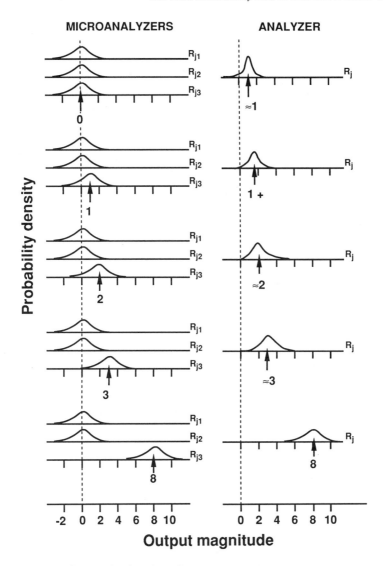

FIG. 8.1 Probability density functions for the random variables (R_{j1}, R_{j2}, and R_{j3}) representing the three microanalyzers' outputs (left) and their maximum (R_j), representing the analyzer output (right). (Certain features have been emphasized in this drawing.) Density functions are shown in response to five different stimulus intensities, those intensities producing (from top to bottom, respectively) mean outputs in the sensitive microanalyzer (R_{j3}) of 0 unit, 1 unit, 2 units, 3 units, and 8 units, respectively. The standard deviation of all microanalyzer outputs' distribution is 1 unit.

microanalyzers (R_{j3}) is sensitive to the stimulus corresponding to analyzer j; note that its mean increases as stimulus detectability increases. The other two microanalyzers are not and their means are always zero.

The right column of Fig. 8.1 illustrates the probability density function of the analyzer ($M_j' = 3$ for this analyzer). Since the analyzer's output R_j is the maximum of the three microanalyzers' outputs, none of the density functions in the right column is exactly a Gaussian; its exact form must be determined by a computation and was only approximately determined for the figure here. (A number of exact computations of the density function of an analyzer's output are illustrated in Fig. 5a of Pelli, 1985 for $R_j' = 1$ and $M_j' = 1, 10, 100, 1000,$ or $10,000$ microanalyzers. See note 1.)

Central Tendency of the Analyzer's Output. Note first that at zero intensity, the means and medians of the three microanalyzers' outputs in Fig. 8.1 are zero, but the mean and median of the analyzer's output are greater than zero. At all intensity levels, in fact, the mean (respectively median) of the analyzer's output must actually be higher than the mean (respectively median) of any of the microanalyzer's outputs. (For the maximum of three random variables is always as high or higher than each of the three. So when the three are independent, as they are here, the maximum will have a higher mean and median than each of the three.)

At the high-intensity levels, however, the maximum output from the three microanalyzers is almost always equal to the one sensitive microanalyzer's output (microanalyzer R_{j3} in this example). Hence the mean (respectively median) of the analyzer's output is almost exactly equal to that of the one sensitive

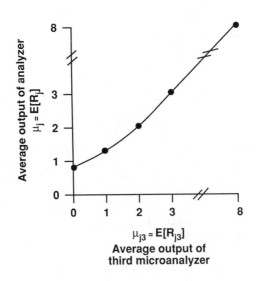

FIG. 8.2 The means of the analyzer density functions shown in the right part of Fig. 8.1 (means of R) plotted as a function of the means of the sensitive microanalyzer's density functions (means of R_{j3}).

microanalyzer's output. Figure 8.2 sketches the mean of the analyzer's output (vertical axis) as a function of the mean of the one sensitive microanalyzer's output (horizontal axis). Note that the function accelerates at low values and then becomes linear (has a unit slope which, if extended, would go through the origin).

Variance of the Analyzer's Output. Some further reflection shows that the variance of the analyzer output R_j increases as the mean of R_j increases, at least for low values. For example, the maximum of three random variables, all of which have the same distribution (top sketch Fig. 8.1), has to be less variable than the maximum of three random variables two of which have that same distribution but the third of which is translated (e.g., second sketch Fig. 8.1). For high enough values of the mean of R_j (e.g., bottom sketch of Fig. 8.1), the variance will remain almost constant for further increases in the mean. The functions in Fig. 5a of Pelli (1985) clearly show this increase in variance.

8.1.4 An Alternative Derivation of Intrinsic-Uncertainty Independent-Analyzers Model

This subsection can be skipped with little loss of continuity.

This intrinsic-uncertainty version of the independent-analyzers model could have been obtained from the original assumptions by another route. Instead of making the assumption about a new probability-distribution family (Assumption 66), we could have modified just one assumption—the perfect monitoring assumption (Assumption 51)—in the manner stated here as Assumption 67. When this new monitoring assumption is combined with the assumption of constant-variance Gaussians and the maximum-output rule along with the remainder of the independent-analyzers assumptions in section 7.3, the predictions are exactly identical to that of the version above (except that what were called microanalyzers in the preceding subsection are called analyzers in the beginning part of this subsection).

The modified monitoring assumption necessary for this alternative set of assumptions would be:

Assumption 67. Monitoring Insensitive Analyzers. *For each far-apart simple stimulus in an alone condition, the observer monitors not only the one analyzer sensitive to that stimulus but also a number of insensitive analyzers with the following conditions: (a) The same number of irrelevant analyzers must be modified for each simple stimulus; (b) the sets monitored for different far-apart stimuli are disjoint (i.e., no analyzer monitored in the alone condition for one of the far-apart stimuli is also monitored in the alone condition for another); (c) the analyzers monitored in an intermixed condition or in a compound condition are the union of the analyzers monitored in the alone conditions for the intermixed or component simple stimuli.*

This alternative version of the intrinsic-uncertainty model using Assumption 67 may seem easier to state than the microanalyzer version of Assumption 66.

Further, it makes this intrinsic-uncertainty model's relation to our previously suggested modification of the monitoring assumption (section 7.4.8 and Assumption 65) clearer. The modification of the intrinsic-uncertainty model (Assumption 67) implies that M' (the number of stimuli monitored in an intermixed block) is greater than M (the number of simple stimuli in an intermixed block) but always by the same factor. The earlier modification (Assumption 65) required that the ratio M'/M change.

However, there is one strong reason for preferring the original microanalyzer version (Assumption 66) to the modified monitoring version (Assumption 67)—namely, it makes easier the application to this intrinsic-uncertainty model of our previously gained knowledge about the effect of changing probability distribution families on the predictions of independent-analyzers models. So we will return now to the microanalyzer terminology.

How General Is the Intrinsic Uncertainty Embodied in the Model Here? It is easy to think of ways in which intrinsic uncertainty could work in a more general way than that embodied in the intrinsic-uncertainty versions just given. For example, individual microanalyzers might not have constant-variance Gaussians; the maximum-output decision variable might not be the right rule (especially not for compound-alone conditions); M' might not be proportional to M; the sets of irrelevant microanalyzers monitored for different far-apart stimuli might not be disjoint (especially when the stimuli are not too far away). All of these are plausible and probably worth investigating, but we will not do so here. Qualitatively, the predictions of many of them can be deduced from information given above and below.

8.1.5   Predicted ROC Curves

For this discussion it will be useful to define two new quantities. Let M'' be the total number of monitored microanalyzers in all the monitored analyzers, that is,

$$M'' = \sum_{j=1}^{M'} M'_j$$

and let P'' be the total number of microanalyzers (in all the monitored analyzers) that are sensitive to the stimulus in question.

Figure 8.3 shows some ROC curves (on normal-normal coordinates) predicted by the intrinsic-uncertainty version of the independent-analyzers model (from Nolte and Jaarsma, 1967). The number written next to each curve is M''. For each curve, P'' was equal to 1.0. The mean of the one sensitive microanalyzer's distribution was taken to equal 1.41 times its standard deviation for the predictions in the left panel and 4 times its standard deviation for the predictions in the right panel.

These ROC curves in Fig. 8.3 can be considered to be predictions for the simple-alone condition; in that case all of the microanalyzers are contained in the one monitored analyzer, that is, $M'' = M'_1$.

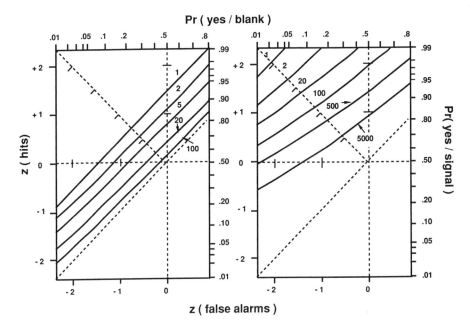

FIG. 8.3 ROC curves calculated from the maximum of M'' microanalyzers (where M'' is written next to each curve) where exactly one of the microanalyzers is sensitive to the stimulus under consideration. The mean of the one sensitive microanalyzer's signal distribution is 1.414 times (left) or 4 times (right) its standard deviation. [The curves are those shown as dashed lines in Figure 4, panels (b) and (c) of Nolte & Jaarsma, 1967; used by permission.]

Or the ROC curves in Fig. 8.3 can be considered to be predictions for a particular simple stimulus in an intermixed condition. In this case the one sensitive microanalyzer and some of the insensitive microanalyzers are contained in the relevant analyzer (the analyzer sensitive to that particular simple stimulus). But all the other microanalyzers are contained in irrelevant analyzers.

When only the one sensitive microanalyzer is monitored (top curve each panel Fig. 8.3), the predicted ROC curve is a straight line on normal-normal coordinates with slope 1; this is just the standard prediction for signal and noise distributions that are Gaussian functions with the same variance. When insensitive microanalyzers are added to this one sensitive microanalyzer, the ROC curve moves down toward the positive diagonal (detectability decreases) and the ROC curves become shallower (the variance of the decision variable on signal trials relative to that on noise trials increases). This decrease in slope is a good deal more pronounced in the right panel than in the left. Notice that a very large increase in number of microanalyzers is necessary to produce a small change in predicted slope.

The changes in predicted ROC curves in Fig. 8.3 accord well (as they must) with the changes in the predicted output density functions like those shown in Fig. 8.1 and in Pelli (1985 Fig. 5a). In particular, as the number of insensitive microanalyzers increases, the signal density functions for high signal strengths are little changed, but the noise density function becomes narrower (its standard deviation decreases), and the distance decreases between the means of the noise and signal density functions (for a given signal strength).

How many microanalyzers are needed to make the predicted slopes from the intrinsic-uncertainty model agree with the generalization from empirical data that the reciprocal of the ROC slope equals 1.0 plus 0.25 times the estimated d' (Fig. 7.9)? Of the predicted curves shown in the right panel of Fig. 8.3, the one for 500 microanalyzers has slope and horizontal intercept closest to the empirical generalization, but the curve for 100 microanalyzers is really quite close and the curve for 20, given the sparsity of the current data base, may be satisfactory as well.

In short, the ROC curves for the simple-alone condition predicted by the intrinsic-uncertainty probability-distribution family for any of a large range of intermediate uncertainties (from something like 20 to something like 500 insensitive microanalyzers) are much like those predicted by the exponential and increasing-variance Gaussian families.

For very low values of uncertainty (very few insensitive microanalyzers), the predicted ROC curves are more like those for the equal-variance Gaussian family.

For very high values of uncertainty, the predicted ROC curves will become as shallow as those for the high-threshold model. Also, at very high levels of uncertainty, the ROC curves are not only shallow but somewhat curved upward. (See, for example, the "5000" curve in right panel.) The ROC curves of the high-threshold model are also curved upward on normal-normal coordinates.

8.1.6   *Predicted Results of Summation and Uncertainty Experiments*

Remember that the predicted results of summation and uncertainty experiments involving far-apart components are completely determined by the ROC curves for the simple-alone condition when the observer's decision variable is the maximum of the analyzer outputs.

Consequently, the predictions of the intrinsic-uncertainty version of the independent analyzers model for summation and uncertainty experiments will be:

1. Very like those of the constant-variance Gaussian family (curve e in Figs. 7.6, 7.7, and 7.8) when very few insensitive microanalyzers are contained in each analyzer.
2. Very like those of the exponential and increasing-variance Gaussian families (curves c and d in Figs. 7.6, 7.7, and 7.8) when intermediate numbers of insensitive microanalyzers—about 10 to 500—are contained in each analyzer.
3. Very like those of the high-threshold family (curve a in Figs. 7.6, 7.7, and 7.8) when very high numbers of insensitive microchannels are contained in each analyzer.

8.2 ADDING ANALYZERS' TRANSDUCER FUNCTIONS TO INDEPENDENT-ANALYZERS MODELS

8.2.1 Relationship Between ROC Curves and Psychometric Functions

The top of Fig. 8.4 shows hypothetical ROC curves for three stimuli: the blank (lower curve, circles), a barely detectable stimulus of intensity *a* (middle curve, triangles), and a somewhat more detectable stimulus of intensity *b* (top curve, squares). The symbols are plotted on those curves at three different false-alarm rates (open symbols at false alarm rate of 0.05, open with dot inside at false-alarm rate of 0.25, and closed at false-alarm rate of 0.45).

The same nine points are plotted in the bottom of Fig. 8.4, but now as psychometric functions with the hit rate plotted against stimulus intensity. Each of the three psychometric functions is for a different false-alarm rate. Only three stimulus intensities and three false-alarm rates are specifically represented by the

ROC curves for three stimulus intensities

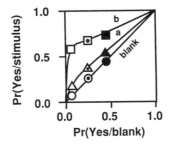

Psychometric functions at three false-alarm rates

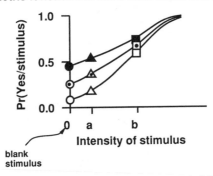

FIG. 8.4 Relationship between a family of ROC curves for different stimulus intensities and a family of yes-no psychometric functions for different false-alarm rates. Top panel shows hypothetical ROC curves for three stimuli. Bottom panel shows hypothetical psychometric functions, one for each of three false-alarm rates. The same nine points from the top panel are replotted in the bottom panel.

points in Fig. 8.4, but if one had a complete family of ROC curves for all levels of detectability one could use them to plot a complete family of psychometric functions for all false-alarm rates, or vice versa. The only aspect of the psychometric functions in the bottom of Fig. 8.4 that was not determined by the ROC curves in the top of Fig. 8.4 is the spacing of the stimulus intensities on the horizontal axis. Although intensity b is plotted as about three times intensity a, that spacing is arbitrary. How the intensities labeled b and a relate to each other is information that is not given anywhere in the top plot.

If the top plot represents experimental information, one could presumably recover the stimulus intensity from knowledge of the experiment. If the top plot represents ROC curves predicted by some version of the independent-analyzers model above, however, actual stimulus intensity is totally unrecoverable. For, in those models, no assumption was made about how the signal strength parameter is determined by stimulus intensity. In other words, no assumption was made about the analyzer's transducer function.

In general, therefore, the family of ROC curves for different intensities of a stimulus gives exactly the same information as the family of yes-no psychometric functions at different false-alarm rates for that same stimulus, except that the psychometric functions also tell how detectability depends on actual stimulus intensity. Note that this statement is true for a stimulus in any experimental condition (e.g., an alone condition or an intermixed condition).

8.2.2 Deducing an Analyzer's Transducer Function From Empirical Results

One consequence of the relationship between ROC curve families and psychometric-function families is this: If any model correctly predicts the families of ROC functions, that model can also be made to correctly predict the families of psychometric functions by adding to the model the appropriate assumption about how the signal strength parameter depends on stimulus intensity (about the analyzer transducer function).

What is the "appropriate" assumption? An example may be more understandable than a general statement. Consider the situation shown in Fig. 8.4. Suppose the ROC curves happened to be curves predicted by a sum-of-outputs exponential model for a simple-alone condition. Suppose the curves are those predicted when the analyzer's stimulus-strength parameter (k' in this case) was set equal to 0.15 (for curve a) and 0.6 (for curve b); that is, a factor of 4 apart.

Suppose now that these two predicted curves matched empirically measured curves when the stimulus intensities were contrasts of 0.025 (for curve a) and 0.05 (for curve b). Now, to make the model predict this relationship one could simply add an assumption that a contrast of 0.025 produces a k' of 0.15 and a contrast if 0.05 produces a k' of 0.6. The more stimulus intensities one knew about, the more complete one could make this description of this transducer function relating k' to contrast.

Of course, one would hope that some simply stated function (rather than a simple pairing of many values) would suffice. The following function would do for the above example:

$$k'_i = \left| \frac{c(\text{stim})}{0.065} \right|^2$$

where the denominator is the stimulus contrast producing a k' value of 1.0.

Since forced-choice performance is just equal to the area underneath the predicted ROC curve (see section 7.6.2), the transducer function could be deduced from forced-choice data in the analogous way: The values of the model's stimulus-strength parameter that predicted certain proportions correct would be associated with the stimulus intensities that produced those proportions correct in experimental data.

If an independent-analyzers model predicts the families of ROC functions (in all experimental conditions) correctly, then with a transducer function added, as in the above example, it will also predict the families of psychometric functions (in all conditions) correctly. The question of just how well any of these independent-analyzers models with added transducer function can predict the full families of psychometric functions or ROC functions for visual patterns (in even the simple-alone condition, much less in all conditions) is still far from settled, however. In the remaining sections of this chapter (which can be skimmed or skipped with little loss of continuity) we will look further at several particular independent-analyzers models with transducer functions added that have appeared in the pattern vision literature.

8.3 HIGH-THRESHOLD VERSION WITH TRANSDUCER FUNCTION

8.3.1 Quick Pooling Model

In Chapter 4 we have already met an example of an independent-analyzers model with a transducer function added. The Quick pooling model was simply a high-threshold independent-analyzers model with the added assumption that the signal strength parameter depended on stimulus intensity in the way specified by the Quick psychometric function (Assumption 43; see section 4.8.2 for discussion).

As we have already seen, the high-threshold version of the independent-analyzers model is inadequate for explaining pattern vision, in several ways: Its predictions for ROC curves and the corresponding psychometric function families are wrong (section 4.7.4); it predicts no extrinsic-uncertainty effect; and, an interrelated fact, it may predict too much summation in blocked-summation experiments (section 7.4.8).

It does a wonderful job, however, at predicting the results of intermixed-summation experiments on many dimensions of pattern vision (see Chaps. 4, 5, and 6). And its prediction for contrast thresholds in intermixed-summation experiments (the Quick pooling formula) is easy to use as well as accurate. A very desirable goal, therefore, is a model that will accurately predict ROC families (and psychometric function families) and extrinsic-uncertainty effects and yet also produce predictions for intermixed-summation experiments that are indistinguisable from the Quick pooling formula.

8.3.2   With Log-Normal Transducer Function

Wilson and Bergen (1979) considered another function relating an analyzer's probability of being in the detect state to stimulus intensity—the cumulated lognormal distribution. (The log-normal distribution is an extension of the normal—Gaussian—distribution in which the logarithm of z rather than z itself is normally distributed.) Like the Quick function (and unlike the cumulative normal distribution, for example), the cumulative log-normal distribution function is zero for zero contrasts (as must be true for any candidate transducer function for high-threshold independent analyzers since, by definition, there is zero probability of a high-threshold analyzer being in the detect state on a blank trial).

No explicit comparisons of this model's predictions with psychometric functions were shown by Wilson and Bergen (1979). And, of course, the high-threshold model with this transducer function added will fail in the same way that other high-threshold models do at explaining the shape of empirical ROC curves and extrinsic-uncertainty effects for sinusoidal gratings of different spatial frequency. For intermixed-summation experiments measuring contrast thresholds, however, this model should do quite well, as the calculations of Wilson and Bergen (1979) show. When the parameters of the log-normal distribution have been set appropriately, the predictions of this model for contrast thresholds in intermixed-summation experiments are very like those of the Quick pooling formula with an exponent of about 4 (somewhat less for small numbers of far-apart components, somewhat greater for large numbers).

8.4   GAUSSIAN VERSION WITH POWER FUNCTION TRANSDUCER

Whenever a model assuming constant-variance Gaussians (or, less frequently, unequal-variance Gaussians or spread exponentials) is fit to data from detection of visual patterns and a transducer function is found relating signal strength parameter (d' or k') to stimulus intensity, then the transducer function is typically described as a power function (as in assumption 92) with exponent larger than 1.0, like that in the equation of section 8.2.2 (e.g., Blackwell, 1963; Cohn et al., 1975; Foley & Legge, 1981; Nachmias & Kocher, 1970; Nachmias & Sansbury, 1974; Stromeyer & Klein, 1974; Tanner, 1961). Such power functions are nonlinear functions of contrast, accelerating with contrast throughout the near-threshold range of contrasts. (For higher contrasts the transducer function is presumably not described by the accelerating power function any longer, but psychometric functions and ROC curves cannot, perforce, give valid information for contrasts very far above threshold.)

The value of the exponent b estimated by fitting a power function to a particular empirical psychometric function turns out to be about 0.8 times the value of the exponent k obtained by fitting a Quick psychometric function (a Weibull function) to the same data (Pelli, 1985, 1987; see also Wilson, 1980b).

With constant-variance Gaussians (no matter what the transducer function), an independent-analyzers model cannot account for the shallow ROC slopes typically found for visual patterns. With increasing-variance Gaussians or exponentials, an independent-analyzers model can account for these slopes, and therefore, with a power-function transducer, presumably could predict both psychometric functions and ROC curves. Such a model (with either the sum-of-outputs or maximum-output decision rules) may also predict extrinsic-uncertainty effects and intermixed-summation effects on the spatial-frequency dimension well, although to my knowledge, such predictions have not been directly compared with empirical results or with predictions from the Quick pooling formula.

For blocked-summation experiments, an approximate formula for the predictions of a sum-of-outputs constant-variance Gaussian model has been developed (Mayer & Tyler, 1984, and personal communication, 1984) starting from the following points: (a) The d' Euclidian sum formula of section 7.6.5, which is appropriate for blocked-summation experiments and implies the use of a sum-of-outputs or equivalent decision variable. (b) Wilson's (1980b) derivation of approximate forced-choice psychometric functions from constant-variance Gaussian versions with nonlinear transducers. The resulting approximate formula is

$$S_{obs}(\text{cmpd}) \text{ proportional to } M^{1/2b}$$

where M is the number of equally stimulated independent and nonoverlapping analyzers (responding to M equally detectable far-apart components).

Compare this with the Quick pooling formula prediction for a similar experiment, namely (see, e.g., Eq. 4.13 in section 4.9.2),

$$S_{obs}(\text{cmpd}) \text{ proportional to } M^{1/k}$$

Since the estimated value of b is about 0.8 times the value of k estimated by fitting a Quick function to the same data, the sum-of-outputs Gaussian model predicts that the sensitivity of the observer should increase as M is increased a good deal more slowly than predicted by the Quick pooling model. In fact, the predicted logarithm of the sensitivity of the observer plotted against the logarithm of the number of components will have a slope about half as great ($\frac{1}{2}b$, which is approximately $\frac{1}{2}$ of the $1/k$ slope predicted by the Quick pooling formula).

This is another reflection of the fact that Gaussian models predict a good deal less blocked summation than do high-threshold models (see Fig. 7.7 for example), but this time expressed in terms of contrast thresholds rather than performance at a given contrast level.

8.5   THE QUICK POOLING FORMULA WITHOUT A HIGH THRESHOLD

There is a maximum-output version of the independent-analyzers model that is not the high-threshold version but still will predict exactly the Quick pooling formula (Eq. 4.9) for yes-no intermixed-summation experiments. No such version predicting the Quick pooling formula seems possible for forced-choice intermixed-summation experiments, however (Nachmias, 1981).

In this version the probability density function and the transducer function characterizing an individual analyzer are such that

Assumption 68. Quick Function With Interdependent Parameters.   *The probability that the ith analyzer's output is less than criterion is given by*

$$\Pr[R_i(\text{stim}) < \lambda] = (1 - g_i(\lambda)) \cdot 2^{-\langle c(\text{stim}) \cdot S_i(\text{stim},\lambda)\rangle k(\lambda)}$$

where the three parameters of the Quick function—the sensitivity parameter S, the false-alarm rate parameter g, and the steepness k—depend on the criterion λ. Two of the three (S and g) also depend on i (i.e., on which analyzer is under consideration).

If one lets the slope parameter k also depend on i, the result we are aiming at cannot be derived. The sensitivity parameter S will also depend on the stimulus, of course.

Then, letting the observer's sensitivity be

$$S_{\text{obs}}(\text{stim},\lambda,M') = \left| \sum_{i=1}^{M'} S_i(\text{stim},\lambda)^{k(\lambda)} \right|^{\langle 1/k(\lambda)\rangle}$$

one can show that (see 8.10.2), with the maximum-output detection rule,

$$\Pr_{\text{obs}}(\text{no}\,|\,\text{stim},\lambda,M') = 2^{-|c(\text{stim})S_{\text{obs}}(\text{stim},\lambda,M')|k(\lambda)} \cdot \Pr_{\text{obs}}(\text{no}\,|\,\text{blank},\lambda,M')$$

where $\Pr_{\text{obs}}(\text{no}\,|\,\text{stim},\lambda,M')$ is the probability that an observer says no to a stimulus given that the criterion equals λ and that M' analyzers are being monitored in an intermixed condition.

As this last equation shows, the observer's psychometric function has the form of a Quick function, where the sensitivity of the observer is playing its usual role.

Further, this equation says that the sensitivity of the observer can be computed as the power sum of the sensitivities of the analyzers, that is, that the Quick pooling formula (Eq. 4.9) applies.

When far-apart stimuli are under consideration, this version of the Quick pooling formula—which contains unobservable quantities—can be turned into forms containing only observable quantities, just as was done in Chapter 4.

In the predictions of this model, however, in contrast to the use of the Quick psychometric function and Quick pooling formula in Chapter 4, the sensitivity, slope, and guessing parameters of the observer's psychometric function are interdependent because they all depend on the criterion λ. They can, therefore, be assumed to vary in the way necessary to fit empirical yes-no psychometric functions (with both slope and threshold increasing as false-alarm rate decreases; Nachmias, 1981). This means, of course, that the predicted amount of summation, which is given by $1/k(\lambda)$, will depend on λ (and therefore on false-alarm rate) in just the same way that the reciprocal of the steepness parameters of psychometric functions do. In particular, if false-alarm rate is very low there should be less summation (a steeper psychometric function) than if it is higher (Nachmias, 1981). Such a prediction, which will also be made by any other version of the maximum-output independent-analyzers model that comes close to predicting the Quick pooling formula, has never been verified empirically to my knowledge.

An Aside. Note that the use of the same criterion for every analyzer's output, which follows from the assumption that the observer's decision is based on the maximum output, is not necessary in the preceding derivation. If one instead had a decision rule according to which every analyzer's output was separately compared with its own criterion and the observer detected a stimulus if and only if at least one of the analyzer's outputs was larger than its own criterion, the same predictions would result.

As this model incorporates "true false-alarms," that is, each analyzer's output is sometimes greater than criterion even when the blank is presented, it will predict decrements due to extrinsic uncertainty.

8.6 INTRINSIC-UNCERTAINTY VERSION WITH LINEAR MICROANALYZER TRANSDUCER

8.6.1 *Linear Microanalyzers Imply Nonlinear Analyzers*

There is a particularly attractive way to add a transducer-function assumption to the intrinsic-uncertainty version of the independent-analyzers model. And it leads to very interesting predictions. The assumption is exactly what would be true if each microanalyzer were a mechanism with photon noise (as in section 8.1.2).

Assumption 69. Linear Transducer Functions for Microanalyzers. *The mean of the Gaussian distribution characterizing any microanalyzer's output is proportional to stimulus intensity.*

(If a microanalyzer is not sensitive to the stimulus under consideration, the constant of proportionality is zero.)

According to this assumption, the intensity levels used for the various rows of Fig. 8.1 must be 0, 1, 2, 3, and 8 units of normalized intensity, where 1 unit of normalized intensity is that intensity producing a d' of 1.0 in the sensitive microanalyzer. Thus, the horizontal axis in Fig. 8.2, which is currently labeled as the average output from the sensitive microanalyzer, could be relabeled normalized stimulus intensity, and then Fig. 8.2 shows the transducer function of the analyzer.

Four Parameters of Intrinsic-Uncertainty Model. Only four parameters need be specified to calculate the predicted detectability of a given stimulus in either alone or intermixed conditions and in either yes-no or forced-choice experiments from the full intrinsic-uncertainty version of the independent-analyzers model (the version with this last transducer function assumption added). The four are (Pelli, 1985):

1. M'', the total number of monitored microanalyzers in all the monitored analyzers, which thus incorporates both extrinsic and intrinsic uncertainty.
2. P'', the total number of monitored microanalyzers that are sensitive to the given stimulus.
3. λ, the criterion for yes-no.
4. The factor relating normalized intensity to physical intensity.

Accelerating Analyzer Transducer Function. The important consequence of Assumption 69 is illustrated in Fig. 8.2. Namely, given a linear transducer function for each microanalyzer, the implied transducer function for the analyzer (the function relating the analyzer output to stimulus intensity) is accelerating at low intensities before becoming linear at high intensities. As mentioned in section 8.4, an accelerating nonlinearity in the analyzer output function is the kind of behavior necessary to describe the empirical detection of visual patterns. It is, in fact, this property of models embodying intrinsic uncertainty that has frequently motivated their use (e.g., Pelli, 1985; Tanner, 1961), because it allows one to assume linear transducer functions for the basic units in the model (the microanalyzers) and yet predict the nonlinearity evident in the data.

8.6.2 *Predicted Psychometric Functions*

The question remains, however, just how well this model can quantitatively predict empirical results. Extensive calculations [most recently and exhaustively by Pelli (1985)] are quite encouraging.

Psychometric Functions. Pelli (1985) derived a number of interesting and useful quantitative relationships between the four parameters of the intrinsic-uncertainty model and both yes-no and forced-choice psychometric functions, including relationships between this model's parameters and the parameters of Quick psychometric functions fit to this model's predicted psychometric functions. See the original article for the precise relationships; these relationships are summarized only qualitatively here.

With reasonable choices of parameters, the intrinsic-uncertainty model can predict not only the empirically obtained decrease in ROC slope with increased detectability (see section 8.1.5) but also—with the linear microanalyzer-transducer assumption added—the change of slope of yes-no psychometric functions with criterion (as described by Nachmias, 1981). It also predicts forced-choice psychometric functions very well, which is not too surprising given their close theoretical relationship to yes-no functions (but see note 2 for a general failure of signal-detection models to properly account for the relationship between yes-no and forced-choice results).

Change of Forced-Choice Psychometric Function Slope with Uncertainty. One prediction of some interest is that, as uncertainty increases (in the sense that M'' increases while P'' remains the same), forced-choice psychometric functions are predicted by this model not only to move to the right but to become steeper on a horizontal logarithmic contrast axis. Pelli (1985) showed some such calculations and also proved that the effect of increasing uncertainty M'' past a constant factor (once M'' is greater than $P'' + 100$) is like subtracting a constant amount of contrast. It is straightforward to apply this prediction to extrinsic-uncertainty experiments as well (where the increase in M'' is due to the observer's monitoring more analyzers in the intermixed-condition and therefore more microanalyzers). In fact, however, although psychometric functions for sinusoidal gratings have been measured many times in the alone condition (e.g., some in Robson & Graham, 1981) versus the intermixed condition (e.g., Fig. 4.10 with the same observers in similar conditions), no steepening has been obvious. Perhaps, however, one should not really expect to see the steepening in an extrinsic-uncertainty experiment even if this kind of model were correct. For suppose one considers raising the uncertainty by a factor of 3, starting from a level that produces psychometric function slopes like those observed. Suppose one starts with $M'' = 300$, for example, which leads to a slope parameter k of 3.28. Approximately tripling M'' to 1000 will only raise the slope parameter to 3.72 (Pelli, 1985, Table 1). This small an increase would be very difficult to tell from the usual kind of data.

One visual study (Cohn & Lasley, 1974; the stimuli varied on the temporal-position dimension) did find a steepening of psychometric function slope, but that experiment may have been more like an intensity discrimination experiment (since a background of lights at all four temporal positions appeared on every trial). However, let's consider these results for the moment. Interpreting the obtained psychometric function slopes using Pelli's Table 1, one would probably conclude that $M'' = 1$ in the alone condition and increases to about $M' = 10$ when four different temporal positions were intermixed ($P'' = 1$ throughout). That is, an increase in M from 1 to 4 produces an increase in M'' from 1 to 10. (Compare section 7.4.8 and Assumption 65.)

Uncertainty's Effect on Yes-No Psychometric Functions. The effect of uncertainty (changing M'' while keeping P'' constant) on yes-no psychometric functions is very different from that just described for forced-choice functions. After the yes-no predicted functions have been "corrected for guessing" (as in section 7.6.6), neither their slopes (with a horizontal logarithmic intensity axis) nor their horizontal positions are affected. (Before correction, however, both slope and position are; e.g., Cohn, 1981.) These parameters are not affected because all the effects of uncertainty are absorbed by the guessing or false-alarm rate parameter [the estimated value of Pr(no/blank)]. For a given criterion λ (and therefore a given slope of yes-no psychometric function), the false-alarm rate increases as uncertainty (M'') increases. The false-alarm rate "absorbs" not only the extra false alarms on the blank (due to monitoring of more microanalyzers) but also the extra hits in response to the nonblank stimulus (spurious hits due to monitoring of more insensitive microanalyzers). A more rigorous argument to this point is given in Pelli (1985).

8.6.3   More Predictions and Summary

Intermixed-Summation. We showed earlier that intermixed-summation results are less sensitive to assumed probability distribution than are blocked-summation or extrinsic-uncertainty experiments (e.g., section 7.4.3). Thus it is not too surprising when any one of the independent-analyzers models predicts intermixed-summation effects much like those of the high-threshold version. But the agreement between the intrinsic-uncertainty model's predictions (with the linear microanalyzer-transducer function) and the high-threshold predictions (with the Quick psychometric function) is more than good—it is extremely good—in Pelli's 1985 calculations, which show both sets of predictions for a couple of sets of experimental results. The intrinsic-uncertainty model accounts very well for intermixed-summation effects measured as contrast thresholds, therefore, since its predictions seem quite indistinguishable from those of the Quick pooling model.

Pedestal Effect in Intensity Discrimination. The intrinsic-uncertainty model also can predict the "pedestal effect" in contrast discrimination experiments—the fact that discrimination is sometimes better than detection. See section 10.8.2.

Open Questions. A serious question remains as to whether the intrinsic-uncertainty model could predict all the results it does if the values of the parameters were kept constant. The parameters in Pelli's (1985) calculations varied rather a good deal, but the experimental results they were chosen to fit were collected on different observers with different patterns and so on.

Although the general results of Chapter 7 can be used to guess quite well at the predictions of the intrinsic-uncertainty model for extrinsic-uncertainty and blocked-summation designs, it would be preferable to calculate some predictions and test them against experimental results.

8.7   A PHYSIOLOGICAL ASIDE—THE PROBABILITY DISTRIBUTION OF SINGLE NEURONS' OUTPUTS

Given the possible correspondence between cortical neurons and mechanisms in the psychophysical multiple-mechanisms model, it is natural to wonder whether visual cortical neurons have the properties postulated of the analyzers or microanalyzers in this and the previous chapter. Both the similarities and differences are intriguing.

Means and Variance of Neuronal Firing Rates. When simple and complex neurons in area 17 of the cat and V1 of the monkey respond to drifting sinusoidal gratings, the variance of their firing rate is generally found to be directly proportional to the mean and somewhat larger than the mean (median factor of 1.76). Both the mean and variance tend to increase linearly with the contrast of gratings once a criterion or threshold contrast level has been exceeded. The mean response to a blank is usually zero for simple cells but will be greater than zero for complex cells. The distribution of the response magnitudes is neither Gaussian nor Poisson (Dean, 1981a, 1981b; Tolhurst & Thompson, 1981, Tolhurst et al., 1983).

This neuronal behavior is quite different from that of the microanalyzers of the intrinsic-uncertainty model. The neuronal behavior is somewhat more similar to that of the exponential or increasing-variance Gaussian versions of the analyzers but is far from identical. The neuronal variance grows too quickly with mean, for one thing, and then (see below), the shape of the neuronal psychometric functions does not seem to be affected by changes in criterion (here taken as number of spikes) in the way that yes-no psychometric functions do.

Psychometric and ROC Functions. The responses of simple and complex neurons in area 17 of the cat and V1 of the monkey to sinusoidal gratings have been analyzed in ways analogous to those used for human psychophysical data (Tolhurst et al., 1983). The responses of a single neuron to gratings of various intensity levels can be described as psychometric functions by plotting the probability that the neuron fires more than a criterion number of spikes. These neuronal psychometric functions are well described by Quick psychometric functions, which suggests a correspondence with human results. Similarly, if a family of ROC functions for different intensities is plotted and the area under the ROC function at each intensity is computed, then a plot of the area (equivalent to forced-choice percent correct according to signal-detection theory) versus stimulus intensity is well fit by a Quick function.

However, when the criterion number of spikes is varied for the neuronal psychometric functions, the slope of these functions stays the same (unlike the slopes of yes-no human psychometric functions at different criteria).

And perhaps more dramatically, the slopes of these neuronal psychometric functions (even when every effort has been made to estimate them over a very short period of time to avoid the shallowing effect of changes in sensitivity) are quite shallow, with slope parameters k ranging generally from 1.25 to 2.5 with a logarithmic mean of 1.82. (These parameters are approximately the same for cat or for monkey, for simple or for complex cells.) Even when corrected for slow fluctuations in sensitivity over time, the slope parameters are only about 25% higher (and thus range from about 1.65 to 3.1 with a geometric mean of about 2.3). These are a good deal shallower than those typically reported for human observers (see Chap. 4) or for monkey observers, which gave estimates of k from 2.4 to 5.7 with a logarithmic mean of 4.2 (data from W. H. Merigan and R. Harwerth as analyzed and reported by Tolhurst et al., 1983).

If the responses of two to eight neurons are combined by the rule that the overall response occurs only if *all* two to eight respond and if all two to eight are assumed to be probabilistically independent, then the resulting psychometric function is still well described by a Quick function, but now has an exponent in the range agreeing with human and monkey behavioral data (Tolhurst et al., 1983). Thus one might wish to suggest that a group of two to eight neurons is the substrate for one analyzer in the models we have been discussing, although the combination rule over a group making up an analyzer must then be different from the combination rule over the analyzers (and see the comments about correlation among neurons in section 5.4.4).

Why Are Neurons and/or Psychophysical Mechanisms Variable? Due to the photon nature of light, different presentations of a nominally identical visual stimulus are not the same, and thus some variability in response to different presentations of a given visual pattern is inevitable. (Thus, the high-threshold model could not be absolutely correct in any case; for, with some probability, a presentation of a blank field will produce the same set of photons at the eye as does a presentation of an above-zero-contrast pattern.)

It is far from clear that most variability has this source, however, and the question remains as to the source of the other variability. Is it just that the biological cost of building a noise-free system is too great to have produced one? Or is the variability actually serving some useful purpose? One such purpose that has been suggested is that the variability ensures that the average firing of a group of neurons adequately encodes the time course of a stimulus in spite of the fact that each neuron's spikes must come at discrete intervals (Knight, 1972; Stein, 1970). Perhaps, also, the nonlinear pooling across analyzers that are differentially responsive to the stimulus (the *probability summation effect*) is of some value to the organism (e.g., in some sense matching the properties of the system to an arbitrary stimulus, as in section 6.7.4).

8.8   ATTENTIONAL CONTROL AND INDIVIDUAL DIFFERENCES

This section discusses a number of issues relevant to the notion of "monitoring" used in the independent-analyzers model here. It can be skipped with little loss of continuity.

8.8.1   *How Many Analyzers Can Be Monitored Simultaneously?*

That the size of the uncertainty effects can be accounted for by independent-analyzers models is consistent with the perfect monitoring assumption used in those models, and therefore suggests that the observer can monitor perfectly the several analyzers sensitive to stimuli in the intermixed condition. It would be interesting to find out just how many analyzers an observer can monitor perfectly, but in the spatial-frequency domain, there is a limit to how many stimuli affecting completely separate analyzers one can find. (If the stimuli do not stimulate completely separate analyzers, the predictions are much harder to compute and depend crucially on parameters like bandwidth, about which we are not certain.) In any case, the greatest number of far-apart spatial frequencies that has been used is five (Davis et al., 1983).

Fast enough switching among different analyzers would, of course, be indistinguishable from simultaneous monitoring of several.

The independent-analyzers models also assume that the observer is able to selectively monitor fewer analyzers when it is appropriate, as in the alone condition. And the tuning of the uncertainty effect when unbalanced-intermixed blocks contain a preponderance of one spatial frequency suggests that observers can monitor a limited set of analyzers in that condition also. Increasing the proportion of trials on which the primary spatial frequency was presented in the unbalanced-intermixed condition of the primary-plus-probe experiments did seem to decrease the range of spatial frequencies and thus perhaps the number of analyzers being monitored (Davis & Graham, 1981). One wonders how narrow a range might be monitored in the extreme.

8.8.2 Conscious Rejection or Preconscious Selection

The question naturally arises as to what process controls which analyzers an observer monitors at any one time. The answer is necessarily complicated, as the huge psychological literature on attention testifies. The experimental results here have little bearing on the answer to this question. Either very late (postconscious) or very early (preconscious) selection or anything in between is consistent with all the experimental results. But the introspective reports of formal and informal observers (described at slightly greater length in Graham et al., 1985) suggest that earlier rather than later selection occurs most of the time in extrinsic-uncertainty experiments on the spatial-frequency and spatial-position dimensions. The same conclusion has been reached for auditory frequency (Scharf et al., 1987).

8.8.3 Effect of Cues

Here we will present a partial experimental answer to one particular question about the process controlling attention—a question about the temporal characteristics of the process. Will cueing the observer shortly before or after a forced-choice trial—where the cue indicates which nonblank stimulus occurs on that trial—improve performance in the intermixed condition?

In intermixed blocks where the spatial frequencies are precued by auditory signals coming 0.75 second before the first of the two intervals in the forced-choice trial, performance is identical to that in alone blocks. In other words, precueing completely eliminates the uncertainty effect (Davis et al., 1983). Observers have reported, in fact, that stimuli in precued intermixed blocks are more salient than stimuli in alone blocks; this suggests that nonasymptotic measures of performance, for example responses required in a certain time interval, might have shown better performance in precued conditions than in alone. Percent-correct detection is, however, equal (within experimental error) in the two conditions.

As the time of the cue is moved later in the trial, the improvement produced by the cue decreases, although some remains even for postcues coming 500 milliseconds after the end of the second interval (Kramer, 1984).

Precueing auditory frequency has been reported to eliminate (Gilliom & Mills, 1976) or reduce (Swets & Sewall, 1961) the uncertainty effect for auditory frequency.

Precues also improve detectability of random-dot patterns of differing direction of motion (Ball & Sekuler, 1981b). Postcues, however, actually hurt performance in this situation. (The difference in effectiveness of cues may well be related to the fact that the uncertainty effect in this situation is much larger than that for gratings of different spatial-frequency, being consistent with a single attention-band model in fact; Ball & Sekuler, 1980).

8.8.4 Individual and Situation Differences

If observers can and do monitor different sets of analyzers depending on what they know about the situation (e.g., monitoring a stationary single analyzer or small groups of analyzers in alone conditions and in the primary-plus-probe unbalanced intermixed condition, but monitoring all relevant analyzers in an ordinary intermixed condition), there is every reason to suppose that differences may exist among individuals in the same experiment as well as between experimental situations. Perhaps some observers' visual systems cannot selectively monitor the outputs of low-level analyzers. Perhaps some observers simply do not do so. They may not have paid enough attention (at a much higher cognitive level) to the information the experimenter gave them about the stimuli that might be presented. They may simply be too occupied with other thoughts (or lazy or forgetful) to change their monitoring strategy from block to block in an experiment (even though the cueing experiments suggest that some observers can do it within a second). Thus they may always monitor all analyzers, thereby erasing the usual uncertainty effect by reducing performance in the alone condition to the level of performance in the intermixed condition. Or they may only sporadically monitor all analyzers in the intermixed condition, tending to concentrate instead on one or two of their favorites, thereby producing a much larger than usual uncertainty effect. The *true* magnitude of the uncertainty effect may therefore be only a "typical" or "usual" quantity for the typical or usual experiment on typical or usual subjects.

Indeed, in our laboratory we have seen occasional (two or maybe three) individuals who produce much smaller uncertainty effects than typical. One individual produced results that varied from session to session more dramatically than most observers' results do, but turned out to have an uncorrected visual deficit that caused her substantial discomfort. Another observer, however, produced results showing typical intersession variability and yet showed no uncertainty effect in either of two groups of six sessions. (Each session contained alone, simple-intermixed, precued-intermixed, and postcued-intermixed conditions for three spatial frequencies—1, 4, and 16 cpd. One group of sessions used feedback, one did not.) This observer disappeared from our laboratory thereafter, however, due to the demands of school work, so we were unable to follow up on possible explanations.

Ball and Sekuler (1981b) also reported individual differences in the effect of uncertainty about the direction of motion of random dots.

Apparently minor differences in experimental situations might also affect the quality of monitoring for most or all individuals. For example, the shorter the block of trials, or the less the observer knows about the experiment, the less likely the observer may be to adopt the "appropriate" or typical monitoring strategy. Feedback or other payoff for correct answers may be more likely to force "optimal" behavior (and therefore the simultaneous monitoring of all analyzers in the intermixed condition and the monitoring of only the one analyzer in the alone condition) unless it backfires and the observer acts less than optimally in a vain attempt to outguess the random sequence of the intermixed block (as in the old probability learning experiments).

8.8.5 Can an Observer Simultaneously Monitor Many Analyzers in More Complicated Tasks Than Detection?

The conclusion that observers in near-threshold detection tasks (like those in summation and extrinsic-uncertainty experiments) can simultaneously monitor all (and only) the relevant analyzers should not be expected to generalize to more complicated tasks. The question of whether it generalizes to near-threshold identification tasks is taken up in section 10.1.4.

Tasks using suprathreshold stimuli are not in general considered in this book, but the following caveat is worth making. Both alternatives of a typical suprathreshold discrimination task overlap heavily along many dimensions (e.g., in spatial position or in spatial frequency) as well as both being far above threshold. According to a multiple-mechanism model of pattern vision, therefore, many of the same mechanisms will produce large outputs in response to both alternatives. With such substantial overlap in what mechanisms respond, any simple rule (like the sum-of-outputs or maximum-output rules used earlier) may well be far from optimal for suprathreshold discriminations (although being close to optimal for near-threshold tasks like those considered here). It is quite likely, therefore, that our nervous systems undertake further and more complicated processing of the mechanisms' outputs in order to make these suprathreshold discriminations. It seems entirely plausible that, in the complicated calculations required to make suprathreshold discriminations effectively, only some of the mechanisms' (analyzers') outputs can be dealt with simultaneously. One might even argue that preconscious selection occurs in near-threshold experiments (see section 8.8.2)—although the observers in those experiments could monitor all analyzers and consciously reject false alarms—because in more ordinary suprathreshold situations costs are incurred if all mechanisms' outputs are allowed upstream.

8.8.6   Selective Attention to Avoid False Alarms

Several functions of selective attention are commonly discussed (e.g., Kahneman & Treisman, 1984): prevention of perceptual overload (as implied in the last paragraph), prevention of memory overload, prevention of paralysis resulting from response competition. The monitoring done by observers in extrinsic-uncertainty experiments has another function, however: that of avoiding false alarms. Many important components of visual scenes (very high spatial frequencies at the fixation point, not so very high spatial frequencies a few degrees out) are at or below their contrast threshold, a range where noise appears to limit detectability. Thus the avoidance of false alarms is an adaptive function of selective attention that could be of considerable importance, not only in the alone conditions of uncertainty experiments but in ordinary visual perception.

8.9   SUMMARY

A new version of the independent-analyzers model—called the *intrinsic-uncertainty model*—postulates that each analyzer is composed of microanalyzers, only some of which are sensitive to the stimuli of the task at hand. These insensitive microanalyzers may be a good model of uncertainty intrinsic to the observer and may reflect the observer's uncertainty about just which microanalyzers (e.g., mechanisms in a multiple-mechanisms model) ought to be monitored in a given task. In the calculations discussed here, these insensitive microanalyzers are assumed to be characterized by constant-variance Gaussian distributions and to be mutually probabilistically independent.

Which of the independent-analyzers models from the previous chapter is most like this intrinsic-uncertainty model depends on the number of sensitive and insensitive microanalyzers. For quite a wide range of parameters, this intrinsic-uncertainty version will make predictions like the exponential and increasing-variance Gaussians of the previous chapter.

A transducer assumption can always be added to any independent-analyzers model. If the appropriate transducer function is added to a model that correctly predicts the ROC curves for different stimulus intensities, then this augmented model will now also predict the empirical psychometric functions correctly.

Examples of transducer function assumptions added to the high-threshold model (in particular, the Quick pooling model) and to the constant-variance

Gaussian models are presented. A maximum-output model that is not a high-threshold version but still predicts exactly the Quick pooling formula for yes-no intermixed-summation experiments is also presented.

With the intrinsic-uncertainty model, an interesting transducer function assumption is that each microanalyzer's mean output is assumed to grow linearly with stimulus intensity; then each analyzer's output has an accelerating nonlinearity at low intensities. This model seems able to predict correctly an impressive variety of empirical facts on the spatial-frequency dimension (Pelli, 1985).

8.10 APPENDIX

8.10.1 Computation of the Intrinsic-Uncertainty Probability Distribution

The following equations calculate $F_j(z\,|\,\text{stim})$—the distribution function for the jth analyzer—from the $F_{ji}(z\,|\,\text{stim})$—the distribution functions for the microanalyzers in the jth analyzer.

$$F_j(z\,|\,\text{stim}) = \prod_{i=1}^{Mj} F_{j,i}(z\,|\,\text{stim}) = |F_{j,1}(z\,|\,\text{stim})|^{P'}\,|F_{j,1}(z\,|\,\text{noise})|^{Mj-P'}$$

Notice that this computation is exactly like that of the general method for calculating the distribution of the observer's maximum-output decision variable from the distributions characterizing the analyzers (section 7.6.3) except that quantities for the analyzers there have been replaced by quantities for microanalyzers here, and quantities for the observer there have been replaced by quantities for the analyzer here.

For the computation here, the distribution functions $F_{ji}(z\,|\,\text{stim})$ are always cumulative Gaussians with the same variance (but potentially different means).

One calculates the density function $f_j(z\,|\,\text{stim})$ for the analyzer's output by differentiating the distribution function $F_j(z\,|\,\text{stim})$.

8.10.2 Derivation From a Maximum-Output Model That Is Not a High-Threshold Model of the Quick Pooling Formula for Yes-No Intermixed-Summation Experiments (Section 8.5)

The equation that follows (see section 7.6.3) gives the predicted probability that the observer says no to a stimulus in an intermixed condition in which M' channels are being monitored and the criterion is λ:

$$\text{Pr}_{\text{obs}}(\text{no}\,|\,\text{stim},\lambda,\text{mix}) = \text{Pr}(R < \lambda\,|\,\text{stim},\text{mix}) = \prod_{i=1}^{M'} \text{Pr}[R_i(\text{stim}) < \lambda]$$

$$= \prod_{i=1}^{M'} [1 - g_i(\lambda)] \cdot 2^{-[c(\text{stim})\cdot S_i(\text{stim},\lambda)]k(\lambda)} = 2^{-|c(\text{stim})k(\lambda)\Sigma S_i(\text{stim})k(\lambda)|} \cdot \prod_{i=1}^{M'} [1 - g_i(\lambda)]$$

This last expression can be simplified by first applying it to the blank stimulus (the contrast of which is zero) to show that

$$\mathrm{Pr}_{\mathrm{obs}}(\mathrm{no} \,|\, \mathrm{blank},\lambda,\mathrm{mix}) = \prod_{i=1}^{M'} (1 - g_i(\lambda))$$

and then substituting the left side of this last equality for the right side above.

Finally, defining the sensitivity of the observer as in section 8.5 and substituting it in the expression above gives the desired result presented in section 8.5.

Notes

1. *Pelli's terminology.* In Pelli's (1985) terminology, microanalyzers are samples; different analyzers are not discussed at all. The total number of microanalyzers is called M by Pelli. It corresponds to the total number of microanalyzers monitored, the quantity called M'' here. The number of microanalyzers sensitive to the stimulus in question is called K by Pelli. It corresponds to P'' here, or, if just one analyzer is being monitored, P'_j).

2. *Discrepancy between yes-no and forced-choice results.* Empirically, the percent correct measured in a two-alternative forced-choice procedure may be consistently larger than the area underneath the ROC curve from yes-no or rating-scale procedures (Nachmias, 1981). This discrepancy is impossible for any of the independent-channels models to predict as is. There are at least two attractive explanations for this discrepancy (Nachmias, 1981). These two explanations could, in principle, be incorporated into any model, although they have not been in any quantitative way.

1. Observers may engage in suboptimal strategies in yes-no or rating-scale procedures but not in forced-choice procedures. An obvious candidate is differential criterion fluctuations: trial-to-trial variations in the observer's criterion when a yes-no procedure is being used, but no such variation (or much smaller variation) in a forced-choice procedure, in which the criterion is somehow less arbitrary. (In a forced-choice procedure, the observer may simply say whichever interval produced the biggest response—that is, a criterion of zero difference between intervals). Although criterion fluctuations are not often considered in signal-detection theory because they are yet one more complication, some discussion of their effects can be found (e.g., Nachmias & Kocher, 1970; Treisman & Williams, 1984; Wickelgren, 1968).

2. The values of the decision variable on the two intervals of a two-alternative forced-choice trial may be positively correlated with each other, whereas the values on a typical signal and a typical noise trial of a yes-no block may not (since they occur farther apart in time).

V
IDENTIFICATION

9
Discrimination

9.1 INTRODUCTION

In identification (or recognition—see note 1) experiments, an observer is asked to identify which of several nonblank stimuli has been presented. In other words, the observer is asked to *discriminate* among several nonblank stimuli. In the adaptation, summation, and uncertainty experiments discussed earlier, the observer was asked only to detect the stimuli (to discriminate between any non-blank stimulus and the blank stimulus). In this book, we will discuss only those identification experiments using stimuli at intensities so low that the stimuli themselves are imperfectly detectable—that is, at intensities near detection threshold or, for short, "near threshold."

9.1.1 Some Typical Value-Selective Results

Figure 9.1 shows some typical value-selective behavior in an identification experiment using simple stimuli that vary along some dimension of interest. The vertical axis shows the amount of confusion between two stimuli, one having a value V_0 (marked by an arrow on the horizontal axis) and the second having a value V (plotted on the horizontal axis). Confusability is the opposite of iden-tifiability; particular operational definitions of confusability will be given later. As Fig. 9.1 shows, when the value V equals V_0, the two stimuli are identical and thus the observer must show complete confusion between the two. When the value V is far enough from V_0, however, the observer may show little or no confusion between the two stimuli. Such value-selective behavior is consistent with the existence of multiple analyzers on the dimension of interest, but there are, as usual, problems of interpretation.

9.1.2 Intuitive Argument for Multiple Analyzers From Identification Experiments

Far-Apart Values. Consider an observer asked to identify which of several near-threshold nonblank stimuli has been presented. Suppose that (a) the stimuli are far enough apart that each excites a different analyzer (or group of analyzers) and (b) the outputs of the analyzers are well enough labeled that higher levels of processing can tell which analyzer a given output came from.

What should happen according to these assumptions? Roughly, whenever the observer is able to detect that some nonblank stimulus has been presented, we know that the appropriate analyzer (or analyzers) has produced a large enough

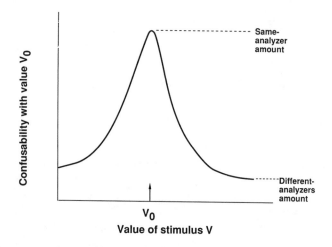

FIG. 9.1 Typical results of an identification experiment showing value-selective behavior. Some measure of confusability between two values is plotted as a function of the second value. The first value is V_0 and indicated by an arrow.

output. Since the analyzers' outputs are assumed to be labeled, the higher stages in the visual system know which of the analyzers produced the large-enough output. Thus the higher stages can identify the stimulus. In short, for far-apart stimuli and labeled analyzers, whenever the observer can detect that a nonblank stimulus has occurred, the observer ought to be able to identify which nonblank stimulus it is. (To make this argument rigorous and produce precise predictions, a complete model is needed; see below.)

Close Values. If, however, the several stimuli all excite the same analyzer or analyzers, then the mere fact that that particular analyzer has produced a large output may not provide sufficient information to identify which of the stimuli caused the output.

Importance of Labeled Outputs. Notice that, if analyzers do not have labeled outputs—that is, if the levels of processing upstream cannot tell which analyzer an output came from—an observer might be unable to identify even very-far-apart stimuli. Thus, if analyzers exist on some dimension but do not have labeled outputs, value-selective behavior might show up in adaptation and summation experiments but not in uncertainty experiments or identification experiments. The eye-of-origin may be an example of such a dimension (see Chap. 12).

9.1.3 Identification Based on Output Magnitudes Instead of on Analyzer Identity

If stimuli cause different magnitudes of output from the same analyzer, these different magnitudes might be used by the higher levels of processing to identify the stimuli. To avoid identification that is based on output magnitudes rather than on which analyzer responded, either of two experimental strategies can be adopted: The intensities of the stimuli can be adjusted to be equally detectable (that is to cause, presumably, the same average magnitude of output from the analyzers responsive to them) or the intensities of the different stimuli can be randomly varied from trial to trial.

9.1.4 *Identification Based on Analyzers on Some Other Dimension*

A subtler problem in interpretation can occur if analyzers on some other dimension are able to contribute to the identification of stimuli on the dimension of interest. For example, consider spatial-frequency analyzers that are channels—are arrays of neurons having receptive fields of the same size but at different spatial positions. Then, even though two stimuli affect only a single spatial-frequency analyzer and are equated for detectability, they may still elicit responses from that single spatial-frequency analyzer that differ in some respect sufficient to allow identification. If the stimulus is a sinusoidal grating, for example, the output profile from this spatial-frequency channel will be a sinusoidal function of spatial position with a period reflecting the period of the grating. If higher levels of the visual system can extract the period in the output profile of a single analyzer, the observer could discriminate spatial frequency quite well even though both gratings affected the same spatial-frequency analyzer. In this example, the observer is using information from receptive fields at different spatial positions (i.e., different analyzers on the spatial-position dimension) to make a discrimination on the spatial-frequency dimension. Thus, this is an example of a complication in interpretation in which value-selective behavior on one dimension may reflect the behavior of analyzers on another dimension.

9.2 DISCRIMINATION AND CLASSIFICATION PARADIGMS

In this chapter we will consider three closely related paradigms for studying identification when only two stimuli are involved—a task that is often called discrimination between two stimuli and to which we will refer simply as *discrimination*. The two stimuli could be far above detection threshold, and often are (e.g., Campbell, Nachmias, & Jukes, 1970), but in this book we are interested only in experiments where they are near threshold.

The three discrimination paradigms considered here are diagrammed in Fig. 9.2 and described below.

A variety of other paradigms for discrimination between two stimuli have been used in the study of various sensory/perceptual dimensions, although not widely in pattern vision. (Presentation of some of these paradigms can be found in Chap. 10 and in, for example, Creelman & Macmillan, 1979; K. O. Johnson, 1980a, 1980b; Luce, 1963; Luce & Green, 1974; Macmillan, Kaplan, & Creelman, 1977. The identification paradigms in Chapter 10 can also be considered

DISCRIMINATION BETWEEN TWO STIMULI

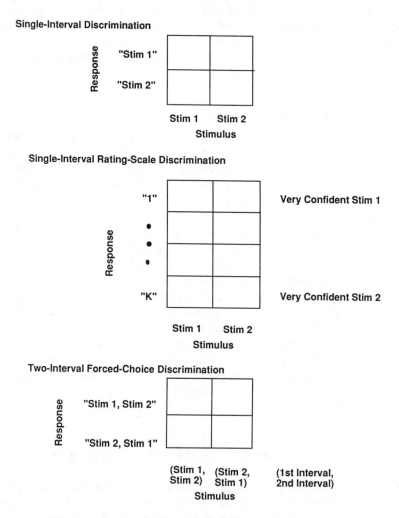

Single-Interval Discrimination

Single-Interval Rating-Scale Discrimination

Two-Interval Forced-Choice Discrimination

FIG. 9.2 Diagram of three kinds of discrimination experiments.

to measure the discriminability between pairs of stimuli, although they are more involved than the paradigms considered in this chapter.)

9.2.1 *Single-Interval Discrimination*

In single-interval discrimination between two stimuli (top of Fig. 9.2), one of two stimuli is presented randomly on each single-interval trial and the observer is to say which was presented.

9.2.2 Rating-Scale Discrimination

In single-interval rating-scale discrimination between two stimuli (middle of Fig. 9.2), each trial again contains a single interval presenting one of two stimuli. Now, however, the observer must use a rating scale ranging from "very confident stimulus 1 was presented" (rating category 1) through "unsure which stimulus was presented" to "very confident stimulus 2 was presented" (rating category k).

9.2.3 Forced-Choice Discrimination

In two-interval forced-choice discrimination (bottom of Fig. 9.2), one interval of each trial contains stimulus 1 and the other stimulus 2. (Which stimulus is in the first interval is chosen randomly). The observer must say which order was used (that is, which stimulus was in the first interval).

9.2.4 The Classification Paradigm

It will be useful to know that two of the three discrimination paradigms in Fig. 9.2 (the single-interval and the forced-choice) are examples of a more general paradigm (illustrated in Fig. 9.3) that we will call the *classification paradigm* here. (It is sometimes called the *complete identification paradigm,* e.g., Bush, Galanter, & Luce, 1963.) In a classification experiment, the N possible stimuli (stim i, $i = 1,N$) and the N possible observer responses (saying stim i, $i = 1,N$)

THE CLASSIFICATION PARADIGM
(COMPLETE IDENTIFICATION)

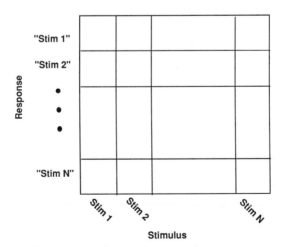

FIG. 9.3 Diagram of classification paradigm.

are in one-to-one correspondence. That is, the observer's response indicates which of the N possible stimuli he or she thinks has been presented. When the single-interval discrimination paradigm is considered as a classification paradigm, the stimuli in the latter correspond to the stimuli in the former and N equals 2. When the forced-choice discrimination paradigm is considered as a classification paradigm, N again equals 2 but now the "stimuli" in the classification interpretation correspond to the two different trial types (stimulus 1 in the first interval vs. stimulus 1 in the second interval) in the discrimination interpretation.

Notice that not all discrimination experiments are classification experiments (e.g., the rating-scale version is not), and vice versa.

For classification experiments there are some equivalences among decision rules (sections 9.4.2 and 9.4.3) that will prove useful here for discrimination paradigms. They will be useful again when applied to the more general identification paradigms that happen also to be classification experiments (see Chap. 10).

9.2.5   *Discrimination When One Stimulus is a Blank*

When one of the two stimuli is a blank, these three discrimination paradigms are equivalent to detection paradigms and are frequently called from top to bottom, respectively: *yes-no* (or *single-interval*) *detection; rating-scale detection;* and *two-alternative forced-choice detection.*

9.3   REVIEW OF PREVIOUS ASSUMPTIONS OF INDEPENDENT-ANALYZERS MODELS

We will start out with the same assumptions that were used in section 7.3 for an independent-analyzers models, and then add assumptions when necessary. We will particularly need to add assumptions describing the transformation from analyzer outputs to observers' responses in identification experiments. The assumptions used in this chapter are the following (number and short title only):

Assumption 25. Single-Number Outputs
Assumption 34. Multiple Analyzers
Assumption 35. Nonoverlapping at Far-Apart Values
Assumption 36. Ineffective Stimulus Rule
Assumption 37. Noninteracting Analyzers
Assumption 38. Probabilistically Independent Analyzers
Assumption 40. Maximum-Output Detection Rule
Assumption 41. Yes-No Rule
Assumption 42. Forced-Choice Rule
Assumption 51. Perfect Monitoring
Assumption 52. Probabilistically Independent Trials

Assumption 53. One Analyzer per Stimulus
Assumption 54. Identical Probability Distribution Families
Assumption 55. High-Threshold Family
Assumption 56. Spread-Exponentials Family
Assumption 57. Increasing-Variance Gaussians ($r = \frac{1}{8}$)
Assumption 58. Increasing-Variance Gaussians ($r = \frac{1}{4}$)
Assumption 59. Constant-Variance Gaussians ($r = 0$)
Assumption 60. Shifted Double-Exponentials Family
Assumption 61. Sum-of-Outputs Detection Rule
Assumption 62. No Criterion Variance
Assumption 63. Hybrid Decision Rule
Assumption 64. Likelihood-Ratio Decision Rule

Of course only one of the six alternative probability distribution family assumptions (Assumptions 55 through 60 in the list) and only one of the four alternative decision rules (Assumptions 40, 61, 63 and 64) is used at any one time. An additivity assumption (e.g., Assumption 36) is necessary only when compound stimuli are included. The assumption that exactly one analyzer is sensitive to each of several far-apart stimuli (Assumption 53) is made for convenience in some places, although with little loss of generality (see discussion in sections 4.7.5, 7.3.6, and 9.6). Further, in this chapter and the next we will frequently drop this assumption and explicitly represent many analyzers per stimulus. Such explicit representation of many analyzers per stimulus is easy to do when constant-variance Gaussians and certain kinds of decision rules are assumed (see section 9.6) and, as it happens, these are the assumptions most frequently made in the identification literature.

9.4 CLASSIFICATION DECISION RULES

We will start with decision-rule assumptions that can be applied to all classification experiments (see Fig. 9.3), including some of the experiments discussed in Chapter 10. In this section we will be applying them to the single-interval discrimination and forced-choice discrimination paradigms (Fig. 9.2). We will also describe some other decision rules for the discrimination paradigms of Fig. 9.2 that cannot be applied to all classification experiments.

9.4.1 Some Definitions and the Closest Stimulus Rule

Several definitions are useful in describing these rules.

Analyzer-Output Space. For single-interval trials, the *analyzer output space* is the space in which each dimension gives the magnitude of the output of one analyzer. Thus the dimensionality of this space for single-interval trials is the number of analyzers. For two-interval trials, each dimension corresponds to the magnitude of the output of one analyzer in a given interval. Thus the dimensionality of the space is twice the number of analyzers.

The Expected Vector—The Stimulus Point. For each possible stimulus in a classification experiment, there is a point in the analyzer-output space that gives the expected output of each analyzer to that stimulus, or, in the case of two-interval trials, the expected output of each analyzer in each interval to that stimulus. For readers familiar with vectors, it will be useful to consider the vector from the origin to this point rather than just this point. Readers unfamiliar with vectors will not go far wrong just thinking about points and skimming over all references to vectors. There is a brief appendix about vectors at the end of this chapter.

We will use the following terms interchangeably: *expected point, expected vector, stimulus point,* and *stimulus vector.* Indeed, we will sometimes talk as if the stimulus itself occupied that point in analyzer-output space.

When it is necessary to refer to these stimulus (or expected) vectors in symbols, we will often observe the following conventions to keep the symbols conveniently short. The stimuli—which up to this point have been numbered—will also be called by uppercase letters used in alphabetical order. For example, stimulus 1 will also be called stimulus A, stimulus 2 will also be called stimulus B, and so on. Then the expected (average) output of analyzer i to stimulus A can be called A_i for short, that is (for example)

$$A_i = E[R_i \text{ (stimulus A)}] \quad \text{and} \quad B_i = E[R_i \text{ (stimulus B)}]$$

And the stimulus vectors for stimuli A and B can be called **A** and **B** that is,

$$\mathbf{A} = (A_i, i = 1, M') \quad \text{and} \quad \mathbf{B} = (B_i, i = 1, M')$$

where M' is the number of monitored analyzers. When appropriate, these vectors are expanded to be of dimensionality $2M'$ by including the expected output of each analyzer twice, once for each interval.

The Observed Vector—The Analyzer-Output Point. The outputs from all the analyzers on any single-interval trial (or from all the analyzers in both intervals on any two-interval trial) also correspond to a point or vector in the analyzer-output space. We will use the following terms interchangeably for this point: *observed vector, observed point, analyzer-output vector,* and *analyzer-output point.* In symbols, that vector will be denoted **R**,

$$\mathbf{R} = (R_i, i = 1, M')$$

For two-interval trials, this vector has $2M'$ dimensions to include the outputs of each analyzer in both intervals of a two-interval trial.

The Difference Between the Observed and an Expected Vector—The Distance Between a Stimulus and the Analyzer Outputs. The Euclidian (ordinary) distance in this analyzer-output space between the stimulus point and the observed analyzer-output point will sometimes be referred to here as the *distance between the analyzer outputs and the stimulus.* This distance is the length of the difference vector between the expected or stimulus vector (**A**) and the observed or analyzer-output vector (**R**). The difference vector is

$$\mathbf{A} - \mathbf{R} = (A_i - R_i, i = 1, M')$$

and its length will be denoted $|\mathbf{A} - \mathbf{R}|$.

The Closest Stimulus Rule. We are now ready to state a very common and useful identification decision rule:

Assumption 70. Closest Stimulus Classification Rule. *The observer's response on each trial is the stimulus that is closest (as measured by Euclidian distance) in analyzer-output space to the observed analyzer outputs on that trial.*

Figure 9.4 illustrates the closest stimulus classification rule for the case of a two-dimensional analyzer-output space (R_1 and R_2) and two far-apart simple stimuli. The stimulus points corresponding to those two stimuli are in the center of the circles on the horizontal and vertical axes. If the observed point on a given trial falls below the positive diagonal, the closest stimulus is the one on the horizontal axis (stimulus 1). Thus, according to Assumption 70, the observer's

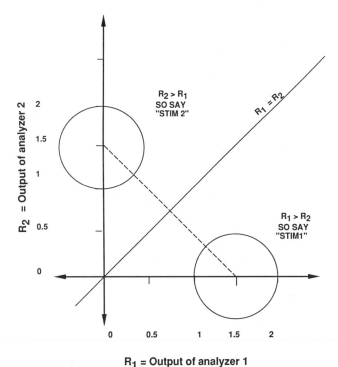

FIG. 9.4 Maximum-output and closest-stimulus rules for two far-apart equally detectable simple stimuli.

response would be "stimulus 1." If the observed point falls above the positive diagonal, the closest stimulus is stimulus 2.

9.4.2 Maximum-Likelihood Decision Rules

The probability that a particular set of analyzer outputs will occur on a trial given that a particular stimulus is presented is called a *likelihood*. In symbols, where k indicates a particular stimulus, the likelihood for stimulus k is

$$\text{Pr}[\mathbf{R}(\text{stimulus } k)] = \text{Pr}[R_i(\text{stimulus } k), i = 1, M']$$

Consider computing this likelihood for all the stimuli k in the experiment under consideration. According to the next assumption, the observer's identification response is determined (not necessarily consciously of course) by whichever of these likelihoods is largest.

Assumption 71. Maximum-Likelihood Classification Rule. *The observer's identification response is the stimulus (indexed by k) for which the likelihood that the observed analyzer outputs were produced is greatest, that is, the k for which the following quantity is greatest:*

$$\text{Pr}[R_i(\text{stimulus } k), i = 1, M']$$

(In case of ties, the observer chooses between outputs without bias.)

Optimal Behavior. As mentioned earlier for detection experiments (section 7.4.7), the maximum-likelihood classification rule produces optimal behavior under some circumstances. If all stimuli are presented equally often, then the maximum-likelihood classification rule is equivalent to maximizing the a posteriori probability, that is, to assuming that the observer's response is whichever stimulus has the highest probability of having occurred on that trial given the analyzer outputs observed on that trial.

If there are symmetric payoffs (the payoffs for all correct answers are the same and the payoffs for all incorrect answers are the same), then maximizing the a posteriori probability maximizes the expected (average) payoff.

Maximizing percent-correct classification—maximizing the total proportion of all trials in which the observer's response corresponds to the stimulus actually presented—is an example of maximizing payoff in a symmetric situation. For computing the percent correct is like giving all correct answers the same payoff ($+1$) and all incorrect answers the same payoff (zero).

In general, however, for unequal presentation probabilities or asymmetric payoffs, maximizing likelihood is not equivalent to maximizing a posteriori probability or payoffs. (For more introduction and discussion see, e.g., Chap. 6 of Coombs et al., 1970; Green & Swets, 1966 or 1974.)

Equivalence to Closest Stimulus Classification Rule for Constant-Variance Gaussians. For constant-variance Gaussians, the closest stimulus classification rule can be shown to be equivalent to the maximum-likelihood classification rule and thus to produce optimal behavior for equal presentation probabilities and symmetric payoffs. This is not true in general for other probability distributions.

9.4.3 Maximum-Output Identification Rule for Simple Stimuli

In a classification experiment (Fig. 9.3) in which the stimuli are all simple stimuli, the following rule seems plausible. According to it, an observer identifies a stimulus on the basis of which one of the M' monitored analyzers gives the maximum output:

Assumption 72. Maximum-Output Identification Rule for Simple Stimuli. *The observer's response is the one stimulus (of all the stimuli used in the experiment) to which the maximally responding analyzer is most sensitive.*

Guessing. In the case of discrete density functions, it is possible that the outputs of several analyzers are tied at the maximum. The observer is then assumed to guess among those analyzers (with equal probability).

Notice that, according to this maximum-output identification decision rule, the observer's response depends on *which* of the random variables R_i produced the maximum output, and not on the magnitude of that maximal output. The maximum-output detection rule (Assumption 40) uses the magnitude of the maximal output.

When the Closest Stimulus Classification Rule and the Maximum-Output Identification Rule Are Equivalent. The closest stimulus classification rule and the maximum-output identification rule are equivalent when the simple stimuli are equally detectable and far-apart and each excites only one analyzer.

To understand this, consider again the case shown in Fig. 9.4 for two equally detectable, far-apart simple stimuli and two analyzers. The mean output of one analyzer to the "other" stimulus is shown as zero, as this illustration is for the case of two far-apart stimuli (nonoverlapping analyzers). The circle around the point for either stimulus contains the central part of the probability distribution, that is, the area of the diagram in which the two analyzers' outputs will fall some given proportion of the time. As these probability distributions are shown as circular, they illustrate the case of independent noise in the two analyzers. Further, as the points representing the analyzers' mean outputs to the two stimuli are equidistant from the origin and the probability distributions are identically shaped, the two stimuli are equally detectable.

Now, according to the maximum-output identification rule, the observer's response will be stimulus 1 (that stimulus 1 was presented) if and only if R_1 was greater than R_2. That happens if and only if the point plotting the observed analyzer outputs falls below the positive diagonal in Fig. 9.4, since on the positive diagonal the difference $R_1 - R_2$ equals zero. But this behavior is exactly that produced by the closest stimulus classification rule, as was discussed earlier (section 9.4.1).

Even when there are more than two stimuli—as long as they are equally detectable and far-apart and excite only a single analyzer each—this equivalence holds. For the stimulus (expected) points in the analyzer-output space are (a) all on the axes of the analyzer-output space and (b) equally far from the origin. And thus the stimulus closest to the analyzer-output point is also the stimulus corresponding to the maximally responding analyzer.

When these conditions are not met, however, and the stimuli are not equally detectable and/or not equally far-apart and/or excite more than a single-analyzer, the closest stimulus classification rule and the maximum-output identification rule are not equivalent at all.

9.5 DISCRIMINATION DECISION RULES

9.5.1 *The Closest Stimulus Classification Rule for Classification of Two Stimuli*

The closest stimulus classification rule can be stated in a different way for discrimination experiments that are also classification experiments (single-interval or forced-choice discrimination paradigms in Fig. 9.2). Consider the line connecting the two stimulus points in analyzer-output space. Consider the plane that is perpendicular to and bisects this line connecting the two stimulus points. The dimension of this plane is one less than that of the analyzer-output space. Thus this plane is a line if the analyzer-output space has only two dimensions, as in Fig. 9.4. We will call this plane the *bisector*. In Fig. 9.4 the dotted line connects the two stimulus points; the solid line perpendicular to and bisecting this line is the bisector. Then, as is clear in Fig. 9.4 (but also applies to the general case of any two stimuli in any dimensionality of analyzer-output space), the closest stimulus classification rule becomes

Assumption 73. Bisector Rule. *The observer says whichever stimulus is on the same side of the bisector as the observed point (the point representing the analyzer outputs on that trial).*

No Bias. This rule predicts that there be no bias toward one alternative over another. When applied to the single-interval discrimination paradigm (top Fig. 9.2), for example, it predicts that the probability of the observer saying stimulus 1 when stimulus 1 is presented is the same as the probability of the observer saying stimulus 2 when stimulus 2 is presented, and thus either probability equals the overall probability of correct identification. When applied to forced-choice discrimination (bottom Fig. 9.2), the bisector rule predicts that there be no "interval bias," that is, the observer is no more likely to be correct when stimulus 1 is in the first interval than when it is in the second interval.

In experimental results, however, bias is sometimes observed. Further, neither of these rules can be applied to the rating-scale discrimination paradigm, because in that paradigm there are more observer responses than there are stimuli.

9.5.2 *Difference-of-Outputs Discrimination Rules*

To deal with these latter complications is relatively straightforward for discrimination between two stimuli. One generalizes the bisector rule by constructing a decision variable that, as usual in signal-detection theory, is compared with a criterion. We will introduce the general decision variable by first illustrating it for the case of two analyzers and discrimination between two equally detectable far-apart stimuli (Figs. 9.4 and 9.5).

For all points on the perpendicular bisector in Fig. 9.4 (the positive diagonal in this case) the difference between the two analyzers' outputs ($R_1 - R_2$) equals zero. Thus, the closest stimulus classification rule for this case can be reworded as: The observer says stimulus 1 if and only if the difference between the analyzers' outputs in the direction favoring stimulus 1 was greater than zero, that is, if and only if $R_1 - R_2$ was greater than zero.

This rewording suggests using the difference between the two analyzers' outputs as a decision variable that determines the observer's response according to standard signal-detection assumptions (see section 9.5.3 for a review). When stimulus 1 is presented, the decision variable $R_1 - R_2$ will tend to be large (very positive), but when stimulus 2 is presented, $R_1 - R_2$ will tend to be small (very negative). As illustrated in Fig. 9.5, the decision variable $R_1 - R_2$ is constant on

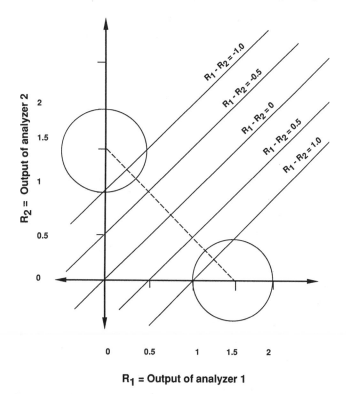

FIG. 9.5 Criterion lines for difference-of-outputs decision variable.

any line that is perpendicular to the line joining the two stimulus points (alternately, on any line parallel to the positive diagonal). Thus, any criterion used with the decision variable $R_1 - R_2$ corresponds to a line that is perpendicular to the line joining the two stimulus points. For example, the criterion $+0.5$ in "Say stim 1 if and only if the decision variable is greater than $+0.5$") corresponds to the line $R_1 - R_2 = 0.5$ shown in Fig. 9.5. We will list this decision variable as a possible assumption before moving on to a still more general one:

Assumption 74. Difference-of-Outputs Discrimination Rule.   *The observer uses the difference between the two analyzers' outputs, $R_1 - R_2$, as the decision variable in the way dictated by standard signal-detection theory where larger (positive) values favor a response of stimulus 1.*

This rule as stated is appropriate for discrimination between two equally detectable simple stimuli.

This rule can be easily generalized to a discrimination between any two stimuli A and B in an analyzer-output space of any dimensionality as follows. One finds the line joining the two stimuli's points **A** and **B** in analyzer-output space and then uses a decision variable for which the criterion planes are perpendicular to this line. These criterion planes will have one less dimension than does the analyzer-output space itself. The decision variable will always be simply a linear combination (a weighted sum or difference) of the various analyzers' outputs, since it is constant on each of the criterion planes. A number of linear weighted combinations could serve as the decision variable. We will use the following one:

Assumption 75. Generalized Difference-of-Outputs Discrimination Rule.   *The decision variable used by the observer is*

$$\mathbf{R} \cdot (\mathbf{A} - \mathbf{B}) = \sum_{i=1}^{M'} R_i \cdot (A_i - B_i)$$

It is used in the standard manner of signal-detection theory where large values of this decision variable are taken to favor the first stimulus (stimulus A).

For those who care about details, this decision variable is the numerator of an expression giving the length of the component of vector **R** that is in the direction of the difference vector $(\mathbf{A} - \mathbf{B})$. (See section 9.11, the appendix on vectors.)

9.5.3   *Standard Assumptions Linking Decision Variables to Observers' Responses in Discrimination Experiments*

Let DV be the symbol for a decision variable (e.g., the difference-of-outputs variables above) with large values favoring stimulus 1. The usual rules of signal-detection theory for using such a decision variable in the three discrimination paradigms of Fig. 9.2 are as listed in the following. Versions of the first and third were stated earlier for detection experiments as Assumptions 41 and 42. The relationships between discrimination and detection will be discussed further in section 9.5.4.

Assumption 76. Using Decision Variables in Single-Interval Discrimination.
The observer says that stimulus 1 (rather than 2) was presented if and only if the decision variable DV was greater than some criterion.

Assumption 77. Using Decision Variables in Rating-Scale Discrimination. *The greater the value of the decision variable, the more confident the observer is that stimulus 1 (rather than stimulus 2) has been presented.*

Or, in symbols, set $k + 1$ criteria ($c_i, i = 0, k$) where $c_i + 1 > c_i$ for all i. Then the observer gives a confidence rating corresponding to the ith category if and only if the decision variable falls between the two corresponding criterion, that is:

$$\text{Observer says } i \quad \text{if} \quad c_{i-1} < \text{DV} \leq c_i$$

Assumption 78. Using Decision Variables in Forced-Choice Discrimination. *A large value of the decision variable in the first interval relative to the second is evidence that stimulus 1 was presented in the first interval. Thus, the observer says that stimulus 1 was presented in the first interval if and only if*

$$\text{DV (first interval)} - \text{DV (second interval)} > 0$$

The rule just stated predicts that there will be no "interval bias"—that is, the observer is no more likely overall to say interval one than interval two overall. To extend the forced-choice rule to allow for interval bias, one allows a value different from zero on the righthand side of the preceding equation. (One can rephrase this rule in terms of one decision variable, comparing the results from both intervals. See note 2.)

9.5.4 Standard Assumptions Applied to Detection Experiments

Often discrimination between two nonblank stimuli is compared with detection of each of those stimuli. The following paragraphs discuss which of the various detection decision rules previously considered correspond to the discrimination rules just discussed.

Detection of a Simple Stimulus. In Fig. 9.6 (top left panel), the two solid circles represent the probability distribution and mean outputs to the blank (lower left circle) and to simple stimulus 1 (lower right circle). Criterion lines are drawn for a decision variable that is just the output of the first analyzer. In this case, this decision variable is equivalent to both the maximum-output and the sum-of-outputs rules as long as the observer is monitoring only a single analyzer, as perfect monitoring and an alone condition would dictate according to our assumptions (see section 9.3). These criterion lines are clearly perpendicular to the line joining the two stimuli's points, and thus this decision variable is equivalent to the generalized difference-of-outputs discrimination rule (Assumption 74). (Ignore the top right panel of Fig. 9.6 for the time being.)

Suppose, however, that the observer is monitoring both analyzers (as should happen in intermixed detection according to our perfect-monitoring assumption and might happen in a simple-alone condition if perfect-monitoring were

RELEVANT ANALYZER'S OUTPUT

SUM OF OUTPUTS

MAXIMUM OUTPUT

LIKELIHOOD RATIO-GAUSSIAN
KNOWN INTENSITY

LIKELIHOOD RATIO-GAUSSIAN
UNKNOWN INTENSITY

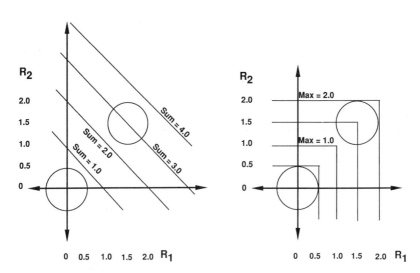

FIG. 9.7 Sum-of-outputs and maximum-output decision rules for detection of a compound (discrimination of a blank from a compound stimulus).

dropped as an assumption). The bottom four panels of Fig. 9.6 show the criterion lines (more generally, curves) for four decision variables that the observer might use in this case. The sum of outputs from both analyzers is in the middle left panel, and the maximum output from the two analyzers is in the middle right panel. The bottom two panels show the likelihood-ratio decision rule appropriate for a condition where two far-apart equally detectable simple stimuli (the one shown and another one having a point located on the vertical axis) are intermixed and the observer is simply to say whether a blank or a nonblank was presented. The probability distributions are assumed to be constant-variance Gaussians, and the intensity of the simple stimuli is assumed to be either known exactly (lower left) or not known exactly (lower right, from Klein, 1985). Notice how similar the criterion lines for the maximum-output decision rule (middle right) are to those for the likelihood-ratio decision rule (lower panels). This is another indication that the maximum-output rule will be close to optimal for simple-intermixed detection.

Detection of a Compound Stimulus. Figure 9.7 shows two diagrams for the

---

FIG. 9.6 Several decision rules for detection of a simple stimulus (discriminating a blank from a simple stimulus). R_1 is the output of the analyzer sensitive to the simple stimulus. R_2 is the output of another independent nonoverlapping, noninteracting analyzer.

detection of a compound stimulus. On the left are some criterion lines for the sum-of-outputs decision rule; the sum of R_1 and R_2 is constant along any line having slope equal to -1. The right diagram shows the criterion lines for the maximum-output decision rule; the maximum of R_1 and R_2 is constant along curves consisting of two half-lines—one vertical and one horizontal—meeting in an upper right corner.

Notice now that the sum-of-outputs detection rule (Assumption 61), illustrated in the upper left of Fig. 9.7), is also a generalized-difference discrimination decision variable (Assumption 75), since the criterion lines are perpendicular to the lines joining the two stimuli to be discriminated (in this case, the blank and the compound having equally detectable far-apart components).

This observation suggests that one could generalize the sum-of-outputs detection rule (Assumption 61) to the case of arbitrary numbers of analyzers with arbitrary sensitivities to the two components A and B of a compound. One could do this by finding the decision variable for which the criterion planes are perpendicular to the line joining the compound of A and B to the blank (zero). One gets, then,

Assumption 79. Generalized Sum-of-Outputs Detection Rule. *The decision variable (used in the standard way of signal-detection theory) is*

$$\mathbf{R} \cdot (\mathbf{A} + \mathbf{B})$$

where high values favor the presence of a signal (usually a compound containing A and B) rather than a blank.

This generalized sum-of-outputs detection rule is exactly equivalent to the generalized difference-of-outputs rule (Assumption 75) applied to the task of discriminating a compound of A and B from a blank. Or, to put it another way at the risk of some terminological confusion, the sum $\mathbf{A} + \mathbf{B}$ here in Assumption 79 is playing the role of $\mathbf{A}$ in Assumption 75, and the zero vector here is playing the role of $\mathbf{B}$ in Assumption 75.

Thus this rule is the optimal rule for the compound detection task when the constant-variance Gaussian probability distribution family is assumed. It can, however, be used for other tasks (just as the original sum-of-outputs detection rule was used for simple-intermixed detection), and we will do so later, but it will not then be optimal.

9.5.5   *Applied to Masking Tasks*

Figure 9.8 summarizes a number of discrimination tasks that are of interest. The diagrams show the probability distributions in response to four stimuli: a blank, two equally detectable simple stimuli, and the compound composed of those two simple stimuli. In the left panel the two stimuli are far enough apart to stimulate separate analyzers (which we are assuming are noninteracting) and in the right panel the two stimuli are close enough together to affect each other's ana-

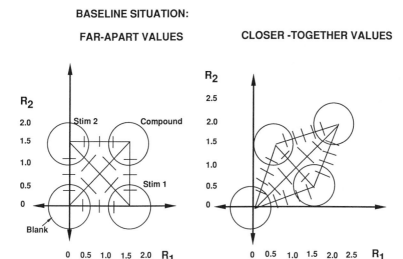

FIG. 9.8 Baseline situation for far-apart (left) and closer together (right) pairs of simple stimuli and their compound.

lyzers. The outputs to the compound are at the upper right corner of a parallelogram; thus complete additivity is assumed (Assumption 27; in the far-apart case, the assumption that ineffective stimuli are ineffective in compounds—Assumption 36—will do).

Because there are four different stimuli, there are six possible pairs that could be used in a discrimination experiment. We have discussed four of those pairs (discrimination between two simple stimuli in Fig. 9.5, detection of each of the simple stimuli in Fig. 9.6, and detection of the compound in Fig. 9.7). For these four, the criterion lines corresponding to a generalized-difference rule (criterion lines perpendicular to the line joining the points) are indicated in Fig. 9.8; only brief segments of these lines are shown to avoid visual confusion.

The remaining two pairs each involve one simple stimulus and the compound of the two simple stimuli. The discrimination between a pair of this sort is often called a *masking task*. For it is a discrimination between a masker (the simple stimulus that is present both by itself and in the compound) and a masker-plus-test (the compound stimulus where the test is the other simple stimulus). In general, masking tasks are beyond the scope of this book, but in these particular cases the masker and the masker-plus-test are both still near threshold.

For these masking tasks in the far-apart case (left panel Fig. 9.8), the generalized-difference decision variable is simply the output of one analyzer (the analyzer sensitive to the test). This decision variable has often been used to model masking experiments. Notice, however, that in the close-together case (right panel Fig. 9.8), the generalized difference-of-outputs decision variable is not just a single analyzer's output (e.g., the analyzer sensitive to the test, as is often assumed) but a linear combination of both analyzers' outputs.

9.6   COMPOSITE ANALYZER COMPOSED OF MULTIPLE ENTITIES

We previously (sections 4.7.5 and 7.3.6) discussed some cases in which a model assuming one and only one analyzer sensitive to each simple stimulus was, in fact, more general—that is, equivalent to models allowing more than one analyzer to be sensitive to each of the simple stimuli. This section discusses one further case [in the spirit of Klein (1985) or Thomas (1983), for example], a case that is of particular use in discussing identification results. This section can be skipped with little loss of continuity as long as the reader is prepared to believe subsequently that restricting the model to only one analyzer per simple stimulus is not too much of a restriction.

9.6.1   Rotating the Analyzer-Output Space

Suppose we start out with a model like the independent-analyzers model in section 9.3 but with more than one analyzer per simple stimulus in the experiment. Consider the analyzer-output space having as many dimensions (N') as there are analyzers. The upper left panel of Fig. 9.9 shows an example where $N' = 3$. Lower case letters r_i are used for the three analyzer outputs in that figure, to save the uppercase symbol R_i for the final composite analyzers. Consider the M points representing the outputs of the N' analyzers in response to the M simple stimuli in some experiment under consideration. $M = 2$ in the upper left panel of Fig. 9.9; the two stimuli will be called A and B. The point for stimulus A is on the "floor" of the drawing; the point for stimulus B is on the "left wall."

Now rotate the space in the upper left panel of Fig. 9.9 (keeping the origin steady) until the point for stimulus A is directly on the horizontal axis. (Algebraically, any such rotation is accomplished by letting each of the new dimensions be a prescribed linear weighting of the values on the old dimensions, that is, by multiplication by the appropriate matrix.) The points representing the $M - 1$ other stimuli may still be in any of a variety of positions. So now further rotate the space while keeping the origin and the point for the first stimulus steady (that is, rotate the space around the horizontal axis) until the point for the second stimulus is on the plane formed by the horizontal and vertical axes (e.g., on the front wall of the drawing as shown in the upper right panel of Fig. 9.9).

For the example of Fig. 9.9, where there are only two stimuli, the process is now finished. The quantities plotted on the first and second new dimensions are called R_1 and R_2, respectively, and are said to be the outputs of the first and second analyzers in a new model; the other dimensions in the new space are ignored.

For the more general case of M stimuli, one continues the process until the points for all M stimuli lie within the first M dimensions of the rotated analyzer-output space.

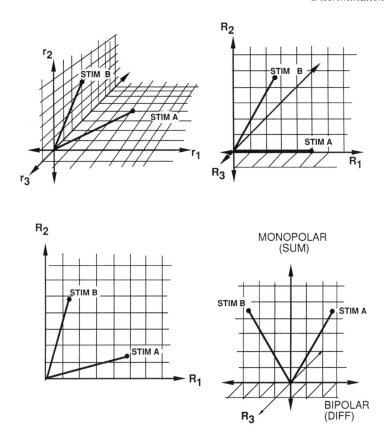

FIG. 9.9 Three ways in which two vectors in three-dimensional space (upper left) can be rotated into a two-dimensional space (the frontal plane in the upper right, lower left, and lower right). The coordinates of the stimulus A and stimulus B vectors in the upper left panel are (3, 0, 4) and (0, 4, 3). In the upper right panel they are (5, 0, 0) and (2.4, 4.4, 0). In the lower left panel they are (1.24, 4.84) and (4.84, 1.24). In the lower right panel they are (2.6, 4.3) and (-2.6, 4.3).

9.6.2   The Multivariate Probability Distributions Have to Be Rotated and Collapsed

It might be best to make explicit that in this rotation process the multivariate probability distributions characterizing the probabilities that the different analyzers in the original model produce various outputs are assumed to rotate appropriately along with the dimensions of the space. Then, when the extra dimensions—those beyond the first M—in the new analyzer-output space are ignored, the probability distributions are collapsed from N'-variate distributions to M-variate distributions by appropriate integration.

Thus the form of the probability distribution characterizing the outputs of the new analyzers may not be identical to that of the old. The new ones will still be

Gaussians, however, if the old ones were. For the new analyzer outputs (the new dimensions) are simply linear combinations of the old, and linear combinations of Gaussian distributions are still Gaussians. Further, if the original analyzer outputs were characterized by the constant-variance Gaussian families (with all analyzers' outputs having the same variance as we have been assuming), then so will the new analyzer outputs be. It is in conjunction with an assumption of constant-variance Gaussian distributions that this rotation approach has been used (e.g., Klein 1985; Thomas, 1983), but it could be used more generally as long as one keeps track of the fact that the probability distribution families characterizing the new analyzer outputs may not be identical to those characterizing the old.

9.6.3 Two More Interesting Rotations for Equally Detectable Stimuli

Monopolar and Bipolar Analyzers (Sum and Difference Analyzers). The lower right panel of Fig. 9.9 shows another possible rotation of the two stimulus points into the frontal plane. Now the vertical axis bisects the angle between them. Klein (1985) has called the resulting analyzers *bipolar* (the horizontal axis) and *monopolar* (the vertical axis). The bipolar analyzer's output says how much of the original analyzers' outputs is in the direction of the difference between the stimulus vectors, and the monopolar analyzer's output says how much is in the direction of the sum. That is, in terms of the stimulus vectors **A** and **B** and the analyzer-output vector **r** from the original space of N' dimensions,

$$\text{Bipolar} = \frac{(\mathbf{A} - \mathbf{B}) \cdot \mathbf{r}}{|\mathbf{A} - \mathbf{B}|}$$

$$\text{Monopolar} = \frac{(\mathbf{A} + \mathbf{B}) \cdot \mathbf{r}}{|\mathbf{A} + \mathbf{B}|}$$

The bipolar analyzer's output can be either positive or negative; it discriminates between the two stimuli in question. The monopolar analyzer's output is generally positive; it indicates how much of either stimulus is present but cannot discriminate between them. See Klein (1985) for further discussion. Cohn and Lasley (1975, 1976) also have considered a pair of analyzers, one summing and one differencing.

Two Symmetric Analyzers. The lower left panel of Fig. 9.9 shows still another rotation in which the positive diagonal bisects the angle between the two stimulus vectors. For the case of equally detectable stimuli, this makes the two resulting analyzers symmetric in the following sense: The expected output of the first analyzer to stimulus B is the same as the expected output of the second analyzer to stimulus A, and the expected output of the first analyzer to stimulus A is the same as the expected output of the second analyzer to stimulus B. This transformation is simply a 45-degree (one-eighth turn) clockwise rotation from the sum and difference analyzers.

If the two stimuli A and B are so far apart that no analyzer in the original space responds to more than one of them, then the cross-dot product $\mathbf{A} \cdot \mathbf{B}$ will be zero (it may be zero in other situations as well) and the stimulus vectors in the symmetric-analyzer space will be on the axes. In this case the rotations in the upper right and lower left of Fig. 9.9 are equivalent.

9.6.4 Relations Between the Original and the Rotated Models Depend on the Decision Rules

The question now becomes, under what assumptions does one of the new models (one that is formed by rotating the old analyzer-output space until there are just as many analyzers as there are simple stimuli) lead to the same predictions as the old model (the one with N' analyzers)? The answer depends on just what the assumptions are.

The Generalized Difference-of-Outputs, Closest Stimulus, and Probability-Based Rules. First an example of a discrimination rule under which rotating the analyzer-output space makes no difference: the generalized difference-of-outputs discrimination rule (an assumption appropriate when the observer knows exactly which two stimuli he or she is trying to discriminate between). The line between the two points in the original space rotates into the line between the two points in the new space. And therefore the criterion planes in the original analyzer-output space, which are planes perpendicular to the line between the stimuli, rotate into planes that are still perpendicular to that line in the new space. Thus with the generalized difference-of-outputs discrimination rule, the new model, with only as many analyzers as simple stimuli, will lead to the same predictions as the old model, with many more analyzers. The generalized sum-of-outputs detection rule (Assumption 79) is an example of such a rule.

The observer's responses using the closest stimulus classification rule will also obviously remain the same after rotation.

Also, if the decision rule is stated in the form of a rule using the full multi-variate probability distributions (which have been correctly rotated and collapsed in going from the old to the new), the old and new model will lead to the same predictions.

The Maximum-Output Detection Rule. Now for an example where rotation and collapse into smaller dimensionality does make a difference. The criterion planes for the maximum-output decision rule in the original analyzer-output space (e.g., if 3 dimensional as in Fig. 9.9, the back, upper and right faces of a cube) will *not* rotate and collapse into criterion lines for the maximum-output decision rule in the new space of smaller dimensionality (e.g., the upper and right edges of a square in two-dimensional space as in the right of Fig. 9.7). Thus the new and old models—both with the maximum-output detection rule—do not lead to the same predictions.

The Maximum-Output Identification Rule and the Closest Stimulus Classification Rule. In the case of far-apart equally detectable simple stimuli, either the rotation shown in the upper right of Fig. 9.9 or that shown in the lower left will put the points for the simple stimuli onto the axes of the new space. Calculations in the original space using the closest stimulus rule will be identical to calculations in the new space using either the closest stimulus classification rule or the maximum-output identification rule.

9.7   PREDICTIONS OF SOME MULTIPLE-ANALYZERS MODELS FOR DISCRIMINATION

Much of the quantitative work for identification experiments has been done assuming the constant-variance Gaussian probability distribution family in a multiple-analyzers model with the generalized difference-of-outputs decision rule. In this case precise results are relatively easy to derive, as will be outlined in section 9.7.2. First, however, section 9.7.1 attempts to provide some insight into these predictions. Finally, section 9.7.3 discusses qualitatively the predictions that would result if various assumptions were loosened.

9.7.1   *When Probability Distributions Are Circularly Symmetric and of Constant Variance*

As it happens, much of the tractability of models assuming the constant-variance Gaussian family comes from the fact that the resulting multivariate probability distributions in analyzer-output space are of the same variance for all stimuli and are, further, circularly symmetric. By circularly symmetric we mean that every isodensity contour (the locus of all points for which the probability density is a given constant value) is a circle in the case of two-dimensional space, a sphere in the case of three-dimensional space, and so on, where circle, sphere, and so on are defined using ordinary euclidian distance. (See note 4 for the possibility of generalizing these arguments to non-Gaussian probability distributions and to noneuclidian metrics.)

This section presents three predictions of multiple-analyzers models that can easily be seen to follow from the generalized difference-of-outputs discrimination rule coupled with constant-variance circularly symmetric probability distributions.

The first two predictions are important in themselves but also serve as an introduction to the third one, which is a generalization that actually includes the first two.

Consider Fig. 9.5 (illustrating a discrimination between two far-apart equally detectable simple stimuli) and the top left panel of Fig. 9.6 (illustrating the simple-alone detection of one of those stimuli). Make the explicit assumption (not made in our earlier use of these figures) that the joint probability distributions for the analyzer outputs R_1 and R_2 are always (as they happen to be drawn) circularly symmetric and of the same variance. Remember that the criterion lines in each diagram are perpendicular to the straight line that connects the two distributions (representing the generalized-difference discrimination rule).

The distributions for discrimination (Fig. 9.5) are further apart than are the ones for detection (Fig. 9.6—by a factor of the square root of 2 in the illustrated case).

Consider what would happen (illustrated by the transformation from the upper left to the upper right panel of Fig. 9.6) if you (a) changed the simple-alone diagram in the upper left panel of Fig. 9.6 by pulling the lower right probability distribution over to the right by a factor of the square root of 2, which corresponds to the use of a simple stimulus of some higher intensity (how much higher depends on the transducer function), and then (b) rotated the expanded simple-alone diagram clockwise by 45 degrees. Now the two distributions and the criterion lines in the diagram for simple-alone detection (upper right panel Fig. 9.6) would look like those in the diagram for discrimination (Fig. 9.5) in the following crucial aspects: The distributions would be the same distance apart in the two diagrams as well as of the same shape and variance, and the criterion lines would run in the same direction. Since these are the only aspects that enter into determining the observer's performance, the following is predicted to hold: Performance measured in the same way should be identical in both the original discrimination task (Fig. 9.5) and in the increased-intensity detection task (upper right Fig. 9.6). The performances can be measured in the same way by running the experiment the same way (e.g., both by single-interval paradigm), or—if the experiments are run differently—performance in one method can be theoretically converted to performance in the other by the appropriate calculation (e.g., forced-choice percent correct equals the area under the rating ROC curve according to the standard signal-detection assumptions).

If one compares the detection task at the original intensity (upper left panel Fig. 9.6) with discrimination (Fig. 9.5), one gets the following prediction:

Prediction 1. Discrimination Better Than Simple Detection for Far-Apart Values. *Discrimination between two simple stimuli (of far enough apart values to stimulate nonoverlapping analyzers) should be better than simple-alone detection of either one (at the same intensity). Discrimination should be better than simple-intermixed detection as well (since simple-intermixed detection is less than or equal to simple-alone detection).*

Now consider rotating the lefthand diagram of Fig. 9.7 (compound detection, sum-of-output decision rule) clockwise or counterclockwise a quarter turn (by 90 degrees). It will be like the diagram for discrimination between the two simple components (Fig. 9.5) in the following respects: The distributions are the same distance apart in both diagrams and are identical in shape and size; the criterion lines run in the same direction. Hence,

Prediction 2. Compound Detection Equals Component Discrimination for Far-Apart Values. *The detection of a compound containing two equally detectable far-apart simple stimuli is predicted to be identical to the discrimination between those simple stimuli.*

This is an elegantly simple prediction that Olzak and Thomas (1981) pointed out and have made good use of.

More generally, whenever (a) the probability distributions are circularly symmetric and of constant variance and (b) the criterion lines are perpendicular to the line connecting the centers of the distributions (the generalized difference-of-outputs discrimination rule),

Prediction 3. Discrimination a Monotonic Function of Euclidian Distance in Analyzer-Output Space. *Performance in discriminations is completely determined by the distance between the two stimuli's points in analyzer-output space. For a given shape and size of probability distribution, the farther apart the two stimuli are in analyzer-output space, the better the observer is able to discriminate between them.*

Note that the two probability distributions need not be centered on the original two axes. Nor does this relationship between performance and distance depend on there being only two analyzers, although that is all the figures illustrate. If there are N' analyzers, the outputs to the two stimuli under consideration can be represented as two points in N' dimensional space, and performance on any two stimuli will be a monotonic function of Euclidian distance. To believe this, simply rotate the two points into the frontal plane, as previously discussed and as shown in Fig. 9.9.

9.7.2   When the Probability Distributions Are Constant-Variance Gaussians

When the constant-variance Gaussian family characterizes individual analyzers' outputs, the probability distributions are circularly symmetric and of constant variance, as in the last section. For this case it is also easy to derive a number of useful quantitative predictions (e.g., Green & Swets, 1974; Klein, 1985; Thomas 1985). These predictions are summarized in the rest of this section and can be omitted with little loss of continuity. In understanding these predictions it is important to remember that, since the generalized difference-of-outputs discrimination rule is a linear combination (a weighted sum) of the individual analyzers' outputs, the probability distribution of the decision variable is Gaussian with constant variance (the same variance in response to any stimulus).

Optimality. For this Gaussian case, optimal discrimination between any two stimuli is achieved using the generalized difference-of-outputs discrimination rule—that is, using criterion lines perpendicular to the line joining the centers of the two distributions in N'-dimensional space where the N' dimensions represent the outputs of all the N' analyzers.

Performance (Measured Appropriately) Equals Distance (Prediction 3 Applied to Gaussians). Let "normalized distance" be the distance between the two stimulus points in analyzer-output space divided by the standard deviation of the probability distribution (where the standard deviation is measured in the distribution collapsed into a plane, as in section 9.6.2). The normalized distance will be represented by the symbol $D(\text{stim } 1, \text{stim } 2)$. For simple-alone detection, the normalized distance reduces to the mean of the signal distribution minus the mean of the noise distribution divided by the standard-deviation—the same quantity called d' in Chapter 7.

Consider the ROC curve from single-interval or rating-scale discrimination experiments; it is formed by plotting the probability of the observer's saying stimulus 1 in response to stimulus 1 (a hit if stimulus 1 is arbitrarily taken as signal and stimulus 2 as noise) against the probability of saying stimulus 1 in response to stimulus 2 (a false alarm). The general Prediction 3 of the last sub-section becomes more precise for this case and says that distance equals performance measured appropriately:

$$D(\text{stim 1, stim 2}) = z(\text{``stim 1''/stim 1}) - z(\text{``stim 1''/stim 2})$$

$$= z(\text{``stim 1''/stim 1}) + z(\text{``stim 2''/stim 2})$$

For detection experiments, this is equivalent to the well-known relationship

$$d' = z(\text{hit rate}) - z(\text{false alarm rate})$$

Negative-Diagonal Relationships (Predictions 1 and 2 Applied to Gaussians). It is often useful to consider the point on the ROC curve at the negative diagonal, the point where there is no bias toward one stimulus or the other so that

$$\text{Pr}(\text{``stim 1''/stim 1}) = \text{Pr}(\text{``stim 2''/stim 2})$$

For the constant-variance Gaussian distribution, the negative-diagonal point on the ROC curve is generated when the criterion line is halfway between the two stimuli's points. For discrimination between two simple stimuli, this unbiased criterion seems quite a natural criterion. If the rotation into a symmetry arrangement has been done (lower left Fig. 9.9), it is equivalent to the maximum-output identification rule (say whichever stimulus corresponds to the analyzer producing the maximum output).

Let z^* denote a z score for the point on the negative diagonal. The last equations imply

$$D(\text{stim 1, stim 2}) = 2 \cdot z^* (\text{``stim 1''/stim 1})$$

For a detection experiment, this can be rephrased as

$$d' = 2 \cdot z^* (\text{hit rate})$$

Now let z^* (simple disc), z^* (simple-alone detect), and z^* (cmpd-alone detect) be symbols for the z scores on the negative diagonals in the indicated tasks, that is, where the two stimuli are the two far-apart simple stimuli for simple discrimination; are one simple stimulus and the blank for simple-alone detection; and are the compound and the blank for compound-alone detection. Then Prediction 1 of the last subsection becomes "discrimination is better than simple detection by the square root of 2 when both are measured by z^*", that is,

$$z^* \text{ (simple disc)} = 2^{1/2} \cdot z^* \text{ (simple-alone detect)}$$

And Prediction 2 of the last subsection becomes

$$z^* \text{ (simple disc)} = z^* \text{ (cmpd-alone detect)}$$

Predicted Relationship Among Performances in the Three Discrimination Paradigms. Performance in the three discrimination paradigms of Fig. 9.2 can be quantitatively related under the assumptions of constant-variance Gaussians and generalized difference-of-outputs discrimination rule. Let AREA be the area underneath either a rating-scale discrimination ROC curve (middle panel Fig. 9.2) or underneath an ROC curve generated by running a number of single-interval discrimination tasks (top panel Fig. 9.2) and inducing different criteria using different payoffs, instructions, and so on. Let FCC be the proportion correct in forced-choice discrimination (bottom panel Fig. 9.2). Let z^* ("stim 1"/stim 1) be the negative-diagonal z score from the single-interval discrimination task (top panel Fig. 9.2). Then (derivation given in note 3)

$$z(\text{AREA}) = z(\text{FCC}) = 2^{0.5} \cdot z^* \text{ ("stim 1"/stim 1)}$$

9.7.3 Predictions From More General Independent-Analyzers Models

For convenient reference, let's repeat here in a slightly different arrangement all the necessary assumptions for the three predictions given in section 9.7.1. These necessary assumptions are illustrated in Fig. 9.8 (left panel), which will be called *the baseline situation* below.

1. The distributions must be located at the four corners of a square, which requires that the stimulus values be far apart, that the analyzers be non-overlapping and noninteracting at far-apart values (Assumptions 35 and 37), and that ineffective stimuli are ineffective in compounds (Assumption 36).
2. The distributions must be circularly symmetric distributions of the same variance. For this it is sufficient to have probabilistically independent analyzers (Assumption 38) with the constant-variance Gaussian family (Assumption 59). See note 4 for discussion.
3. The decision rule must be the generalized difference-of-outputs decision rule (Assumption 75) and the observer's criterion must stay constant throughout the block of trials over which performance is measured (Assumption 62).

Figures 9.10, 9.11, and 9.12 illustrate the consequences of relaxing these assumptions one at a time (with all the others still as in the baseline situation on the left of Fig. 9.8).

Interactions and/or Overlap. The left panel of Fig. 9.10 shows inhibitory interactions between analyzers—the output of one analyzer to the other analyzer's stimulus is negative. (The outputs to the compound stimulus are shown here as being the sum of the outputs to the components, so although the four distributions no longer mark the corners of a square, they still mark the corners of a parallelogram). Everything else staying constant (e.g., circularly symmetric con-

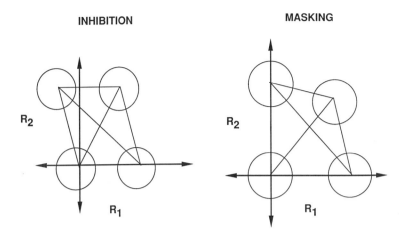

FIG. 9.10 Inhibition (left) and masking (right).

stant-variance Gaussian distributions, generalized difference-of-outputs discrimination rule), it is clear from the left of Fig. 9.10 that inhibition increases the discriminability of the two simple stimuli from one another relative either to each one's detectability or to the detectability of the compound. That is, D(stim 1, stim 2) gets larger relative to D(blank, stim 1) and to D(blank, cmpd).

On the other hand, overlap between the two analyzer's sensitivities or excitatory interactions between them (e.g., as shown previously in right panel Fig. 9.8) would decrease discriminability (increase confusability) relative to detectability. As values on a dimension get closer together, increased overlap is expected and hence increased confusability, as shown in Fig. 9.1.

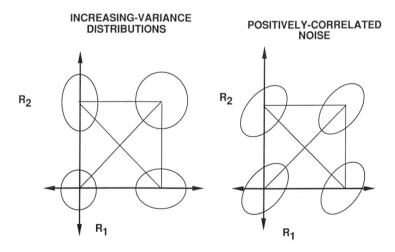

FIG. 9.11 Increasing-variance probability distributions (left) and positively correlated noise (right).

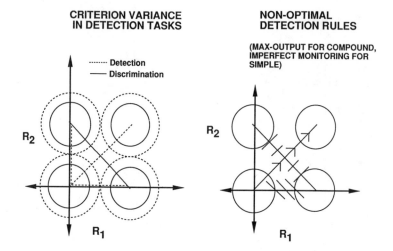

FIG. 9.12 Criterion variance in detection tasks (left) and nonoptimal detection rules (right).

Masking. The right panel of Fig. 9.10 shows a case for far-apart simple stimuli where not only is there not complete additivity but there is not even the weaker property that an ineffective stimulus is ineffective in a compound. Instead, each analyzer's output to the compound is smaller than its output to the one component it responds to. To put it another way, although in this example a component is ineffective by itself in stimulating a given analyzer, it "masks" the other component when the compound is presented to the analyzer. This masking decreases detectability of the compound relative either to discriminability of the simple stimuli from one another or to detectability of the simple stimuli.

For closer together values on many dimensions (e.g., spatial-frequencies, orientations, directions of motion, temporal frequencies, this kind of masking (i.e., less than complete additivity) between different values is expected to occur as a result of probability summation across spatial position or temporal position.

Other Probability Distribution Families. The left panel of Fig. 9.11 shows probability distributions in which variance increases with mean. Note, for example, that although the distance between the points for the simple stimuli (along the negative diagonal) equals the distance between the blank's and the compound's points (along the positive diagonal), the various distributions do not have the same shape, and thus equal distance does not guarantee equal performance.

The ratio of simple discrimination to simple-alone detection performance, and also the ratio of simple discrimination to compound detection performance, has been calculated for the six probability families in Assumptions 55 through 60 (Graham, et al., 1987).

The ratio of z^* (simple disc) to z^* (simple-alone detect)—which is always 1.414 for the constant-variance Gaussian case—varied from about 1.20 to 1.50

depending on the probability distribution family and on the level of detectability. It was greater than 1.41 only for the high-threshold distribution and very low detectability. In general the ratio gets lower as simple-alone detectability gets higher.

The ratio of z^* (simple disc) to z^* (cmpd-alone detect)—which is always 1.0 for the constant-variance Gaussian case—varied from about 0.7 to 1.0 (respectively 1.4) when the sum-of-outputs (respectively maximum-output) rule was used. In general, this ratio gets lower as one moves to distributions having shallower ROC curves.

Positively Correlated Noise. The right panel of Fig. 9.11 shows positively correlated analyzer outputs. The bivariate distributions are not circular but are elongated on the positive diagonal. The standard deviation of these distributions along the negative diagonal, which is the standard deviation relevant for the discrimination between the two simple stimuli, is clearly smaller than that along the positive diagonal, which is the one relevant to the detection of a compound. Hence positively correlated noise improves simple-discrimination performance relative to compound-detection performance. The improvement relative to simple-detection performance will be much smaller. Negatively correlated noise would have the opposite effect.

Some positive correlation between different analyzers' outputs seems almost unavoidable for a variety of reasons, such as slow drifts in sensitivity over time (discussed, for example, by K. O. Johnson, 1980a; Robson & Graham, 1981).

Criterion Variability. The left panel of Fig. 9.12 shows a situation where the criteria for compound detection and simple-alone detection tasks are assumed to vary from trial to trial while the criterion for the simple-discrimination task is assumed to be constant. In the figure, the dotted circles and lines represent the distributions and criteria for detection, and the solid circles and lines represent those for discrimination between the two simple stimuli. Criterion variability is equivalent to added noise. Hence the distributions for detection are shown as more variable (the circles are larger) than those for identification. It has sometimes been argued that differential criterion variability would be more likely to occur in detection tasks where the criterion is essentially arbitrary than in either the single-interval or forced-choice discrimination paradigms where the observer could use the natural criterion of zero, that is, choose whichever output is larger [Klein, 1985 (Klein discussed these discrimination tasks under the heading "Separate Runs" as the simple discrimination and simple or compound detection performances are measured in separate experimental runs); Yager et al., 1984]. Such differential criterion variability would increase simple-discrimination performance relative either to compound-alone detection or simple-alone detection.

Nonperpendicular Criterion Lines. The right panel of Fig. 9.12 shows criterion lines that are not always perpendicular to the line joining the center of the two stimuli to be discriminated. In other words, it shows criterion lines for decision variables other than generalized difference of outputs. Specifically, the decision variable for the compound-alone detection task is shown as the maximum of the two relevant analyzers' outputs (rather than the sum, as in the baseline situation), and the decision variable for the simple-alone detection task is shown as the sum of the two analyzers' outputs (rather than the output of the one relevant analyzer, as in the baseline situation).

The use of nonperpendicular criterion lines for some tasks but not for others will change the predicted relative performances. For example, for the situation shown in the right of Fig. 9.12 with the assumption that the distributions are constant-variance Gaussians, the predicted ratios of z^* (simple disc) to z^* (cmpd-alone detect) and to z^* (simple-alone detect) are increased about 20% over the values of 1 and 1.414 predicted when all criterion lines are perpendicular (as in section 9.7.2). [Some calculations assuming constant-variance Gaussians are available in Klein (1985) and assuming all six distributions are available in Graham et al. (1987).]

Johnson (1980a) (in a discussion most naturally applied to intensity discriminations, however) also considered the effect of nonoptimal decision rules in several discrimination paradigms.

Memory. At least one other factor—memory loss for the first interval in two-interval designs—has also been considered in modeling sensory discriminations. Specific attempts to include variance due to memory processes in signal-detection models can be found in several places (e.g., Durlach and Braida, 1969; Johnson, 1980a; Macmillan, 1987), although these discussions have centered on cases like intensity discrimination (cases where the discrimination is handled by differences in the magnitude of outputs rather than by differences in the pattern of activity across two or more analyzers).

One Warning. As the values of two simple stimuli become closer together on the dimension of interest, the ratio of their discriminability to detectability typically decreases (i.e., confusability increases), as shown in Fig. 9.1. This increase in confusability has typically been attributed to overlapping analyzers (excitatory interactions) at close values (as in right panel of Fig. 9.8).

Sometimes confusability is even less at far-apart values than is predicted by the baseline situation for independent noninteracting analyzers. The temptation then is to attribute this additional decrease in confusability to inhibitory interactions at far values (as in left panel of Fig. 9.10). Given the multiplicity of other factors that might contribute to changes in the discriminability/detectability ratio, however, any such conclusion should be treated with caution, at least until evidence from other sources converges on the same conclusion.

9.8   DISTANCE (NONPROBABILISTIC, GEOMETRIC, VECTOR) MODELS

Another class of models [called expected-distance by Thomas (1985) and geometric or vector by Wandell (1982)] directly relates the discriminability of any two stimuli to distance in an analyzer-output space very like that just discussed except that the output of the analyzers is deterministic. These models have been particularly common for wavelength (color) discriminations.

9.8.1 Distinguishing Assumptions

The important assumption distinguishing this class from the independent-analyzers class is an assumption like the following, which replaces all the previous assumptions linking analyzer outputs to observer responses.

Assumption 80. Discriminability of Two Stimuli Determined by Distance. *Two pairs of stimuli—one pair A and B and the other C and D—are equally discriminable if the distance between the points representing one pair equals the distance between the two points representing the other pair, that is, if*

$$d(\mathbf{A}, \mathbf{B}) = d(\mathbf{C}, \mathbf{D})$$

where d is some distance measure. Generally, discriminability between two stimuli A and B is assumed to be a monotonic function of distance in analyzer-output space.

More specific versions of this assumption use particular definitions of distance:

Assumption 81. The Minkowski Metric. *Like Assumption 80 except that the distance between the points for the two stimuli A and B is*

$$d(\mathbf{A,B}) = \left| \sum_{i=1}^{M'} |A_i - B_i|^k \right|^{1/k}$$

and discriminability is determined by distance.

Three values of k are worth individually discussing: These are 1, 2, and infinity.

Assumption 82. The City-Block (Sum-of-Absolute-Differences) Metric. *Like Assumption 80, but distance is specified by the Minkowski metric with k = 1, or*

$$d(\mathbf{A,B}) = \sum_{i=1}^{M'} |A_i - B_i|$$

and discriminability is determined by distance.

Assumption 83. The Euclidian Metric. *Like Assumption 80 but distance is specified as the Minkowski metric with an exponent of 2; equivalently, the distance equals the length of the difference vector or*

$$d(\mathbf{A,B}) = |\mathbf{A} - \mathbf{B}|$$

and discriminability is determined by distance.

Assumption 84. The Maximum-of-Absolute-Differences Metric. *Like Assumption 77 but distance is specified as the Minkowski metric with an exponent of infinity; equivalently the distance equals the largest absolute difference between individual analyzers' responses to the two stimuli, that is*

$$d(\mathbf{A,B}) = \underset{i=1}{\overset{M'}{\text{MAX}}} \, |A_i - B_i|$$

and discriminability is determined by distance.

Relation to Previous Detection Rules. If B is taken to be the blank stimulus, the sum-of-absolute-differences and the maximum-of-absolute differences assumptions (Assumptions 82 and 84) are related to the sum-of-outputs and maximum-output detection rules (Assumptions 61 and 40) earlier. They are not identical rules, however. The assumptions here use absolute values and, probably more important, apply to deterministic analyzer outputs (or to the expected values of the analyzer outputs) rather than to outputs that vary from trial to trial.

Incidentally, it should be clear from the above development that other probabilistic detection rules between the maximum output and the sum of outputs could be constructed simply by varying the exponent in an expression like the right side of Assumption 81.

9.8.2   Advantages of the Euclidian Distance Model

The Euclidian distance model is in many ways much easier to use than other geometric or probabilistic models. Since it assumes discriminability is a monotonic function of vector length, one can use well-known and powerful methods of computation with matrices and vectors, as beautifully described and illustrated by Nielson and Wandell (1988). They argued that although the Euclidian distance model is, for example, not quite correct for detection (e.g., the summation-experiment results in Figs. 4.10 and 4.11 require an exponent distinctly bigger than 2), perhaps it is a good enough approximation to use for many purposes. For example, the Euclidian model may allow direct computation, from measured contrast thresholds, of estimates of the spatial/temporal weighting functions of the analyzers rather than having to compute predictions from many possible weighting functions and then find out which ones best fit the measured thresholds. These estimates will not be perfect (since this model is not), but the ease of obtaining them may outweigh their imperfections.

9.8.3   Relationships Between the Probabilistic (Trial-by-Trial) and Geometric (Distance) Classes of Models

In general, for a model of one class there is not necessarily any model of the other class that makes the same predictions.

We have already seen some equivalences, however. For detection experiments, the probabilistic high-threshold model with a Quick psychometric function leads to the Quick pooling formula. This pooling formula has an alternative interpretation—the Minkowski distance between the origin (the blank stimulus) and the point representing the responses of different analyzers to the stimulus under consideration. Under this interpretation the exponent is thought to be between 3 and 5 (see section 4.8.5). In Chapter 7 we met other versions of independent-analyzers models that make predictions for detection experiments very well described by the Quick pooling formula and, therefore, by a geometric model.

As discussed earlier in this chapter (section 9.7.2), and as Thomas (1983, 1985) has emphasized, the probabilistic model with constant-variance Gaussian probability distributions and with the generalized difference-of-outputs discrimination rule has the property that the discriminability of two stimuli is a monotonic function of the Euclidian distance between the centers of the distributions. See also note 4 for possible generalizations to other probability distributions and other metrics.

Wandell (1982) discussed at some length both the similarities and differences between these two general classes of model (called statistical vs. geometric or vector by him) as applied to discrimination of color differences.

9.8.4   Identification Experiments Using More Than Two Stimuli

Extending the distance assumption (Assumption 80) to directly predict performance in tasks involving more than two stimuli (e.g., the simple identification and concurrent detection tasks described in the next chapter) is not straightforward. One could convert the results for any two stimuli in such a task to some measure of discriminability and then see if those pairwise discriminabilities are accounted for by the geometric model.

9.9   NEAR-THRESHOLD DISCRIMINATION OF SPATIAL FREQUENCY

Many spatial-frequency discrimination experiments have used suprathreshold gratings and will not be considered here. A few, however, have used near-threshold gratings in the paradigms of Fig. 9.2.

9.9.1   Far-Apart Spatial Frequencies

The single-interval rating-scale discrimination paradigm (middle Fig. 9.2) was used to study (a) discrimination between two simple stimuli containing far-apart spatial frequencies, (b) the detection of each simple stimulus, and (c) the detection of the compound made up of the two simple stimuli (Olzak & Thomas, 1981). The results were compared with the predictions in section 9.7.2, assuming constant-variance Gaussians.

When the two spatial frequencies were a factor of 2 apart (3 and 6 c/deg):

discrimination was better than simple detection (z scores related by a factor of 1.4) and discrimination and compound-detection performances were identical. As the spatial-frequency ratio increased still further to 3 (3 and 9 c/deg) and 4 (3 and 12 c/deg), however, discrimination performance increased relative to both compound-detection and simple-detection performances. Inhibitory interactions or positive correlation (as suggested by the original authors) or criterion variability or nonoptimal decision variables caused perhaps by attending to irrelevant analyzers (as suggested by Klein, 1985) could explain these results (see section 9.7.3). Most peculiar, perhaps, was the behavior as the frequency ratio was increased still further to 6 (3 and 18 cpd). Now the ratio of discrimination to simple detection was as expected, but both were too good relative to compound detection. (See section 4.9.7 for discussion of this behavior).

9.9.2   Close Spatial Frequencies

Thomas (1981) reported results from discrimination between pairs of very close spatial frequencies (4 vs. 5 c/deg was the largest difference used) as measured in all three paradigms of Fig. 9.2. Discriminability was compared with detectability of either simple stimulus by itself. As one expects for close values (right panel Fig. 9.8), the discrimination performance was much poorer than detection performance.

In another study (Lennie, 1980a), whether the fixed standard frequency was 0.5 or 8.0 c/deg, the observer's forced-choice discrimination performance was the same when plotted as a function of ratio of variable to standard frequency. A ratio of 1.3 in spatial frequency produced about 80% correct discrimination when the contrasts of the stimuli were just at threshold. At twice threshold contrast, a ratio of 1.1 was sufficient.

As Lennie discussed, this finding that discrimination was as good at 0.5 as at 8.0 c/deg qualifies the interpretation of one aspect of reported perceived appearances. At threshold, gratings of low spatial frequency are sometimes said to look less patterned (less "spatial") than gratings of high spatial frequency. The discrimination results show that although they may look less patterned, spatial-frequency discrimination (as a function of spatial-frequency ratio) is just as good.

The finding that spatial-frequency discrimination depends primarily on ratio of spatial frequencies (rather than difference, for example) will be repeated in a number of identification paradigms in this book, and suggests once again that bandwidth is equal on a logarithmic frequency axis.

9.10   SUMMARY

Discrimination experiments are identification experiments involving only two stimuli. Three different kinds of discrimination experiments—single interval (dichotomous judgment), single-interval rating scale, and two-interval forced choice—are described here.

Classification experiments (sometimes also called *complete identification experiments*) are those in which responses are in one-to-one correspondence with the stimuli. Some but not all discrimination experiments are classification experiments, and vice versa.

One common decision rule for classification experiments is the closest stimulus rule. For certain situations, this rule is also optimal.

A number of other decision rules for discrimination experiments are described and their relationships to one another discussed.

The "baseline" independent-analyzers model is one in which there are non-interacting, independent, and additive analyzers with probability distributions that are circularly symmetric and of constant variance—that is, the constant-variance Gaussian family—and with a decision rule by which performance depends on distance in an analyzer-output space (e.g., the closest stimulus rule, the generalized difference-of-outputs rule).

This baseline model predicts that discrimination of two far-apart equally detectable simple stimuli (a) should be better than detection of either one, but (b) should equal detection of the compound.

The effect of a number of changes in the baseline model—nonadditivity, inter-actions, probabilistic dependence, distributions that are not circularly symmetric, nonoptimal decision rules, and criterion variance—on the above predictions are considered.

9.11   APPENDIX. ABOUT VECTORS

Consider two vectors $\mathbf{A} = (A_1, A_2, \ldots, A_N)$ and $\mathbf{B} = (B_1, B_2, \ldots, B_N)$. Graphically, any vector can be represented as an arrow from the origin of the graph to the point having the coordinates. Starting at the origin is not critical, however. Any arrow having the same length and direction as the one starting at the origin is equally good as a representation of the vector.

9.11.1   Sums

The sum of the two vectors is $\mathbf{A} + \mathbf{B} = (A_1 + B_1, A_2 + B_2, \ldots, A_N + B_N)$.

Consider drawing a parallelogram by starting with two sides equaling the original vectors $\mathbf{A}$ and $\mathbf{B}$ and then completing it by drawing in two more parallel sides. Then draw in the two diagonals. The diagonal that starts at the origin of the graph and terminates at the far corner of the parallelogram is a graphical representation of the vector $\mathbf{A} + \mathbf{B}$.

For example, consider the specific vectors $\mathbf{X} = (3,4)$ and $\mathbf{Y} = (5,6)$. Then the sum of $\mathbf{X}$ and $\mathbf{Y}$ is $(8,10)$. If you are not familiar with vectors, it might be useful to actually draw the parallelogram and see.

9.11.2   Differences

To be consistent with the definition of a sum, the difference between $\mathbf{A}$ and $\mathbf{B}$ must also be defined in terms of the differences between the coordinates—that is, $\mathbf{A} - \mathbf{B} = (A_1 - B_1, A_2 - B_2, \ldots, A_N - B_N)$. In the example, $\mathbf{X} - \mathbf{Y} = (-2, -2)$. Graphically, the difference vector is represented by an arrow joining the tips of the arrows representing the original vectors.

9.11.3   Dot Products

The dot product of two vectors is a single number

$$\mathbf{A} \cdot \mathbf{B} = \sum_{i=1}^{N} A_i \cdot B_i$$

This is also known as the *inner product* or the *scalar product*. For our example, $\mathbf{X} \cdot \mathbf{Y} = 3 \times 5 + 4 \times 6 = 15 + 24 = 39$.

9.11.4   Vector Lengths

Notice that $\mathbf{A} \cdot \mathbf{A}$—the dot product of a vector with itself—is just the square of the ordinary Euclidian length of the vector. That is, if one denotes the length of the vector $\mathbf{A}$ by $|\mathbf{A}|$, then

$$|\mathbf{A}| = (\mathbf{A} \cdot \mathbf{A})^{1/2}$$

In our example $|\mathbf{X}|$ equals the square root of $(3 \times 3 + 4 \times 4)$ and thus equals 5, and $|\mathbf{Y}|$ equals the square root of $(5 \times 5 + 6 \times 6)$ and thus equals 7.81. (Again, if you aren't familiar with vectors, measuring the length of a drawn example might be useful.)

9.11.5   Angles Between Vectors

More generally, there is a useful relationship between the dot product of any two vectors and two geometric properties: the vectors' lengths and the angle between them. Call that angle φ. Then

$$\cos(\varphi) = \frac{\mathbf{A} \cdot \mathbf{B}}{|\mathbf{A}| \, |\mathbf{B}|}$$

In our example, therefore, the cosine of the angle between $\mathbf{X}$ and $\mathbf{Y}$ equals $39/(5 \times 7.81) = 0.998$, so the angle is 2.9 degrees. To put it another way, the vectors $\mathbf{X}$ and $\mathbf{Y}$ run in almost the same direction.

In Fig. 9.9 another example of the relationship between the dot product and the angle and lengths can be found. All four figures there show two vectors of length 5 with an angle between them (in the three-dimensional space, not necessarily in the picture plane) of 61.3 degrees (the cosine of 61.3 degrees equals 0.48). But the vectors are represented by different coordinates in each panel because the space has been rotated. If you calculate the dot product for the coordinates given in each panel, you will see it equals the cosine of 61.3 degrees.

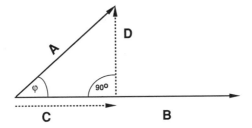

FIG. 9.13 Vector **C** is the component of vector **A** in the direction of vector **B**.

9.11.6 Component of One Vector in the Direction of Another

Consideration of the definitions of vector sums shows that any vector can be decomposed into (i.e., is equal to the sum of) any one of many pairs of other vectors. More particularly, the two vectors in the pair can be at right angles to one another. Look at Fig. 9.13. The vector **A** is equal to the sum of **C** + **D** (equivalently, the vector **D** equals the difference **A** − **C**). **C** and **D** are at right angles to each other. The vector **C** is often called *the component of* **A** *in the direction of* **B** because the vectors **C** and **B** go in the same direction, and the vector **C** plus another vector at right angles to **C** (that is, **D**) sum up to **A**.

If φ is the angle between **A** and **C** (or equivalently between **A** and **B**), then the lengths of **C** and **D** can be expressed in terms of that angle and the length of **A**. In particular

$$|\mathbf{C}| = \cos \varphi \cdot |\mathbf{A}|$$

For the length of **D** one uses the sine instead of the cosine.

In light of this, it is interesting to rearrange the definition of the dot product slightly to give the length of the component of **A** in the direction of **B** (that is, to give $|\mathbf{C}|$) in terms of the dot product between **A** and **B**:

$$|\mathbf{C}| = \cos \varphi \cdot |\mathbf{A}| = \frac{\mathbf{A} \cdot \mathbf{B}}{|\mathbf{B}|}$$

Notes

1. *Some terminology.* The experiments called identification experiments here (see sect. 9.1) have frequently been called "recognition" experiments. But the word "recognition" has connotations both in everyday language and in the technical language of literature on memory that seem less appropriate here than the connotations of "identification."

2. *Forced-choice decision variables.* The forced-choice discrimination rule stated in section 9.5.3 as Assumption 78 is in terms of the same decision variable DV that was used in the rules for the two single-interval paradigms. Accordingly, DV corresponds to a line

in the analyzer-output space having one dimension per analyzer. This forced-choice discrimination rule can be restated in terms of a decision variable—call it DVFC—corresponding to a line in the expanded analyzer-output space having two dimensions per analyzer, one for each interval. DVFC corresponds to the line between the points in this space corresponding to the two orderings of stimuli in the intervals: (stim 1, stim 2) and (stim 2, stim 1). DVFC is equal to the difference between the values of DV in the two intervals, that is:

$$DVFC = DV \text{ (1st interval)} - DV \text{ (2nd interval)}$$

If you find this note more confusing than helpful, forget it.

3. *Derivation.* The derivation of the last relationship in section 9.7.2 is as follows. First we will restate for general discrimination experiments the fact we met before, that the area under the yes-no or rating-scale detection ROC curve is the percent correct in two-alternative forced-choice detection (assuming, of course, that the decisions in the different tasks were made on the basis of the same decision variable and according to standard signal-detection theory reviewed above): No matter what the probability distribution of the decision variable (Green & Swets, 1974)

$$AREA = FCC$$

For the constant-variance Gaussian (e.g., Green & Swets, 1974)

$$z(AREA) = z(FCC) = \frac{D(\text{stim 1, stim 2})}{2^{1/2}}$$

Combining this with the equation

$$D(\text{stim 1, stim 2}) = 2 \cdot z^* \text{ ("stim 1"/stim 1)}$$

gives the desired result.

4. *About circular symmetry and more general metrics.* The important property leading to the predictions in section 9.7.1 is the circular symmetry of the probability distributions and not the probabilistic independence.

When the measure of distance is Euclidian and the random variables are independent, the only probability distribution leading to circularly symmetric joint probability density functions is the Gaussian. (A circularly symmetric multivariate probability density is one having isodensity contours that are circles in two-dimensional space, spheres in three-dimensional space, etc. Some people prefer to call this property *radial symmetry.* Proof of this statement is implied by the proof of a more general statement below.)

In general, however, if the random variables are not independent, there are an infinite number of circularly symmetric joint probability distributions.

Generalizing to other Minkowski Metrics. Further, if the case of any Minkowski metric is considered, the only univariate probability density function $f(x)$ that can produce circularly symmetric joint multivariate density functions if the random variables are independent is the density function that is proportional to

$$\exp(-|x|^k)$$

where k is the power characterizing the metric (e.g., see Assumption 81). The proof of this—kindly shown me by David H. Krantz—involves noting the following.

By the circular-symmetry condition, the multivariate density depends only on the sum of each of the variables raised to the power appropriate to the metric. For example, in the two-dimensional case, since f is constant on a circle there exists a function g such that

$$f(x, y) = g(x^k + y^k)$$

(We are assuming for ease that f is centered at the origin.)

The independence condition coupled with circular symmetry further requires that the multivariate density depend on the product of identical univariate functions. For example, in the two-dimensional case, there exists a function h such that

$$f(x, y) = h(x) \cdot h(y)$$

The combination of the preceding two equations are suggestive of the functional equation for an exponential. Indeed by defining

$$\theta(u) = \frac{f(0, u^{1/k})}{f(0, 0)}$$

you can show that

$$\theta(u + v) = \theta(u) \cdot \theta(v)$$

which is exactly the functional equation for an exponential. Hence θ is an exponential; with a little more work tidying up constants you get the desired result.

Using this result, it would be interesting to try to generalize the results of section 9.7.1 and 9.7.2 to these other probability distributions and other Minkowski metrics. (Some care would be required since, for example, the Minkowski distance between two points does not in general remain the same when the axes of the space are rotated, except when $k = 2$.)

10

Three More Paradigms
and Transducer Functions

In this chapter we will discuss three more identification paradigms, each of which has its advantages (and disadvantages) for studying various aspects of multiple analyzers. We will continue to use all the assumptions of the independent-analyzers model of the previous chapter. For the first of the three paradigms considered here we will even be able to borrow a decision rule from the previous chapter. For the second and third paradigms, however, we will have to use new decision rules.

10.1 SIMPLE DETECTION AND IDENTIFICATION PARADIGM

10.1.1 Description of Experimental Procedure

Figure 10.1 illustrates the stimuli and responses in what we will call the *simple detection and identification paradigm* (sometimes known as *detection and recognition,* e.g., Green & Birdsall, 1978). Look first at the diagram in the upper left; the other diagrams illustrate alternative ways of thinking about the paradigm and will be discussed later.

Single-Interval Trials with Simple Stimuli. Each trial contains a single interval in which either the blank stimulus or one of a set of simple stimuli is presented (labels across bottom front of diagram in upper left Fig. 10.1). The number of different simple stimuli will be called M, and so the total number of different stimuli is $M + 1$.

This is the only identification paradigm we will explicitly look at where experiments involve more than two simple stimuli, that is, where $M > 2$. Thus this is the only paradigm where two important questions will be addressed: systematic confusion among different alternatives and uncertainty effects as the number of alternatives is increased.

Although the two other paradigms discussed in this chapter could be used with $M > 2$, they have not been to any extent.

Another type of single-interval identification experiment uses compound stimuli as well as simple stimuli. This type is called *concurrent identification* here and is the third and final paradigm discussed in this chapter.

Detection Response. On each trial the observer is asked to make two kinds of response—a detection response and an identification response. The detection

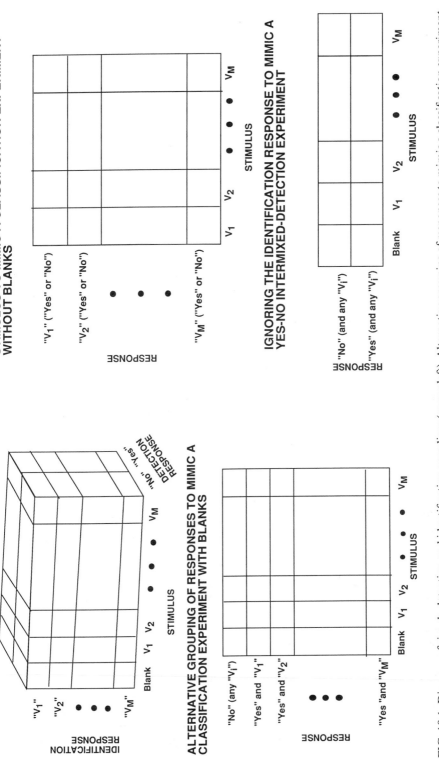

FIG. 10.1 Diagram of simple detection and identification paradigm (upper left). Alternative grouping of responses to mimic a classification experiment with blanks (lower left). Ignoring the detection response and the blank stimulus to mimic a classification experiment without blanks (upper right). Ignoring the identification response to mimic a yes-no intermixed-detection experiment (lower right).

response is to say either yes (indicating a nonblank stimulus) or no (indicating the blank stimulus). These two possible detection responses are indicated in the upper left diagram of Fig. 10.1 by labels on the z axis (the axis supposed to be going directly away from the viewer).

Identification Response. Whether the detection response was yes or no, the observer is also asked to make an identification response on each trial. This response indicates which of the nonblank stimuli the observer thinks was presented. These M possible identification responses are indicated in the upper left diagram of Fig. 10.1 by labels on the vertical axis.

Simple Detection and Identification with Responses Regrouped to Mimic a Classification Experiment. The bottom left diagram of Fig. 10.1 regroups the responses from the top left of Fig. 10.1 into responses that plausibly correspond one to one with the stimuli and thus mimic a classification experiment (with M + 1 different stimuli—one blank and M simple stimuli). The no detection response (paired with any identification response) plausibly corresponds to the blank stimulus; the yes detection response paired with any particular identification response (e.g., saying the stimulus has the first value V_1) plausibly corresponds to that particular stimulus (V_1).

Of course, in spite of the plausibility, the results when asking the observer to make two separate responses on each trial (yes vs. no, and then to name one of the nonblank stimuli, as in the simple detection and identification paradigm) might turn out to be systematically different from those when asking the observer to make only one response on each trial (naming the stimulus, either blank or one of the values, as in a standard classification experiment).

Running the experiment as a simple detection and identification experiment seems preferable, at least in many cases. In particular, it provides more information: The identification responses on blank trials can be used to deduce the criteria in each of several different analyzers (see below).

Separate Detection and Identification Runs. Rather than requiring the observer to make both detection and identification responses on each trial, the detection responses might be collected in one experimental session and the identification responses in another [as in what Klein (1985) called the *separate-runs* paradigm]. The identification run would usually not include the blank stimulus. Many of the analyses of results from the simple detection and identification paradigm just described are identical to those done when the detection and identification responses are obtained in separate runs. That is, the responses from the simple detection and identification paradigm can be regrouped, as shown in the right half of Fig. 10.1, into identification responses to the nonblank stimuli (upper right) or detection responses (lower right). In this regrouping, the identification part is a classification experiment using M simple stimuli and no blank (an experiment sometimes called *pure recognition*); this is a generalization to M stimuli of the single-interval discrimination paradigm (top Fig. 9.2). And the detection part is a yes-no simple-intermixed-condition detection experiment.

10.1.2 Assumptions and Decision Rules

The assumptions of independent-analyzers models reviewed in section 9.3 will be used again here—including the detection decision rules, particularly the maximum output and the sum of outputs (Assumptions 40 and 61)—except that there is no need for the weak additivity assumption (Assumption 36), because compound stimuli are not used in this paradigm.

The identification decision rule will be the maximum-output identification rule for simple stimuli (Assumption 72). This is equivalent to the closest stimulus classification rule (Assumption 70) when the simple stimuli are equally detectable and far apart and there is only one analyzer sensitive to each stimulus (see section 9.4.3).

10.1.3 Response Biases and Confusions—Predictions and Results on the Spatial-Frequency Dimension

This model (section 10.1.2) leads to two interesting predictions about the relative frequencies of the different possible identification responses to any one stimulus.

When the stimulus is the blank, the observer ought to be no more likely to call the blank one value than any other. For, on average, the blank evokes the same output from every analyzer, and the maximum output identification rule as stated makes no allowances for biases in the observer's responses. This lack of response bias was nearly although not exactly found in a simple detection and identification experiment run with gratings of different spatial frequency by Yager et al. (1984).

Second, if the values of stimuli in a simple identification experiment are far enough apart to stimulate completely separate analyzers, there ought to be no systematic confusions among them. That is, when an observer is wrong about the value of a simple stimulus, he ought to be no more likely to call it a near value than a far value.

The results of Yager et al. (1984) when spatial frequencies were a factor of 2 apart showed substantial systematic confusions for one observer (EG), some systematic confusions for a second observer (PW), and none for a third observer (DY). There were no systematic confusions for either of two observers (DY or PW) when spatial frequencies were a factor of 3 apart. These results were consistent with the second prediction above if the following subsidiary assumptions are made about analyzers' spatial-frequency bandwidths: Bandwidths for observer EG are wide enough that an individual analyzer responds significantly to frequencies a factor of 2 apart; those for observer PW are somewhat narrower but still encompass frequencies a factor of 2 apart; and those for observer DY are narrow enough that frequencies a factor of 2 apart fall in different analyzers.

Needless to say, this is not the only interpretation of the individual differences apparent in these confusion results. An interesting alternative candidate is that the bandwidths of the lower level analyzers are the same and very narrow for all three observers but the maximum-output identification rule is violated in the following way: Labeling is quite sloppy for observer EG, so higher levels confuse outputs coming from nearby analyzers; the labeling is somewhat sloppy for observer PW; and the labeling is very clean for observer DY.

These two possibilities could never be distinguished on the basis of this kind of evidence alone. Had we other kinds of experimental evidence on these three observers yielding, for example, bandwidths from adaptation or summation experiments, some conclusion might be drawn.

10.1.4   Probability of Correct Identification—Uncertainty Effects

The previous subsection discussed the relative frequencies of different identification responses to one stimulus; this subsection and the next two examine the probability of correct identification over all the simple (nonblank) stimuli in a given condition. See the appendix (section 10.10.1) for more details of these calculations.

When the number of alternative far-apart simple values in an identification experiment is varied, one can ask about the existence and size of uncertainty effects for identification, just as we did for detection. Are any effects observed, and if so are they small enough to be explained simply by the monitoring of extra noisy analyzers—as were the detection uncertainty effects on the spatial-frequency dimension (Chap. 7)—or is there evidence for imperfect monitoring (attention capacity limitations) in the potentially more complicated task of identification?

Figure 10.2 shows the predicted percentage correct in simple identification experiments of one set size ($M = 4$) plotted against that in another set size ($M = 2$) as the value of the signal-strength parameter is changed for several independent-analyzers models using the maximum-output identification rule and each of several probability distributions (labeling the curves). The perfect-monitoring assumption is being applied here. (This figure could apply either to the identification responses in a simple detection and identification experiment or to a pure identification experiment as long as some procedure is used to ensure that the M simple stimuli are equally detectable).

The solid line labeled "no uncertainty effect" is the positive diagonal. For simple identification experiments, however, one would be quite surprised to find performance on this line. Even if the observer never looked at any stimulus and answered on the basis of nonvisual input (e.g., guessing), he or she would be correct more often in the smaller set size than in the larger. For example, when $M = 2$, the observer will be correct by chance 50% of the time, but when $M = 4$, he or she will be correct by chance only 25% of the time.

The predictions of the high-threshold model are simply a straight line running from perfect performance in both set sizes (when the signal strength is so high that the probability that the analyzer sensitive to the stimulus goes into the detect state equals 1.0) down to chance performance in both set sizes (when

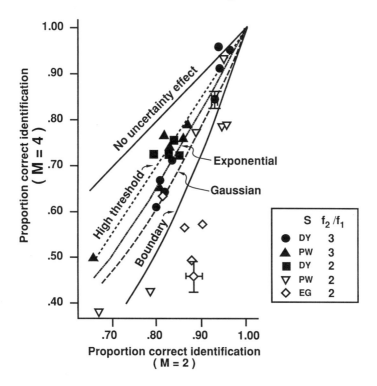

FIG. 10.2 Proportion of correct identification with four values intermixed ($M = 4$) versus proportion of correct identification with two values intermixed ($M = 2$). The curves show theoretical predictions and the points show results from an experiment on the spatial-frequency dimension. The two points with error bars illustrate ± 1 standard error computed from the binomial distribution. (Figure 3 in Yager, Kramer, Shaw, & Graham 1984; used by permission.)

the signal strength is so low that the probability that the analyzer sensitive to the stimulus goes into the detect state equals 0.0).

The predictions of the exponential and constant-variance Gaussian probability distributions are curves slightly below that. The predictions of the different distributions (including increasing-variance Gaussian and double-exponential although these are not shown in Fig. 10.2) are again ordered as they were in Chapter 7 for uncertainty effects in detection: The steeper the slope of the ROC curve for detection in the simple-alone condition, the greater the predicted uncertainty effect in identification experiments.

Shaw's Boundary Theorem. An infinite number of additional probability distributions might be considered in an independent-analyzers model. Although it is impossible to calculate predictions for all of them individually, it is possible to compute a bound on their predictions for uncertainty effects in simple identification experiments (Shaw, 1980). The lowest curve in Fig. 10.2 is Shaw's calculated lower boundary for the region in which all independent-analyzers models' predictions fall no matter what continuous probability distribution is assumed (assuming one analyzer for each simple stimulus, that the same probability-distribution family holds for all analyzers, that all stimuli are equally detectable and stimulate nonoverlapping, noninteracting, probabilistically independent analyzers, and that the maximum-output identification rule determines the observer's response).

The data points on Fig. 10.2 will be discussed in section 10.1.6.

10.1.5   Comparison of Detection and Identification Performances

Simple-Alone Detection Versus Identification. First consider the case where the intensities of the two simple stimuli in an $M = 2$ identification experiment were chosen so that the stimuli would be equally detectable in simple-alone forced-choice detection experiments. Then the probability of correct identification (in the $M = 2$ intermixed identification experiment) would exactly equal the probability of detection (for each simple stimulus in the simple-alone forced-choice detection experiment). Notice that probability distribution would make absolutely no difference in the predictions of identification performance, therefore!

(To see why probability of correct identification would exactly equal probability of detection in this circumstance, consider the following: Both the two-alternative simple identification experiment and the two-alternative forced-choice detection experiment can be seen as forced choices between two alternatives, where one alternative is represented by a random variable having a signal distribution and the other by a random variable having a noise distribution. Thus performance in both would be the same.)

In general, probability distribution makes less difference in predictions of identification performance from simple-alone detection performance than it does in the predictions we looked at earlier for detection uncertainty effects or identification uncertainty effects. When detectability is equated for some other way than in two-alternative forced choice, however, or when measuring identification with $M > 2$, probability distribution does have an effect on the comparisons between simple-alone detection and identification, but the effect is slight. [A case where the stimuli were equated for detectability measured as negative-diagonal d' is shown in Fig. 3 of Graham et al. (1987).]

Intermixed Detection Versus Identification. The predicted relationship between detection performance in intermixed conditions and identification performance (necessarily in intermixed conditions) does depend on probability distribution in a systematic way. This effect is primarily determined by the fact that larger detection uncertainty effects dominate the smaller identification uncertainty effects. When detection performance in an intermixed block is equated for, the best identification performance (in the same set size M as for the detection performance) is predicted by the double-exponential distribution and the worst by the high-threshold distribution. The differences predicted when the sum-of-outputs detection rule is used are somewhat greater than those predicted with the maximum-output rule (since the sum-of-outputs rule predicts bigger detection uncertainty effects).

10.1.6 Simple Detection and Identification of Spatial Frequency

Four models have been compared with the results of simple detection and identification of far-apart spatial frequencies: the exponential and constant-variance Gaussian combined with the maximum-output and sum-of-outputs detection rules (Yager et al., 1984).

Figure 10.2 shows some of these results when comparing identification in one condition ($M = 4$) with that in another ($M = 2$). The solid points are cases (observers and frequency ratios) for which there was no systematic confusion (see section 10.1.3). In these cases, the identification uncertainty effect can be explained by models of the independent-analyzers class, as evidenced by the fact that all these points are above Shaw's boundary line. The open data points—from the cases where there were systematic confusions—however, tended to fall below the boundary line, indicating a violation of the independent-analyzers model in consideration here (section 10.1.2). One possible violation would be a limitation to attention capacity, that is, imperfect monitoring. As mentioned in section 10.1.3, however, these stimuli may be so close they are stimulating the same analyzers, or there may be confusions among neighboring analyzer outputs at higher levels of the visual system. In either case, points in Fig. 10.2 might fall below the boundary line, since in the four-frequency intermixed block a middle frequency has two neighbors, whereas in the two-frequency intermixed block each frequency has only one neighbor. Thus, there seems no need to postulate limited capacity in the identification of spatial frequency, just as there was no need in the detection of stimuli varying in spatial frequency.

In the comparison of detection with identification results from this study, one systematic (although small) deviation between the predictions of the independent-analyzers models and the results was obtained even for the cases where there were no systematic confusions. In particular, in the prediction of identification performance from simple-alone detection performance, the models predicted that such performance should be somewhat greater than it is (about 0.1 on the probability-of-correct scale). [This is in a sense opposite to the kind of result reported by Olzak and Thomas (1981), where discrimination was too good relative to simple detection.] The comparisons between intermixed detection and identification accorded with the independent-analyzers models' predictions.

Overall, comparisons *not involving* the alone condition were all consistent with an independent-analyzers model predicting relatively small uncertainty effects—that is, the maximum exponential model. Conversely, comparisons involving the alone condition were not consistent with that same model but required a model predicting larger uncertainty effects.

In summary, all the comparisons among experimental conditions (with far-apart spatial frequencies) are within the range of predictions from the class of independent-analyzers models. (See note 1.) On the other hand, some modification of assumptions is necessary before a perfect fit can be found between any one version of the model and the results. Some possible modifications were already discussed in Chapter 7. Further discussion can be found in Yager et al. (1984).

10.2   2 × 2 PARADIGM

10.2.1   Experimental Procedure

Figure 10.3 shows two alternative diagrams of the 2 × 2 paradigm. Each trial contains two intervals. In one interval a blank stimulus is presented and in the other interval one of two nonblank patterns is presented. There are thus four different trial types (labeled along the bottom of the diagrams in Fig. 10.3). The patterns are called A and B in Fig. 10.3 rather than 1 and 2 to avoid confusions later; the word *stimulus* will be reserved in this paradigm for the whole two-interval presentation of a blank and a nonblank pattern. The interval presenting the nonblank pattern varies randomly from trial to trial. The observer makes two responses on each trial. The detection response indicates which of the two intervals the nonblank pattern was presented in, and the identification response indicates which of the two nonblank patterns was presented. The upper panel in Fig. 10.3 illustrates this paradigm, using separate axes for the detection and identification responses. The lower panel illustrates a regrouping of the detection and identification responses onto one dimension to show that this 2 × 2 paradigm can be viewed as a classification experiment, since there is a one-to-one correspondence between the four possible stimuli and the four possible conjunctions of detection and identification responses.

Considering Only the Detection Response. Suppose the observer made only the detection response. Then this experiment would be exactly the same as a forced-choice two-intermixed-stimuli detection experiment (e.g., see Chap. 7), where the stimuli intermixed are the two nonblank patterns.

Considering Only the Identification Response. Suppose the observer made only the identification response. Then this experiment would be similar to (but not exactly like) a single-interval identification experiment. The two are similar in that, on each trial, there is only a single interval containing a nonblank pattern to be identified. They differ in that here the observer also sees a blank on each trial—and doesn't know which interval contains the blank.

An M × 2 Paradigm. The use of *M* different nonblank patterns in an *M* × 2 paradigm would be perfectly possible, but I know of no such study.

TWO- BY- TWO PARADIGM

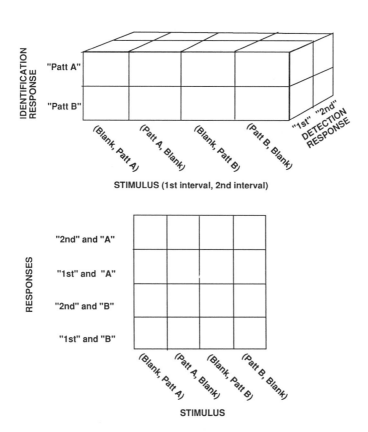

FIG. 10.3 Diagram of 2 × 2 paradigm (upper). Responses regrouped to show paradigm as a classification experiment (lower).

10.2.2 Assumptions and Decision Rules

The assumptions reviewed in section 9.3 will be used here with the following exceptions. The detection decision rules do not apply directly and so will not be used in that form. We will drop the assumption that only one analyzer is sensitive to each of a set of far-apart stimuli (Assumption 24) and allow an indefinite number (except where noted). The probability-distribution family will usually be constant-variance Gaussian (Assumption 59), although occasionally the high-threshold distribution (Assumption 55) is considered.

Four Decision Rules. Figure 10.4 (adapted from Klein, 1985) illustrates the action of three of the four 2 × 2 decision rules that will be presented in the subsequent sections. For this figure, two equally detectable far-apart simple pat-

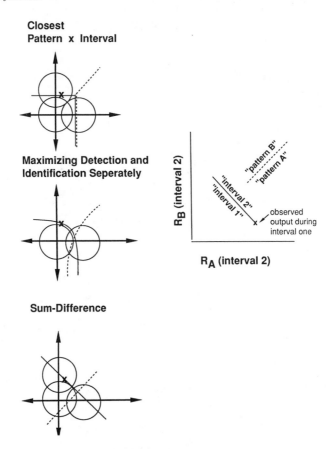

FIG. 10.4 Illustration of three decision rules for 2 × 2 paradigm showing criterion lines for detection (dashed) and identification (solid) responses on a plot giving the possible outputs of the two analyzers in the second interval (horizontal and vertical axes). The outputs of the two analyzers during the first interval are indicated by the X. (Adapted from Klein, 1985.)

terns are assumed. Only two analyzers are shown in this figure, although they may be viewed as resulting from the appropriate rotation of a space showing many more analyzers (see Fig. 9.9 and section 9.6). Even assuming that only two analyzers are involved, a complete diagram of the decision-rule criteria for this 2 × 2 paradigm would require four dimensions—each analyzer in each interval of the trial. Each panel in Fig. 10.4 shows only two of the necessary four dimensions—those for the second interval. The horizontal axis gives R_A (interval 2), the output of the analyzer sensitive to pattern A during the second interval. The vertical axis gives R_B (interval 2), the output of the analyzer sensitive to pattern B during the second interval. The three circles in each of three panels of Fig. 10.4 show central portions of the probability distributions of the outputs to each of three stimuli during the second interval. Those three stimuli are the two far-apart simple patterns (upper left and lower right circles) and the blank (lower left circle). The point marked by the X indicates the hypothetical analyzer outputs during the first interval. (In this figure, the X indicates outputs that are most likely to have been produced by the simple pattern B, but they could have been produced by the other simple pattern or by the blank.) The solid and dotted lines in each panel are the criterion lines for the detection and identification responses, respectively, and will be explained in detail in subsequent sections. If (as indicated in the right panel of Fig. 10.4) the two analyzers' outputs in the second interval lie to the lower left of the solid line, then interval 1 is the detection response; otherwise, interval 2 is. If the two analyzers' outputs in the second interval lie to the lower right of the dashed line, then pattern A is the identification response; otherwise pattern B is.

10.2.3   Closest Pattern-by-Interval Decision Rule

Viewing the 2 × 2 paradigm as a classification experiment involving four stimuli (bottom Fig. 10.3) suggests using the closest stimulus classification rule (Assumption 70) applied to the relevant space, which has twice as many dimensions as there are analyzers (each analyzer's output in the first interval and in the second interval output). Or, rephrased in terms of this paradigm.

Assumption 85. Closest Pattern × Interval Decision Rule (for the 2 × 2 Paradigm). *The stimulus (the pattern and interval combination) for which the expected M′ × 2 outputs (M′ analyzers in 2 intervals) are closest to the observed outputs (Euclidian distance) dictates both the detection response (the interval the observer says contains the nonblank pattern) and the identification response (the nonblank pattern the observer says was presented).*

The criterion lines for the second interval for this rule are illustrated in the top panel of Fig. 10.4.

Applying to this case a number of equivalences presented in the earlier discussion of closest stimulus rules (section 9.4) leads to the following facts. For the case of constant-variance Gaussian distributions (as assumed by Watson, 1983, and Klein, 1985), the above closest pattern × interval decision rule for the 2 × 2 paradigm is equivalent to the corresponding maximum-likelihood rule—that is, to choosing whichever of the four pattern × interval combinations has the highest likelihood of producing the analyzer outputs that actually occurred in the two intervals. (This equivalence holds for close as well as for far-apart values, incidentally.)

Equivalent to Maximizing Proportion Doubly Correct. When the presentation probabilities of the four stimuli (pattern × interval combinations) are equal (as they usually are), then—no matter what the probability distribution assumed—maximizing a likelihood is equivalent to maximizing the corresponding percent correct. In this application, *correct* means correct both about the interval and the pattern, that is, both correct detection and correct identification, or *doubly correct*. [This is goal 4 in Klein (1985) and the goal of Watson (1983).]

The closest pattern × interval rule has been used to analyze the results of 2 × 2 experiments using both far-apart and close-together spatial frequencies (Watson, 1983).

10.2.4   *The Maximum-Output Rule for the 2 × 2 Paradigm*

A general maximum-output rule has also been used to calculate predictions for 2 × 2 experiments involving both close and far-apart values (Thomas & Gille, 1979). According to this rule, both the detection and identification responses are based on the maximum of the $M' \times 2$ outputs (M' analyzers in each of two intervals) in the following way:

Assumption 86. Maximum-Output 2 × 2 Decision Rule.   *If the maximum of the $M' \times 2$ outputs occurs during the first interval, the observer's detection response is "interval one"; otherwise it is "interval two." If the maximum output is from an analyzer that is more sensitive to stimulus A than to stimulus B, the observer's identification response is "pattern A"; otherwise it is "pattern B."*

When the Closest Pattern × Interval Decision Rule Is Equivalent to the Maximum-Output Rule.   When the two nonblank patterns used in a 2 × 2 experiment are equally detectable far-apart simple patterns (the special case of Fig. 10.4), the points representing the four pattern × interval combinations lie in perpendicular directions in the relevant analyzer-output space and are equally far from the origin. Let us rotate the space so the four stimulus points lie on the first four dimensions (and ignore the rest of the dimensions), or equivalently, assume there are only two analyzers—one sensitive to each of the two far-apart patterns. Then (see section 9.4.3) the closest pattern × interval rule is equivalent to an appropriate maximum-output rule—finding the one of the first four dimensions on which the biggest activity occurs and using it in the "natural" way to determine both the detection and identification responses. For example, if on a given trial the analyzer A-interval two dimension has the biggest output, the observer gives an identification response of "pattern A" and a detection response of "interval two." Consistent with this equivalence, notice that the detection criterion line shown in Fig. 10.4 (top panel) for the closest pattern × interval decision rule is just like that for the maximum-output detection rule (the upper right corner of a square) (compare Fig. 9.6 middle right).

10.2.5   *Maximizing Detection and Identification Performances Independently of Each Other*

Although the closest pattern × interval decision rule maximizes the proportion doubly correct at least for the case of constant-variance Gaussians (section 10.2.3), it does not maximize either the proportion-correct detection (counting up the trials on which the detection response was correct whether or not the identification response was correct) or the proportion-correct identification. To maximize these quantities [goal 1 of Klein (1985)], another decision rule is needed. In this new rule, subrules for detection and identification are stated completely independently of one another. Since presentation probabilities are equal in the 2 × 2 paradigm, the desired subrules are those that maximize the corresponding likelihoods. Thus

Assumption 87. Maximizing Detection and Identification Independently in the 2 × 2 Paradigm. *The rules for detection and identification are stated independently of each other. Let "observed outputs" mean the M′ × 2 outputs produced by all analyzers on both intervals of the trial in question.*

Detection Subrule. *The observer's detection response is the interval (i = 1 or 2) for which the value of the following probability is bigger:*

Pr(observed outputs | nonblank pattern in interval i)

Identification Subrule. *The observer's identification response is the nonblank pattern (k = A or B) for which the value of the following probability is bigger:*

Pr(observed outputs | nonblank pattern k)

It might help to describe these subrules as procedures that could be followed step by step. The detection subrule would be: Compute the probability that the outputs that were observed on this trial would have been produced if the nonblank pattern had been presented in the *first* interval (and the blank in the other interval, of course) no matter which nonblank pattern it was. Do the same computation except with *second* substituted for *first*. Choose the bigger of the two computed probabilities. The detection response is whichever interval produced this bigger value.

The identification subrule should be: Compute the probability that the outputs that were observed on this trial would have been produced if the nonblank pattern had been pattern A (no matter which interval the nonblank pattern was presented in). Do the same computation with B substituted for A. Choose the bigger of the two computed probabilities. The identification response is whichever pattern produced the bigger value.

The criterion lines maximizing these likelihoods are not the same for all assumed probability distributions (nor are they generally easily computable). The ones for constant-variance Gaussian distributions (from Klein, 1985) are shown in Fig. 10.4.

Since, had the observer given only the detection response, the 2 × 2 paradigm would be exactly equivalent to the forced-choice intermixed-detection paradigm, the detection subrule is exactly the same as the rule that maximizes percent-correct detection in straight forced-choice detection experiments. The criterion lines for that decision variable were shown in Fig. 9.6 (bottom part) for equally detectable far-apart simple patterns and constant-variance Gaussians. The halfway criterion is the one used for forced-choice experiments with no interval bias.

This rule maximizing detection and identification independently has never been applied to results from 2×2 experiments to my knowledge, but some calculations appear in Klein (1985).

10.2.6 Difference-Identification and Sum-Detection Decision Rule (Maximizing Ratio of Doubly Correct to Doubly Wrong)

When the probability distributions are constant-variance Gaussians, the decision rule illustrated in the bottom panel of Fig. 10.4 maximizes the probability that both the detection and the identification responses are correct divided by the probability that both are wrong (Klein, 1985). As the bottom panel of Fig. 10.4 shows, the criterion lines for the detection task are those appropriate to a sum-of-outputs decision rule and those for the identification task are appropriate to a difference-of-outputs decision rule. This is equivalent to the Thomas et al. (1982) decision model. More specifically, the following assumption is made:

Assumption 88. Sum-Detection and Difference-Identification in the 2×2 Paradigm. *The rules for detection and identification are independent of each other.*

Detection Subrule. *The observer responds "interval one" if and only if the generalized sum of outputs in interval one is greater than in interval two, that is, if and only if*

$$(\mathbf{A} + \mathbf{B}) \cdot \mathbf{R} \text{ (interval 1)} - (\mathbf{A} + \mathbf{B}) \cdot \mathbf{R} \text{ (interval 2)} > 0$$

This rule can also be written out in terms of the individual analyzers as follows: the observer's response is interval one if and only if

$$\sum_{i=1}^{M'} A_i R_i \text{ (interval 1)} + \sum_{i=1}^{M'} B_i R_i \text{ (interval 1)} - \sum_{i=1}^{M'} A_i R_i \text{ (interval 2)}$$

$$- \sum_{i=1}^{M'} B_i R_i \text{ (interval 2)} > 0$$

Since the detection task here is a simple-intermixed detection task rather than a compound-detection task, this sum-of-outputs detection subrule is not the optimal detection rule.

Identification Subrule. *The observer responds "pattern A" if and only if the generalized difference of outputs in the first plus that in the second interval is greater than zero, that is,*

$$(\mathbf{A} - \mathbf{B}) \cdot \mathbf{R} \text{ (interval 1)} + (\mathbf{A} - \mathbf{B}) \cdot \mathbf{R} \text{ (interval 2)} > 0$$

This last expression can be written out in terms of the individual analyzers as

$$\sum_{i=1}^{M'} A_i R_i \text{ (interval 1)} - \sum_{i=1}^{M'} B_i R_i \text{ (interval 1)} + \sum_{i=1}^{M'} A_i R_i \text{ (interval 2)}$$

$$- \sum_{i=1}^{M'} B_i R_i \text{ (interval 2)} > 0$$

Note that the generalized difference-of-outputs rule for discrimination experiments (Assumption 75) did not sum the differences over two intervals as this last subrule does. Although Assumption 75 was optimal for those simpler experiments, this last subrule is not optimal for identification responses in 2 × 2 experiments.

10.2.7   Other Possible Decision Rules

Klein (1985) analyzed three other decision rules: (a) minimizing the number of doubly-wrong responses, (b) the detection rule that maximizes correct detections (as in the second rule above) with an identification rule that maximizes correct detections contingent on correct identification, and (c) the identification rule that maximizes correct identifications (as in the second rule above) with a detection rule that maximizes correct identifications contingent on correct detections.

A large number of other rules could undoubtedly be suggested.

10.3   PREDICTIONS OF INDEPENDENT-ANALYZERS MODELS FOR 2 × 2 PARADIGM

10.3.1   For Far-Apart Equally Detectable Simple Stimuli

The following simple prediction is made by a number of independent-analyzers models:

Prediction: For Far-Apart Values, Identification Performance Equals Detection Performance in 2 × 2 Paradigm. *When the two nonblank patterns are far-apart, equally detectable simple patterns, identification percent-correct equals detection percent-correct in the 2 × 2 paradigm.*

In the discrimination paradigms of the last chapter, discrimination (which was identification of two alternatives) was predicted to be better than detection (prediction 1 of section 9.7.1). In the 2 × 2 paradigm, however, both intervals of the trial provide information relevant to the detection response, but only the nonblank interval provides information relevant to the identification response. Hence, compared with the discrimination paradigm, identification performance in the 2 × 2 paradigm is diminished relative to detection performance. As it happens, it is diminished by just the right amount to equalize identification and detection performance according to many (but not all) combinations of probability-distribution and decision-rule assumptions in independent-analyzers models.

The Closest Pattern × Interval Decision Rule with the High-Threshold or the Constant-Variance Gaussian Distributions. To see why this prediction holds when using the closest pattern × interval decision rule (Assumption 85) with some probability distributions, consider the following: On some trials, the closest pattern × interval combination will be the "right" combination—the one corresponding to the pattern and interval that was actually presented. Then both the observer's detection and identification responses will be correct.

On other trials, the closest pattern × interval combination will be one of the three possible "wrong" ones (ones that were not actually presented that trial). Of these three wrong combinations, one leads to the wrong detection response but to the right identification response, one to the wrong identification response but to the right detection response, and one to both wrong responses. When the probability distributions are high threshold or constant-variance Gaussians (still assuming the outputs of different analyzers in different intervals are probabilistically independent), these three wrong combinations are equally likely. Thus, on the trials where the closest pattern × interval combination is a wrong one, the detection response is no more or less likely to be wrong than is the identification response.

(In the case of high-threshold distributions, the closest combination will be the right one whenever a detect state occurs in one or more analyzers. When no detect state occurs, the observed analyzer outputs are all not-detect, that is, at the origin of the analyzer-output space. The origin is equally far-away from all the stimulus points, since these are equally detectable patterns. Then the observer must "guess" which the closest is and all three wrong ones are again equally likely.)

Since detection and identification percent-correct are equal both on trials where the closest stimulus is right and on trials where it is wrong, overall detection and identification performances will also be equal.

Constant-Variance Gaussians and Two Other Decision Rules. Percent-correct identification is also predicted to equal percent-correct detection (for far-apart equally detectable stimuli) for the constant-variance Gaussian distribution combined with two other decision rules—maximizing detection and identification performances independently (Assumption 87) and sum-detection and difference-identification (Assumption 88) as discussed in Klein (1985) and in Thomas et al. (1982).

General Independent-Analyzers Models. All the factors (illustrated in Figs. 9.10, 9.11, and 9.12) that can disturb the predicted relation between identification and detection in the discrimination paradigms can disturb it here as well. The operation of most of them in the 2 × 2 paradigm is quite similar to that in the preceding paradigms. Two of the factors merit some further discussion.

Different Decision Rules. What kind of decision rule would predict that identification and detection performances *not* be equal for far-apart stimuli in this 2 × 2 paradigm? If the observer adopts a "better" identification rule than he or she does detection (e.g., optimizing identification but using sum-of-outputs detection), discrimination will be improved relative to detection. Two of the six rules considered by Klein (1985) but not discussed in detail here (those maximizing one kind of response contingent on a correct response of the other kind) lead to predictions, in fact, of unequal performance on identification and detection.

Limited Attention. Imperfect monitoring will also affect the predictions. In the case of the 2 × 2 paradigm where the observer has to make two different responses, one might argue that he or she is overburdened and might ease the load by monitoring only one analyzer some of the time (e.g., Klein, 1985). If so, detection performance will be decreased (as in the singleband model of Chap. 7). Identification performance need not be affected nearly as much, however, if the observer uses the following reasonable strategy: Respond with the stimulus appropriate to the unmonitored analyzer whenever the monitored analyzer's output is below some criterion (Klein, 1985; Shaw, Mulligan, & Stone, 1983). Thus, the monitoring of only a single analyzer may decrease detection performance much more than identification performance.

10.3.2 Comparison of Predictions with Identification of Far-Apart Spatial Frequencies

A number of studies have shown that, once spatial frequencies are a factor of 2 or 3 apart, identification is just as good as detection (Furchner, Thomas, & Campbell, 1977; Nachmias & Weber, 1975; Barker, 1979, published in Thomas et al., 1982; Watson & Robson, 1981). As in the simple detection and identification results (Yager et al., 1984), however, there are individual differences, some subjects requiring a factor of only a little more than 1.5 (Furchner et al., 1977; Thomas et al., 1982). Temporal conditions probably matter as well, with a larger factor being required at higher temporal frequencies (Watson & Robson, 1981).

One study has systematically investigated spatial frequencies that are very far apart in a 2 × 2 paradigm (Olzak, 1985). The results are very like those described earlier for discrimination experiments with very-far-apart frequencies (section 9.9.1): Namely, identification is actually better than detection when 3 and 9 c/deg or 3 and 12 c/deg are used but not when 3 and 6 c/deg or 3 and 18 c/deg are used. Whether the increased discrimination performance for 3 and 9 c/deg and 3 and 12 c/deg should be attributed to one or more of the following is unclear, however: inhibitory interactions, noise correlations, imperfect monitoring, decision rules.

10.3.3 Identification Performance When Wrong Interval Is Chosen

One way of distinguishing among versions of the independent-analyzers model is to consider identification performance on trials where the detection response was wrong. Assuming the high-threshold probability distribution, for example, the only detect states will occur in the interval during which the nonblank pattern was actually presented and by analyzers that are sensitive to that pattern. Thus, by any reasonable decision rule, if the observer is wrong about the interval there must have been no detect states at all on that trial. And therefore his or her identification performance will be chance.

The same prediction—chance identification performance when the detection response is wrong—is also made by any model in which the identification response is based only on the analyzer outputs during the interval specified by the detection response (e.g., independent-analyzers models using the closest pattern × interval or the maximum-output decision rules, Assumptions 85 and 86).

Many other models, however, sensibly integrate information across intervals in specifying the identification response and predict, therefore, that identification performance will be better than chance even when the detection response is wrong (e.g., independent-analyzers models using the decision rule that maximizes detection and identification performance separately, or the sum-detection and difference-identification decision rule—Assumptions 87 and 88).

Experimental tests of this prediction are difficult and have been somewhat inconclusive (King-Smith & Kulikowski, 1981; Thomas et al., 1982), but identification performance is probably better than chance even when the detection response is wrong (Thomas et al., 1982).

10.3.4 Predictions for Close Stimuli

Analyzer bandwidths can be estimated from the confusion between close-together stimuli in the 2 × 2 paradigm, but (as always) the estimated bandwidths will depend on many assumptions. For a number of different independent-analyzers models, Table 10.1 summarizes how far apart two stimuli have to be (expressed as a percentage of the half-amplitude full-bandwidth) in order that $z(\text{ident})/z(\text{detect})$ be 0.5, where $z(\text{ident})$ and $z(\text{detect})$ are the z scores corresponding to predicted probability of correct identification and detection, respectively. For all the models of Table 10.1, the analyzers were assumed to be probabilistically independent noninteracting and characterized by the constant-variance Gaussian distribution. The decision rule, the number of analyzers, and the shape of the analyzers' sensitivity functions varied, however, as is briefly indicated in Table 10.1 and described further here. The necessary stimulus separation varies from about two thirds of the bandwidth down to about one sixth!

Sum-Detection and Difference-Identification Rule and Vectors in Analyzer-Output Space. Use of the sum-detection and difference-identification decision rule allows the following very interesting equation to be derived (Thomas et al., 1982; see section 10.10.2):

$$\frac{z(\text{ident})}{z(\text{detect})} = \frac{|\mathbf{A} - \mathbf{B}|}{|\mathbf{A} + \mathbf{B}|} = \tan\frac{\varphi}{2}$$

where $\mathbf{A}$ and $\mathbf{B}$ are the vectors (in the M'-dimensional analyzer-output space) representing the average outputs of the M' monitored analyzers to the two non-blank patterns A and B and φ is the angle between $\mathbf{A}$ and $\mathbf{B}$. Notice that we are not assuming only one analyzer per stimulus for this equation.

This relationship between the angle φ and the ratio $z(\text{ident})/z(\text{detect})$ is quite linear (see Fig. 5 in Thomas et al., 1982). An angle φ of 53 degrees corresponds to a ratio of 0.5 (identification half as good as detection). When φ is 90 degrees, that is, when the vectors $\mathbf{A}$ and $\mathbf{B}$ are perpendicular (orthogonal), the ratio of

TABLE 10.1. The Separation Between Two Stimulus Values (Expressed as a Proportion of the Half-Amplitude Full-Bandwidth) That Will Make z(ident)/z(detect) Equal 0.5 in a 2×2 Experiment.

Model	Separation	Reference
Sum-Detection/Difference-Identification		
Two symmetric analyzers where the shape of sensitivity function is:		
Triangular	0.67	Section 10.10.2
Half-cosine-cycle	0.58	Section 10.10.2
Many analyzers where the shape of sensitivity function is:		
Triangular	0.58	*Thomas, Gille, and Barker 1982
Half-cosine-cycle	0.48	*Thomas, Gille, and Barker 1982
Maximum-Output		
Many analyzers,		
Half-cosine-cycle	0.33	*Barker reported in Thomas and Gille 1979
Closest-Pattern-by-Interval		
Many Gabor-type mechanisms with half-amplitude full-bandwidth =		
One octave (spatial frequency)	0.20	Watson 1983
38 degrees (orientation)	0.15	Watson 1983

* Augmented by personal communications from J. Thomas 1986

z(ident) to z(detect) is 1.0, as in the prediction of section 10.3.1 for far-apart values. A special case of orthogonality is when patterns A and B are far apart, that is, when they affect completely different sets of analyzers: then, for each analyzer i, either A_i or B_i is zero.

The angle φ—although related to bandwidth—does not directly give us the bandwidths of individual analyzers. To find those bandwidths requires more assumptions about how many analyzers there are and their sensitivity functions.

Two, Symmetric Analyzers Case. Let us start with a very simple model, one in which there are only two analyzers and these analyzers are symmetric (in the sense shown in the lower left panel of Fig. 9.9). To find the half-amplitude full-bandwidth for two symmetric analyzers (see section 10.10.3 for more details), you find the difference in values for which φ is 37 degrees (or equivalently, for which z(ident)/z(detect) is 0.33) and double that value. Alternatively, as in Table 10.1, one can ask at what stimulus separation φ will equal 53 degrees (equivalently, z(ident)/z(detect) will equal 0.5). To answer this question, one needs to know the shape of the function relating each analyzer's sensitivity to value on the dimension of interest. Table 10.1 gives the answers for a triangular analyzer sensitivity function and for a cosine-shaped one.

Many Analyzers on the Dimension of Interest. Thomas and Gille (1979) did calculations assuming many analyzers on the dimension of interest. The exact number of analyzers turned out to matter little as long as the analyzers were spaced more closely than four per half-amplitude full-bandwidth. Thomas and Gille used three different functions to describe the sensitivity of each analyzer to values on the dimension of interest: a half-cycle of a cosine, a triangle, and a function even more concave than a triangle. Their calculations were done with a slightly different model that did not handle the "uncertainty" (the fact that if observers monitor analyzers for both stimuli all the time, noise from the irrelevant analyzer produces a decrement in performance); thus one must modify their theoretical predictions (e.g., Fig. 5 of Thomas & Gille, 1979) to make bandwidth estimates 20% narrower (personal communication, J. Thomas, April 1986, revising the comment in Thomas et al., 1982, p. 1647).

As reported in Table 10.1, this modification shows that the difference in values giving a z(ident)/z(detect) ratio of one half is approximately 0.48 of the half-amplitude full-bandwidth of an individual analyzer, assuming that each analyzer's sensitivity as a function of value was half a cycle of a cosine. Assuming that the shape was triangular leads to a value of 0.58. (See note 2.)

The Maximum-Output Decision Rule. Thomas and Gille (1979) also reported some calculations of Barker's using the maximum-output 2 × 2 decision rule with the same analyzers just described (and handling uncertainty correctly). For this model to produce z(ident)/z(detect) = 0.5, the necessary difference in values is about 0.33 of the half-amplitude full-bandwidth.

Closest Pattern × Interval Decision Rule and Multiple Receptive Fields. Unlike the predictions just described, the analyzers in Watson's 1983 model were not just specified by their sensitivity function on the dimension of interest, but were individual mechanisms ("sensors," in Watson's terminology) having receptive fields at different spatial positions and differing in their orientation and the width of their excitatory and inhibitory sections at each spatial location. Thus they were described not only by their sensitivity on the spatial-frequency dimension but by their sensitivities on the spatial-position and orientation dimensions. See section 6.9.2 for a fuller description of Watson's 1983 sensors.

Also unlike the above calculations, Watson's 1983 model assumed the closest pattern × interval decision rule.

Like the above calculations, Watson's 1983 calculations assumed constant-variance Gaussian distributions as well as noninteracting, probabilistically independent analyzers.

The half-amplitude spatial-frequency bandwidth of the mechanisms (sensors) in Watson's model was one octave and the half-amplitude orientation bandwidth was 38 degrees. Thus both Watson's spatial-frequency and orientation bandwidths were a good deal broader than the bandwidth estimates just given.

To calculate the entry for Watson's model in Table 10.1: The model predicts that z(ident)/z(detect) of 0.5 occurs at a spatial-frequency ratio of about 1.20 or 1.25, which is a frequency difference less than one fourth of the sensor's half-amplitude bandwidth. It also predicts a z(ident)/z(detect) ratio of about 0.5 for an orientation difference of about 5 degrees, which is less than one seventh of the half-amplitude bandwidth.

10.3.5 *Estimates of Bandwidth From 2 × 2 Experiments on the Spatial-Frequency Dimension*

Rather extensive results from 2 × 2 experiments on the spatial-frequency dimension can be found in Thomas et al., (1982) and Watson and Robson (1981). Both studies showed equivalent behavior at low and high spatial frequencies when spatial frequency is plotted on a logarithmic scale. [Spatial frequencies an octave apart could be perfectly discriminated throughout the range from 0.25 to 30 c/deg in Watson and Robson (1981).] This equivalence once again suggests that spatial-frequency bandwidths are constant on a logarithmic frequency axis.

At very low spatial frequencies (near 0.25 c/deg), the identification/detection results suggest even broader estimates on the log-frequency axis (Furchner et al., 1977).

The actual bandwidth estimates will vary depending on the model used to estimate them. Figure 7 of Thomas et al. (1982) shows that spatial-frequency ratios between 1.2 and 1.4 (depending on observer) produce an angle φ of 53 degrees (a z(ident)/z(detect) ratio of 0.5). As can be seen in Table 10.1, these ratios might correspond to as little as 0.20 or as much as 0.67 of the spatial-frequency half-amplitude full-bandwidth, thus yielding bandwidths as great as one to two octaves (depending on observer) or as little as 0.33 to 0.66 octave (depending on observer).

Similarly, Fig. 6 of Thomas et al. (1982) shows that orientation differences between 3 and 7 degrees (depending on observer) produce a z(ident)/z(detect) of 0.5, thus leading to bandwidths as great as 18 to 42 degrees (depending on observer; Watson's model has 38 degrees) or as little as 4.5 to 10.4 degrees (depending on observer).

See Chapter 12 for dependence of these bandwidth estimates on other parameters (e.g., temporal frequency).

10.4 CONCURRENT PARADIGM

This paradigm has been optimistically described as "advantageous precisely because it displays the underlying cognitive quirks used by the observer" (Klein, 1985). It has been touted as the paradigm "most useful for investigating independence-related concepts" (Ashby & Townsend, 1986). Most certainly, this paradigm provides rich experimental results on which a large variety of different analyses can be done for fun and, potentially, for scientific profit.

No name for this paradigm, either in the pattern-vision literature or elsewhere, has become standard; some alternatives are given in note 3.

10.4.1 Experimental Procedure

Stimuli. Figure 10.5 (upper left) shows the stimuli of the concurrent paradigm. They can be represented as an $N \times N$ matrix where the rows give the intensity levels in one component B and the columns give the intensity levels in the other component A. The lowest intensity levels C_1 and C_1' are always zero. Hence the lower left cell in the matrix represents the blank stimulus; the bottom row represents different simple A stimuli at different intensities and the left column represents simple B stimuli. All the other cells represent compound A + B stimuli.

On each single-interval trial, one of these $N \times N$ stimuli is shown at random (usually with equal presentation probabilities).

TWO-VALUE CONCURRENT EXPERIMENT

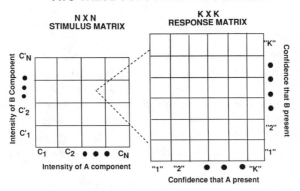

ALTERNATIVE REPRESENTATION

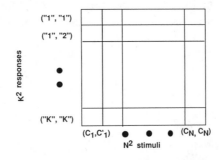

FIG. 10.5 Separate stimulus and response matrices for a concurrent experiment involving two values (top). Alternative representation in one matrix (bottom).

Responses. On each trial the observer makes two confidence ratings, one giving confidence that component A was present (at above zero intensity) and the other giving confidence that component B was present (at above zero intensity). To put it another way, the observer answers two questions: "Is stimulus A present?" and "Is stimulus B present?" If the answers are given on a K-category confidence rating scale, the responses can be represented as a $K \times K$ matrix (shown in Fig. 10.5 upper right).

An alternative representation of a concurrent identification experiment with the K^2 possible response combinations labeling the rows and the N^2 stimuli labeling the columns is shown in the bottom of Fig. 10.5. If there are the same number of categories in the confidence rating scales (K) as there are intensity levels in the component stimuli (N), then there are the same number of responses as stimuli. Observers may establish the natural one-to-one correspondence between confidence ratings and stimuli (trying to give the lowest category on both rating scales to the blank, etc.), either on their own or because of explicit instructions from the experimenter. Then this concurrent paradigm becomes an example of a classification experiment.

Extension to More Values. Concurrent experiments can be run using three components (e.g., Pohlman & Sorkin, 1976; Wickelgren, 1967), four (e.g., Townsend et al., 1984), or more (in principle). In that case the stimulus and response matrices must include three, four, or more dimensions instead of the two illustrated in Fig. 10.5.

Response Variants. The number of categories in the confidence rating scale may vary. Further, for any given number of categories, the observer might be asked to give responses in several different ways that seem identical formally but might produce different results empirically. As an illustration of some of the possibilities, consider the case where there are only two intensity levels in each of two components and only two categories (no and yes) in each of the two confidence rating scales. (a) The observer might be asked to say the two ratings out loud, each one being no or yes. (b) The observer might be asked to push one of each of two pairs of buttons, each pair representing the no versus yes answers for one component. (c) The two categories on each of two scales might be combined to give four names—blank, A (meaning A only), B (meaning B only), and A + B—and the observer might be asked to say one of these names out loud. (d) The observer might be asked to push one of four buttons representing the four names.

Single-Task Control. A variant of the above concurrent paradigm is to use the same set of stimuli but to ask the observer to give only one of the confidence ratings on a trial (e.g., the one about A).

10.4.2 Assumptions and Decision Rules

The assumptions of the independent-analyzers models reviewed in section 9.3 will be used here except that the detection decision rules are largely irrelevant, the one-analyzer-per-stimulus assumption will often be explicitly loosened, and alternatives to the perfect-monitoring assumption will be explicitly considered. We will need to use an additivity assumption here, using the assumption that ineffective stimuli are ineffective in compounds (Assumption 36) for far-apart values but considering an assumption of complete additivity to a compound (Assumption 27) when close-together values are at issue.

We will make only one kind of formal decision rule for this paradigm (in several versions, next subsection)—the kind that has most often been considered—and then informally we will consider how other kinds of decision rules might affect the predictions.

10.4.3   Noninteracting (Direct) Reports

The class of decision rules we will formally consider assumes that the observer's confidence that one component has been presented depends only on the outputs of the analyzers sensitive to that particular component. In particular, it does not depend on the outputs of analyzers that are sensitive to the other component(s) used in the experiment but not to the one about which confidence is being rated. We will call this kind of decision rule *noninteracting reports* or *direct reports*. Several versions of this sort of assumption are possible. If, for example, we allow for multiple analyzers per stimulus, we might assume:

Assumption 89. Direct Reports of Analyzers' Outputs.   *The decision variable that the observer uses in giving a confidence rating about one component is the maximum of the outputs from the analyzers sensitive to that component.*

Note that in this and the following decision rules the observer is assumed to use the decision variable for each component in the standard way for rating responses (Assumption 77).

If all the analyzers sensitive to a particular component are grouped into a "composite analyzer"—so there is only one analyzer per component used in the experiment—and if that analyzer has a single-number output, then the following form of the noninteracting report assumption might be used:

Assumption 90. Direct Reports of the Relevant Analyzer's Output.   *The decision variable used by the observer in rating confidence about one component is the output of the one analyzer sensitive to that component.*

This last assumption is equivalent to the previous one if the output of the composite analyzer is taken to be the maximum of the outputs of the analyzers and (as is assumed true for far-apart components) the analyzers themselves are probabilistically independent, noninteracting, and nonoverlapping.

Some criterion lines for the decision variables in the one-analyzer-per-stimulus version (Assumption 90) are shown in Fig. 10.6 for far-apart components (left and close components (right). The output of the one analyzer sensitive to the first component is shown on the horizontal axis and the output of the analyzer sensitive to the second component is shown on the vertical axis. The circles

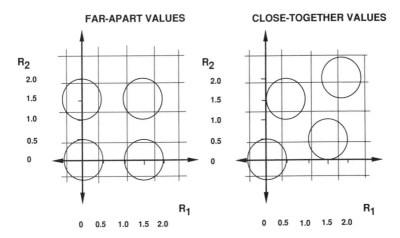

FIG. 10.6 Illustration of criterion lines in a concurrent experiment on the assumption of direct (noninteracting) reports for far-apart values (left) and close-together values (right).

represent the central parts of the probability distributions in response to four stimuli: the blank (lower left), each of two simple stimuli (upper left and lower right), and the compound (upper right). Notice that the criterion lines are perpendicular to the two axes (and therefore to each other), since the decision variable always equals the value plotted on one axis or the other. The placement of the distribution for the compound assumes complete additivity (Assumption 27), so that the four points form a parallelogram. (For presentation of vector sums and parallelograms see section 9.11.)

Rather than viewing Fig. 10.6 as showing the outputs of exactly two analyzers, one might consider it the result of rotating an M' dimensional analyzer-output space in the proper way so as to put the two vectors for the two simple stimuli in the frontal plane (and thereby automatically putting the one for the compound distribution in the frontal plane if there is additivity). Then the following assumption will lead to the criterion lines shown in that figure:

Assumption 91. Direct Reports Using Perpendicular Criteria. *The criterion planes for the decision variable used by the observer in giving a confidence rating about one component in a concurrent experiment are perpendicular to the criterion planes for the other decision variable(s) used to give the confidence rating(s) about the other component(s).*

10.4.4 Interacting (Nondirect) Reports

The observer's confidence that one component was presented may depend not only on the analyzer (analyzers) sensitive to that component but also on the analyzer (analyzers) sensitive to the other component. If so, the criterion lines will no longer be perpendicular to the axes. (An example that will be discussed later is shown in the right of Fig. 10.10.)

10.5   PREDICTIONS FOR CONCURRENT EXPERIMENTS

10.5.1   *Computing d' Values (More Generally, Signal Strength Parameters) Separately for Each Question*

This section describes one way of analyzing the results from concurrent experiments in order to compare them with the predictions of independent-analyzers models. Alternative analyses—directed at testing many of the same predictions—can be found in Ashby and Townsend (1986), Olzak and Wickens (1983), and Sorkin and Pohlman's papers (e.g., Pohlman & Sorkin, 1976; Sorkin et al., 1973, 1976). A modification of the analysis discussed here (from Klein, 1985) will be discussed in section 10.7.2.

An Example. Consider the question for each component separately (e.g., Is component A present?) and compute from the answers to it the d' for each of the stimuli (always taking the blank as noise). This calculation is illustrated in Fig. 10.7 for hypothetical results from a concurrent experiment with a 2 × 2 stimulus matrix (two intensity levels in each of two components A and B) and a 2 × 2 response matrix (yes and no being the two categories in each confidence rating scale). The 2 × 2 response matrices for each stimulus (labeled above the matrix) are shown in Fig. 10.7. The numbers inside each matrix are the proportions of all trials of that stimulus on which the indicated response was given (e.g.,

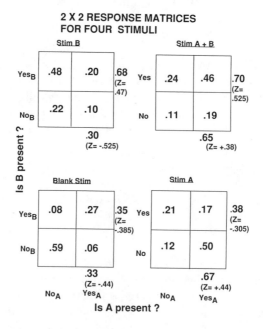

FIG. 10.7 Example of calculation of d' values from the two confidence ratings in a concurrent experiment.

on 0.48 of trials of stimulus B the observer said "Yes, B was present" and "No, A was not present"). The total proportions of yes answers to each question (regardless of the answer to the other question) are given in the margins of the response matrices with the corresponding z score in parentheses underneath. The question from which a d' value is computed will be indicated by subscripts on d'. Consider, for example, the computation of d'_A (stim A + B), which is the d' value computed from the answer to the question, "Is A present?" when the stimulus was the compound A + B. The computation is done in the standard way for yes-no experiments by computing z(hits) minus z(false alarms), which in this case is z (yes A|stim A + B) minus z(yes A|blank) or $+0.38 - (-0.44) = 0.82$. (Notice that the d' values for the blank must necessarily be zero.)

Generally. The example computation assumes that the constant-variance Gaussian family was the appropriate characterization of the decision variable underlying the answer to each question, but this assumption can easily be replaced and the signal-strength parameters appropriate to any other distribution family be used instead as discussed further in note 4. For convenience we will continue to talk about d' values, however, rather than signal-strength parameter values.

One the assumption of direct reports from the relevant single analyzer (Assumption 90), the decision variable underlying the answer to a given question is just the relevant single analyzer's output. On this assumption, therefore, the computed d' is proportional (except for sampling variability) to the relevant analyzer's average output. More precisely, the computed d' is an estimate of the relevant analyzer's expected output to the stimulus minus its expected output to the noise divided by the standard deviation of its output to the noise. Therefore, as is done in Fig. 10.8 for the example computation, it is interesting to plot the d' values computed from the answer to one question (say the question about A) on the horizontal axis and the d' values computed from the answer to the other question (say the question about B) on the vertical axis. (The ellipses will be discussed in section 10.5.5.) This kind of plot represents the estimated outputs from the two relevant analyzers in the same form we have often used to discuss theoretical questions (e.g., Fig. 10.6)—the estimated expected output from one analyzer is on one axis and that from the other analyzer is on the other axis. [Nachmias (1974) may have been the first to use this kind of plot.]

This d'-d' plot remains interesting even if, instead of assuming direct reports from relevant single analyzers (Assumption 90), one assumes direct reports using perpendicular criteria (Assumption 91). For then this d'-d' plot is a picture of estimated stimulus vectors rotated into the frontal plane.

10.5.2 Bandwidth and the Angle Between the Simple-Stimulus Vectors

For far-apart stimuli, the d'-d' plot should look like the left panel of Fig. 10.6 on either of the direct reports assumptions (90 or 91) coupled with the other independent-analyzers models assumptions; in particular, the estimated stimu-

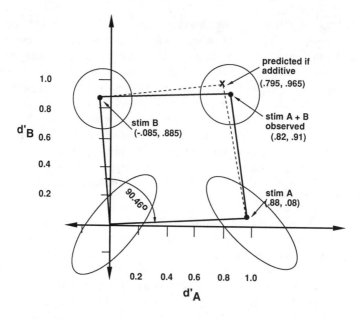

FIG. 10.8 Plot of the d' values from the example in Fig. 10.7.

lus vectors for the simple stimuli should fall on the axes (except for sampling variability). As the simple stimuli get closer together, the vectors should move closer together (e.g., right of Fig. 10.6). The angle φ between the two vectors from the simple stimuli is a useful way to summarize the degree of overlap of the analyzers' outputs to the two stimuli. Use of that angle to estimate bandwidth of the underlying analyzers will depend on how many analyzers are assumed and on the shape of the functions relating sensitivity to value, just as it did for the 2 × 2 paradigm (see section 10.3.4). Calculations relating the angle to analyzer bandwidth for the two-symmetric-analyzers case are given in section 10.10.3.

10.5.3   Additivity and Masking in Results for the Compound Stimulus

Since the d'-d' plots mirror the plots of analyzer outputs, one can make interesting predictions about the results for the compound stimulus.

If there is complete additivity to the compound (Assumption 27 or 47), the point for the compound stimulus should be the fourth corner of the parallelogram generated by the blank and the two simple stimuli, whether those simple stimuli are close or far, as in Fig. 10.6 left or right. If A and B are far apart, complete additivity is not needed for this prediction; it is sufficient to assume that an ineffective stimulus is ineffective in a compound (Assumption 36). Algebraically one can write the prediction as

$$d'_A(\text{stim A} + \text{B}) = d'_A(\text{stim A}) + d'_A(\text{stim B})$$

$$d'_B(\text{stim A} + \text{B}) = d'_B(\text{stim A}) + d'_B(\text{stim B})$$

If, however, as is more reasonable for close-together values on the spatial-frequency dimension because of spatial probability summation, each analyzer's output to the compound is less than the sum of its outputs to the two components, the point for the compound will fall somewhat inside the parallelogram extrapolated from the points for the components.

In the example of Figs. 10.7 and 10.8, completing the parallelogram formed by the vectors for the simple stimuli (dotted lines) gives a "predicted" point for the compound that is shown by an X on the figure. The observed d'-d' point is slightly removed from the predicted one. Depending on the number of trials that entered into the computation, however, the discrepancy between the X and the observed point for the compound may or may not be anything more than sampling error.

Subadditivity and Masking. We will say there is subadditivity when the d' value observed for the compound is less than that predicted from additivity. For example, for the A response there is subadditivity when

$$d'_A(\text{stim A} + \text{B}) < d'_A(\text{stim A}) + d'_A(\text{stim B})$$

Subadditivity might also be called *masking,* as the above equation is equivalent to

$$d'_A(\text{stim A} + \text{B}) - d'_A(\text{stim B}) < d'_A(\text{stim A})$$

In this last equation the left side gives (for the A response) the discriminability between the test stimulus A and a mask-plus-test stimulus A + B, or what is sometimes called *the detectability of A in the presence of a mask B.* The right side gives the unmasked detectability of A. So the equation says that the detectability of A is decreased by the presence of a mask B. This decrease is often called masking.

Masking d' Values. In fact, some authors compute d' values for the compound stimulus not as we did above (using the blank stimulus as noise) but instead using one of the component stimuli, for example,

$$z(\text{yes}_A | \text{stim A} + \text{B}) - z(\text{yes}_A | \text{stim B})$$

I will call d' values computed this way *masking d' values,* because they reflect the discriminability of a test plus mask (stim A + B) from a mask (stim B).

For yes-no scales, as trivial algebra will show, a masking d' will always just equal the difference between our d' for the compound and our d' for the component being used as the mask (e.g., B above). For example, the difference between z scores in the last equation also equals

$$d'_A(\text{stim A} + \text{B}) - d'_A(\text{stim B})$$

For confidence rating scales containing more than two categories, this equivalence will hold also except for artifacts encountered in fitting ROC curves.

10.5.4   *Perfect Monitoring Versus Limited Capacity*

The analysis so far could have been carried out even if the two questions had been asked on different trials or different blocks; it used only the total proportions of yes answers to each question regardless of the answer to the other. Thus, the same analyses can be carried out on results from single-task control experiments.

The perfect-monitoring and direct-reports assumptions—coupled with the other assumptions of the independent-analyzers models—make the following prediction: The d' values computed for a single-task control experiment asking a particular question should be the same (within measurement error) as the d' values for that question in the full concurrent experiment.

If they are not the same we presume that some aspect of our assumptions is wrong. It might be limited attention capacity, limited ability to make direct reports, interactions among analyzers, and so on (see a similar brief summary in a different style in Sperling, 1984, pp. 124–125).

10.5.5   *Correlation Between the Answers Across Trials of a Given Stimulus*

To use the rest of the information available from a concurrent experiment—that information that is not available from single-task controls—one can compute the correlation between the answers given to the two questions across all trials of any given stimulus. If one uses the ordinary Pearson product-moment correlation, one must assign numbers to the categories in the confidence-rating scales; which numbers one assigns (if there are more than two categories) will make some difference. One wishes the calculated correlation to reflect the correlation between two analyzers' outputs. Simply numbering the categories consecutively may be sufficient. [For when the placement of the criterion lines dividing categories has been examined—in unpublished data from the Hirsch et al. 1982 study—the lines seem to be evenly spaced along the axis representing analyzer output; one manifestation of this is that average confidence rating when categories are numbered consecutively is straight-line function of d' computed from those ratings. See Hirsch (1977) for examples.] In any case, simply numbering the categories consecutively will be sufficient to reveal whether there is probabilistic independence between the two answers, as no numbering scheme can introduce a correlation where there is probabilistic independence between the decision variables. That is, the following prediction follows from the direct reports and probabilistic assumptions coupled with the other assumptions of the independent-analyzers model:

Prediction 2.   *If no analyzer is sensitive to both A and B, then the correlation should be zero between the confidence ratings for A and for B across trials of any stimulus in a concurrent experiment.*

Given an assignment of numbers to categories (0 and 1 in the case of two categories, as in the example results of Fig. 10.7), the correlations can be directly

computed from the response matrices. For the example in Fig. 10.7, these correlations are approximately zero for B and for A + B but positive for the blank
(more double no's and double yes's tend to be given than combinations of a no
and a yes) and negative for stimulus A. Circles and ellipses roughly representing
these correlations have been drawn on Fig. 10.8. (See Olzak, 1986, for other
examples from actual experimental results.)

Again, whether or not these correlations are significantly different from zero
depends on the number of trials entering into the analysis. And the fact that
these categories are discrete requires consideration in calculating exact significance values. Furthermore, using estimators that are meant for discrete data
(e.g., the tetrachoric r suggested by Pearson rather than the more commonly used
Pearson product-moment correlation coefficient) should provide more accurate
estimates (see e.g., simulations in Ashby 1988).

10.6   COMPARISON OF INDEPENDENT-ANALYZERS MODELS' PREDICTIONS WITH SPATIAL-FREQUENCY RESULTS

The results of concurrent experiments on the spatial frequency dimension are
much as predicted by the independent-analyzers model above. The d'-d' plots
are close to parallelograms, the angle between vectors increases as the spatial
frequencies get farther apart, and the correlations between the two ratings are
low or zero (Hirsch et al., 1982; Graham et al., 1985; Nachmias, 1974; Olzak,
1986). Single-task controls have not been adequately done (note 5). Some systematic, although small, deviations exist, however. These will be discussed in
section 10.6.2 after presentation of the basic confusion results. Possible explanations for these deviations are discussed in section 10.7.

10.6.1   Angle Between Vectors

The estimated angle between the simple-stimulus vectors is shown in Fig. 10.9
from concurrent experiments varying spatial-frequency ratio over the range
from 1 to 3 (Nachmias, 1974; reanalysis of results published in Hirsch, et al.,
1982). (The estimation method is described in note 6.) As is certainly expected,
confusion between two components increases (the angle decreases) as their values get closer together.

Confusion in the concurrent paradigm depends primarily on the ratio between
the two spatial frequencies (as plotted on the horizontal axis of Fig. 10.9) rather
than on spatial-frequency difference. For example, the squares in Fig. 10.9 are
for a lower spatial frequency of 3 c/deg compared with the upward pointing triangles, which are for a lower spatial frequency of 15 c/deg. As usual, this suggests
that spatial-frequency bandwidth (in this spatial-frequency range from 3 to 15
c/deg in any case) is approximately constant on a logarithmic spatial-frequency
axis.

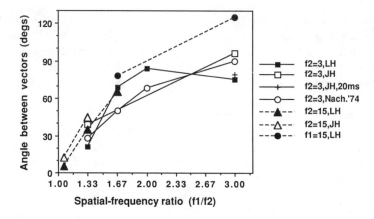

FIG. 10.9 The angle between the estimated simple stimulus vectors in d'-d' plots from concurrent experiments on the spatial-frequency dimension as a function of spatial-frequency ratio. For each curve either the lower (f2) or the higher (f1) spatial frequency was kept constant at the value (in c/deg) indicated in the figure inset where the observer is also indicated. JH and LH are the observers reported in Hirsch, Hylton, and Graham (1982). The cross shows results from two sessions with observer JH, where the exposure duration was only 20 milliseconds. The open circle shows results from the observer reported by Nachmias 1974.

Comparison with 2 × 2 Results. The angle φ computed from available results on the 2 × 2 paradigm may be larger than in the concurrent paradigm. At a spatial-frequency ratio of 1.33, the angles measured in the concurrent paradigm range from 20 to 45 degrees (Fig. 10.9), for example, but those in the 2 × 2 paradigm range from 40 to 65 degrees (Thomas et al., 1982, Fig. 7). Although the same subjects and same conditions (e.g., time course, mean luminance) were not used in the same conditions in the two paradigms, the difference is large enough that one is tempted to say (in an admittedly loose and vague manner) that the greater complexity of the concurrent paradigm may simply make it more "confusing" to the observer, where the confusion is at some higher level of processing than represented by the bandwidth of the analyzers in our model.

10.6.2 Three Systematic Deviations

This section describes three systematic deviations between experimental results and independent-analyzers models' predictions. Section 10.7 discusses possible explanations of these deviations for far-apart values.

Deviation One. Simple Stimulus Points Not on Axes. The simple stimulus vectors for far-apart values seem to not lie exactly on the axes of the d'-d' plot. For very-far-apart frequencies (a factor of 4 or 6) the angle φ may be greater than 90 degrees (Olzak, 1986; Olzak & Kramer, 1984). This wide angle correlates with the analogous aspect of the results in discrimination and 2×2 experiments for the same spatial frequencies, that is, better discrimination between simple stimuli (relative to the detectability of either one) than is predicted by independent-analyzers models. This wide angle φ is not always to be found, however, even for these same spatial frequencies. One of the three subjects in Olzak's study (1986), for example, has an angle φ between vectors of about 78 degrees (for 3 and 12 c/deg) and 83 degrees (for 3 and 18 c/deg).

A rotation counterclockwise in the results for far-apart frequencies is also seen occasionally, that is, a rotation toward the higher spatial-frequency axis. This kind of asymmetry in the degree to which one of the observer's confidence ratings is sensitive to the other component is visible in five of the six conditions (two pairs of frequencies by three observers) published by Olzak (1986). This kind of rotation also showed up in three of the five conditions studying spatial frequencies a factor of 3 apart in Fig. 10.9 and in four of the four conditions of another study (Haber, 1976, briefly described in Graham et al., 1985).

Deviation Two. Nonadditivity. A second systematic deviation may be some nonadditivity even for far-apart spatial frequencies (Nachmias, 1974). Of the nine conditions studying spatial frequencies a factor of 3 apart in Fig. 10.9 and in Haber (1976), five showed subadditivity (masking) but one showed superadditivity and three showed no consistent deviation from additivity at all. Similar mixed results can be seen in Olzak (1986). In any case, the subadditivity is not great. The median difference between the observed d' and the predicted d' is at most 0.25 of a d' unit.

Deviation Three. Nonzero Correlations. The third systematic deviation is that, even for far-apart spatial frequencies, the correlations between the confidence ratings given in answer to the two questions across trials of the same stimulus are consistently found to be unequal to zero (Hirsch et al., 1982; Olzak, 1986). For the blank (or barely detectable stimuli), the (Pearson-product-moment) correlation is consistently greater than zero. For example, for eight of the nine cases a factor of 3 apart in Fig. 10.9 and in Haber (1976), the median correlation on the blank was positive. Again, however, it would be a mistake to overemphasize the degree of this correlation. The largest median found on the blank for the nine conditions was 0.40. Therefore "the amount of variance accounted for" was 0.2. To a good first approximation the two answers even to the blank are probabilistically independent.

The probabilistic dependence to the nonblank stimuli is even less pronounced. In fact, many of the conditions seemed to demonstrate a graded decrease in correlation with increased detectability of stimuli, often ending up in negative correlations for the most detectable stimuli. This trend was particularly apparent for simple stimuli, less clear for compound.

Close-Together Values. Variants of the above three kinds of "deviations" for far-apart spatial frequencies are also found for close-together spatial frequencies.

For close spatial frequencies, however, their interpretation is different as they are not necessarily deviations from predictions of independent-analyzers' models. One expects the stimulus vectors to be inside the axes for close values (and they are—see Fig. 10.9—rotations are sometimes found and sometimes not). Subadditivity is expected on the basis of spatial probability summation (and found frequently; in Haber, 1976; Hirsch et al., 1982, Nachmias, 1974, although again it was small). Some correlation is expected as the analyzer outputs overlap, although the fact that the correlations differ with detectability of the stimulus (as they did for far-apart values) is somewhat puzzling.

10.6.3 Effects of Experimental Procedure and Practice

No Effect of Number of Stimuli or Feedback. One unpublished study from our laboratory manipulated several aspects of the concurrent paradigm (Haber, 1976). The number of stimuli (2×2 vs. 3×3 stimulus matrices) did not make a measurable difference (although it was not studied extensively enough to have revealed any minor effects). Neither did the kind of feedback—partial versus complete or complete versus none—although again it was not studied extensively nor with every possible response variant (see the following).

Effect of Response Variant. The only consistent effect in that study was an effect of the form of response. In some sessions the observer had to make two separate confidence ratings each on a 5-category scale (called *component rating* below), and in other sessions the observer had to indicate a single one of four names—blank, low, high, both (called *stimulus naming* below). With stimulus naming—which might be taken to be the easier response variant—observers showed absolutely no confusion between spatial frequencies an intermediate distance apart (a factor of 1.67 apart), but with component rating they showed considerable confusion. For far-apart spatial frequencies (a factor of 3 apart), however, the response variant did not matter; the observers never showed any confusion.

One might explain these results informally by saying that the harder response variant (component rating) puts a burden on the observer's higher levels of processing, and that this burden was large enough to show up as worse performance in the harder task (discriminating spatial frequencies a factor of 1.67 apart) but not in the easier (discrimination spatial frequencies a factor of 3 apart). Alternatively one might say that the stimulus-naming response variant exerted a stronger covert demand on the observers to be correct than did the component rating. Hence the observers' stimulus naming was less directly influenced by analyzer outputs and more influenced by higher level strategies than were the component ratings.

Response variant had a somewhat different effect in a concurrent study using four components on a higher order shape dimension (different shapes of lines which could be either absent or present in a figure): There was more correlation when names were given than when confidence ratings were made to each component separately (Townsend et al., 1984). Due to the nature of the components, the results of this study may well reflect higher level processing than intended in this book, but in any case this second effect of response variant suggests caution in using and interpreting the concurrent paradigm.

Improvement with Practice. The interesting and important question of whether observers show improvement with practice is difficult to answer from studies in our laboratory, which always included a number of informal initial sessions in order to find the right contrast levels and familiarize subjects with the procedure. I always got the impression, however, particularly at intermediate spatial-frequency ratios (e.g., 1.67), that observers were showing improvement with practice.

A suprathreshold discrimination study (Fiorentini & Berardi, 1981) did document some learning in discriminations. This learning occurred for suprathreshold discriminations involving at least one compound grating but not in those involving only simple gratings of different spatial frequencies. Much of the learning went on in the first 40 trials. Further, the learning would transfer only to patterns of similar spatial frequencies (within 0.50 octave) or orientations (within 30 degrees), not to more disparate patterns (one octave or 90-degree rotations).

This learning, as it seems to asymptote after relatively few trials, probably presents no interpretational problems in the data analysis. But the fact that it occurs is of interest in itself.

10.7   PREDICTIONS OF MORE GENERAL INDEPENDENT-ANALYZERS MODELS

To explain the systematic deviations presented in section 10.6.2, one might modify the baseline independent-analyzers models in either (or both) of the following ways: (a) Change the assumptions about the analyzers themselves, (b) change the assumptions about the transformation from analyzer outputs to observer responses.

10.7.1   Modifying the Assumptions About the Transformation From Stimulus to Analyzer Outputs

The results of *any* single concurrent experiment can always be explained by changes in the assumptions about the transformation from stimulus to analyzer outputs. One simply assumes that, rather than being nonoverlapping, noninteracting, and probabilistically independent, the analyzers have whatever properties are revealed by the observer's responses, on the assumption that the observer's responses are direct reports of the analyzers' outputs. In other words, one just assumes that the plot of analyzer outputs looks exactly like the d'-d' plot of concurrent results. For example, to explain angles φ that are larger than 90

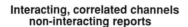

**Interacting, correlated channels   Non-interacting, independent channels
non-interacting reports   interacting reports**

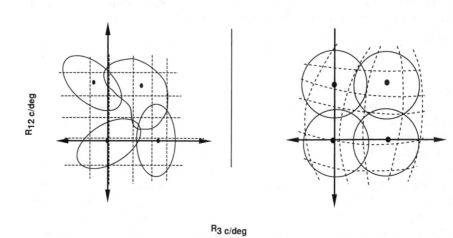

R₃ c/deg

FIG. 10.10 Two alternative explanations of the same set of results from a concurrent experiment: noninteracting reports but interacting and dependent analyzers (left) or interacting reports with noninteracting and independent analyzers (right). (Adapted from Klein, 1985.)

degrees, inhibition is assumed (e.g., Fig. 9.10 left). To explain correlations between the answers to the two questions over trials of the same stimulus, the outputs of the analyzers are assumed to be correlated in whatever way is necessary (e.g., Fig. 9.11 right). To explain subadditivity, each analyzer is assumed to be subadditive (Fig. 9.10 right).

Examining Response Matrices More Carefully. A rather sophisticated version of this kind of explanation is illustrated in the informal drawing from Klein (1985) of the analyzer outputs necessary to account for one set of 3 and 12 cpd results from Olzak (1986) (Fig. 10.10 left. The points in Fig. 10.10 indicate means of analyzer outputs, and the closed curves indicate the central part of the bivariate probability distributions.) This left panel looks rather similar to the data plot itself in Olzak (1986), except that Klein—on the basis of the full response matrices themselves—thought that the distribution of outputs to the compound stimulus looked like a boomerang rather than a bivariate Gaussian function. This boomerang shape will figure prominently again in this chapter in another kind of explanation. It would be very interesting to know if the response matrices to compound stimuli in other concurrent studies were also consistent with a boomerang shape.

Implications of This Type of Explanation. If one explains the deviations in the concurrent results in terms of interacting, correlated analyzer outputs (on the assumption of noninteracting, direct reports), one must go back to the other paradigms (e.g., summation experiments, the results of which were consistent with nonoverlapping, noninteracting, and probabilistically independent analyzers) and ask whether the degree of interaction and probabilistic dependence one postulates here (particularly in the case of far-apart spatial frequencies) would be consistent with those other paradigm's results. To do so is not an easy task, and it has certainly not been done conclusively.

10.7.2 Interacting Reports (Nonperpendicular Criterion Lines)

In any case, the direct-reports and perfect-monitoring assumptions are at least as suspect as the analyzer-output assumptions. Indeed, the somewhat greater confusability between spatial frequencies in the concurrent paradigm than in the 2 × 2 paradigm, the effect of response variant, and the improvement in discrimination involving compound gratings with practice (see section 10.6) all shed doubt on the complete adequacy of these two assumptions.

The right panel of Fig. 10.10 (from Klein, 1985) shows some possible nonorthogonal criterion lines to explain the same results explained in the left panel by interacting dependent analyzers. For example, instead of a rotation counterclockwise of the 12-cpd stimulus point in Fig. 10.10 (left) (and in the d'-d' plot of the experimental results), the criterion lines near the simple 12-cpd distribution in Fig. 10.10 right are rotated in the opposite direction.

In fact, Klein (1985) argued that a change in any one of the following three factors—(a) analyzer overlap and interactions (the positions of the stimulus points in analyzer-output space), (b) correlations among noise sources (the shape of the bivariate probability distributions), and (c) the position and shape of nonorthogonal criterion lines—can be perfectly imitated by a combination of the other two factors. (See Fig. 9 of Klein, 1985, for a demonstration of how inhibition and nonorthogonal criterion can mimic positive correlation.)

One can imagine many reasons why the criterion lines should not be perpendicular or even straight. For example, any attempt by an observer to maximize the degree to which certain pairs of stimuli are discriminable in his or her responses may produce criterion lines for the two responses that are not perpendicular to each other.

However, interacting reports are not a guaranteed cure-all in the way the interacting, dependent analyzers were. For the nonorthogonal criterion lines appropriate to account for peculiarities in the observers' response matrix for one stimulus (e.g., one of the simple stimuli) may not simultaneously explain the observer's response matrix to another stimulus (e.g., the compound stimulus).

Klein's 1985 Algorithm. It would be ideal, therefore, to have a way of finding out whether any set of nonorthogonal criterion lines exists that could explain the results of a given concurrent experiment (while still postulating nonoverlapping, noninteracting, and probabilistically independent analyzers). Klein (1985) presented an algorithm that goes part way toward this goal. The algorithm takes the two-dimensional response matrices for a pair of stimuli (e.g., blank vs. compound) and then searches for the placements of the criterion lines that will maximize the discriminability of those two stimuli (given certain restrictions against wild gerrymandering by the criterion lines). It then repeats this procedure for each pair, producing a d' value for each pair. It would be better if the criterion lines were found for all stimuli simultaneously—which seems not to be the case—but this is a start. Klein analyzed some of Olzak's (1986) results with this algorithm (those for 3 and 12 c/deg and 3 and 18 c/deg) and suggested that there is no need to postulate any inhibition or correlated noise in these results if one allows interacting reports. The subadditivity was still present, however, in this analysis.

10.7.3   Imperfect Monitoring—Intrinsic Uncertainty

A possible modification of the perfect monitoring assumption is to incorporate intrinsic uncertainty in the following way: Assume that the (composite) analyzer for a given simple stimulus contains not only the analyzers sensitive to that simple stimulus but also some insensitive ones. Suppose that some of the same insensitive analyzers are present in the composite analyzers for both simple stimuli. On trials of the blank stimulus, therefore, the outputs of the two composite analyzers would be positively correlated to some extent as a result of the shared insensitive analyzers; hence there would be some positive correlation between the answers of the observer to the two questions (about the two components). However, as stimulus detectability increases, the shared insensitive analyzers become less and less important in determining the output of the composite analyzers. Hence, if the sensitive analyzers in the two composite analyzers are nonoverlapping and probabilistically independent (as for far-apart values), there should be less and less correlation between the outputs of the two composite analyzers as the level of detectability increases. Notice that this decrease in correlation (as detectability rises) will be tied to an increase in the variance of the composite analyzers' outputs (as detectability rises). Quantitatively, furthermore, the decrease in correlation seems about right for the increase in variance that is reflected in the slope of ROC curves (see note 7 for more details). This kind of intrinsic uncertainty does not explain any of the other deviations, however.

10.7.4   Imperfect Monitoring—Contingent Analyzer Interference

Another quite different kind of attentional effect—interference in one analyzer contingent on activity in the other—is illustrated in Fig. 10.11. That figure is modeled most closely after Klein's (1985) suggestion, but similar suggestions were made earlier by Sorkin and Moray and their colleagues on the basis of their work in audition (Moray, Fitter, Ostry, Favreau, & Nagy, 1976; Ostry, Moray, & Marks, 1976; Pohlmann & Sorkin, 1976; Sorkin et al., 1973, 1976; or see summary on p. 194 of Wickelgren, 1979). According to explanations of this kind, the

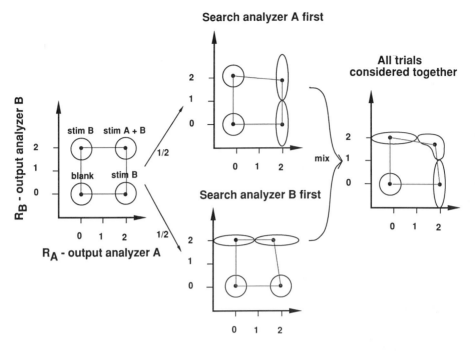

FIG. 10.11 Diagram of contingent analyzer interference.

fact that an observer monitors two analyzers does not in itself produce any deficits relative to monitoring one analyzer. But as soon as there is activity in one analyzer monitored by the observer, then there will be a deficit in the observer's response to the other analyzer. The interference seems to have been attributed to a number of quite different causes, for example, deficits in attention, changes in response bias, low-level effects on the analyzer outputs themselves.

Figure 10.11 shows a particular version of this explanation in which the observer sequentially searches both analyzers. If activity is found in one of the analyzers, the output of the other analyzer is detrimentally affected. The left panel of Fig. 10.11 shows the original analyzer output distributions. The middle panel shows the effective distributions on trials when analyzer A is searched first (top panel) and on trials when analyzer B is searched first (bottom). Consider what happens when analyzer A is searched first (top middle). On trials of the blank (lower left probability distribution) and on trials of the simple B stimulus (upper left probability distribution), there is usually very little activity in the A analyzer and hence the probability distributions for both analyzers are usually unaffected. On trials of the simple A stimulus (lower right probability distribution) or of the compound (upper right probability distribution), however, there is usually a good deal of activity in the A analyzer and hence the outputs of the B analyzer are detrimentally affected. In the figure, two kinds of detrimental effects are shown: The mean output of the B analyzer in response to stimulation is lowered, and also the variability of the B analyzer output is increased whether it is stimulated or not.

The right panel of Fig. 10.11 shows the analyzer-output distributions pooled across all trials. Notice the boomerang shape of the distribution to the compound and the subadditivity—the fact that the mean output of either analyzer to the compound is slightly less than its mean output to the appropriate component. To the extent that these two effects are found consistently in concurrent results, this kind of contingent-interference explanation becomes attractive. (Of course, one has to assume some decision rule to find the analyzer outputs from the experimental results; the direct-reports assumption is being made implicitly here.)

By itself, however, this contingent interference will not explain the positive correlation on the blank or the asymmetries. One could always throw in a little intrinsic uncertainty and interacting reports to explain those effects.

The possibility of contingent interference is one reason why the single-task control experiment would be interesting to do. In the single-task control, the subadditivity (masking) might disappear if the observer were able to selectively attend only to the relevant analyzer. (Of course, the observer might not be able to block out the stimulation on the wrong analyzer that caused the interference, in which case the subadditivity would remain.)

10.7.5   Imperfect Monitoring—Fluctuations in Confidence or Attentiveness

The observer's response might be affected by the feeling/knowledge of how fully he or she was attending to the pattern on that trial, as Klein (1985) pointed out. Consider, for example, trials of the blank stimulus. On trials when the observer was sure of full attention and yet seemed to see nothing, he or she might be willing to give a (0,0) confidence rating (very confident that neither component was present). On trials when attention seemed to have wandered, however, the observer might be less confident that it was really a blank even when he or she got the same "perception" (same set of analyzer outputs), and thus might say (1,1) or (2,2). In either case the observer would be unwilling to give unequal numbers, however, since the perception was the same for both components. This behavior would produce a positive correlation between the responses pooled over all trials of the blank stimulus. Similar behavior would produce positive correlation on trials of the compound. Over all trials of a simple stimulus, however, this kind of behavior might produce negative correlations with the observer saying, for example, (5,1) when in a state of full attentiveness but only (4,2) when unsure of attentiveness.

This suggestion appeals to me, because it accords with my intuitions as an observer in concurrent experiments. To model this behavior completely would be rather complicated, however. One might have several different analyzer-output diagrams (one giving analyzer outputs on trials when the observer was fully attending, one when his or her mind was wandering, etc.) and then the overall analyzer-output diagram (including criterion lines) would be a mixture of the ones for different states of attentiveness.

A short-cut to modeling this behavior would simply be to assume a set of nonorthogonal criterion lines reflecting the biases introduced by the above strategy (e.g., reflecting positive correlation). Klein (1985) discussed some of these. It is not yet clear to me just how many of the aberrations discussed above could be successfully explained by this approach.

10.7.6   Bringing the Factors Influencing Higher Level Processes under Experimental Control

One can argue that concurrent experiments ought not to be done at all (at least not for the study of low-level processes) if all these higher level factors are going to contaminate the results. On the other hand, one can argue (with Klein, 1985) that the same factors may contaminate the results of the other simpler paradigms but may simply be undiscoverable there because the simpler structure of the observer's responses reveals less information; one can argue that the concurrent paradigm affords a better opportunity for analyzing the influence of those factors either to learn about those higher level factors directly or to be able to discount them in order to draw conclusions about low-level processes. In either case, manipulating these higher level factors directly (in the ways fancied by cognitive psychologists, for example) instead of letting the individual idiosyncracies of laboratories or observers determine them would probably be a good idea (cf. Sperling, 1984, p. 124).

10.8   ADDING A TRANSDUCER FUNCTION

A complete multiple-analyzers model for identification would include a transducer function. This section briefly discusses two aspects of transducer functions as they affect results of identification experiments.

10.8.1   Improvement in Detection and in Identification of Value as Intensity Increases

Each panel of Fig. 10.12 shows hypothetical analyzers' outputs to two patterns (numbered 1 and 2), each at two different intensities (indicated by letters *a* and *b*). The intensities are supposed to have been chosen so that the two patterns at a given intensity level (1*a* and 2*a*, for example) are equally detectable. The distance from the origin of the pair of points at intensity *a* (respectively *b*) is 0.75 (respectively 1.5). Although the transducer function cannot be shown explicitly on figures of this kind, certain points about transducer functions can be made clear.

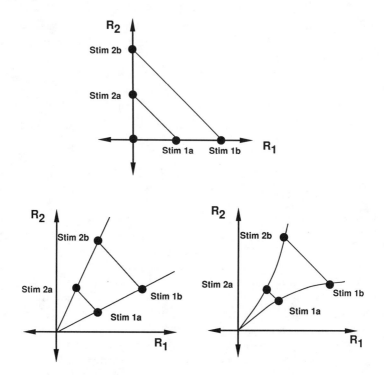

FIG. 10.12 Outputs of two analyzers to four stimuli (two values on a dimension of interest each at two contrast levels). The top panel shows far-apart values. The bottom panels show two hypothetical situations for closer together values.

Far-Apart Values. On the independent-analyzers assumptions, the vectors for two far-apart stimuli must always be perpendicular (e.g., top panel Fig. 10.12). Hence the distance between the two patterns will always increase proportionately to the distance between each pattern and the blank.

Close-Together Values. Transducer-function assumptions can change the diagram for close-together values, however, as illustrated in the two bottom panels of Fig. 10.12. In the left diagram, increasing the intensity of any simple stimulus only increases the distance from the origin without changing the angle it makes with the axes. This can only happen if the transducer functions in different analyzers are related to each other appropriately. In particular, the average response of each of the two analyzers to a simple stimulus must increase by the same factor when the intensity of the stimulus is raised. When this is the case the discriminability of two stimuli grows in proportion to their detectability.

In general, one might get something else, as in the situation shown in the right bottom diagram. Here, as intensity is changed, the output of the analyzer that is more responsive to the stimulus (the output plotted on the axis closer to the circle representing the stimulus) grows faster with intensity than does the output of the other analyzer. Hence the discriminability of the two stimuli grows faster than does their detectability.

Close-Together Spatial-Frequency Results. For a variety of pairs of spatial frequencies near the peak of the contrast sensitivity function (in the range from 3.84 to 5.50 cpd), the bottom left diagram of Fig. 10.12 is the appropriate description; that is, the discriminability of any pair of spatial frequencies (contrasts chosen so that the two were equally detectable) increased in proportion to detectability (Thomas, 1983; using single-interval rating scale and forced-choice discrimination paradigms as well as the 2×2 paradigm).

Further, the discrimination and detection performances increased in a way consistent with the following assumptions (Thomas, 1983). First, the probability distribution family was taken to be Gaussian with increasing variance. This is like the increasing-variance Gaussian families we have been using except that the parameter r may be other than 0.25 or 0.33; in fact, the estimated r values varied from 0.05 to 0.14. Second, the average analyzer output was assumed to grow in proportion to the square of intensity, with a constant of proportionality determined by the sensitivity of the analyzer to the stimulus (S_i). That is, the transducer function was assumed to be a power function with a power b equal to 2:

Assumption 92. Power Function Transducer. *The mean output of each analyzer is a power function of the stimulus intensity times sensitivity:*

$$E[R_i(c)] = (c \cdot S_i)^b$$

Some evidence suggested the exponent may be higher for higher spatial frequencies.

The precise predictions that followed from these assumptions and were confirmed by the results are briefly described in the next few paragraphs.

For the unequal-variance Gaussian model, detection and discrimination performance will depend not just on the average output of the analyzers but also on the standard deviations. Thus, if z(task, c) is performance on a certain task at intensity c measured as the z score corresponding to the point on the negative diagonal or the percent correct, then performance for patterns at intensity c is proportional to the mean at intensity c divided by the standard deviation at intensity c. (The constant of proportionality depends on the task.)

At low intensities, since average output was assumed to increase proportionately to the square of intensity and variance is changing very slowly, the z-score measure of performance is predicted to increase with the square of intensity. This positive acceleration at low intensities agrees with many other estimates of the transducer function from the growth of detectability with intensity (see Chap. 8).

At higher intensities, however, the growth in variance begins to catch up with the growth in mean, so the z-score measure of performance is predicted to slow down its rate of growth and finally level off at an asymptotic high performance. The use of difficult discrimination tasks (discriminating between two close spatial frequencies) allowed Thomas (1983) to go up to much higher intensities than possible with detection tasks (since very high proportions cannot be measured accurately without vast numbers of trials). The predicted asymptote was found.

One piece of evidence is inconsistent with the above assumptions. If the variance continues to grow up to higher intensities as postulated by Thomas (1983), the slopes of the ROC curves for suprathreshold discriminations should be shallower than 1. Some evidence suggests they are not, however (Gouled-Smith, 1986; Nachmias & Kocher, 1970).

10.8.2   Discrimination Between Near-Threshold Intensities—Facilitation or the Pedestal Effect

Identification of stimuli that are identical except for intensity has been studied using stimuli on many different sensory/perceptual dimensions. Although other identification paradigms have sometimes been used, discrimination between two stimuli of differing intensity (contrast discrimination in the context of pattern vision) is the most frequently used paradigm (see Chap. 9 for a description). Discrimination between suprathreshold intensities is beyond the scope of this book, but discrimination between near-threshold intensities is not. And one quite interesting phenomenon is found for near-threshold intensities. Look at the plot in the top of Fig. 10.13 showing typical results from intensity discrimination experiments. The just-discriminable intensity difference—call it Δc—is plotted as a function of the lesser of the two intensities (call it c, often known as the pedestal or background). As the lesser intensity is increased from zero, the just-discriminable difference actually decreases before beginning its expected increase. Thus, in the top of Fig. 10.13 for example, an intensity difference of 0.002 is sufficient to allow an observer to discriminate between intensities of 0.004 (the background marked by the arrow on the horizontal axis) and 0.006 (the background plus 0.002), but an observer cannot discriminate between intensities of 0.0 and 0.002 (since, as shown on the graph, Δc is greater than 0.002 when the background is 0.0). This phenomenon is sometimes called *facilitation* or the *pedestal effect*. Or, as is sometimes said, "contrast discrimination is better than contrast detection."

(The graph in the top of Fig. 10.13 shows idealized results, using 3-cpd gratings, from Nachmias & Sansbury, 1974. Other results can be found in that article and in Foley & Legge, 1981, for example.)

The kind of explanation often offered for this phenomenon (e.g., Nachmias & Kocher, 1970) is sketched in the bottom panel of Fig. 10.13. (The horizontal intensity axis is expanded compared with that in the top panel to show the intensities of interest here more clearly.) The vertical axis shows the expected output of an analyzer. The difference between two intensities is assumed to be just discriminable to the observer whenever the difference in the outputs of the analyzer to those two intensities is equal to some criterion difference ΔR_i (at least approximately; see discussion below). In the bottom panel of Fig. 10.13, the difference between two intensities Δc (marked by a horizontal double-headed arrow) nec-

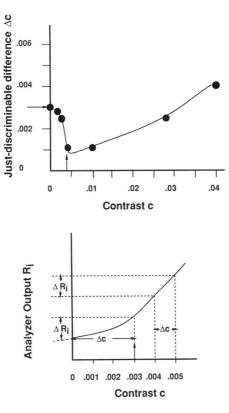

FIG. 10.13 Discrimination on the intensity dimension. The top panel shows some idealized results (after those in Nachmias & Sansbury, 1974), plotting the just noticeable difference in contrast as a function of the lower of the two contrasts. The bottom shows hypothetical analyzer output as a function of contrast. Note that the scale on the bottom panel's horizontal axis is expanded relative to the scale on the top panel's horizontal axis.

essary to get a criterion difference between the analyzer outputs ΔR_i (marked by a vertical double-headed arrow) is shown for two background intensities: 0.0 and 0.004. Notice that, as a result of the positive acceleration in the analyzer-output-versus intensity function, the intensity difference necessary to evoke a criterion ΔR_i is much larger when the pedestal is at zero intensity than when it has an intensity in the positively accelerating region (e.g., 0.004). [Neurons in monkey V1 cortex may show a positive acceleration in output versus contrast functions (Barlow, Kaushal, Hawken & Parker, 1987).]

If the analyzer's output has a constant-variance Gaussian distribution and if only one spatial frequency is investigated in a block so that the decision variable is the output of that one analyzer, the above argument applies exactly, since the just-discriminable intensity difference will correspond exactly to a given difference in analyzer output (to a given difference in d').

For other models, not only the expected output of the analyzer but also its variance matters [see, for example, the preceding discussion of Thomas (1983)]. In general, in fact, the whole shape of the distribution matters. The basic intuition seems to remain valid, however: If the expected analyzer output accelerates positively with intensity to any extent, facilitation will be predicted.

Of particular interest, the intrinsic-uncertainty model (see Chap. 8) has a positively accelerating nonlinear relationship between analyzer output and intensity (Fig. 8.2). Although the probability distribution of the analyzer output is not Gaussian and has increasing variance, it predicts Foley and Legge's (1981) near-threshold intensity discrimination results very well indeed (Pelli, 1985, 1987). See note 8 for a comparison of this prediction to explanations couched in terms of a "reduction in uncertainty."

10.9 SUMMARY

The simple detection and identification paradigm uses one-interval trials; on each trial a blank stimulus or else one of M simple stimuli is presented. As M increases, independent-analyzers models predict that the proportion-correct identification should decrease, that is, there should be uncertainty effect just as there was in detection, because the observer must monitor more different analyzers.

Uncertainty effects for identification on the spatial-frequency dimension are consistent with these predictions.

The 2×2 paradigm also measures detection and identification simultaneously but uses two-interval trials. One interval contains a blank and the other contains one of two possible nonblank patterns. If the two patterns are simple stimuli of far-apart values, a number of different independent-analyzers models predict that proportion-correct identification should equal proportion-correct detection. On the spatial-frequency dimension, this equality seems to hold whenever two spatial frequencies are a factor of 2 or more apart.

The concurrent paradigm uses one-interval trials (like simple detection and identification) but uses compound stimuli as well as their simple components (and a blank). This paradigm requires the observer to indicate separately whether each component was present in the stimulus on a given trial. This provides a richly structured set of data.

If one is willing to assume that an observer can directly report the outputs of analyzers and also can perfectly monitor all relevant analyzers, the data from a concurrent experiment are sufficient to test the assumptions of additivity, of independence, and of noninteraction. On the spatial-frequency dimension these assumptions are approximately upheld, although certain systematic deviations have been reported.

Unfortunately, these deviations can be explained not only by modifications of the additivity, independence, and noninteraction assumptions but also by modifications of the direct-report or perfect-monitoring assumptions. Untangling these two explanations will require evidence from other experiments.

The discrimination from one another of two visual patterns that are identical except for contrast (one of contrast c and the other of contrast $c + \Delta c$) is often easier than the detection of a single pattern of contrast Δc. A nonlinear transducer function may explain this effect.

10.10 APPENDIX. METHODS FOR CALCULATING PREDICTIONS

10.10.1 Calculating the Predicted Probability of Correct Identification in the Simple Detection and Identification Paradigm

The probability of correct identification in the simple detection and identification paradigm will be defined as equal to the proportion of nonblank trials on which the observer's identification response corresponds to the stimulus presented (e.g., a response of "V_2" given to stimulus V_2). In the diagram in the upper right of Fig. 10.1, it is the total number of trials falling in the diagonal squares divided by the total number of trials in the whole matrix (since blank trials are excluded from this matrix). The symbol $I(M)$ will be used for this quantity. The following paragraphs describe the calculation of $I(M)$ as predicted by independent-analyzers models for the special case of M equally detectable and far-apart simple stimuli.

Under the assumptions of the independent-analyzers model in section 10.1.2 the probability that the observer identifies a stimulus correctly equals the probability that the maximum of the M monitored analyzers' outputs comes from the one analyzer that is most sensitive to the stimulus. Call that the signal analyzer, because that particular analyzer's output has a signal probability distribution while the other M-1 monitored analyzers' outputs have noise probability distributions (because we are assuming far-apart stimuli). Thus, the probability that the observer identifies a stimulus correctly equals the probability that the maximum of M random variables (one having a signal distribution and the others having a noise distribution) comes from the one having a signal distribution. One way to calculate this quantity is the following:

1. For each possible real number λ, calculate the probability that the signal analyzer's output exceeds that criterion λ and call this probability $y(\lambda)$. In the case of continuous probability distributions:

$$y(\lambda) = \int_{\lambda}^{\infty} f_1(z \,|\, \text{signal}) \, dz$$

where $f_1(z \,|\, \text{signal})$ is the density function of a single analyzer's output to signal. (Since all analyzers are assumed to be characterized by the same probability distribution family, we will just use the subscript 1.)

2. Also calculate the probability that a nonsignal analyzer's output exceeds the criterion λ and call that probability $x(\lambda)$:

$$x(\lambda) = \int_{\lambda}^{\infty} f_1(z \mid \text{noise}) \, dz$$

where $f_1(z \mid \text{noise})$ is the density function of a single analyzer's output to the blank.

3. The joint probability that the signal analyzer's output exceeds λ while the other analyzers' outputs do not is $y(\lambda)$ times $[(1 - x(\lambda))$ raised to the $(M - 1)$ power].

4. So the joint probability that the signal analyzer's output exceeds all the other analyzers' outputs is the integral over all values of λ of the probability in 3, that is:

$$\int_{-\infty}^{+\infty} y(\lambda)[1 - x(\lambda)]^{M-1} \, d\lambda$$

It is this last quantity that is predicted to equal $I(M)$ by the independent-analyzers models.

(The above applies strictly only to the case of continuous probability density functions. For discrete probability density functions, ties need to be taken into account. For the discrete probability function of interest here—the high-threshold one—it is straightforward to algebraically calculate the probability of correct identification. It equals the probability that the correct analyzer is in the detect state plus the probability that no analyzer is in the detect state but the observer guesses correctly.)

Relationship Between Identification and Simple-Alone Detection (Area Theorem). Remember that the three detection rules—maximum output, sum of outputs, and hybrid (Assumptions 40, 61, and 63)—are equivalent for the simple-alone condition. The predicted relationship between the proportion correct identification $I(M)$, when M far-apart and equally detectable stimuli are intermixed, and the ROC curve for detection in the simple-alone condition ($M = 1$) is well known (e.g., Green & Birdsall, 1978; Green & Swets, 1974, pp. 45–51) and follows directly from the integral above. First notice that the $x(\lambda)$ and $y(\lambda)$ are also equal to the probabilities of false alarms and hits, respectively, in the simple-alone condition with criterion λ. Since both x and y are monotonic functions of λ, either one can be taken to be a function of the other. Then the independent-analyzers model of section 10.1.2 (with any continuous probability density function) predicts

$$I(M) = \int_{0}^{1} (1 - x)^{M-1} \, dy$$

This relationship is often known as the *area theorem* since, when $M = 2$, this integral is equivalent to the integral of y with respect to x, that is, to the area underneath the ROC curve in the simple-alone condition. Although true in general only for continuous probability density functions, the same relationship is easily shown to hold for the high-threshold distribution.

For the Gaussian density functions, the values of these integrals must be obtained numerically. They have been tabled for the equal-variance case (Elliot's table in Green & Swets, 1974; recently improved by Hacker & Ratcliff, 1979) and an algorithm for extending them has been suggested by J. E. K. Smith (1982).

For the exponential, the integral can be done analytically (see Yager et al., 1984).

Identification and Simple-Intermixed Detection (Starr, Metz, Lusted, and Goodenough Theorem). Another more recent theorem gives $I(M)$—proportion-correct identification in an intermixed condition—in terms of the ROC curve for detection in that same intermixed condition (Starr, Metz, Lusted, & Goodenough, 1975; presented and discussed in, for example, Green & Birdsall, 1978; Swenson & Judy, 1981). This theorem makes a prediction for the joint probability both of saying yes and of correctly identifying conditional on the presence of the signal and on a particular criterion λ. This theorem holds for any continuous probability distribution family, for the case of M equally detectable stimuli affecting independent and nonoverlapping analyzers, the maximum-output detection rule (with the same criterion in each analyzer), and the maximum-output identification rule, or equivalently for this case, the closest stimulus rule (i.e., the model of section 10.1.2).

Notice that the use of this Starr, Metz, Lusted, and Goodenough theorem to calculate the predictions from the various probability distributions above necessarily leads to the same predictions as those done directly from the simple-alone ROC curves by the area theorem above. No assumption about the distribution is needed in using either the area theorem or the Starr, Metz, Lusted, and Goodenough theorem, because the distribution is, in effect, deduced from the detection ROC curve.

10.10.2 Calculations for the 2 × 2 Paradigm and the Sum-Detection and Difference-Identification Decision Rule

Assumptions in Brief. There are M' monitored analyzers where A_i is the mean output of analyzer i to pattern A and B_i is the mean output of analyzer i to pattern B. The analyzers are probabilistically independent and noninteracting. (The assumption of one analyzer per simple stimulus is not necessary. Nor is any form of additivity assumption necessary, since compound stimuli are never presented.) The probability distribution family is constant-variance Gaussian and identical for all analyzers. The decision rule is the sum-detection and difference-identification rule.

Relation Between Identification and Detection Performances and the Angle Between the Stimulus Vectors. The following prediction, where the middle term

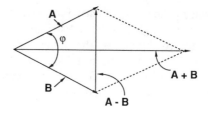

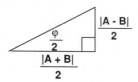

FIG. 10.14 The top panel shows two vectors, the angle between them, their sum, and their difference. The bottom panel shows the upper-left portion of the drawing in the top panel.

is appropriate only for equally detectable simple stimuli, is derived in Thomas et al., 1982:

$$
\frac{z(\text{ident})}{z(\text{detect})} = \left| \frac{\sum_{i=1}^{M'} (A_i^2 - A_i B_i)}{\sum_{i=1}^{M'} (A_i^2 + A_i B_i)} \right|^{1/2} = \frac{|\mathbf{A} - \mathbf{B}|}{|\mathbf{A} + \mathbf{B}|}
$$

Figure 10.14 (top) shows the two vectors **A** and **B** (rotated into the plane of the paper), their difference vector (the vector between the endpoints of **A** and **B**), and their sum vector (the other axis of the parallelogram having sides **A** and **B**). From the foregoing equation, it is easy to show that the $z(\text{ident})/z(\text{detect})$ ratio can also be expressed in terms of the angle φ between the vectors **A** and **B** when the two simple stimuli are equally detectable. For then the vectors **A** and **B** are of equal length, and their difference and sum vectors cross at right angles to one another (as drawn in the upper panel of Fig. 10.14), forming right triangles, one of which is shown in the lower panel with the length of its sides marked. It is clear in that triangle that the tangent of $\varphi/2$ is equal to half the length of the vector difference divided by half the length of the vector sum, thus equaling by the previous equation the $z(\text{ident})/z(\text{detect})$ ratio:

$$
\tan \frac{\varphi}{2} = \frac{|\mathbf{A} - \mathbf{B}|/2}{|\mathbf{A} + \mathbf{B}|/2} = \frac{z(\text{ident})}{z(\text{detect})}
$$

(An alternative formula using the sine of φ rather than the tangent is derived in Thomas et al., 1982.)

*10.10.3   Two Symmetric Analyzers. Relation of Angle Between Stimulus
           Vectors to Analyzer Bandwidths*

Suppose there are only two analyzers and these analyzers are symmetric in the
sense shown in the lower left panel of Fig. 9.9. Then, since φ is the angle between
the two stimulus vectors, $(90 - \varphi)/2$ is the angle between **A** (which has the coordinates A_1 and A_2) and the horizontal axis. Remember that, by the symmetry of
the two analyzers, $A_2 = E[R_2(\text{pattern A})] = B_1 = E[R_1(\text{pattern B})]$. Then

$$\tan \frac{90 - \varphi}{2} = \frac{A_2}{A_1} = \frac{B_1}{A_1}$$

But B_1/A_1 is just the sensitivity of the first analyzer to pattern B divided by its
sensitivity to pattern A. Thus, assuming that the first analyzer's peak sensitivity
is to pattern A, B_1/A_1 is the analyzer's relative sensitivity to pattern B. If one
finds the two stimuli for which the relative sensitivity is 0.5, the difference
between the values of those two stimuli on the dimension of interest is the half-
amplitude *half*-bandwidth of the relevant analyzer. One doubles that difference
to find the half-amplitude *full*-bandwidth. By the above equation for the two-
symmetric-analyzers model, a relative sensitivity of 0.5 corresponds to an angle
φ of 37 degrees. Thus, to find the half-amplitude full-bandwidth one finds the
difference in values for which φ is 37 degrees and doubles it. The experimental
results could come either from the 2 × 2 paradigm (using equation at end of
section 10.10.2) or from the concurrent paradigm (see sections 10.5.1 and
10.5.2).

To calculate the top two entries in Table 10.1 one notes that in the 2 × 2
paradigm $z(\text{ident})/z(\text{detect}) = 0.5$ when $\varphi = 53$ degrees (by equation at end of
section 10.10.2). This corresponds to $(90 - \varphi)/2 = 18.5$ degrees and, therefore,
(see above equation) to a B_1/A_1 of 0.33. The stimulus separation giving $B_1/A_1 =
0.33$ is obviously a bit greater than that giving $B_1/A_1 = 0.5$ (the latter being the
half-amplitude *half*-bandwidth, see preceding paragraph). But to know exactly
how much greater, one needs to know the function giving an analyzer's sensitivity as a function of value. If you assume the function is a symmetric triangle
peaked at the stimulus, for example, then $B_1/A_1 = 0.33$ at a stimulus separation
34% greater than that at which $B_1/A_1 = 0.50$. So the entry in Table 10.1 is 1.34
times the half-amplitude *half*-bandwidth, or 0.67 the half-amplitude *full*-band-
width. An analogous calculation produces an answer of 0.58 when sensitivity as
a function of value has the shape of one-half cycle of a cosine.

Notes

1. *Rating-scale identification paradigm.* Just as the single-interval discrimination paradigm (top Fig. 9.2) can be generalized to more than two stimuli (e.g., the upper right of
Fig. 10.1), so can the rating-scale discrimination paradigm (middle of Fig. 9.2). The results
of a rating-scale experiment using five disks of different diameter seemed consistent with
the existence of multiple spatial-frequency analyzers having bandwidths like those typi-

cally found and having labeled outputs (Thomas & Shimamura, 1974; also presented in Thomas, 1985), as do the results with gratings summarized in section 10.1.6.

2. *Entries in Table 10.1.* All the entries in Table 10.1 (described in section 10.3.4), except those for the two-symmetric-analyzers case, involved reading from graphs and thus are only accurate to about 2% W.

The 0.58 in the third row is derived as follows: Thomas and Gille (1979) reported that bandwidth estimates using a triangular function were proportional to those using the half-cosine shape within error of measurement. The half-amplitude bandwidth estimates were reported as only about 0.83 as large (Thomas & Gille, 1979, p. 657). Thus the point at which a given identification/detection ratio is reached must be 1/0.83 as large. And 0.48/0.83 = 0.58.

3. *Concurrent identification: Terminology and other studies.* The experiments described in section 10.4 are called *concurrent* experiments here following Sperling's (1984) and Sperling and Dosher's (1986) terminology, since the subject is carrying out two or more tasks concurrently; each task is the detection of a single component. Sperling contrasted these tasks to "compound" tasks (of which the simple-intermixed detection condition is an example), and pointed out that the concurrent tasks (when compared with single-task controls) allow a test of the perfect monitoring assumption (a test for possible attention limitations) that does not require quantitative comparisons depending on particular probability distributions (see discussion of single-task control in section 10.7 and note 5).

No terminology for this experiment in the sensory literature has become standard. Concurrent experiments have also been called "two-frequency, two response" (Hirsch, 1977), "simultaneous recognition of two components" (Hirsch et al., 1982), "two-response rating-paradigm" (Olzak, 1985), "double-judgment double-knob rating-scale experiments" (Klein, 1985), "multiple detection" (Wickelgren, 1967), "simultaneous n-channel detection" and "inclusive-or detection" (e.g., Sorkin, Pohlman, & Gilliom, 1973; Sorkin, Pohlmann, & Woods, 1976), and "the complete identification experiment in which the stimulus ensemble is created by factorially combining several levels of two or more physical components" (Ashby & Townsend, 1986) which is shortened to "feature-complete factorial" (Townsend, Hu, and Kadlec, 1988).

Other studies using this paradigm include Nachmias (1974); studies by Nachmias, Kramer, and Haber reported in Graham et al. (1985); Townsend, Hu, and Ashby (1981); and Townsend, Hu, and Evans (1984).

4. *More general signal strength parameter versus signal strength plots from concurrent experiments.* The constant-variance Gaussian assumption used in section 10.5.1 could be dropped, at least on the assumption of direct reports from relevant analyzers' outputs. From the confidence ratings given in answer to one question about one stimulus, points on the ROC curve can be plotted. (The number of points will be the number of categories in the rating scale minus 1.) In principle, one can find the theoretical ROC curve from a given family (e.g., the exponential) that is the best fit to these empirical points. The best-fitting theoretical ROC curve gives an estimate of the appropriate signal-strength parameter. (It is d' for Gaussians or k' for exponentials—their values will be practically identical—and can be estimated as -1 times the value at the horizontal intercept of the ROC curve plotted on normal-normal coordinates.)

In cases where only two-category rating scales are used (yes and no), there is only enough information to plot one point on the ROC curve. From that point, a signal strength parameter can always be calculated if one assumes any one-parameter family of probability distributions (e.g., making an assumption about the ratio of the signal and noise variances in a Gaussian family).

In practice the ROC curves from concurrent experiments on the spatial frequency dimension seem to be consistent with exponential or increasing-variance Gaussian families (see Fig. 7.9 and accompanying discussion). Thus, in principle, one ought to compute k' from the exponential or d' from the increasing-variance Gaussian families rather than d' from the constant-variance Gaussian family, as done in the above example. In practice, however, this nicety probably makes little difference at this point in the game.

5. *Single-task controls.* I know of no published experiments on the spatial-frequency dimension using a single-task control. (Other results for spatial frequency are given in section 10.6.) Some unpublished experiments by Nachmias are inconclusive, although they suggest that the decrement in the single-task control (if there is one) is no greater than can be compensated for by an increase in contrast of 10 or 20%. A similar conclusion could be drawn from an experiment on the spatial-position dimension (in Graham et al., 1985). When single-task controls are used with more complicated stimuli, decrements are often found. See Sperling (1984) for a review of some.

6. *Angle between simple-stimulus vectors.* To estimate the angles plotted in Fig. 10.9 and discussed in section 10.6.1, $d'-d'$ plots were made for each condition where a separate point was plotted for each stimulus from each session. A line was fit (see next paragraph) to the points for each simple stimulus. (If two contrast levels were used with the same spatial frequency, the same line was fit to points from both contrast levels.) The angle made by each fitted line with the horizontal axis was measured. The difference between the angles for the lines for the two simple values is what is plotted on the vertical axis of Fig. 10.9.

The lines that were fitted were what could be called *median spokes.* A median spoke is a line through the origin rotated until half the experimental points are on one side of the line (and close to the line) and half on the other. (Since the points always form a rather compact cluster, this is a sensible procedure. No point was more than 90 degrees from the median spoke.) When there are an even number of points so there is a range over which the median spoke could be positioned, it is taken to bisect that range.

7. *Re intrinsic-uncertainty and concurrent experiments.* Following a suggestion of Bernice Rogowitz's on examining Hirsch's (1977) and Haber's (1976) results, she and I did some sample calculations that are the basis for the comment in section 10.7.3 to which this is a note. This calculation assumed (a) that two analyzers' outputs in response to the blank stimulus have a positive correlation of about 0.2 (as do observer's responses to the blank in concurrent experiments) and (b) that all the *extra* variance in any analyzer's output as the stimulus intensity increases is independent of every other analyzer's extra variance. This extra variance is estimated from the decrease in ROC slope as detectability rises. See Fig. 7.9 and accompanying discussion. Then calculations showed that, as the detectability level of stimuli increases, the calculated correlation between analyzer outputs decreases, much like the correlation observed between observer's responses in concurrent experiments does (within the very considerable error of measurement). In particular, the calculated correlation between the two analyzers' outputs decreases to effectively zero by a d' level of between 2 and 3.

8. *Pedestal effect (facilitation) and reduction of uncertainty.* One other common verbal explanation of the pedestal effect discussed in section 10.8.2 is that it results from a "reduction in uncertainty." The observer is presumed to monitor some insensitive analyzers when there is no background (pedestal), but somehow the background is supposed (in spite of the fact that the background is at or below threshold) to reduce the observer's uncertainty so that the observer monitors only sensitive analyzers. This has always seemed slightly peculiar to me.

It is interesting to note, however, that the nonlinearity between contrast and analyzer output in the intrinsic-uncertainty model (illustrated in Fig. 8.2)—the nonlinearity that causes that model to predict the pedestal effect—could be described as the result of a reduction in uncertainty or, perhaps better, as a reduction in "effective" uncertainty. According to the intrinsic-uncertainty model, this reduction in effective uncertainty occurs as intensity is raised for the following reason: At low intensities all the microanalyzers contribute to the analyzer's output on one trial or another. As intensity becomes higher, however, the sensitive microanalyzer(s) becomes more and more likely to determine the analyzer's output on every trial, and thus the fact that insensitive microanalyzers are being monitored becomes insignificant. That is, it is not that the observer monitors fewer analyzers when a pedestal is present but that the extra analyzers that are monitored become insignificant when a pedestal is present.

VI
MULTIPLE DIMENSIONS

11
Some General Considerations

11.1 REVIEW AND PREVIEW

11.1.1 Preview of This and Next Two Chapters

Chapter 12 briefly presents conclusions from four kinds of analyzer-revealing experiments (adaptation, summation, uncertainty, and identification) done on each of the pattern-vision dimensions. A rather extensive and organized list of references comprises the second half of Chapter 12 so that the interested reader can pursue particular topics and arrive at his or her own conclusions.

Chapter 13 similarly summarizes the conclusions from parametric experiments and also includes an organized list of references.

First, however, this chapter discusses the issues that arise when more than one dimension (e.g., spatial frequency, orientation, and spatial position) are involved in a study—issues that must be considered before arriving at conclusions of the kind presented in Chapters 12 and 13. Most of the material in Chapter 11 applies to other sensory and perceptual domains as well as to pattern vision. For the reader interested primarily in pattern vision, Chapter 11 could be omitted with little loss of continuity (but with, perhaps, a loss of caution).

11.1.2 Review of Logic of Four Analyzer-Revealing Paradigms

In previous chapters we have examined in detail four kinds of analyzer-revealing near-threshold experiments: adaptation, summation, uncertainty, and identification. Although the precise assumptions used in interpreting each kind of experiment are crucial in drawing any detailed conclusions about analyzers from the experimental results, the overall logic applied to each type can be summarized as follows.

The basic form of each kind of experiment uses two simple, nonblank stimuli: (a) An adaptation experiment uses an adapt stimulus and a test stimulus. (b) A summation experiment use two simple component stimuli (as well as the compound stimulus containing both). (c) Uncertainty experiments use two simple stimuli (in intermixed and in alone conditions). (d) Identification experiments use two simple stimuli that are to be identified (discriminated) as well as detected.

Interaction Between Stimuli. If these two simple stimuli show no "interaction" in the experiment (where interaction in the experiment must be defined separately for each kind of experiment), the stimuli are presumed to affect completely separate (nonoverlapping and probabilistically independent) analyzers. If two stimuli interact, however, they are presumed to stimulate the same analyzer (s) to some extent. And, the more they interact, the more the analyzers they affect are presumed to overlap. To briefly review the meaning of interaction in each kind of experiment:

1. In adaptation experiments, interaction means threshold elevation.
2. In summation experiments, interaction means summation between components.
3. In uncertainty experiments, interaction means the *absence* of a decrement when comparing intermixed with alone conditions. (Calling such an absence interaction may seem a bit strained, but it is the proper direction.)
4. In the identification experiments, interaction is confusability (lack of discriminability) between stimuli.

Caveat. As discussed in detail in earlier chapters, the exact interpretation of any of the types of experiments is still incompletely understood. For example, the selective threshold elevation after adaptation may result from fatigue caused by the previous excitation or from inhibition among analyzers. This incomplete understanding certainly limits the conclusions that can be drawn from any of these four types of experiments. A priori, changing any of the assumptions of a model might change the conclusions drawn about any other aspect of the model. When, however, there is agreement among many results (as summarized in Chap. 12), I suspect that the general conclusions will be little affected by details of the models (except where noted).

11.1.3   Some Definitions: Experimental and Auxiliary Dimensions, Joint Experiments

Experimental Dimension. If the two simple stimuli in an experiment differ only in their value along one dimension (e.g., two gratings differing in spatial frequency), that one dimension will be called the *experimental dimension* and the experiment will be said to be an experiment on that dimension (e.g., a spatial-frequency experiment).

Not all of the 15 pattern dimensions are equally well suited to serve as experimental dimensions. See discussion in section 11.8 of special features in the interpretation of experiments on each dimension.

Joint Experiments. In principle, although infrequently in fact, the two simple stimuli used in an experiment could differ along two dimensions (e.g., in both orientation and spatial frequency). Such experiments will be said to be joint experiments on both dimensions (e.g., joint orientation and spatial-frequency experiments).

Auxiliary Dimensions. A given type of experiment along a given dimension (e.g., an adaptation experiment along the spatial frequency dimension) could be done at each of a large number of values along some other dimension (e.g., at each of a number of different temporal frequencies). For example, one might first adapt to 3 cpd and test with many spatial frequencies using gratings all drifting at 2 Hz, and then one might repeat the experiment using gratings drifting at 18 Hz.

What information might running an experiment at several values on an auxiliary dimension give? Suppose the experiments are to be taken as evidence for analyzers on the experimental dimension (spatial frequency in this example). Then running the experiment at several values on an auxiliary dimension can tell whether the analyzers along the experimental dimension (spatial frequency in this example) have the same characteristics (in particular, bandwidth) at the two values along the auxiliary dimension (2 Hz and 18 Hz in this example). One might find, for example, that the bandwidths deduced from threshold-elevation curves at one value (18 Hz) were somewhat broader than those at the other (2 Hz).

More Complicated Dependencies Still. In principle, one might find that the way in which results on the one experimental dimension (e.g., spatial frequency) depended on the value on a second, auxiliary dimension (e.g., temporal frequency) depended on the value on a third, auxiliary dimension (e.g., spatial position). Perhaps in the fovea spatial-frequency selectivity might depend on temporal frequency, as in the above example, but in the periphery there might be no such dependence on temporal frequency. Very few of these nested dependencies have been discovered or looked for or even discussed in pattern vision but, a priori, they are not only possible but even likely.

11.1.4 Problems in Interpreting Analyzer-Revealing Experiments

If experiments on a given dimension show interaction for close-together values with less and less interaction as the values become further apart, we will say there is value-selective behavior on that dimension. In general, value-selective behavior in experiments on a given dimension can be explained by postulating analyzers selectively sensitive on that dimension.

However, a number of problems arise in interpreting the results of these analyzer-revealing experiments. The first part of this chapter discusses three such problems that apply rather generally: (a) Are analyzers selective on only one dimension at a time, or are they selective along several dimensions simultaneously (section 11.2)? (b) Is there covariation between the peak sensitivities of a group of analyzers on one dimension and the peak sensitivities on another that is being hidden by the use of broad-band stimuli and suggesting misleading conclusions (section 11.3)? (c) Is an analyzer's sensitivity along one dimension (e.g., spatial frequency) the same at all values along some other dimension (e.g., orientation)? In other words, is an analyzer's joint sensitivity to two dimensions separable into two sensitivity functions for each dimension individually (section 11.4)?

Two other problems of interpretation seem more easily presented in the context of particular pattern dimensions and so are postponed until the third part of this chapter (section 11.8; Figs. 11.5 and 11.6). These are both examples of the general problem that value-selective behavior on one dimension—although it can be explained by analyzers selective on that dimension—can often also be explained by analyzers selective on some other dimension. Then the question of deciding which interpretation is better becomes important. Unfortunately, this question can be very difficult to answer, requiring at the least extensive calculations.

11.1.5   Preview of This Chapter

The first part of this chapter (sections 11.2–11.4) discusses the three general problems just mentioned. The next rather brief part of this chapter introduces parametric experiments (section 11.5) and the logic of their interpretation.

These first two parts would apply to other domains just as they do to pattern vision.

The third part of this chapter (sections 11.6–11.8) discusses the dimensions of pattern vision in particular, raising certain issues that need to be considered before the results of analyzer-revealing and parametric experiments on these dimensions can be interpreted correctly.

11.2   DOUBLY VERSUS SINGLY SELECTIVE ANALYZERS

Figure 11.1 illustrates two quite different schemes in which there are multiple analyzers along each of two dimensions. Each ellipse or circle in the figure encloses the range of values to which a single analyzer is sensitive at greater than half-peak sensitivity.

If, as in the left half of Fig. 11.1, each analyzer is sensitive to a narrow range of values along one dimension but to the full range of values along the other, the analyzers will be called *singly selective* (sometimes called *single duty*). In postulating singly selective analyzers along each of two dimensions, one is postulating that there are multiple (two, to be precise) bandwidths of analyzers along each of the two dimensions; one of the two bandwidths is very narrow and the other is as wide as the visual system's sensitivity along that dimension. Although not easy to indicate directly on the left half of Fig. 11.1, we will also assume that, where two ellipses intersect, the sensitivities of the two corresponding analyzers are equal.

If, as in the right half of Fig. 11.1, each analyzer is sensitive to narrow ranges along both dimensions, the analyzers will be called *doubly selective* (also called *double duty* in some literature).

With three or more dimensions, one could have triply selective analyzers, and so on.

Figure 11.1 also indicates by crosshatching which analyzer(s) responds to each

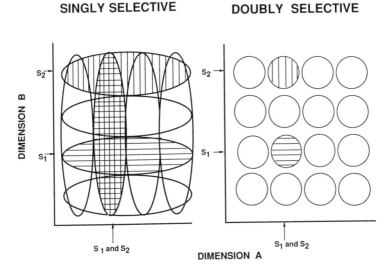

FIG. 11.1 Singly selective analyzers (left) and doubly selective analyzers (right). Values on dimensions A and B are plotted on the horizontal and vertical axes, respectively. Each ellipse or circle is a constant-sensitivity (e.g., half-peak) contour of a different analyzer. The analyzers affected by stimulus S_1 are horizontally crosshatched; those affected by S_2 are vertically crosshatched.

of two stimuli—S_1 and S_2. These stimuli have the same value on dimension A (indicated by an arrow on the horizontal axis) but different values on dimension B (indicated by arrows on the vertical axis). The horizontal crosshatching indicates analyzers sensitive to S_1 and the vertical indicates analyzers sensitive to S_2.

In earlier chapters, a simple stimulus was often represented by a V for its value on the dimension of interest. In this chapter, however, more than one dimension is of interest, so a stimulus will be represented by an S (which, unfortunately, is also the letter used for sensitivity, e.g., section 11.4).

11.2.1   A Possible Advantage of Singly Selective Analyzers

The singly selective case postulates fewer total analyzers than the doubly or more selective case (8 vs. 16 in Fig. 11.1) but still allows the identification of the stimulus along those two dimensions. The numerical advantage can be considerable when larger numbers of values on each dimension or larger numbers of dimensions are considered. Suppose, for example, one considers the case of seven values on each of five dimensions. There would need be only 35 (seven times five) singly selective analyzers, but there would be 16,807 (seven to the fifth power) multiply selective channels.

11.2.2   Conclusions to Be Drawn From Analyzer-Revealing Experiments on Each Dimension Separately

The next several subsections discuss how well each of the four kinds of analyzer-revealing experiments can distinguish between doubly and singly selective cases. We will assume throughout that analyzers are noninteracting for far-apart values. We will consider both the assumption of no pooling across analyzers (i.e., the observer's threshold is determined by the single most sensitive analyzer) and the assumption of pooling across analyzers (i.e., probability summation due to independent variability or equivalent nonlinear pooling like that in the Quick pooling formula).

The conclusions from the next several subsections are easy to summarize in one way: In general, the predictions depend quite heavily on whether there is pooling across analyzers or not, but in general summation experiments are the best experiments for distinguishing between singly and doubly selective analyzers.

Summary Figure. Figure 11.2 summarizes the conclusions from the next several subsections by showing, for each kind of analyzer-revealing experiment

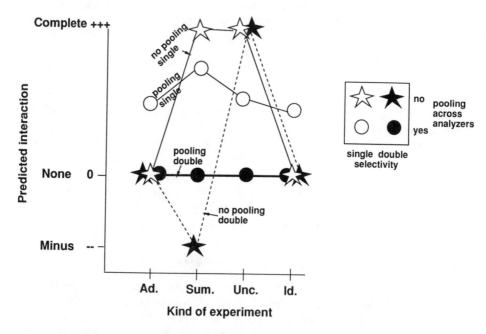

FIG. 11.2 The amount of interaction between far-apart stimuli on one dimension predicted by singly selective (open symbols) or doubly selective (closed symbols) analyzers when there is (circles) or is not (stars) pooling across analyzers (i.e., independent variability in the outputs of different analyzers). The horizontal axis shows the four kinds of analyzer-revealing experiments. The vertical axis shows amount of interaction on a rough scale described in the text.

(horizontal axis), the amount of interaction predicted to occur between two stimuli that are far apart on the experimental dimension but of the same value on the other dimension (like S_1 and S_2 in Fig. 11.1) according to various assumptions. The open and closed symbols are for the singly and doubly selective cases, respectively. The circles and stars are for the assumptions that there is and there is not, respectively, pooling across different analyzers.

The predicted interaction is shown on the vertical axis on the following ordinal scale: *Complete* interaction is the amount of interaction predicted to occur between two stimuli when only a single analyzer is involved (i.e., when both stimuli affect the same analyzer and only that analyzer); *zero* interaction is taken to be the amount predicted when two stimuli affect two nonoverlapping analyzers and there is pooling across analyzers (the case indicated by the closed circles in Fig. 11.2); *minus* interaction is interaction on the other side of zero from complete (e.g., facilitation rather than elevation in adaptation experiments).

11.2.3 Adaptation Experiments

Suppose fatigue is the mechanism of adaptation. Let S_1 be the adapting stimulus and S_2 the test stimulus where, as in Fig. 11.1, they are to be far apart on dimension B but identical on dimension A. After adaptation to S_1, only the analyzers indicated by the horizontal (with or without vertical) crosshatching in Fig. 11.1 will be less sensitive than they were before.

Consider the assumption of no pooling across analyzers first. On either the singly or doubly selective scheme, the observer's thresholds for S_2 will be unaffected. For, even with singly selective analyzers, there is an unadapted analyzer [indicated by vertical (without horizontal) crosshatching in Fig. 11.1] able to detect S_2 after adaptation. (Remember that the sensitivity of two analyzers where they intersect is assumed to be identical in the singly selective case.) Hence on the assumption of no pooling across analyzers, these adaptation experiments cannot distinguish between singly selective and doubly selective schemes at all. (The open and filled stars on the left edge of Fig. 11.2 both indicate no interaction.)

If, however, there is pooling across analyzers, adaptation experiments can distinguish between the singly selective and doubly selective cases. (The open circle is somewhat above the filled circle on the left edge of Fig. 11.2.) The doubly selective scheme predicts no threshold elevation for S_2 after adaptation to S_1. The singly selective scheme predicts a small amount of threshold elevation, since now one of the two analyzers that were originally equally sensitive to S_2 is much less sensitive than it used to be.

11.2.4 Summation Experiments

Summation experiments' ability to distinguish between the singly selective and doubly selective schemes was briefly mentioned in Chapter 5.

The discussion here is predicated on the assumption that individual analyzers show additivity to a compound (complete, as in Assumption 27—or at least substantial). There are some dimensions on which you do not expect much additivity (as will be discussed in points 3 and 4 at the beginning of section 11.8) and for which, therefore, this discussion is less relevant.

What happens if there is pooling across analyzers (probability summation)? The doubly selective case predicts what is called zero interaction in Fig. 11.2, that is, the compound should be slightly more detectable than the components by the amount expected by pooling across two nonoverlapping, probabilistically independent analyzers. The singly selective scheme will predict even more summation than this, however. For, in the singly selective scheme, not only is there pooling across two separate analyzers (indicated by the two horizontally elongated ellipses in Fig. 11.1 left) but the third singly selective analyzer (indicated by the vertically elongated ellipse in Fig. 11.1 left) is actually more sensitive to the compound than it is to either component.

Suppose now that there is no pooling across analyzers (i.e., the observer's threshold equals the threshold of the most sensitive analyzer). In the doubly selective case, the compound would be no more detectable than the most detectable component because no analyzer is sensitive to both components; that is, there would be even less summation than in the pooling-across-analyzers case (so the closed star in Fig. 11.2 for summation experiments is at minus interaction). In the singly selective case, however, the compound would be considerably more detectable than either component because the analyzer indicated by the vertically oriented and crosshatched ellipse in the left of Fig. 11.1 would be much more sensitive to the compound than to either component (and is just as sensitive to each component as is the analyzer indicated by the appropriate horizontally oriented ellipse); hence this one analyzer's thresholds would equal the observer's threshold and there would be complete summation.

11.2.5   Uncertainty Experiments

If one assumes that uncertainty effects in pattern vision are due to independent variability (as in the models of Chap. 7) and then assumes there is no pooling across analyzers (thereby assuming there is no independent variability), then no uncertainty effects are predicted by either the singly or doubly selective case. That is, complete interaction is predicted (the same result as if both stimuli affected only a single analyzer), as shown by the stars for uncertainty experiments in Fig. 11.2.

If, however, there is independent variability (and hence pooling across analyzers), then being forced to monitor for two stimuli on a given dimension (as in an intermixed condition) will produce a deficit compared with monitoring for only one (as in an alone condition) for either doubly selective or singly selective schemes. The doubly selective case will predict a somewhat bigger deficit, however (that is, will predict less interaction), than the singly selective case, if additional reasonable assumptions are made. For, in the doubly selective scheme, the observer might reasonably be assumed to be monitoring two analyzers in the intermixed condition compared with only one in the alone condition. But in the singly selective scheme, the observer might be monitoring three analyzers in the intermixed condition compared with two in the alone condition.

11.2.6 Identification Experiments

If analyzers are labeled according to their sensitivities but there is no independent variability in their outputs (and hence no pooling across analyzers), the observers could identify whether the stimulus was S_1 or S_2 whenever the stimulus was detected (whenever it was above detection threshold criterion) in either the singly selective scheme (where both singly selective analyzers would be responding since their sensitivities are assumed equal) or in the doubly selective scheme (where the label on the one doubly selective analyzer would be sufficient to identify the stimulus).

If there is independent variability in the output of the two analyzers, the two stimuli S_1 and S_2 should be somewhat more confusable (at detection threshold) in the singly selective scheme than in the doubly selective scheme. For in the singly selective scheme, the stimulus will sometimes be detected by the analyzer corresponding to the vertically oriented ellipse in Fig. 11.1, and that analyzer responds to both S_1 and S_2 and thus cannot distinguish between them.

Concurrent identification experiments are discussed in section 11.2.7.

11.2.7 Why Are Summation Experiments Best at Distinguishing Between Singly and Doubly Selective Analyzers?

As Fig. 11.2 summarizes, if there is no pooling across analyzers, only summation experiments can distinguish between the doubly and singly selective schemes at all (closed vs. open stars). If there is pooling across analyzers, all four can distinguish between the two schemes (closed vs. open circles), but the summation experiments will probably make the distinction more easily (given the properties of the independent variability deducible from spatial-frequency experiments, for example). Why are summation experiments better for this job? Notice that the crucial difference between the singly and doubly selective schemes is the singly selective analyzer sensitive to both S_1 and S_2 (the vertically oriented ellipse in the left of Fig. 11.1). Only in summation experiments is this analyzer given a chance to dominate the other two by the use of a compound that raises its sensitivity relative to that of the other two analyzers (assuming substantial additivity to a compound).

Compound stimuli are also used in concurrent experiments, and these experiments also could distinguish well between singly and doubly selective analyzers on any of a number of reasonable assumptions relating analyzers' outputs to observers' responses.

11.2.8   Joint Experiments

In general, experiments done jointly on two dimensions give information about the sensitivity of an individual analyzer along both dimensions. Put this way, it might seem as if joint experiments could be used to answer the singly selective versus doubly selective question above. But the singly selective versus doubly selective cases have analyzer sensitivities that differ only along lines parallel to the axes in Fig. 11.1, and so the interesting joint experiments to differentiate these two cases are the same as experiments done on one dimension at a time.

11.2.9   Caution About Suprathreshold Results

Double rather than single selectivity is suggested by most near-threshold experiments in pattern vision (see Chap. 12). This result should not be extrapolated casually to suprathreshold tasks, however. For one thing, singly selective analyzers that are less sensitive than the doubly selective ones might show up in suprathreshold effects. More important, however, the observer's responses in suprathreshold tasks may almost always be strongly affected by higher level stages of processing than the low-level analyzers. The outputs of these higher level stages may well depend on quite complicated interrelationships among different low-level analyzers' outputs; thus the properties of individual low-level analyzers may not show up clearly in suprathreshold results.

For example, although near-threshold psychophysical results (and physiological results from neurons in V1 and V2) strongly suggest double selectivity for orientation and spatial frequency, the following two suprathreshold results have been reported (both are kinds of results that have frequently been interpreted as showing single selectivity): (a) Suprathreshold discriminations between values on the spatial-frequency dimension are not any better when both stimuli have the same orientation than when they have perpendicular orientations (Burbeck & Regan, 1983). (b) Observers are not able immediately to segregate different regions containing single sinusoidal patches where the different regions are defined by conjunctions of spatial frequency and orientation (Walters, Biederman, & Weisstein, 1983). For the second result, a counter-argument and demonstration have been published suggesting that low level analyzers are doubly selective for spatial frequency and orientation (Sagi 1988).

11.3   COVARIATIONS HIDDEN BY BROAD-BAND STIMULI ON A NONEXPERIMENTAL DIMENSION

11.3.1   Covariations Between Analyzers' Sensitivities Along Two Dimensions

The axes of Fig. 11.3 again give values of the stimuli along two dimensions (A and B), and each circle or ellipse encloses the values to which an analyzer has

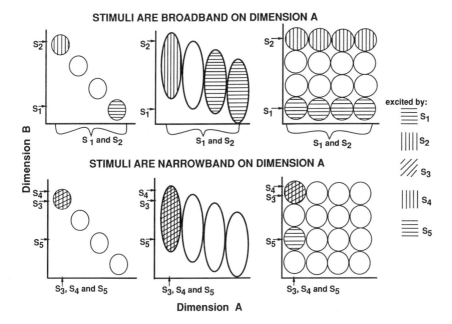

FIG. 11.3 Three patterns of joint selectivity by multiple analyzers (left, middle, and right). Stimuli are narrow band along the experimental dimension B. In the top row, the stimuli are broad band along the nonexperimental dimension A. In the bottom row, the stimuli are narrow band along this dimension. The values of the stimuli are indicated along the axes. Crosshatching indicates which analyzers responded to each stimuli (see inset).

greater than half-peak sensitivity. The left and middle panels in this figure each illustrate a particular kind of covariation (a trade-off) between the values on dimensions A and B to which the analyzers are sensitive: The values to which a given analyzer is sensitive on one dimension tend to be high when the values on the other dimension are low.

11.3.2   The Terminological Problem Presented by Covariation

When there are trade-offs and other covariations, the following terminological problem arises: Should one describe these situations as having multiple analyzers on each dimension? Let's take dimension B. Now, if you consider all analyzers, no matter what their sensitivities along dimension A, in the left or middle sections of Fig. 11.3 you would say, "Yes, there are multiple B analyzers, that is, there are several analyzers selectively sensitive to different ranges of values on dimension B." But if you consider only a single value on dimension A, you would say, "No, there are not multiple B analyzers, that is, there is only a single analyzer on dimension B at any given A value."

In the top left panel of Fig. 11.3, the situations for the A and B dimensions are identical. (The nonuniform single spatial-frequency analyzer model of Chap. 4 is a model of this sort, where dimensions A and B are spatial frequency and spatial position, respectively.) And, in my opinion at least, whether you wish to say that there are multiple analyzers on each dimension or not is entirely a matter of convention.

In the top middle panel of Fig. 11.3, however, there are multiple analyzers on the A dimension at many (although not all) values of the B dimension, while there are never multiple analyzers on the B dimension at any single value on the A dimension. So it seems more natural to describe the top middle panel of Fig. 11.3 as showing multiple analyzers on dimension A but not dimension B with some trade-off between peak value on the A dimension and the range of values on the B dimension. The joint selectivity of temporal frequency (as dimension B) and spatial frequency (as dimension A) has sometimes been suggested as like that in the middle panels of Fig. 11.3.

The right panel shows a clear-cut situation where there are multiple analyzers on each dimension at every value on the other (doubly selective analyzers in particular), and I think everyone would say in this case that there are multiple analyzers on both dimensions.

11.3.3   The Problems Introduced by Broad-Band Stimuli on the Nonexperimental Dimension

Whatever one decides about the terminological question, one might want to know which (if any) of the situations in Fig. 11.3 correctly describes joint selectivity on a given two dimensions. The top row in Fig. 11.3 illustrates what happens with stimuli S_1 and S_2 that are far apart and narrow band on the experimental dimension (B) but broad band on the nonexperimental dimension (A). In each situation, nonoverlapping analyzers respond to the two stimuli, and therefore the experiment should show the noninteraction (e.g., lack of threshold elevation in an adaptation experiment) typical of separate analyzers. Thus, in spite of frequent explicit or implicit attempts to do so, one cannot distinguish among the three situations in the top row of Fig. 11.3 using stimuli broad band on dimension A.

Two places where confusion of this kind has arisen in the pattern-vision literature are (a) temporal-frequency experiments (section 12.3) using spatially aperiodic stimuli that are broad band on the spatial-frequency dimension, and (b) spatial-frequency experiments using full-field gratings that are thus broad band on the spatial-position dimension (section 4.5).

11.3.4   Using Stimuli That Are Narrow Band on the Nonexperimental Dimension

A way to distinguish among these three situations is to use stimuli that are narrow band on the nonexperimental dimension A as well as on the experimental dimension B (e.g., S_3, S_4, and S_5 in the bottom row of Fig. 11.3). In the trade-off situations of the left and middle, both stimuli (e.g., S_3 and S_4) will now affect the same analyzer if they affect the visual system at all (which S_5 would not in the left situation) and will interact (e.g., threshold elevation after adaptation). In the clear-cut multiple-mechanism case of the right bottom panel, however, once the values are far-enough apart (e.g., S_3 and S_5), the experiment should show noninteraction, although the visual system is still responding to both stimuli.

11.4 SEPARABILITY

Figure 11.4 illustrates a question not about the interrelationships among different analyzers but about the properties of a single analyzer. One can ask whether the sensitivity of a single analyzer as a function of value on one dimension is independent (in a sense to be made precise) of the value on the other dimension. The sense of independence meant here is usually described by the word *separable* and is the following: The sensitivity to both dimensions can be expressed as the product of sensitivities to each dimension separately. Algebraically, letting $S(V_A, V_B)$ be the sensitivity of the analyzer to a stimulus having values V_A and V_B on dimensions A and B, respectively, then the function S is separable if and only if there exist two other functions $S_A(V)$ and $S_B(V)$ such that

$$S(V_A, V_B) = S_A(V_A) \times S_B(V_B)$$

When an analyzer's sensitivity along two dimensions is separable in this sense, its relative sensitivity to two values on one dimension (the ratio of its sensitiv-

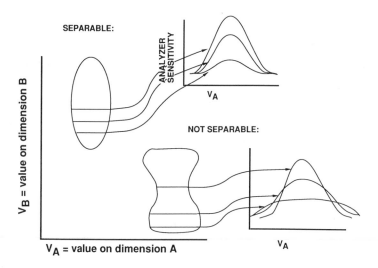

FIG. 11.4 Constant-sensitivity contours of two analyzers are plotted in the graph in the left. The little graphs to the right show the sensitivity of each analyzer as a function of value on dimension A, where different curves are for different values on dimension B.

ities to those two values) will be independent of value on the other dimension. The upper analyzer in Fig. 11.4 is separable, as illustrated by the inset on the upper right showing its sensitivity as a function of value on dimension A for each of 3 fixed values on dimension B. (If sensitivity had been plotted on a logarithmic scale in that inset, the three curves would have been vertical translations of one another.)

The lower analyzer in Fig. 11.4 is nonseparable. It is sensitive to a much wider range of values on dimension A at certain values on dimension B than at others. (There are many other ways for a function to be nonseparable, of course.)

To discover whether individual analyzers' sensitivity functions are separable on a given pair of dimensions requires doing rather extensive and very precise joint experiments on those two dimensions. Even then, particularly in the presence of other analyzers, it may be difficult to get precise enough measurements to decide the question.

11.5   PARAMETRIC CONTRAST SENSITIVITY EXPERIMENTS

Many of the experiments done using near-threshold stimuli fall into a fifth class, which we will call *parametric contrast sensitivity functions* or simply *parametric* experiments. These are essentially different from all four analyzer-revealing types of experiment in that they provide little if any evidence about whether there are multiple analyzers on a dimension. They provide other useful information, however, as discussed here.

11.5.1   The Experiments

In parametric experiments, the observer's detection performance (usually threshold intensity—contrast threshold in the case of pattern vision—or its reciprocal, sensitivity) is measured for simple stimuli as a function of value along some dimension of interest.

Consider an experiment in which contrast sensitivity is measured for sinusoidal patches at a number of spatial frequencies and temporal frequencies (keeping spatial position, spatial extent, mean luminance, etc., constant). The results of this experiment can be equally well plotted as a function of spatial frequency with a different curve for each temporal frequency, or vice versa. (Such plots are shown in Fig. 13.6.) The logical roles of spatial frequency and temporal frequency are equivalent. For comparison, consider a spatial-frequency adaptation experiment done at a number of temporal frequencies. There the roles of the two dimensions cannot be reversed.

Primary and Secondary Dimensions. Of course, investigators have often been primarily interested in one dimension (which will be called primary) and have thus studied many values along it while studying only a few values along another dimension (which will be called secondary). This distinction is, however, of quite a different sort than that for experimental versus auxiliary dimensions in analyzer-revealing experiments.

11.5.2 Interpretation of Parametric Experiments

If there is only a single analyzer on a given dimension, the parametric contrast sensitivity function on that dimension is approximately equal to the one analyzer's sensitivity function. If there are multiple analyzers on a given dimension, the parametric contrast sensitivity function on that dimension is approximately the upper envelope of the analyzers' sensitivity functions. (It would be precisely the envelope if the observer's sensitivity were exactly equal to the most sensitive analyzer's sensitivity.) For example, see Fig. 12.1, where the solid points approximate the upper envelope of the three analyzer curves.

Thus parametric experiments give useful information about the peak sensitivities of different analyzers (on dimensions where there are multiple analyzers) or about the sensitivity function of a single analyzer (on dimensions where there is only a single analyzer).

The exact relationship between the measured parametric contrast sensitivity function and the theoretical sensitivity functions of analyzers depends on other assumptions. For example, it will depend on whether there is independent variability and/or interanalyzer interaction (e.g., inhibition). Further, it will depend to some extent on all analyzers in the full model (particularly in situations like those shown in Figs. 11.3, 11.5, and 11.6).

As discussed in the next subsection, parametric experiments on some dimensions can be viewed as parts of summation experiments on other dimensions (and analyzed accordingly to give other types of information).

11.5.3 Parametric Experiments on Bandwidth-Type Dimensions Are Closely Related to Summation Experiments

Consider a parametric experiment on the spatial-extent dimension, an experiment that measures the visibility of grating patches containing different numbers of cycles all centered at the same position (e.g., Fig. 5.7). Each such patch is a compound stimulus on the spatial-position dimension; the simple components are small patches at different spatial positions. Thus this parametric experiment on the spatial-extent dimension is part of a summation experiment on the spatial-position dimension: In particular, it is the part measuring the sensitivity to compounds. It lacks, however, the measurements of sensitivity for the simple components (which are small patches at many different positions in this example).

The spatial extent of a patch tells how broad the patch is on the spatial-position dimension; in other words, it tells the bandwidth of the patch on the spatial-position dimension. (It also tells the bandwidth of the patch on the spatial-frequency dimension, but that is not relevant here.)

In general, when the value of a stimulus on one dimension can be viewed as the bandwidth of the stimulus on a second dimension, a parametric experiment on the first dimension measures the sensitivity for compound stimuli on the second dimension; such a parametric experiment is, therefore, a subpart of a summation experiment on the second dimension. Explaining the results of parametric experiments on bandwidth-type dimensions is, therefore, a matter of explaining summation experiments on the relevant dimensions. See, for example, the explanation of the growth of sensitivity with spatial extent in terms of summation over spatial positions (Chaps. 5 and 6).

11.5.4   The Subdivision, or "What Travels Together Belongs Together" Argument

Since the parametric contrast sensitivity functions on a single dimension can just as easily be a single analyzer's function as the envelope of multiple analyzers' sensitivity functions, results from parametric experiments do not bear very strongly on the question of whether there are multiple analyzers or not.

From some kinds of parametric results, however—those showing sensitivity while values are varied on at least two dimensions—people do occasionally argue for the existence of multiple analyzers. The argument goes as follows.

Consider measurements of sensitivity on one dimension of interest (e.g., temporal frequency) while values on another dimension or dimensions (e.g., spatial position) are being changed. Suppose the measurements have the following property that I will call the subdivision property:

The Subdivision Property. The first dimension can be subdivided into a number of ranges, such that whenever the value of the stimulus on the other dimension(s) is changed, (a) sensitivities at all values within each range on the first dimension change in the same way but (b) sensitivities at values in different ranges on the first dimension sometimes change in different ways.

For example, sensitivities to a range of high temporal frequencies might stay relatively constant with changes in spatial position while sensitivities to a range of low temporal frequencies might decrease with eccentricity (e.g., Tyler & Silverman, 1983). When the spatial extent of the patches is increased with eccentricity, however (in a way consistent with some version of the size-scaling model described in Chap. 13), sensitivities to the high temporal frequencies might increase with eccentricity while sensitivities to the low temporal frequencies stay relatively constant (Tyler & Silverman, 1983; Tyler 1985, 1987). In this example, you can divide the temporal-frequency dimension into two ranges (called low and high here) such that values within each temporal-frequency range "travel together" (change the same way) with changes in spatial position and spatial extent while values in different ranges do not. Tyler and Silverman 1983 concluded that high and low temporal frequency mechanisms have "separate neural substrates with different scaling characteristics across retinal eccentricity." Clearly a model in which there are two temporal-frequency analyzers (one sensitive to low temporal frequencies and the other to high) at each spatial frequency and spatial position is consistent with these experimental results. More generally, multiple-analyzers models are always consistent with results exhibiting the subdivision property.

But to conclude strongly in favor of a multiple-analyzers model, one needs to argue against a single-analyzer model. That is, the following question needs to be answered negatively, "Is there any single temporal-frequency analyzer model consistent with the changes produced by spatial position and spatial extent?" In fact, the answer depends first on what is meant by a single temporal-frequency analyzer. In particular, what about a trade-off situation like that in the middle of Fig. 11.3, where dimension B is temporal frequency and dimension A is some other dimension (spatial frequency is useful for our current purpose, because this study used stimuli that were broad band on the spatial-frequency dimension)? If we say there is only a single temporal-frequency analyzer in that trade-off situation, then it is trivial to explain the above results with only a single temporal-frequency analyzer. One simply assumes that the temporal-weighting functions associated with different spatial frequency mechanisms change differently with eccentricity (e.g., the ones associated with low spatial frequencies might be the ones sensitive to high temporal frequencies and might change differently with eccentricity than do the temporal weighting functions associated with high spatial frequencies and low temporal frequencies). Thus, on this interpretation of trade-off situations, a single temporal-frequency analyzer (meaning a single one at each spatial frequency) explains the results easily.

Suppose, on the other hand, all trade-off situations like that in Fig. 11.3 middle column are said to demonstrate multiple (rather than a single) temporal-frequency analyzers [as many people—perhaps Tyler and Silverman (1983) among them—would be happy to say]. Is there still something called a single temporal-frequency analyzer model that will explain the results described above? Yes, but then the single analyzer's temporal-frequency sensitivity function must change with value on the spatial-position dimension as the observer's measured sensitivity does. Although logically possible for a single analyzer, such behavior seems quite peculiar and coincidental because of the subdivision property exhibited by the data.

11.5.5 Using a Parametric Sensitivity Function as a Window of Visibility

According to a very broad class of models, the parametric contrast sensitivity functions on various dimensions are useful—regardless of whether they are the approximate envelopes of multiple analyzers or the sensitivity functions of single analyzers—as *windows of visibility* in the following sense (e.g., Watson, Ahumada, & Farrell, 1986). Not only is a single stimulus that lies outside the "window" invisible (that's how the window is defined) but the following property also holds: If the difference between two stimuli (taken literally as the point-by-point difference between the two spatiotemporal luminance profiles) is a stimulus that lies outside the window of visibility, the original two stimuli should be completely equivalent to the observer. An example of an application of this reasoning can be found in the successful prediction of which stroboscopic stimuli should seem identical to smoothly moving stimuli (Watson et al., 1986). There are certainly models, although not perhaps plausible ones, that would not make this prediction.

11.6   HOW VISUAL PATTERN ANALYZERS MIGHT EXIST ALONG 17 DIMENSIONS

The 15 dimensions necessary to specify a sinusoidal-patch visual pattern (see Figs. 2.7, 2.8, and 2.9) are also dimensions along which visual analyzers (e.g., single neurons) are selectively sensitive. They are, therefore, dimensions along which multiple analyzers having different sensitivities might exist. In the next few subsections we discuss how such multiple analyzers on each of these 15 dimensions could be constructed, and then we add two more dimensions. This is a preparation for discussions of the difficulties in interpreting experiments on these dimensions (see section 11.8) and for presentation of conclusions about analyzers on these dimensions (Chaps. 12 and 13).

11.6.1   *Spatial Dimensions, Temporal Frequency, Temporal Extent, and Temporal Phase*

We will first consider all the seven spatial dimensions of Fig. 2.7 and three of the temporal ones in Fig. 2.8 (temporal frequency, temporal extent, and temporal phase). To obtain selective analyzers on these 10 dimensions, one need only consider hypothetical mechanisms (e.g., neurons) that are linear systems. Then the drawings in Figs. 2.7 and 2.8 can be reinterpreted as representations of the mechanisms' spatial or temporal weighting functions. (Note that the temporal weighting function cannot literally be a Gabor function as in Fig. 2.8, for that would require going back an infinite amount of time. But something similar to the central part of Gabor functions would do nicely.)

The change shown between each pair of weighting functions in Figs. 2.7 and 2.8 is the change necessary to produce mechanisms differing in sensitivity along the corresponding dimension; in other words, it is the change necessary to produce multiple analyzers (in particular, mechanisms) on that dimension.

It might be worthwhile to mention that, although it is possible to get selectivity along these dimensions with linear systems, one could easily find nonlinear analyzers sensitive along those same dimensions as well.

11.6.2   *Different Shapes of Sensitivity-Versus-Value Functions*

Although changes in the spatiotemporal weighting function will produce selectivity along the 10 dimensions mentioned in the preceding subsection, the kind of selectivity produced is not always the same. More precisely, the shape of the curve giving sensitivity as a function of value on a dimension will be qualitatively different for different ones of those 10 dimensions.

Peaked Functions. The functions giving sensitivity at each value on a dimension for individual mechanisms will not always be highest at a middle value on a dimension and go to zero for lower or higher values. For example, for the spatial- or temporal-frequency dimensions the sensitivity of individual mechanisms will be highest at some middle value and go to zero for high enough values, but the sensitivity will only go to zero at very low frequencies if the excitation and inhibition in the weighting functions exactly cancel each other out. Unless there is absolutely no inhibition, however, the sensitivity functions on these two dimensions will always have a single peak and decrease on either side. The sensitivity function on the orientation dimension will be peaked also.

Multiphasic. Sensitivity of a single mechanism as a function of spatial position (which function is just the spatial weighting function itself, as shown in Fig. 2.7) will generally contain both peaks and troughs; when useful, we will refer to such a sensitivity function not only as peaked but also as *multiphasic.*

For mechanisms that are linear systems, sensitivity as a function of spatial or temporal phase is even more strongly multiphasic than sensitivity as a function of spatial position. In particular, as the phase of a sinusoidal grating patch (the phase of the sine wave with respect to the window) changes away from that phase that most stimulates the mechanism, the response of the mechanism first decreases through zero to a negative response, then increases again until it is as large as initially (at a phase shift of 360 degrees). In other words, sensitivity as a function of spatial or temporal phase is periodic.

Monotonic. For linear mechanisms having a windowed-sinusoid type of spatial weighting function, the function relating sensitivity to spatial (or temporal) extent is of a still different form: Sensitivity first increases quite dramatically as spatial (or temporal) extent increases from zero and then sensitivity levels off and remains at least approximately constant for all larger spatial extents. This type of sensitivity function will be called *monotonic.*

11.6.3 *Temporal Position*

The temporal position dimension (one of the temporal dimensions in Fig. 2.8) requires slightly more discussion. To explain selectivity on this dimension, one need not postulate literally separate mechanisms on this dimension, which in terms of the possible physiological substrate would mean separate neurons, each one responding at a single moment in time. One ordinarily makes the perfectly reasonable assumption that a single mechanism (neuron) gives different outputs at different moments in time. Selectivity along the temporal-position dimension, as demonstrated in various kinds of experiments (e.g., summation experiments), is presumed to be based on these different outputs. Then the little drawings for temporal position in Fig. 2.8 represent the temporal weighting functions for the response of a mechanism at different moments in time. For simplicity in terminology, we will sometimes call the output of a single mechanism at a single point in time an *element* of the overall multiple-mechanism model (section 1.8).

11.6.4   Direction of Motion

Imagine a drifting grating that is being viewed through a stationary aperture or window. For concreteness' sake, suppose it has vertical bars. From the observer's point of view, this grating will either appear stationary or appear to be drifting rightward or leftward. It never appears to be drifting diagonally up and to the right, for example. Why not? Because a grating that is drifting diagonally up and to the right behind the window is exactly equivalent (produces an identical pattern of light on the retina) to a grating that is drifting straight right behind the window at a somewhat slower velocity (slower by the square root of 2). This exact physical equivalence dictates that the two stimuli must look identical to the observer; that they happen to both look as if they were drifting right is a perceptual fact.

This exact equivalence means that both for stimuli having a windowed-sinusoid type of spatiotemporal luminance profile (what we have been calling grating-patch stimuli) and for linear mechanisms described by a windowed-sinusoid type of spatiotemporal weighting functions, there are really only two distinct values on the direction-of-motion dimension (the last temporal dimension shown in Fig. 2.8). These two values are the two directions perpendicular to the bars of the stimuli or to the elongated flanks of the weighting function.

The Aperture Problem or Direction Ambiguity. An implication of this fact is the following: An individual mechanism can only know one small piece of information about which direction an oriented extended stimulus (i.e., a stimulus having an edge that is longer than the receptive field of the stimulus) is actually moving; it can only know whether it is moving "rightward" or "leftward" with respect to the axis of the field. In this guise, this fact is sometimes known as the *aperture problem.* See discussions in, for example, Adelson and Movshon (1982), Marr (1982), Marr and Ullman (1981), and Watson and Ahumada (1985).

Linear Versus Nonlinear Direction-of-Motion Analyzers. There are linear systems that are selective for the direction of motion of drifting gratings, that is, that respond to one direction but not the opposite (e.g., Watson & Ahumada, 1985). But it is more typical for models of directionally selective mechanisms (neurons) to postulate nonlinear mechanisms. See review by Nakayama (1985) for example.

11.6.5   Contrast, Mean Luminance, and Eye of Origin

Mechanisms (analyzers) can also be selective along the three miscellaneous dimensions of Fig. 2.9.

Contrast. Some selectivity along the contrast dimension can be obtained using mechanisms that are linear systems. Suppose each mechanism is a linear system, but different ones have different constants of proportionality between contrast and output. These mechanisms would show some selectivity in the sense that different mechanisms would have different outputs to the same contrast. But note that each mechanism's output would be proportional to contrast, and the sensitivity function would be strictly monotonic with no leveling off.

With nonlinear analyzers, one could get more dramatic selectivity along the contrast dimension. Let's mention two possible types. (a) Analyzers that respond to patterns within some range of contrasts and not at all to contrasts below or above that range, that is, analyzers with peaked sensitivity functions. (b) Analyzers that each produce zero output to a range of low contrasts, increasingly larger outputs throughout a middle range of contrasts (the location of which changes from analyzer to analyzer), and a constant maximal output to all still-higher contrasts, that is, analyzers with monotonic sensitivity functions that level off (saturate) at high contrasts.

Mean Luminance. Analyzers (e.g., single neurons) sensitive to different ranges of mean luminance—analogous to any of the three types described above on the contrast dimension—might certainly exist as well. Indeed, if some neurons were driven only by rods and some by cones, they would be such analyzers.

Eye. To obtain selectivity on the eye or *eye-of-origin* dimension—a dimension with just two values (right and left)—is easy with linear or nonlinear mechanisms. One just assumes that some mechanisms are sensitive to stimuli in one eye, and others are sensitive to stimuli in the other eye.

11.6.6 Two More Dimensions: Degree of Monocularity and Degree of Direction Selectivity

There are many further ways in which analyzers at early levels of pattern vision could differ one from another, in other words, many other dimensions on which multiple analyzers might exist. The only two we will consider to any extent in this book are closely related to 2 of the 15 dimensions we have already looked at, being measures of bandwidth on those two dimensions.

Degree of Monocularity. One will be called the *degree of monocularity.* Does a mechanism respond only to one eye (complete monocularity), does it respond much more to one eye than to the other (considerable monocularity), or does it respond equally to both eyes (zero monocularity)?

Notice that a value on this new dimension (degree of monocularity) is a measure of bandwidth on the eye-of-origin dimension. If an analyzer is very narrow band, it responds only to one eye and thus has complete monocularity. If it is maximally broad band, it responds equally to both eyes and has zero monocularity.

We could combine this continuously valued degree-of-monocularity dimension with the "eye dimension" (which has only two values, left and right). Then we could have a new bipolar *eye-dominance* dimension that goes from only to the right eye through to both eyes equally to only to the left eye. This combined eye-dominance dimension is the one Hubel and Weisel described cortical neurons in terms of, for example. One can apply the new, single, eye-dominance dimension to stimuli also by allowing sinusoidal patches that stimulated both eyes to occupy middle places on the eye-dominance dimension according to the relative contrasts in the two eyes.

Whether it is more convenient to use two dimensions (a two-valued eye dimension and a continuously valued unipolar degree-of-mononocularity dimension) or one continuously valued bipolar dimension (left through both to right) depends on the particular discussion under way.

We opt here for the two-dimension approach, since the combined one-dimension approach leads to difficulties in exposition later on, not only for the eye case but for the analogous direction-of-motion case we discuss next.

Degree of Direction Selectivity. The second new dimension is *degree of direction selectivity:* Does an (orientation-selective) mechanism respond only to one of the two possible directions (complete direction selectivity), does it respond a good deal more to one than the other (considerable direction selectivity), or does it respond to both equally (zero direction selectivity)? This degree-of-direction-selectivity dimension relates to the two-valued direction-of-motion dimension precisely the way that degree-of-monocularity related to the two-valued eye dimension. It is a measure of bandwidth on the two-valued direction-of-motion dimension.

Remember that the bandwidths on many other of the original 15 dimensions are already included in the original 15 (e.g., spatial extent is effectively bandwidth on the spatial fequency and on the spatial position dimensions). These and related interrelationships among the dimensions are summarized in the next section and are important in interpreting analyzer-revealing experiments.

11.7   INTERRELATIONSHIPS AMONG PATTERN DIMENSIONS

11.7.1   *Any Combination of Values Specifies a Different Stimulus (Analyzer)*

All the pattern dimensions we have now met are logically independent in the following sense: Knowing the value (which means, often, the nominal or central value, since there is often a range of values) of a stimulus or of a visual mechanism on any one dimension does not tell you the value on any other. For example, knowing the spatial frequency does not tell you the orientation, the spatial position, or the spatial extent. To put this point a different way, any arbitrary combination of values on the first 15 dimensions specifies a different sinusoidal patch, and therefore can correspond to the luminance profile of a different visual stimulus. You could add the last two dimensions to this statement also by allowing grating patches stimulating both eyes or containing components moving in both directions. Similarly, any arbitrary combination of values on the 17 dimensions can specify a different visual mechanism (e.g., a visual cortical neuron).

11.7.2 Independence of Dimensions of Excited Analyzers

One might hope that all the pattern dimensions would be completely independent in the following sense also: When two stimuli differed along only one dimension (the experimental dimension), one might hope that the two groups of analyzers (e.g., elements—mechanisms' outputs at single points of time) that responded to those two stimuli would differ only along that experimental dimension. In other words, one might hope that the analyzers differentially excited by the two patterns would differ only along the experimental dimension, not along any of the other dimensions in the model under consideration.

In general, whether one gets this kind of strong independence clearly depends on the model of the analyzers as well as on the dimensions. And, alas, in the case of any reasonable models of pattern vision I know, this strong type of independence does not exist. Much of this lack of independence is a manifestation of the fact that the values on some dimensions are related to the bandwidths on other dimensions.

The All-Possible-Linear-Elements Population. To discuss the dependencies that do exist in at least one family of pattern-vision models, it will be convenient to give a name to the hypothetical population of all possible elements (all possible mechanisms' outputs at single points of time), where the elements are linear systems and have a windowed-sinusoid type of spatiotemporal weighting function. This population would contain a very large number (infinite or effectively so) of elements having spatiotemporal weighting functions at all spatial frequencies, all orientations, all spatial positions, all spatial extents, all spatial phases, all temporal frequencies, all temporal positions, all temporal extents, all temporal phases, both directions of motion, all degrees of direction selectivity, both eyes, and all degrees of monocularity. (We will not, however, consider contrast or mean luminance in the present discussion.) We will call this the *all-possible-linear-elements population.*

Now consider two sinusoidal-patch stimuli identical except in their value on one dimension (the experimental dimension) and ask what two subpopulations of elements in the all-possible-linear-element population are excited by these two stimuli. The subpopulations will often turn out to differ not only along the experimental dimension but also along one (or more) other dimension. When this happens, the experimental dimension and the other dimension(s) will be said to be interdependent (see section 11.7.3 for examples). If, however, stimuli differing only on the experimental dimension excite subpopulations that differ on the experimental dimension but not on a second dimension, the experimental and second dimension will be said to be independent in a very strong sense (see section 11.7.4 for examples).

11.7.3   Interdependent Dimensions

The following list gives the most important interdependencies found among the pattern dimensions within models assuming linear elements (or something close to it), where the kind of independence/dependence under consideration is that described in the previous subsection.

Two sinusoidal-patch stimuli that differ on *any* of the spatial dimensions will differentially excite elements along the spatial-position dimension (with the exception that the two stimuli differing in spatial extent in one direction will not differentially excite along the *perpendicular* spatial-position dimension). An example discussed below is illustrated in Fig. 11.6.

Analogously, two sinusoidal-patch stimuli that differ on *any* of the temporal dimensions will differentially excite elements along the temporal-position dimension.

Notice that two sinusoidal-patch stimuli that differ only in direction-of-motion will differentially excite elements along both the spatial-position and temporal-position dimensions. (Direction-of-motion is most properly thought of as a spatial and temporal dimension, although I usually call it a temporal dimension for simplicity.)

Changing the spatial position of a sinusoidal-patch stimulus changes which spatial phases (spatial symmetries) of elements are stimulated at any particular spatial position, spatial frequency, and so on. (Note, however, that changing the spatial position does not affect any spatial dimensions other than spatial phase.)

Analogously, changing the temporal position of a sinusoidal-patch stimuli changes which temporal phases (symmetries) of elements are stimulated at any particular time. (Note, however, that changing the temporal position does not affect any temporal dimensions other than temporal phase.)

Increasing the spatial extent perpendicular to bars of a sinusoidal-patch stimulus while keeping values on all other pattern dimensions constant has the following effect on the all-possible-linear-elements population: (a) It reduces the range of responding elements along the spatial-frequency dimension. (b) It reduces the range of responding elements along the spatial-phase dimension. (c) It widens the range of spatial positions. (These interrelationships with spatial extent were discussed in Chapters 5 and 6. They are illustrated in Fig. 11.5 and discussed below as well.)

Increasing the spatial extent parallel to bars, (a) narrows the range of orientations and (b) widens the range of spatial positions.

Increasing temporal extent (a) reduces the range of temporal frequencies, (b) reduces the ranges of temporal phases, and (c) increases the range of temporal positions.

And, of course, increasing the degree of monocularity (or, respectively, degree of direction selectivity) reduces the range of values on the eye dimension (or, respectively, the direction-of-motion dimension).

Whether contrast and mean luminance are independent of the other dimensions will depend on how the selectivity for these dimensions is modeled. If the elements are taken to be linear systems, as we are doing in this subsection, contrast and mean luminance will interact with each other but not with the other dimensions. However, linear systems can produce only a rather weak kind of selectivity for contrast and mean luminance, the kind caused by changing the constant of proportionality (see section 11.6.5).

11.7.4 Mutually Independent Dimensions

The following list gives five pattern dimensions that are mutually independent in this very strong sense: If two sinusoidal-patch stimuli differ only in value on one of the five dimensions (call it the experimental dimension), the two subpopulations from the all-possible-linear-elements population that respond to the two stimuli will differ in value along the experimental dimension, but not along any of the other four dimensions:

Spatial frequency
Orientation
Temporal frequency
Direction of motion
Eye

In general, in fact, there is mutual independence in the above sense among all triplets of the following form:

Any spatial dimension
Any temporal dimension
The eye dimension

It is worth emphasizing that, in addition to these sets of mutually independent dimensions, there were some important one-sided independent relationships that appeared in the list of interrelationships above:

Changing spatial position does *not* affect spatial frequency, orientation, or spatial extent.
Changing temporal position does not affect temporal frequency, temporal extent, direction of motion.

11.8 SPECIAL POINTS ABOUT INTERPRETING EXPERIMENTS ON EACH PATTERN DIMENSION

For each of 17 pattern dimensions, this section will describe any features that make interpretation of behavior on this dimension not a straightforward analogue to the models given in Chapters 3, 4, 7, and 9.

These features are of several sorts:

1. As summarized in section 11.7, patterns differing along one experimental dimension may differentially excite analyzers differing along other dimensions as well as the experimental dimension.

2. Visual processes (e.g., light adaptation) other than the low-level pattern analyzers under consideration may be known on other grounds to intrude significantly into the results of certain experiments on certain dimensions.

3. For certain dimensions an analyzer's output to a compound stimulus is expected to be something quite different from the sum of the outputs to the inputs. This, of course, affects the interpretation of summation experiments.

4. Another complication in interpreting summation experiments results from the nature of stimuli varying on certain dimensions. It occurs often enough to be worth describing in the abstract and naming. We will call it the *no-true-compound* problem and describe it further here.

No True Compound (When a Compound Stimulus Is Also a Simple Stimulus). On a number of dimensions, a compound stimulus formed by the sum of two simple stimuli is the same as some other simple stimulus on that dimension. For example, consider two simple stimuli on the contrast dimension, that is, two stimuli identical on all dimensions except in contrast (e.g., two stationary vertical grating patches of 3 c/deg). The compound made by adding these two simple stimuli will be identical to the original simple stimuli except in contrast (e.g., it will be another stationary vertical grating patch of 3 c/deg but still higher contrast), and thus will itself be equivalent to another simple stimulus on the contrast dimension. Of the 17 dimensions we are considering for visual patterns, 6 lack true compounds (more detail given below): spatial phase, temporal phase, degree-of-direction selectivity, contrast, mean luminance, and degree of monocularity.

Thus if you tried to do a summation experiment on one of these dimensions (tried comparing a compound with its two simple components), you would actually be doing a small (three-stimulus) parametric experiment on the dimension.

As described in section 11.6, parametric experiments are not very informative about whether there are multiple analyzers, as any empirically determined function of value on a given dimension could be the approximate envelope of multiple analyzers' functions or could be an individual analyzer's function.

11.8.1 Spatial-Frequency Experiments

The prototypical stimuli would be two spatiotemporal grating patches differing in spatial frequency while being identical on every other dimension. (In this context, "identical in spatial extent" usually means spatial extent measured in degrees of visual angle rather than in number of cycles.)

Patches differing in spatial frequency do excite elements differentially along not only the spatial-frequency dimension but also the spatial-position dimension. The quantitative modeling necessary to get around this problem (e.g., to account for spatial probability summation and spatial nonuniformity) has been described in detail in Chapters 5 and 6.

In practice, the stimuli have rarely had a Gaussian or similar temporal window but have usually been aperiodic in time (have abruptly been turned on, left on for a while, and then turned off) and thus rather broad band on the temporal-position and temporal-frequency dimensions. They have also often been of rather large spatial extent (that is, distinctly broad band in one or both spatial-position dimensions as well). This potentially introduces the interpretational problem discussed at length previously (see Fig. 11.3 and section 11.3, as well as Chapters 5 and 6).

11.8.2 Orientation Experiments

The prototypical stimuli for analyzer-revealing experiments on the orientation dimension would be two spatiotemporal sinusoidal grating patches differing in orientation.

The interpretation of experiments along this dimension is exactly analogous to the interpretation of ones along the spatial-frequency dimension.

Again, stimuli that are broad band on the temporal-position and spatial-position dimensions have frequently been used, introducing interpretational problems like that in Fig. 11.3 (see section 11.3).

11.8.3 Spatial Position Experiments (Two Dimensions)

The prototypical two stimuli would be two spatiotemporal sinusoidal grating patches differing in position in the two-dimensional visual field but identical on all other pattern dimensions.

In fact, such stimuli have rarely been used. More frequently, the stimuli have been spatially and temporally aperiodic (e.g., lines that came on and stayed on for a while) potentially introducing the broad-band interpretational problem of Fig. 11.3.

An additional interpretational problem that arises in summation experiments is that the *compound* stimulus containing stimuli at two spatial positions will excite elements (in the all-possible-linear-elements population) that have different values along the spatial-frequency and spatial-phase dimensions from those excited by either of the two components (e.g., see discussion of frequency spread in section 5.4.1).

Further, even if there were not mechanisms at different spatial positions but only mechanisms having different spatial phases (symmetries) at the same spatial position, stimuli at slightly different spatial positions might affect different symmetries of mechanisms rather than different positions. (This possibility seems unlikely on other grounds, however.)

11.8.4 Spatial Extent Experiments (Two Dimensions)

The prototypical two stimuli for analyzer-revealing experiments on a spatial-extent dimension would be two sinusoidal patches differing in number of bars or length of bars but identical on all other dimensions.

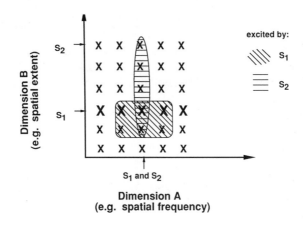

FIG. 11.5 An analyzer is represented here not by a constant-sensitivity contour but by an x marking its values along dimension A and dimension B. The values of the two stimuli S_1 and S_2 are marked by arrows on the axes. The horizontal crosshatching (respectively, diagonal cross-hatching) encloses the analyzers stimulated by S_2 (respectively, S_1). Although both these stimuli have the same value along dimension A, stimulus S_1 (which has a lower value on dimension B than does S_2) affects a broader range of analyzers along dimension A than does S_2

Monotonic, Overlapping Sensitivity Functions. Even for far-apart spatial extents, elements with Gabor-type spatial weighting functions have monotonic (and therefore overlapping) sensitivity functions on this dimension (as mentioned previously in sections 5.5.1 and 11.6.2). The implications of this overlap were discussed in section 5.5 for certain summation experiments and are illustrated more abstractly in Fig. 11.5. In this figure, each symbol x shows the best spatial frequency (horizontal coordinate) and the spatial extent (vertical coordinate) of a single element in the all-possible-linear-elements model. Many x's are shown (although not for all possible elements, obviously). The difference between the smaller and larger x's will be discussed shortly. The arrows on the horizontal and vertical axes indicate the spatial frequency and spatial extent of two sinusoidal patches, one of small extent (perhaps a single bar—S_1) and one of larger extent (many cycles—S_2). The elements in the all-possible-linear-elements population that are excited by the patch of smaller extent (S_1) are shown by the diagonally cross-hatched region while those excited by the patch of larger extent (S_2) are shown by the horizontally crosshatched region. Notice that, even when there are multiple analyzers on the spatial-extent dimension at a single value on the spatial frequency dimension (even when the columns of x's shown in the figure from the all-possible-linear elements population are assumed to exist in a model), some of the same analyzers would be excited by both stimuli, no matter how far apart the stimuli are on the spatial-extent dimension. Thus some interaction is expected even at far-apart values on the spatial-extent dimension (and it is found in experimental results; see section 5.5.1).

Interaction with Spatial Frequency. A second interpretational problem, also illustrated in Fig. 11.5, arises in spatial-extent experiments because of a dimensional interrelationship presented in section 11.7 (and in section 6.7.3). Namely, two stimuli that differ in spatial extent not only stimulate—in the all-possible-linear-elements population—elements differing on the spatial-extent dimension but also stimulate elements differing on the spatial frequency, spatial phase, and spatial position dimensions. Let's consider the subpopulation of elements marked by larger X's in Fig. 11.5 (the second row of elements from the bottom in the figure). Now we are considering multiple analyzers on the spatial-frequency dimension but only a single analyzer on the spatial-extent dimension. However, of these elements, S_1 stimulates three elements but S_2 stimulates only one. Therefore, an experiment may show much less than complete interaction between two stimuli far apart in spatial extent (S_1 and S_2), even if there is only a single spatial-extent analyzer, as long as there are multiple spatial-frequency analyzers (the large X's).

Interaction with Spatial Position. The horizontal axis in Fig. 11.5 could be thought of as spatial position instead of spatial frequency. Then S_1 should represent the patch of larger extent.

11.8.5 Spatial-Phase Experiments

The prototypical stimuli for analyzer-revealing experiments on the spatial-phase dimension would be two sinusoidal patches differing in the phase of the sinusoid that is underneath the window.

No True Compound. On this dimension a compound of two stimuli is a simple stimulus. For adding together two sine waves of the same frequency but at different phases (and different amplitudes) produces another sine wave of the same frequency but at a third phase. As described at the beginning of section 11.8, this lack of a true compound undermines the usefulness of summation experiments.

Two Independent Phases. Further, although of less direct relevance in the interpretation of analyzer-revealing experiments, there are only two completely independent values on the spatial-phase dimension in the following sense: Not only does adding two sine waves of different phases produce a third phase of the same frequency sine wave, but all possible phases can be produced that way. In other words, any phase of sine wave can be formed as a compound of two particular arbitrarily chosen phases (that is, any phase can be constructed by summing together the appropriate amplitudes of sine waves of the chosen two phases). Which two are chosen is arbitrary as long as they are not identical or 180 degrees out of phase with one another.

Interaction with Spatial Position. A major problem in interpreting spatial-phase experiments is that sinusoidal-patch stimuli of different spatial phases (symmetry) excite—in the all-possible-linear-elements population—not only

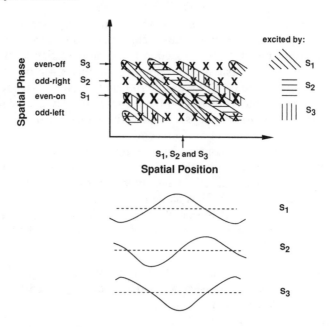

FIG. 11.6 An illustration of the interaction of spatial phase (vertical axis) and spatial position (horizontal axis). As in the preceding figure, each analyzer in this figure is indicated by an x plotted at the analyzer's value on the two dimensions. The four kinds of spatial-phase analyzers illustrated are also named next to the vertical axis. The arrows on the axes indicate the values of three sinusoidal patches all centered at the same spatial position (and having the same spatial frequency, orientation, etc.) but of different spatial phases. The shading, horizontal crosshatching, and vertical crosshatching indicate which analyzers are well stimulated by S_1, S_2, and S_3, respectively. The sketches at the bottom give the luminances of S_1, S_2, and S_3 as a function of spatial position (same horizontal coordinates as in the top graph).

elements of different spatial phase at a given position but also elements of different spatial position.

This problem was described in section 5.6.1, listed in section 11.7.3, and is illustrated more abstractly in Fig. 11.6. In this figure, each symbol x shows the spatial position (horizontal coordinate) and spatial phase or symmetry (vertical coordinate) of a single element in the all-possible-linear-elements model. (All these elements are assumed to be sensitive to the spatial frequency and orientation of the patches being presented.) The arrows on the horizontal and vertical axes indicate the spatial phases and spatial positions of three sinusoidal patches, all centered at the same spatial position but of even symmetry with a bright center (S_1), odd symmetry with the right half excitatory (S_2), or even symmetry with a dark center (S_3). The elements in the all-possible-linear-elements population that are substantially excited by S_1 are shown by the diagonally crosshatched region, those excited by S_2 by horizontal crosshatching, and those excited by S_3 by vertical crosshatching. Even if there is only one analyzer on the spatial-phase dimension (even symmetry, on center, for example, as indicated by the row of large X's in Fig. 11.6)—as long as there are different analyzers on the spatial-position dimension—two stimuli of different spatial phases will excite different analyzers.

Randomizing Spatial Positions and Compound Stimuli. One way of attempting to get around the interaction between spatial phase and spatial position is to randomize from trial to trial the spatial position of stimuli of different spatial phases (symmetries). Sinusoidal-patch stimuli may be used or, more frequently, other kinds of stimuli have been used—gratings containing two spatial frequencies (the relative phase of which is manipulated), aperiodic stimuli like lines (bright vs. dark, a 180-degree phase shift) or edges (left vs. right, another 180-degree phase shift). These stimuli are simple on the spatial-phase dimension but compound (indeed, often broad band) on the spatial-frequency dimension. One hopes that by randomizing the spatial position the observer is prevented from using information from spatial-position analyzers and thereby that one can find out whether multiple spatial-phase analyzers exist.

11.8.6 Temporal-Frequency Experiments

The two prototypical stimuli for analyzer-revealing experiments on this dimension would be two sinusoidal patches differing only in temporal frequency. Such experiments and their possible interpretations are analagous in all respects (except their actual results—see Chap. 12) to those on the spatial-frequency dimension.

11.8.7 Temporal-Position Experiments

Being identical in temporal position means coming at the same time after some relevant zero time in the experiment (e.g., the beginning of the trial). Two prototypical stimuli in analyzer-revealing experiments on this dimension, therefore, would be two sinusoidal grating patches coming at different times after some relevant zero time.

In summation, uncertainty, and identification experiments, the relevant zero time could be taken to be some marked starting point of a trial. The logic of interpreting these temporal-position experiments would be exactly analogous to that of interpreting spatial position experiments. There is again the slight interpretational problem due to the interdimensional relationship between temporal position and temporal phase but, even more so than with the analogous problem between spatial position and spatial phase, the alternative where there are only elements at different temporal phases and not elements at different temporal positions seems unreasonable.

In adaptation experiments, however, the adapting and test stimulus must always differ substantially in temporal position (with respect to the beginning of a trial) or it would not be an adaptation experiment. Further, variations on this temporal-position dimension (e.g. variations in how long after the adapting stimulus the test stimulus comes) seem likely to reveal properties of the fatigue, inhibitory, or other desensitization process rather than having anything to do with temporal-position elements (with responses of mechanisms at different points of time—that is, with the time course of responses of mechanisms to a current stimulus).

11.8.8   Temporal-Extent Experiments

Two prototypical stimuli to use in temporal extent experiments would be sinusoidal patch stimuli identical on all the pattern dimensions except in their temporal duration. With these stimuli, the interpretation of summation, uncertainty, and identification experiments should be much like that of spatial extent.

In adaptation experiments, however, variations on the temporal-extent dimension imply variations in the duration of adapting and test stimuli. These seem more likely to reveal characteristics of the process by which individual analyzers desensitize (be it fatigue, inhibition, or something else) rather than anything about the temporal properties of the analyzers themselves. See similar comments under temporal position.

11.8.9   Temporal-Phase Experiments

Two prototypical stimuli for investigation of the temporal-phase dimension would be two flickering sinusoidal patches differing only in the phase of the temporal sinusoid with respect to the temporal window. The interpretation of these experiments would run into difficulties exactly analogous to those encountered on the spatial-phase dimension (section 11.8.5), including the no-true-compound problem.

11.8.10   Direction-of-Motion and Degree-of-Direction-Selectivity
Experiments

Direction of Motion. The two prototypical stimuli for analyzer-revealing experiments on this dimension would be two sinusoidal patches differing only in that their sinusoidal function is drifting in opposite directions.

If these two stimuli have equal contrast, their compound would just be a flickering patch (since the sum of two gratings of the same contrast, spatial frequency, orientation, etc., but of opposite directions of motion is a flickering grating).

Some models have assumed that the response of a completely directionally selective analyzer to the compound is the same as the response to the one component it is sensitive to (that is, the analyzers are at least additive in the weak sense that an ineffective component is ineffective in the compound, Assumption 36).

Other models have assumed, however, that the directionally selective analyzer is totally insensitive to the flickering compound (e.g., Wilson, 1985) and that only a nondirectionally selective analyzer responds to the flickering compound at all.

Direction of motion and spatial and temporal position are interdependent in the sense that two stimuli differing in direction of motion excite subpopulations of the all-possible-linear-elements population that differ in spatial position and temporal position as well as in direction of motion. But resulting complications (in particular, probability summation across space and time in summation experiments) can be handled as they were with spatial-frequency experiments.

Degree of Direction Selectivity. A simple stimulus on the degree-of-direction-selectivity dimension is a grating patch containing components moving in both directions but not necessarily in equal amounts. Thus, a simple stimulus on the degree-of-direction-selectivity dimension is the same as a compound stimulus on the direction-of-motion dimension.

A compound stimulus on this degree-of-direction-selectivity dimension is, further, identical to some simple stimulus on that dimension. Thus, the no-true-compound problem undermines the usefulness of summation experiments (see beginning of section 11.8).

11.8.11 Eye-of-Origin and Degree-of-Monocularity Experiments

Eye-of-Origin. Sinusoidal patch stimuli can have only two values on this dimension—the left eye or the right eye. A compound stimulus is one that stimulates both eyes (although not necessarily equally in both eyes).

The response of an individual mechanism to a compound has sometimes been assumed to be the sum of its responses to the components, and therefore a completely monocular mechanism's output to a compound would equal its output to the relevant component. But inhibition between eyes might make a monocular analyzer less sensitive to compound than to appropriate component (as with direction of motion).

Degree of Monocularity. A simple stimulus on the degree-of-monocularity dimension is a grating patch stimulating both eyes but not necessarily equally. Thus, a simple stimulus on the degree-of-monocularity dimension is the same as a compound stimulus on the eye-of-origin dimension.

A compound stimulus on this degree-of-monocularity dimension is then identical to some simple stimulus on that same dimension. That is, there are no true compounds on this dimension, which undermines the usefulness of summation experiments.

11.8.12 Contrast

Two prototypical stimuli for analyzer-revealing experiments on the contrast dimension would be grating patches of different contrasts (so one could not measure contrast thresholds; one would have to measure detection and/or identification performance at each contrast level). There are no true compounds on this dimension (see beginning of section 11.8), which undermines the usefulness of summation experiments.

11.8.13   Mean Luminance

Two prototypical stimuli for analyzer-revealing experiments on the mean-luminance dimension would be two grating patches varying in mean luminance but identical on all other dimensions. (A priori, whether one wanted the two patches to be identical in contrast or in luminance difference—that is, maximal minus minimal luminance—might well depend on other theoretical considerations.)

Mean luminance is still another dimension where a compound stimulus (the sum of the two prototypical simple stimuli) is itself a simple stimulus, and the no-true-compound problem complicates interpretation of summation experiments.

11.9   SUMMARY

Summation experiments are better than adaptation, uncertainty, or simple identification experiments at distinguishing between doubly selective and singly selective analyzers (as long as individual analyzers show substantial additivity to compounds).

Using stimuli that are broad band on an auxiliary dimension in an analyzer-revealing experiment has the following unfortunate result: It disguises the differences between different kinds of analyzers' joint sensitivity on the experimental and auxiliary dimensions.

An individual analyzer's sensitivity function along two dimensions is said to be separable if it equals the product of one function along one dimension times another function along another dimension.

Parametric experiments measuring the observer's sensitivity as a function of stimulus value along some dimension are not very useful for distinguishing between single- and multiple-analyzers models. They do give useful information about the peak sensitivities of multiple analyzers or the sensitivity function of single ones.

All the pattern dimensions are mutually independent in the following sense: Specifying the value of a stimulus or an analyzer along any of the 15 pattern dimensions introduced in Chapter 2 plus two more (degree of monocularity, degree of direction selectivity) does not give the value on any other.

One might hope that all the pattern dimensions would also be mutually independent in the following sense: If two patterns differ only along one dimension, the two subpopulations of analyzers they excite would differ only along that dimension and not along a second (or third, etc.) dimension. This kind of independence does hold for a number of pairs of pattern dimensions, but not for others. These dimensional interdependencies produce complications in interpreting the results of analyzer-revealing experiments.

These complications, as well as other features that make interpretation of analyzer-revealing experiments on a given experiment different from a straightforward analogue to that given in earlier chapters (Chapters 3, 4, 7, and 9), are gone through dimension by dimension in the latter part of this chapter as a preparation for the conclusions about analyzers on each dimension that are presented in the next chapter.

12

Results of Analyzer-Revealing Experiments

12.1 INTRODUCTION

This chapter summarizes available evidence from the four kinds of near-threshold analyzer-revealing experiments discussed previously in this book—adaptation, summation, uncertainty, and identification—for each of the 17 pattern-vision dimensions along which multiple analyzers might exist (section 11.6). Occasional references are given in the course of this summary, but the majority of the references are to be found in an organized list of references in section 12.9.

The next chapter will summarize evidence from parametric experiments on these dimensions.

12.1.1   The Three Questions to Be Answered About Each Dimension

A large part of this chapter is devoted to answering the following three questions for each of the 17 possible dimensions

1. Multiple analyzers? Are there analyzers sensitive to different values along that dimension?
2. Bandwidth? If there are such multiple analyzers on a dimension, what is their bandwidth on that dimension? More generally, what is an individual analyzer's sensitivity as a function of value on that dimension?

To answer this question for most dimensions on which there are multiple analyzers, we will assume that the analyzers are mechanisms (section 1.10) and are linear systems (section 2.5). When we make this assumption, the word *mechanism* will be used in the answer to this question in place of *analyzer*.

The reasoning by which one answers the first two questions (on the basis of results from four analyzer-revealing kinds of experiments) was extensively described in Chapters 3 through 10. A summary can be found in section 11.1.2.

3. Labeled? If there are multiple analyzers on a particular dimension, are these analyzers' outputs "labeled"? That is, can the higher stages that compute the decision variable keep track of which output comes from which analyzer?

Value-specific behavior in adaptation or summation experiments can be explained by multiple analyzers even if the outputs of these analyzers are not labeled, that is, even if the subsequent stages of processing know only the magnitudes of the analyzers' outputs without knowing anything about which analyzer produced which output. To explain value-specific behavior in uncertainty and identification experiments, however, seems to require that the outputs of the analyzers be labeled (not necessarily perfectly) by which analyzer produced them (see Chaps. 7 and 9). Therefore, we will conclude here that analyzers' outputs are labeled if and only if value-specific behavior is found in the relevant uncertainty and/or identification experiments.

Correlation and Inhibition. At the end of this chapter a short section summarizes evidence about two further issues—the possible correlation among analyzers and the possible inhibition among analyzers.

12.1.2 Not Summarized in This Chapter

Many features necessary to specify a multiple-analyzers model completely are not discussed in the following summary. Four of the five such features listed below are discussed in earlier chapters, and the fifth is briefly discussed in the next subsection.

1. What is the probability density function describing an individual analyzer's output, and how does it depend on signal strength? (Chaps. 7 and 10.)
2. What is the exact form of the decision variable? Is it, for example, the maximum output or some weighted sum, or the more complicated calculation of likelihood ratio required for an optimal observer? (Chaps. 7 and 10.)
3. Exactly what analyzers (mechanisms, elements) form the subset of analyzers that enter into the decision variable in any given task? What analyzers does the observer "pay attention to" or "monitor"? (Chaps. 7 and 10.)
4. Are the analyzers (mechanisms) linear systems, or, for example, do they embody a compressive or rectifying nonlinearity? Can the nonlinearity be modeled as a point-by-point nonlinearity coming between the luminance profile and a linear system (a filter described by a spatiotemporal weighting function)? (Not discussed in any detail here.) And/or as a nonlinear function acting on the output of the analyzer? (Chaps. 8 and 10.)
5. Exactly how many analyzers are there on a given dimension, and how are they spaced? (Section 12.1.3.)

To calculate quantitative predictions, these features and more must often be specified. Changing any of these features, therefore, might affect the conclusions drawn about any other feature, including the features summarized in this chapter. The attempt in this chapter, however, is only to summarize qualitatively the broad and impressive consistencies found among results from different kinds of experiments done by different investigators. I suspect that these general conclusions will be little affected by details of the other features of the model (with one exception—the decision rule for identification—see section 12.5).

12.1.3 Number and Spacing of Analyzers

The number and spacing of analyzers have often been varied in theoretical calculations and found to have no discernible effect once there were "enough" analyzers. Enough typically turns out to mean one or two every half-amplitude full-bandwidth [at threshold; Klein and Levi (1985) needed even closer spacing for a suprathreshold discrimination]. Thus, from near-threshold experiments of the type described here, there is almost no evidence about the exact number of analyzers. A minimum number can often be estimated, but any more than that minimum would do as well (the sensitivity of each would just have to be reduced correspondingly). That minimum number of distinct analyzers (analyzers having different sensitivity functions) depends crucially on the bandwidth estimate. The wider this width estimate, the smaller the number of distinct analyzers one could assume.

Similarly, there is no good evidence about the exact placements of the peak values of the analyzers along the various dimensions. Basically the analyzers seem to be densely enough spaced on any dimension that their individual placement is hidden (in any of the kinds of experiments considered here at least). For example, sensitivity as a function of value is always a relatively smooth function showing no evidence of peaks due to individual analyzers, a fact that does, however, put constraints on just how far apart analyzers could be placed on a dimension (see, for example, calculations in Watson, 1982a).

12.1.4   Disclaimer—Typical Values on Pattern Dimensions

The total number of different analyzer-revealing experiments that could be done is very large as discussed further in note 1. The conclusions to be given here apply, of course, only within the ranges on each pattern dimension that have been explored to date. The following list attempts to give the range of values on each dimension that has typically been used when that dimension is an auxiliary dimension in analyzer-revealing experiments (summarized in Chap. 12) or a secondary dimension in parametric experiments (summarized in Chap. 13). The full range of values on a dimension has generally been explored when a dimension is the experimental or primary dimension. When values on auxiliary (or secondary) dimensions are not explicitly specified in the text of Chapters 12 and 13, therefore, they will generally be the values given in the list here.

In a very few of the possible combinations of dimensions (e.g., temporal frequency as an auxiliary dimension when spatial frequency is the experimental dimension), enough analyzer-revealing experiments have been done to show conclusively that there is an effect of the auxiliary dimension on the experimental dimension results. Such cases will be explicitly described. The reference list in section 12.10 gives all references I know to such cases. Many more such dependencies are well documented in the case of parametric experiments, as will be summarized in Chapter 13.

12.1.5   Other Disclaimers

For readers interested in the evidence for and against any conclusion, the reference list at the end of the chapter (section 12.10) should provide a starting point.

Typical Parameter Ranges

Spatial frequency	Low to medium (1 to 10 c/deg or aperiodic)
Orientation	Vertical, horizontal
Spatial position	Centered at fixation point
Spatial extent	2 to 6 degrees
Temporal frequency	Low to medium (1–10 c/sec or aperiodic); unstabilized viewing
Temporal extent	Long (many temporal cycles or, if aperiodic, several hundred milliseconds or longer)
Mean luminance	Low to moderate photopic
Binocular viewing	
Miscellaneous	Observer's ordinary refractive correction Broadband white or bluish to yellowish green Young adult to middle-aged (humans)

Inevitably a summary of conclusions like that given in the rest of this chapter is misleading. At its best, it is only adequate when taken as a summary of major effects and when taken in the context of all the remarks made previously (e.g., section 11.8) about difficulties in interpretation.

12.2 ANALYZERS ON SPATIAL DIMENSIONS

12.2.1 *Spatial-Frequency Analyzers*

Many experiments on the spatial-frequency dimension were used to illustrate points in Chapters 3 through 10.

Multiple Analyzers? Yes, multiple analyzers exist on the spatial-frequency dimension. The common use of full-field and temporally aperiodic gratings in experiments on the spatial-frequency dimension, however, leaves open the kind of interpretational problem illustrated in Fig. 11.3. That multiple spatial-frequency mechanisms exist at a single spatial position has been verified by using summation experiments with localized patches to rule out the possibility that the multiple mechanisms revealed by experiments with full-field gratings existed at separate spatial positions (section 4.5). An analogous potential difficulty in interpretation caused by temporal inhomogeneity has been ruled out by experiments varying the relative time of onsets of the components in a compound grating (section 4.5.4).

Bandwidth? Spatial-frequency bandwidths are sufficiently narrow that at least several analyzers with essentially nonoverlapping sensitivity ranges exist along the spatial-frequency dimension. The spatial-frequency bandwidth of individual analyzers seems to increase in proportion to spatial frequency or, in other words, to be approximately constant on a logarithmic spatial-frequency axis. The bandwidth on a logarithmic axis may broaden slightly at very low spatial frequencies (tending toward constancy on a linear spatial-frequency axis).

The exact value of this bandwidth estimate depends, however, a good deal on details of the model. Estimates vary from about 0.5 to 1.5 octaves. (See sections 3.5, 6.4.3, 6.9, 10.3.5, and 10.6.1 for details.)

Spatial-frequency bandwidths seem to be the same (within the precision of current measurements) at different mean luminances, different orientations and different spatial positions. (See section 12.9 for reference list.)

At high temporal frequencies, however, the spatial-frequency bandwidths may be slightly broader. On the spatial-frequency dimension, adaptation (Graham, 1972) and summation (Arend & Lange, 1979a; Pantle, 1973; Thompson, 1981) experiments show only a little broadening of bandwidth as temporal frequency is raised, but identification experiments seem to show a larger increase in bandwidth (Watson & Robson, 1981). This discrepancy is discussed further in section 12.5.

Labeled? Yes. The multiple spatial-frequency mechanisms are labeled in the sense necessary for selective monitoring of spatial frequency in uncertainty experiments and for identification of spatial frequency at detection threshold (see Chaps. 7, 9, and 10).

12.2.2   Orientation Analyzers

Multiple Analyzers? Yes, at least several of which are effectively nonoverlapping in sensitivity.

Bandwidth? The orientation bandwidths (expressed in degrees of rotation) seem to be very similar at all orientations (within the precision of measurement) and spatial frequencies. The exact value of this bandwidth depends on details of the model interpreting any kind of evidence. These estimates (half-amplitude full-bandwidth) vary from as little as 5 or 10 degrees to as much as 40 to 60 degrees, depending on a number of factors. Estimates from summation and 2×2 identification experiments were presented earlier, in sections 6.5 and 10.3.5, respectively. I know of no estimates from uncertainty experiments. The estimates from adaptation experiments made using the equivalent-contrast transformation are between 10 and 20 degrees (Blakemore & Nachmias, 1971; Movshon & Blakemore, 1973). If, however, orientation bandwidth is estimated as twice the orientation differences causing half-maximal adaptation (a procedure that produces estimates close to those of a full Stiles-type model, see section 3.5), the estimates are about 60 angular degrees for low spatial frequencies (up to a spatial frequency of 7 c/deg) and then decrease, reaching about 20 degrees by a spatial frequency of 20 c/deg (using the results from the studies of Blakemore & Nachmias, 1971; Sekuler, Rubin, & Cushman, 1968; and Movshon & Blakemore, 1973).

As just indicated, orientation bandwidth may be smaller at higher spatial frequencies [also suggested by consideration of thresholds for circular vs. rectilinear gratings like the thresholds collected by Kelly (1982a) and by Kelly and Magnuski (1975)].

Results from the one joint orientation and spatial-frequency experiment (adaptation, Blakemore & Nachmias, 1971) suggest that orientation and spatial frequency are separable in the tuning function of single analyzers (but this conclusion is model-bound).

The available evidence, particularly from summation experiments (see section 11.2), indicates that the analyzers are doubly selective for orientation and spatial frequency.

Orientation bandwidth (like spatial-frequency bandwidth) may be broader at higher temporal frequencies, or perhaps more accurately, at high velocities. (See adaptation experiments by Sekuler et al., 1968; Sharpe & Tolhurst, 1973a; Kelly & Burbeck, 1987; see summation experiments of Wilson et al., 1983—Fig. 6.10 here—who found a broader orientation bandwidth when a lower spatial frequency was combined with higher temporal frequencies; also, for orthogonal orientations, see Kelly & Burbeck, 1987).

Mean luminance seems to make no difference in summation of far-apart orientations (Carlson et al., 1977).

Labeled? Yes (e.g., Thomas & Gille, 1979).

12.2.3 Spatial-Position Analyzers (Two Dimensions)

Multiple Analyzers? Yes, as has been assumed for decades. The range of spatial positions to which any one spatial-position analyzer is sensitive is a very narrow subrange of the visible range of spatial positions. Thus there are effectively a great number of analyzers having nonoverlapping ranges on these two spatial-position dimensions.

Bandwidth? Evidence from summation experiments on the spatial-frequency, orientation, and spatial-position dimensions contributes to an understanding of a mechanism's sensitivity as a function of spatial position (which is the same as its two-dimensional spatial weighting function) (See Chap. 6).

First, let's note the following fact: If the spatial weighting functions of different mechanisms (tuned to different spatial frequencies and orientations) all have the same number of excitatory and/or inhibitory regions and also the same length/width ratio (but just come in different overall sizes), then the spatial-frequency bandwidths of different mechanisms would be the same on a logarithmic axis and the orientation bandwidths would be the same in angular degrees of rotation. If, on the other hand, the spatial weighting functions of different mechanisms (tuned to different spatial frequencies and orientations) have the same overall sizes (the same spatial extents measured in degrees of visual angle) but different numbers of regions (equivalently, different regional length/width ratios), then the spatial-frequency bandwidths of different mechanisms would be the same on a linear frequency axis and the orientation bandwidths would be the same when expressed as distance in the two-dimensional spatial-frequency plane. Available evidence from near-threshold psychophysical experiments suggests that the first alternative (that spatial weighting functions all have the same number of regions and the same length/width ratio but differ in overall size) is a much better description than the second one (that weighting functions have the same overall size). When deviations from the first alternative exist, however, they are in the direction of the second alternative.

Each mechanisms's spatial weighting function in the direction perpendicular to the bars seems to contain an excitatory central region, a significant inhibitory surround region, and, perhaps, secondary excitatory regions (e.g., see Fig. 6.9 and section 6.9).

The spatial weighting function parallel to the bars presumably contains only an excitatory portion; evidence about its extent is scanty. In the model of Watson (1983), the two spatial window functions (the one parallel and the one perpendicular to the elongated regions of the receptive field) are taken to be identical, making the length/width ratio of the central excitatory region equal to about 3 (taking the ends of that region to be the points at half-peak sensitivity).

Labeled? Yes (e.g., Davis et al., 1983; Graham et al., 1985; King-Smith & Kulikowski, 1981).

12.2.4 Spatial-Extent Analyzers (Two Dimensions)?

Multiple Analyzers? Probably not, near threshold. Although adaptation and summation experiments using stimuli of different spatial extent show selectivity on both spatial-extent dimensions (e.g., Kulikowski & King-Smith, 1973; Wright, 1982), this observed selectivity with stimuli of different spatial extents does not necessarily require multiple mechanisms of different spatial extents (sections 6.7.3 and 11.8.4). In fact, the success of the predictions for the spatial-extent summation experiments, assuming only mechanisms having different best spatial frequencies (although all of the same spatial extent) but allowing for independent variability in their outputs (see section 6.7.3), provides some evidence *against* the existence of multiple spatial-extents of mechanisms (multiple spatial-frequency bandwidths—near threshold, of course). For, if such mechanisms existed, they should have affected the predictions.

Bandwidth? The presumed spatial extent of a single mechanism has been described under spatial position above (assuming there are not different extents). The sensitivity of such a mechanism to stimuli of different spatial extents can be straightforwardly calculated and is monotonic with spatial extent.

Labeled? This question is not applicable.

12.2.5 Spatial-Phase Analyzers?

Multiple Analyzers? It is unclear whether there are multiple mechanisms near threshold. Few experiments have been done, and the interpretational difficulties (see sections 5.6 and 11.8.5) are great. On the other hand, I know of no good evidence against the existence of multiple spatial phases, and it is an attractive idea. If there is only a single spatial phase, which phase it is is not clear (although it is often assumed to be even-symmetric). So little near-threshold work has been done that some suprathreshold studies are given in the reference list, section 12.10.

Bandwidth? Computable from spatial weighting function (section 12.3.3).

Labeled? Unknown and/or not applicable.

12.2.6 Two Examples of Worked-Out Models and a Word About Modeling

In section 6.9, two different models of multiple analyzers on the spatial pattern dimensions are described in some detail. If one wishes to do some calculations of the outputs of low-level analyzers to spatial patterns, starting with either of these models is reasonable. On the other hand, when doing novel calculations one should always worry about the possible effects of changing some parameter's value. It is possible that a small change—well within the range consistent with available evidence—for example, might make large changes in the predictions for a novel situation. If calculations show this is so, of course, one is in the nice position of being able to test for the correct value of the parameter. (If changing the parameter value within the allowable range does not make a difference, one is in another nice position, that of not having to worry about the exact value of the parameter.)

12.3 ANALYZERS ON TEMPORAL DIMENSIONS

12.3.1 Broad-Band Temporal-Frequency Analyzers

Multiple Analyzers? There are no narrowly tuned temporal-frequency analyzers but probably several broadly tuned ones. In spite of the formal analogy between temporal frequency and spatial frequency and in spite of the similarity between the psychophysical contrast sensitivity functions on those two dimensions, results from analyzer-revealing experiments on those two dimensions are entirely different. (This difference should erase any fears that, in some artifactual way, sinusoids magically generate their own results.) The difference is easy to characterize: There is much less selectivity on the temporal-frequency dimension than on the spatial-frequency dimension. This is true for adaptation (e.g., Moulden, Renshaw, & Mather, 1984; Pantle, 1971; R. A. Smith, 1970, 1971), summation (Watson, 1977) and identification (Mandler & Makous, 1984; Thompson, 1983; Watson & Robson, 1981).

DIRECT COMPARISON OF SPATIAL-FREQUENCY AND TEMPORAL-FREQUENCY DISCRIMINATION. One study (Burbeck, 1981) directly compared spatial-frequency and temporal-frequency discriminations near threshold by finding the minimum contrasts at which a flickering grating (call its spatial and temporal frequencies, respectively, x c/deg and y c/sec) could be discriminated from (a) a blank field (0 c/deg) flickering at the same rate as the flickering grating (y c/sec), or (b) from a steady grating (0 c/sec) of the same spatial frequency as the flickering grating (x c/deg). (Burbeck called this the pattern or flicker threshold, respectively; but these two discrimination thresholds bear no necessary relationships to the appearance thresholds of the two types that we discuss elsewhere.) Perusal of the results show that, whenever $x = y$, the spatial-frequency discrimination between 0 and x c/deg [see (a) above] was always much easier (its contrast threshold much lower) than the temporal-frequency discrimination between 0 and y Hz [see (b) above]. In fact, the two discriminations were equally difficult only when y was much greater than x.

USE OF SPATIALLY APERIODIC STIMULI. Most temporal-frequency experiments have been done using spatially aperiodic stimuli, and thus are open to the interpretational problem illustrated in Fig. 11.3 middle column, where dimension A is spatial frequency and dimension B is temporal frequency. The temporal-frequency selectivity might be a by-product of the existence of multiple analyzers on the spatial-frequency dimension coupled with some interaction between temporal and spatial frequency (e.g., the analyzers sensitive to low spatial frequencies are quite sensitive to high as well as to low temporal frequencies, unlike the analyzers sensitive to high spatial frequencies).

Bandwidth? Some temporal-frequency experiments have, however, been done with spatial sinusoids (e.g., Bowker & Tulunay-Keesey, 1982; Thompson, 1983; Watson, 1977; Watson & Robson, 1981) and do seem to indicate more than a single analyzer at a single spatial frequency.

DISCREPANCY BETWEEN IDENTIFICATION AND ADAPTATION/SUMMATION. On the temporal-frequency dimension (in the typical low-to-middle spatial-frequency range), adaptation and summation experiments show *less* selectivity (almost none in fact) than do identification experiments. This discrepancy between identification experiments on the one hand and adaptation and summation experiments on the other is in the opposite direction from the discrepancy on the spatial-frequency dimension at high temporal frequencies (section 12.2.1). The reason for this discrepancy is not clear; the discrepancy is discussed further in section 12.5.

BROAD BANDWIDTH. Even the temporal-frequency identification results are consistent with very broad bandwidth temporal-frequency analyzers, however. Figure 12.1 shows the sensitivity functions of the three temporal-frequency analyzers used by Mandler and Makous (1984) to predict identification near threshold and various suprathreshold results; the lowest analyzer is lowpass, and the second and third have half-amplitude full-bandwidths of roughly three and two octaves, respectively. (The stimuli were spatially aperiodic, which, given the trade-off between spatial frequency and temporal frequency, is likely to have

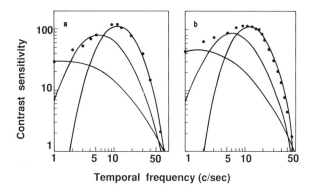

FIG. 12.1 Sensitivity as a function of temporal frequency for the three analyzers in Mandler and Makous' (1984) model. The filled symbols indicate detection thresholds. The two panels are for two different observers. (Figure 2 in Mandler & Makous (1984); used by permission.)

made these estimates of temporal-frequency bandwidths narrower than they should be, if anything.) The question of sustained (lowpass) versus transient (bandpass) analyzers is discussed at some length in note 2.

JOINT TEMPORAL-FREQUENCY SPATIAL-FREQUENCY SENSITIVITY. Temporal-frequency bandwidths seem to get somewhat broader at higher spatial frequencies according to adaptation (Bowker & Tulunay-Keesey, 1983) and identification (Thompson, 1983) results.

Even when adapt and test gratings drift at rather different rates, maximum threshold elevation is found in adaptation experiments when adapt and test spatial frequencies are very close or identical (Kelly & Burbeck, 1980; Tolhurst, 1973). Thus the analyzers are not "velocity analyzers," that is, are not sensitive to a narrow range of velocities over a rather broad range of spatial frequencies and temporal frequencies.

Figure 12.2 shows some candidate arrangements of analyzers' sensitivities on the spatial- and temporal-frequency dimensions. The solid diagonal line marks the line where spatial and temporal frequencies are equal, that is, where velocity equals 1 degree/second for drifting gratings. (The distinction between dashed and solid contours is discussed in sections 12.3.5 and 13.6.3.) Arrangement 4 (lower left) seems to be the most consistent with available experimental results (putting somewhat more weight on the identification than on the adaptation and summation results). The other arrangements suffer from various flaws:

Arrangement 1 (upper left) is clearly incorrect because it shows too little selectivity on the spatial-frequency dimension.
Arrangement 2 probably shows too little selectivity on the temporal-frequency dimension.
Arrangement 3 makes the roles of spatial frequency and temporal frequency quite symmetric, probably simultaneously producing too little selectivity on

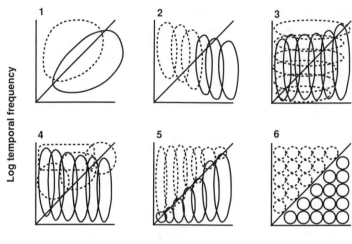

Log spatial frequency

FIG. 12.2 Six possible ways in which analyzers' selectivity for temporal frequency (vertical axis) and spatial frequency (horizontal axis) might be arranged. The straight line on the positive diagonal marks a temporal-frequency/spatial-frequency ratio of 1 degree/second. Each analyzer is represented by a constant-sensitivity contour. The contour is drawn with a dashed line if the analyzer is directionally selective and with a solid line if it is not. Note that the peak sensitivities of the analyzers are, unfortunately, not represented on this graph. Arrangement 4 is most consistent with evidence from near-threshold experiments.

the spatial-frequency dimension and too much on the temporal-frequency dimension. An adaptation experiment that could have confirmed this kind of arrangement strongly disconfirms it (Bowker & Tulunay-Keesey, 1983).

Arrangement 5 probably shows too clear a dividing line (too little overlap) between the two temporal-frequency analyzers at each spatial frequency.

Arrangement 6 (lower right) is clearly incorrect because it shows too much selectivity on the temporal-frequency dimension.

One adaptation study suggests that temporal-frequency selectivity at scotopic levels may be similar to that at photopic (Nygaard & Frumkes, 1985).

Labeled? Yes, temporal-frequency analyzers are labeled in the sense of producing uncertainty effects (Ball & Sekuler, 1980; Sekuler & Ball, 1977; Martens & Blake, 1980) and identification at detection threshold (reference above).

12.3.2   Temporal-Position Analyzers

Multiple Analyzers? Yes, multiple analyzers for temporal position; these are called *multiple elements* in the terminology here. That is, the selectivity for temporal position comes from the fact that a given mechanism (e.g., neuron) has different outputs at different moments in time rather than from literally separate mechanisms (e.g., neurons). All available near-threshold evidence indicates that there is selectivity for temporal position: (a) Two stimuli presented far apart in time do not sum completely in determining threshold, as has been shown in dozens of temporal-summation studies (e.g., Barlow, 1958; Rashbass, 1970; Watson & Nachmias, 1977); (b) an observer can identify at which of several relatively far-apart times a stimulus was presented (as is, in fact, taken for granted by the use of two-interval forced-choice paradigms); (c) uncertainty about temporal position causes a decrement in performance (e.g., Lasley & Cohn, 1981b).

Bandwidth? An element's sensitivity as a function of temporal position is identical to what we have been calling the temporal weighting function of a mechanism (which is closely related to its temporal impulse-response function; see Chap. 2). Summation experiments on both the temporal-frequency and temporal-position dimensions provide information about this function. The considerations necessary to estimate these temporal weighting functions accurately from psychophysical results are, in principle, analogous to those described for the spatial case in Chapter 6. However, the fact that there are only several broadband analyzers on the temporal-frequency dimensions, where there many narrow-band analyzers on the spatial-frequency dimension, has introduced differences in practice.

In fact, I know of only one estimate of temporal weighting functions from near-threshold psychophysical results that takes into account the possibility of multiple temporal-frequency analyzers. That is the estimate derived from the temporal-frequency sensitivity functions used by Mandler and Makous (1984) and shown in Fig. 12.1. Their broad temporal-frequency bandwidths imply temporal weighting functions that have only an excitatory phase (in the lowpass analyzer's case) or an excitatory phase followed by a minor inhibitory phase (in the case of the two- and three-octave temporal-frequency bandwidths of the analyzers centered at higher temporal frequencies). See note 2 for a discussion of lowpass (sustained) versus bandpass (transient) analyzers' temporal weighting functions and responses to a step of light.

Almost all the estimates of temporal impulse-response functions have assumed (usually implicitly) that there was only a single temporal-frequency analyzer (or only a single one at a given spatial frequency). Because the temporal-frequency bandwidths are so broad, you may not go too far wrong using this assumption.

DEPENDENCE ON MEAN LUMINANCE AND SPATIAL FREQUENCY. One estimation procedure based on this assumption is to find a temporal impulse-response function that has a Fourier amplitude characteristic consistent with the observer's sensitivity as a function of temporal frequency (e.g., Kelly 1971a, 1971b; Roufs 1972a, 1972b; Watson 1981, 1982b; Stork & Falk, 1987; Swanson, Ueno, Smith, & Pokorny 1987). To do so, you have to make some assumption about the phase characteristic. Figure 12.3 shows temporal-impulse response functions at two spatial frequencies (a uniform field—roughly 0 c/deg—and a flickering grating

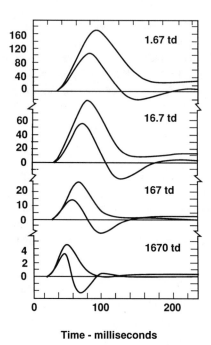

Time - milliseconds

FIG. 12.3 Each panel shows two temporal impulse responses—the monophasic one calculated from results for a counterphase square-wave grating at 3 c/deg and the lower more
oscillatory one from the results for a 7-degree-diameter uniform field. Each panel shows
impulse responses calculated at a different mean luminance (the vertical scales are different for each panel). (Figure 10 in Kelly (1971b); used by permission.)

at 3.5 c/deg). As mean luminance increases, the excitatory phase of the temporal-impulse response shortens and—for the higher of the two spatial frequencies—an inhibitory phase appears. A set of impulse-response functions at different mean luminances that is quite similar to those in Fig. 12.3 was used in a
model of light adaptation processes (Fig. 7, Sperling & Sondhi, 1968); it predicted quite successfully an observer's sensitivity both as a function of temporal
frequency and as a function of temporal extent (for spatially aperiodic stimuli).
The ways these estimated temporal-impulse response functions depend on mean
luminance and on spatial frequency reflect changes in the observer's sensitivity
as a function of temporal frequency; these will be discussed in the next chapter
(sections 13.6 and 13.9.4).

Since there seems to be more than a single temporal-frequency analyzer at a
given spatial frequency, the plots in Fig. 12.3 may show something more like the
upper envelope of the temporal weighting functions of the several analyzers.
Thus individual analyzer's sensitivity functions might show more dramatic
inhibitory phases than are shown here.

Temporal-impulse functions have also been estimated from temporal-position summation experiments. Figure 12.4 shows results of a temporal-position summation experiment (Watson & Nachmias, 1977) using two brief presentations of sinusoidal gratings separated by various amounts along the temporal-position dimension (i.e., there were various onset asynchronies). The results at the lower spatial frequencies (1.75 and 3.5 c/deg) are consistent with a biphasic temporal-impulse response function (and probability summation across temporal position) and those at higher spatial frequencies (7.0 and 10.5 c/deg) are consistent with a monophasic temporal-impulse response function (and probability summation across temporal position.

Several other kinds of experiments have shown the same kind of dependence as that shown in Figs. 12.3 and 12.4—at least qualitatively—of the presumed temporal-impulse response function on spatial frequency. These experiments include (a) sensitivity as a function of the temporal duration of a grating, which is a form of temporal-position summation experiment if one assumes the sen-

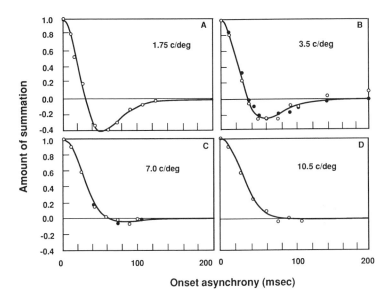

FIG. 12.4 Results of a summation experiment on the temporal-position dimension (Watson & Nachmias, 1977). The two stimuli were two brief exposures of a stationary grating where the time between the onsets of the two exposures is shown on the horizontal axis and the spatial-frequency of the grating is indicated separately for each panel. The amount of summation is indicated on the vertical axis here as a parameter z which comes from considering the full intensity-interrelationships functions. Intensity-interrelationship functions at relatively short onset asynchronies (where the value has not yet asymptoted in the figure here) are well fit by ellipses, and for these cases the summation index equals the square root of $(2 + 2z)$. For intensity-interrelationship functions at long-onset asynchronies, however, the quantity on the vertical axis here equals 0, but the summation index would be a great deal smaller than the square root of 2.0 (more like 1.1 or 1.2). See original paper for details. (Figure 3 in Watson & Nachmias, 1977; used by permission.)

sitivity at each moment in time is equal (many references in list in section 12.10); (b) the form of the distribution of reaction times to near-threshold gratings of different spatial frequency (Harwerth, Boltz, & Smith, 1980; Tolhurst, 1975a); (c) differences in sensitivity for stimuli with specially designed time courses (Gaussian windows versus biphasic blips, as in many studies by Hugh Wilson and his colleagues); ramped or other slow onsets versus abrupt onsets (Breitmeyer & Julesz, 1975; Tolhurst, 1975b; Tulunay-Keesey & Bennis, 1979); (d) interaction between temporal-extent and temporal-position summation experiment (a long-duration and a short-duration flash of grating at different onset asynchronies; Tolhurst, 1975b). Some peculiarities in the results of this latter experiment were also attributed to the existence of more than one temporal-frequency analyzer at a given spatial frequency.

Attempts at quantitative comparisons among the different results often lead to puzzling inconsistencies, but proper comparisons would require collecting the different kinds of results from the same observers in identical experimental conditions and analyzing the results with a full model of multiple mechanisms on many dimensions. Little of this has been done.

Labeled? Yes, outputs at different points in time are labeled in the sense of producing temporal-position uncertainty effects (e.g., Lasley & Cohn, 1981b) and allowing identification of temporal position (e.g., two-interval forced-choice paradigms).

12.3.3   Temporal-Extent Analyzers?

Possible selectivity for temporal extent has been relatively little studied, but one identification experiment reported some selectivity (Zacks, 1970). Interpreting the selectivity, however, runs into a problem analogous to that for spatial extent. Namely, such selectivity might well be due to mechanisms having sensitivites that vary along the temporal frequency and/or to outputs at different temporal positions. Some quantitative predictions will probably be necessary to untangle the answer.

12.3.4   Temporal-Phase Analyzers?

Possible selectivity for temporal phase has been little investigated. Were selectivity found in experiments using stimuli that vary in temporal phase, interpretation would run into problems analogous to those with spatial phase.

12.3.5   Direction-of-Motion Analyzers

Multiple Analyzers? Yes, multiple analyzers at high velocities; no multiple analyzers at low velocities. In experiments using near-threshold stimuli differing in direction of motion, direction selectivity is found at low spatial frequencies and high temporal frequencies (at high velocities for drifting stimuli). Little or no direction selectivity is found at high spatial frequencies and low temporal frequencies (at low velocities). The results of these experiments are displayed in Figs. 12.5, 12.6, and 12.7 with spatial frequency on the horizontal axis and temporal frequency on the vertical axis. Each closed circle shows a result in which there was no direction selectivity. Each open circle shows a result in which there was considerable direction selectivity. The studies from which these figures were compiled are listed in the figure legends. A fourth figure for uncertainty experiments could have been presented but would have shown only one point indicating direction-selective results found, with random dots moving at 4 degrees/second—this stimulus contains a wide range of spatial frequencies, orientations, and temporal frequencies (Ball & Sekuler, 1980; Sekuler & Ball, 1977).

As can be seen in the figures, there is a strong dependence on the ratio of temporal to spatial frequency (on velocity for drifting stimuli) with the boundary region between about 0.5 and 2 degrees/second. Nondirectionally selective

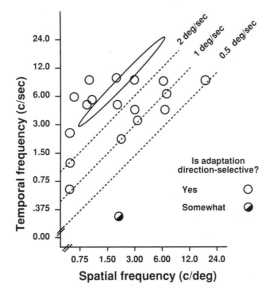

FIG. 12.5 Open symbols indicate that the threshold elevation after adaptation to a moving stimulus (at the spatial and temporal frequency indicated; test and adapt stimuli were identical in everything except direction) was found to be directionally selective, whereas half-filled symbols indicate only a little directional selectivity. Symbols are plotted at the spatial frequency and temporal frequency of the stimulus used. The long diagonal oval indicates a moving stimulus made of random dots (and thus containing many spatial frequencies and temporal frequencies) moving at 4 degrees/second. (The studies contributing points to this figure are: Levinson & Sekuler, 1975a, 1975b; Pantle, Lehmkuhle, & Caudill 1978; Pantle & Sekuler, 1968b, 1969; Sekuler & Ganz, 1963; Sekuler, Rubin, & Cushman, 1968; Sharpe & Tolhurst, 1973a, 1973b; Stromeyer, Madsen, & Klein, 1979; Stromeyer, Madsen, Klein, & Zeevi, 1978; Tolhurst, 1973; and Tolhurst & Hart, 1972.)

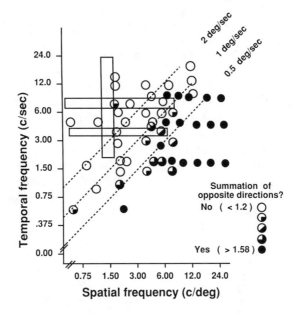

FIG. 12.6 Open (filled) symbols indicate that there was not (was) substantial summation between gratings drifting in opposite directions. The long horizontal (vertical) rectangles in this figure indicate that many spatial frequencies (temporal frequencies) were used in combination with the indicated temporal frequency (spatial frequency). Partially filled symbols indicate partial summation, as shown in the inset. (The studies contributing points to this figure are: Arditi, Anderson, & Movshon, 1981; Kulikowski, 1978; Levinson & Sekuler, 1975a; Murray, MacCana, & Kulikowksi, 1983; Stromeyer, Madsen, Klein, & Zeevi, 1978; and Watson, Thompson, Murphy, & Nachmias, 1980.)

results (closed circles) almost always occur at velocities below this boundary region, and directionally selective results (open circles) almost always occur at velocities above this boundary region. Using equal-velocity stimuli has usually shown some dependence on spatial frequency as well, however (e.g., Arditi, Anderson, & Movshon, 1981).

The role of eye movements in these experiments could be substantial, complicating interpretation considerably by making the temporal characteristics of the stimulus on the retina quite different from the ones specified by the experimenter. One identification experiment compared results for gratings (8 c/deg at 1.5 Hz) that were stabilized on the retina with those for unstabilized gratings and found no difference: observers were unable to identify direction of drift even for the stabilized gratings (Mansfield & Nachmias, 1981).

Dependence on spatial frequency and temporal frequency (on velocity) shows up in two other places described later (sections 12.7.2 and 13.6.3).

This division of the spatial-frequency/temporal-frequency plane into regions

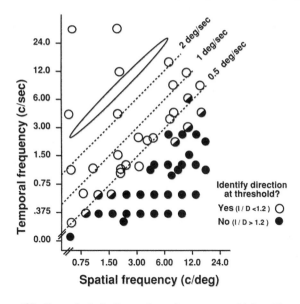

FIG. 12.7 Open (filled) symbols indicate that observers could (could not) identify the direction of motion of a grating at detection threshold. The long diagonal oval in this figure indicates a random-dot pattern moving at 4 degrees/second. (The studies contributing points to this figure are: Ball, Sekuler, & Machamer, 1983; M. Green, 1983; Hess & Plant, 1985; Lennie, 1980a; Mansfield & Nachmias, 1981; Thompson, 1984; and Watson, Thompson, Murphy, & Nachmias, 1980).

of direction selectivity versus nondirection selectivity is what is indicated by the dashed versus solid lines showing the analyzer contours in Fig. 12.2.

It is also interesting to note that, at high velocities, although the effect of adaptation on detection threshold is direction selective, its effect on the pattern-appearance threshold (see Chap. 13) seems not to be (Levinson & Sekuler, 1975a, p. 363; 1980). Further, the effect of adaptation on the pattern-appearance threshold may not be temporal-frequency selective either (Tolhurst, Sharpe, & Hart, 1973).

Bandwidth? At high velocities, an individual mechanism may be completely insensitive to the opposite direction; for example, the amount of summation between opposite directions at high velocities is typically that expected from probability summation between two nonoverlapping analyzers. On the other hand, since there are only two values on this direction-of-motion dimension, you cannot use values even further apart than opposite to help disambiguate the situation. And the small amounts of summation, confusability, and nondirectionally selective adaptation that are often found with opposite directions of motion might be due to individual analyzers' being somewhat sensitive to the unpreferred direction.

Using random-dot patterns rather than gratings, one infers an analyzer's sensitivity to 360 degrees worth of directions of motion, but this measure may be confounding orientation sensitivity with direction-of-motion sensitivity.

Labeled? Yes (at high velocities where direction selectivity is found), as indicated both by uncertainty effects and by good identification of near-threshold stimuli. The uncertainty effect for direction of motion (which has only been published for random-dot patterns to my knowledge) is much larger than that for other pattern dimensions (e.g., Ball & Sekuler, 1980). It is too large to be explained merely as selective monitoring and probabilistically independent noise, in fact, but requires postulating something like limited-capacity attention (e.g., some inability of the observer to monitor all mechanisms at once).

One unpublished study (by P. DeLucia and P. Kramer at Columbia University, New York) measured uncertainty effects with gratings moving in opposite directions at a high velocity (4 degrees/second velocity with a spatial frequency of 2.9 c/deg and a temporal frequency of 11.6 Hz; 600-millisecond exposure of the stimulus; other conditions like those in Kramer et al., 1985). This study found only small effects consistent with selective monitoring and probabilistically independent noise in two analyzers sensitive to opposite directions. Whether this smaller effect of uncertainty is due to using gratings rather than random-dot patterns (which would be somewhat unsettling to the independent-analyzers model—see note 3), to a difference in attention strategies (perhaps due to differences in instructions or observer expectations), or to some other factor is unclear.

12.3.6　Different Degrees of Direction Selectivity?

To decide whether analyzers having different degrees of direction selectivity exist or not would require a good deal of precision in these near-threshold experiments, perhaps more than is plausible. The existence of analyzers having different degrees of direction selectivity is certainly plausible, however. In fact, one of the earlier psychophysical adaptation studies suggested that both nondirectionally selective and completely directionally selective analyzers existed (where the two kinds are in series rather than in parallel). This suggestion was made to explain the finding that directionally selective threshold elevation saturated at a lower adapting contrast than does nondirectionally selective threshold elevation (Pantle & Sekuler, 1969.)

The suggestion has also been made that flickering gratings are detected entirely by nondirectionally selective analyzers, whereas drifting analyzers are detected by directionally selective ones (e.g., Wilson, 1985), a suggestion supported by measurements in visually normal and abnormal cats (Pasternak, 1986).

Much current work on motion perception uses suprathreshold patterns and is, therefore, beyond the scope of this book (e.g., Adelson & Bergen, 1985; Adelson & Movshon, 1981; Burt & Sperling, 1981; Morgan, 1980a, 1980b; Morgan

& Watt, 1983; Nakayama, 1985; Pantle & Picciano, 1976; van Santen & Sperling, 1984, 1985; Watson & Ahumada, 1985).

12.4 THE OTHER DIMENSIONS

12.4.1 Probably No Contrast Analyzers Near Threshold

To what extent—if there were analyzers selectively sensitive to different contrasts in any of the three ways mentioned earlier (section 11.6.5)—would interpreting the analyzer-revealing experiments on the contrast dimension be analogous to interpretations given in Chapters 3, 4, 7, and 9?

If analyzers desensitize after responding, adaptation to one contrast and testing at another might indeed reveal contrast analyzers of any of the above types. Although no one has reported any evidence of such selectivity when testing with contrasts near detection threshold, there is some evidence for analyzers (of type B above) when testing with suprathreshold contrasts (Blakemore, Muncey, & Ridley, 1971, 1973; Georgeson, 1985; Hertz, 1973).

Summation experiments (comparing the detectability of a compound with that of its components) on the contrast dimension reduce to parametric experiments on the contrast dimension, since a compound of the two simple stimuli is just another simple stimulus. As has been shown many times, the detectability of a simple visual pattern (its discriminability from a blank background of the same mean luminance) is always found to increase as contrast increases. Since this is what one expects whether or not there are contrast analyzers, this "summation" result is of no use in revealing contrast analyzers.

Uncertainty experiments might reveal analyzers in the near-threshold contrast range, if such analyzers can be selectively monitored. Since there appears to be no uncertainty effect for contrast, this is some evidence against contrast analyzers in the near-threshold range (Davis et al., 1983).

Identification experiments on the contrast dimension (contrast discrimination) were discussed briefly in section 10.8.2. Typical contrast discrimination results can be (and typically are) modeled as resulting from different magnitudes of output from the same analyzer(s) rather than as resulting from different analyzers. Thus these contrast discrimination results are of little use in deciding whether there are analyzers selectively sensitive to contrast.

12.4.2 Mean Luminance Analyzers?

Analyzers (e.g., single neurons) might certainly exist that are sensitive to different ranges of mean luminance in ways analogous to the three types on the contrast dimension (section 11.6.5). Indeed, rod-driven versus cone-driven systems would be such. However, on the basis of a very large amount of both physiological and psychophysical evidence, one must also presume that there are nonlinear light-adaptation processes quite early in the visual system that affect the response of any single pattern analyzer. Since using two patterns of very different mean luminances is sure to activate these early light-adaptation processes, interpreting any analyzer-revealing experiment on the mean-luminance dimension would require very careful reasoning to discount the effect of these early light-adaptation processes.

12.4.3　Analyzers on the Eye Dimension

Multiple Analyzers? Yes. Both adaptation and summation experiments show selectivity along this dimension: The phenomena known as *incomplete interocular transfer* and *incomplete binocular summation*. These results suggest the existence of multiple mechanisms that are differentially sensitive to inputs from the two eyes.

Bandwidth? Some analyzers apparently respond to both eyes, because partial interocular transfer is typically found (e.g., Blakemore & Campbell, 1969) and the amount of summation is somewhat greater than expected on the basis of probability summation between nonoverlapping analyzers. (The smallest summation index reported is typically about 1.4, substantially greater than that between far-apart spatial frequencies, for example).

The amount of summation between the two eyes is smallest for those spatial-frequency/temporal-frequency combinations where the amount of summation between opposite directions of motion is largest (high velocities; see Fig. 12.8).

Many joint experiments have been done involving the eye dimension (probably more than with any other dimension). In general, dichoptic summation experiments (joint experiments on the eye dimension and a second dimension) give the following result: If the monocular components of the dichoptic compound differ greatly along any one of a number of other dimensions (spatial frequency, orientation, spatial position, spatial phase, temporal phase, temporal position, direction of motion, and perhaps temporal frequency), the resulting dichoptic compound is only slightly more detectable than its monocular components (e.g., Arditi et al., 1981; Bacon, 1976; Blake & Levinson, 1977; Blake & Rush, 1980; M. Green & Blake, 1981). As the values get closer, sensitivity to the dichoptic compound in general increases.

Labeled? No. Although information about which eye produced which response is presumably used in stereopsis, information about which eye is connected to which mechanism seems to be lost upstream. Evidence for this statement comes from both the uncertainty and identification paradigms. Uncertainty about eye of origin does not decrease detectability (e.g., Cormack & Blake, 1980), nor can observers consistently identify eye of origin (particularly not at high spatial frequencies and low temporal frequencies—which is exactly the range where evidence for multiple analyzers from adaptation and summation experiments is strongest; e.g., Blake & Cormack, 1979b). The partial ability of

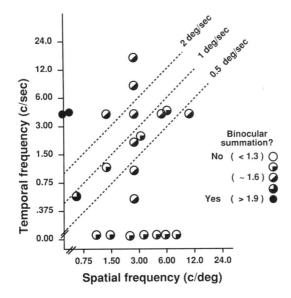

FIG. 12.8 Open (filled) symbols in this figure indicate that there was not (was) substantial summation between gratings stimulating different eyes. (The studies contributing points to this figure are: Arditi, Anderson, & Movshon, 1981; Blake & Cormack, 1979b; Blake & Levinson, 1977; and Lema & Blake, 1977.)

observer's to identify eye of origin that is sometimes reported may be due to other factors (Ono & Barbeito, 1985).

The eye dimension is thus the only dimension on which there is abundant evidence that results from the four kinds of near-threshold mechanism-revealing experiments are dissociated, with two kinds (adaptation and summation) showing selectivity and the other two (uncertainty and identification) not. This particular discrepancy seems reasonably explained by assuming that, although multiple analyzers exist, their outputs are not labeled. Indeed, if the labels used by an observer in identification and uncertainty experiments occur at some level "above" stereopsis (above the level at which the two eyes' outputs are used to compute the depth of objects), it would seem quite sensible to lose information about the eye of origin per se.

12.4.4 *Different Degrees of Monocularity/Binocularity?*

It requires a good deal of precision in near-threshold experiments on the eye dimension to be able to distinguish a multiplicity of bandwidths on the eye dimension (analyzers having different degrees of monocularity or, as is often said, "ocular dominance") from a model in which each analyzer is predominantly sensitive to one eye while partially sensitive to the other. However, experiments measuring not only binocular summation at threshold (for various contrast ratios in the two eyes—that is, measuring complete contrast interrelationship curves) but also the effect of adaptation to a monocular grating on the binocular summation contrast interrelationship plot do suggest a multiplicity of bandwidths on the eye dimension (Anderson & Movshon, 1986, who also studied the effect of masking with correlated and uncorrelated visual noise to support this suggestion), as does an experiment measuring discriminability between equally detectable although different binocular stimuli (e.g., increments in both eyes vs. an increment in one eye and a decrement in the other; Cohn, Leong, & Lasley, 1981).

12.5   ABOUT DISCREPANCIES BETWEEN IDENTIFICATION AND ADAPTATION/SUMMATION RESULTS

Three discrepancies between conclusions from different analyzer-revealing experiments were mentioned in the preceding summary.

On the eye dimension, identification experiments suggest no analyzers in situations where both adaptation and summation experiments suggest analyzers. This discrepancy is easily and naturally explained by assuming that the eye analyzers do not have labeled outputs (section 12.4.3).

On the spatial-frequency dimension, adaptation and summation experiments show only a little broadening of bandwidth as temporal frequency is raised, but identification experiments seem to show a large increase in bandwidth (section 12.2.1). If this discrepancy proves robust—for example, can be found with the same observers in the same conditions—one could explain this discrepancy by saying (in analogy with the explanation for the eye-dimension discrepancy) that, at high temporal frequencies (but not at low temporal frequencies) the narrowband spatial-frequency channels are not well labeled. Postulating unlabeled analyzers seems less natural here than on the eye dimension, however.

In any case, the third discrepancy—one on the temporal-frequency dimension—is in the wrong direction for this explanation. Adaptation and summation experiments show *less* selectivity for temporal frequency than do identification experiments (at least in the typical low-to-middle spatial-frequency range; section 12.3.1).

These so-called discrepancies depend, of course, on all the details of the models used to interpret the adaptation, summation, and identification experiments. And it seems likely that the cause of the second and third discrepancies is with the model used in interpreting identification results, in particular with the simple kind of decision rule used (e.g., the identity of the maximally responding mechanism). The substantial practice and instructional effects that are found in identification experiments (e.g., section 10.6.3) reinforce this not-very-surprising guess. One presumes that all levels of the visual system higher than these pattern analyzers are used for something more complicated than computing the simple decision rules (e.g., maximum output) adequate to quantitatively explain near-threshold behavior. Perhaps the only reason such simple rules work near threshold is that, near threshold, they happen to be near optimal (section 7.4.7).

12.6   CORRELATION AND INHIBITION

12.6.1   *Two Questions to Be Answered*

This section summarizes, for each dimension, the evidence available to answer the following two questions:

1. Probabilistic independence? If there are multiple analyzers on the dimension, are they probabilistically independent (uncorrelated)? (Are the outputs of any pair of analyzers uncorrelated over different presentations of the same stimulus? In still other words, are the noise sources in the two analyzers independent?)

Probabilistic independence among the outputs of different analyzers may show up as probability summation, in summation experiments—that is, sensitivity for a compound containing far-apart values is a little higher than that for either component (Chap. 4); the appropriate size of decrement in extrinsic uncertainty experiments (Chap. 7); and uncorrelated responses by the observer to the two component values in concurrent identification experiments (Chap. 10). Finding any of these effects will be taken as evidence for such probabilistic independence in the following summary.

2. Inhibition (or excitation) among analyzers? If there are multiple analyzers on the dimension, does one analyzer's output ever directly affect (excite or inhibit) another's? Or can each analyzer's expected output to a particular stimulus be computed directly as a function only of the stimulus parameters? The answer to this question is logically independent of the answer to question 1.

Support for the notion of inhibition among analyzers can come from finding—in adaptation, summation, uncertainty, or identification experiments—an effect when far-apart values are used that is the "opposite of" the effect found with very close values. By *opposite* is meant the other side of the baseline case where two stimuli affect two entirely different sets of analyzers and these analyzers do not interact in any way. The baseline depends on many features of the overall model and will not necessarily be the same as "zero" effect in the experiment. Although in adaptation experiments, for example, the baseline is zero so that the opposite effect is the lowering of thresholds after adaptation (e.g., K. De Valois, 1977b), in summation experiments the baseline is the small amount of summation expected from independent variability in separate analyzers (probability summation).

Another piece of evidence suggesting inhibition can come from finding that adapting to a compound stimulus produces less effect than adapting to one of its components (e.g., Levinson & Sekuler, 1975b; Tolhurst, 1972a).

The problem with all the evidence is that there are often reasonable alternative explanations not requiring inhibition (see sections 3.7, 3.8, 9.7.3, 10.3.2, 10.7). Further, the results themselves are often less robust (weaker and less replicable) than many of the other results reported here. Consequently, the psychophysical evidence to date for inhibition on any pattern-vision dimension is, in my opinion, not compelling. In the summary that follows, therefore, a tentatively affirmative answer given to the question about inhibition means only that effects have been reported at far values that are opposite to those at close values. It should not be taken to imply compelling evidence for inhibition.

12.6.2   Answers for Certain Dimensions

Answers are not given for the dimensions in the following list because evidence suggests there are not multiple analyzers on those dimensions and/or because no information is available: spatial extent, spatial phase, temporal frequency, temporal position, temporal extent, temporal phase, degree of direction selectivity, degree of monocularity, contrast, and mean luminance. For the other dimensions, the answers to the two questions just posed are as follows.

12.6.3   Spatial Frequency Analyzers

Probabilistic Independence? Yes, at least to a large extent (e.g., Hirsch et al., 1982; Sachs et al., 1971). See sections 4.7.7, 4.9.4, 4.9.5, 7.4.8, and 10.6.

Inhibition Among Analyzers? Maybe. Some opposite effects have been reported in adaptation experiments (e.g., K. De Valois, 1977b; Tolhurst & Barfield, 1978), in identification experiments (Graham et al., 1985; Hirsch et al., 1982; Olzak, 1981; Olzak & Thomas, 1981) and sometimes in summation experiments (Olzak & Thomas, 1981), but not always (Kramer, 1984). Further, adapting to a compound stimulus produces less adaptation than adapting to either component alone (e.g., Stecher et al., 1973b; Tolhurst, 1972a). See sections 3.7.1, 3.7.4, 3.7.9, 3.8.4, 4.9.7, 9.9.1, and 10.6.2.

12.6.4   Orientation Analyzers

Probabilistic Independence? Yes, apparently (e.g., Kelly, 1982a; Thomas & Gillie, 1979; and section 5.2.3).

Inhibition Among Analyzers? Maybe. Some opposite effects have been reported (e.g., Thomas & Shimamura, 1975; but see Thomas, 1985), although primarily using suprathreshold patterns. See sections 3.7.9 and 5.2.3.

12.6.5   Spatial Position Analyzers (Horizontal and Vertical)

Probabilistic Independence? Yes (e.g., King-Smith & Kulikowski, 1981; Robson & Graham, 1981; and section 5.4).

Inhibition Among Analyzers? Maybe. Some opposite effects have occasionally been reported at far values, but the difficulties in interpretation are numerous (e.g., Graham et al., 1985; H. Wilson et al., 1979).

12.6.6   Temporal-Position Analyzers

Probabilistic Independence? Yes (e.g., probability summation across time—Watson, 1979; Watson & Nachmias, 1977).

Inhibition Among Analyzers? Unknown.

12.6.7   Direction-of-Motion Analyzers

Probabilistic Independence? Probably yes. The directionally selective analyzers are presumably probabilistically independent (at low spatial and high temporal frequencies) because the amount of summation seen between opposite directions in a summation experiment is of the correct order of magnitude for probability summation (e.g., Watson et al., 1980), although that small amount of summation might also be explained by analyzers having some sensitivity to the opposite direction. (See similar discussion on eye dimension below.)

Inhibition Among Analyzers? Maybe (at high velocities). Although little information about possible "opposite" effects is available, the result of adapting to a compound has been reported to be less than that of adapting to a single component (Levinson & Sekuler, 1975b)

12.6.8   Analyzers on the Eye Dimension

Probabilistic Independence? Unclear. The question of whether there is independent variability is hard to answer on the eye-of-origin dimension. A compound pattern stimulating both eyes is always more detectable than either component, often by an amount that might be interpreted as due to independent variability in the two eyes, but usually by a somewhat greater amount than, for example, two far-apart spatial frequencies. As mentioned earlier, this and the partial interocular transfer suggest that most analyzers are somewhat sensitive to both eyes. (You cannot look at values even further apart than "left" vs. "right" to help disambiguate the situation, since there aren't any.) So all the partial summation seen between the two eyes could just as well be due to broadband analyzers having sensitivity to both eyes rather than due to independent variability. Unfortunately, one cannot look to uncertainty and identification experiments on this dimension to disambiguate the situation, since the analyzers do not appear to be labeled (section 12.4.3).

Inhibition Among Analyzers? Unclear for much the same reasons as the answer to the previous question is.

12.7   AN ASIDE ABOUT PHYSIOLOGY—SELECTIVE SENSITIVITY ALONG VISUAL PATTERN DIMENSIONS

Single neurons in the lower levels of the visual cortex (see sections 1.4 through 1.8) are candidates for the physiological substrate of the analyzers suggested by near-threshold psychophysical experiments. It is interesting to compare, therefore, the properties of cortical neurons and of these analyzers. This subsection contains a brief comparison of selectivity on each of the pattern dimensions. Earlier physiological asides (in sections 3.6.1, 3.6.2, 3.7.8, 5.4.4, and 8.7) have discussed transducer functions, selective adaptation, inhibition, probabilistic independence, and probability distributions. Some introductory physiology appeared in sections 1.4, 1.5, 1.6, and 1.7.

When statements in this section are not referenced, they are based on the following studies: Movshon, Thompson, and Tolhurst's (1978a, 1978b, 1978c) study of areas 17 and 18 in the cat cortex; R. De Valois, Yund, and Hepler's (1982) and R. De Valois, Albrecht, and Thorell's (1982) study of area V1 of the monkey; and K. Foster, Gaska, Nagler, and Pollen's (1985) study of areas V1 and V2 of the monkey. See also Schiller, Finlay, and Volman (1976a, 1976b, 1976c).

12.7.1   The Spatial Dimensions

Spatial Frequency. In the lowest levels of the visual cortex (in particular, areas 17 and 18 in the cat, V1 and V2 in the monkey), different cells are tuned to different narrow ranges of spatial frequency (even though sensitive to the same spatial position and orientation). The peak spatial frequencies of all the cells considered together cover almost all of the full visible range for each species (ranging from about 0.2 to 2.0 c/deg in the cat and from about 0.5 to 11 c/deg or greater in the monkey; the rest of the visible range is covered by cells peaking at the highest or lowest spatial frequency). The peak spatial frequencies in area 18 of the cat and area V2 of the monkey, however, tend to be lower (by a factor of 3 or 4) than those in 17 and V1, respectively.

Not only do cortical cells, like the inferred psychophysical analyzers, vary in the ranges along the spatial-frequency dimension to which they are sensitive (at the same spatial position and orientation), but some more subtle trends are also the same for cortical cells as for inferred psychophysical analyzers. The spatial-frequency bandwidth in octaves decreases somewhat at higher spatial frequencies at least in monkey area V1 (e.g., in the studies of De Valois and his colleagues, the average spatial-frequency bandwidth was about 2.2 octaves for cells having peak sensitivity at less than 0.7 c/deg and about 1.2 octaves for cells having peaks at greater than 11 c/deg). Also, the peak spatial frequency tends to be greater for cells sensitive to the fovea than to the parafovea. (Eccentricities were studied out to about 10 degrees in the cat; eccentricities concentrated within about a degree of foveal center and within a degree of the point 5 degrees out were studied in primates by De Valois and colleagues. Most cells were between 2 to 5 degrees from the fovea in the Foster et al. (1985) study of primates, but a small sample of foveal cells was also studied for comparison.)

Orientation. Cells in these low-level cortical areas are also tuned to different narrow ranges of orientation spanning the full 360 degrees (at the same spatial frequency and spatial position).

No information is given directly about variations in orientation bandwidth with peak spatial frequency. Judging from the overall high correlation (+0.5) between spatial-frequency and orientation bandwidth (in the monkey), however, it seems likely. An individual cell's sensitivity to orientation and spatial frequency is usually separable (Webster & De Valois, 1985).

Cells in area MT of the monkey, another cortical area receiving direct input from V1 (as does V2 and V3) are also known to exhibit orientation selectivity (as well as great direction selectivity). These MT neurons tend to respond best to peak spatial frequencies in the range from 0.5 to 5 c/deg.

Spatial Position. Different cortical cells are sensitive to different spatial positions (at the same orientation and spatial frequency), of course, as has been known for almost as long as single cells have been studied.

Spatial Extent. Although the evidence from near-threshold psychophysical experiments is, if anything, against the existence of multiple analyzers on the two spatial-extent dimensions, cortical neurons having different selectivities along these dimensions clearly exist. There are neurons having different spatial-frequency and orientation bandwidths but having the same best spatial frequencies, orientations, and spatial positions. Indeed, spatial-frequency bandwidths at one spatial frequency can vary over a couple of octaves (see references given at beginning of this section; also Mullikin, Jones, & Palmer, 1984). Orientation bandwidths can vary from 10 degrees to 100 degrees (the latter seen quite frequently), and there are some cortical cells that are nonselective for orientation.

One might argue that the narrowest bandwidth cells are those involved in the psychophysical detection experiments (and De Valois et al. do so), but available evidence suggests the argument cannot be based solely on absolute sensitivity, because the correlation between sensitivitiy and bandwidth seems slight.

R. De Valois and his colleagues based their argument on the fact that "orientation and spatial frequency sharpening appear to be the main activities which take place at the level of the striate cortex." Thus the narrow-bandwidth cells "appear to be the end product of striate processing," and it seems more reasonable to incorporate the mostly narrowly tuned cells (both in orientation and spatial frequency) into models of spatial vision. Taking the narrowly tuned subgroup (comprising the 31% of all cells that had both spatial-frequency and orientation bandwidths less than median) gave an average spatial-frequency bandwidth of 1.07 octaves and an average orientation bandwidth of 26 degrees.

Spatial Phase (Symmetry). The receptive fields of cortical simple cells have at least two different symmetries, as has been known since the earliest reports from Hubel and Wiesel and has been studied in some detail recently (Field & Tolhurst, 1986; J. Jones & Palmer, 1987a, 1987b; J. Jones et al., 1987; Pollen & Ronner, 1981).

12.7.2   The Temporal Dimensions

Temporal Frequency. The temporal-frequency sensitivity curves of different cortical cells do differ from one another but in subtler ways than do the spatial-frequency sensitivity curves. These more subtle differences correlate rather well with the differences among analyzers inferred from near-threshold psychophysics. The temporal-frequency sensitivity curves of neurons (e.g., Fig. 15 of Foster et al., 1985), however, may be somewhat more narrow band than those inferred from psychophysical near-threshold experiments (e.g., Fig. 12.1 here, but these are for spatially aperiodic stimuli).

Grouping cells from areas 17 and 18 in the cat or areas V1 and V2 in the macaque monkey together shows a relationship between peak spatial frequency and form of temporal sensitivity. The neurons sensitive to relatively high spatial frequencies tend to have lowpass temporal-frequency sensitivity functions (corresponding to sustained responses to an abrupt step stimulus as described in note 2); the cells sensitive to relatively low spatial frequencies tend to have bandpass temporal-frequency sensitivity functions (corresponding to transient step responses). More details are given in the original papers. There are some differences between the cat and the monkey, which is not surprising given the known differences in projections. For example, the LGN (lateral geniculate nucleus) projections go only to V1 in the monkey and from there to V2, whereas there is some direct projection of LGN Y cells to area 18 in the cat. (If anything, the absence of more differences is rather surprising. A much more dramatic species difference apparently does exist for direction selectivity, as is discussed below.)

The sensitivity functions of low-level cortical neurons on the spatial-frequency and temporal-frequency dimensions seem to be at least approximately separable (as defined in section 11.4) on those dimensions (e.g., Foster et al., 1985; Tolhurst & Movshon, 1975).

Temporal Position. A single neuron responds at more than one moment in time, and thus a single neuron's response at a given moment in time could well be the substrate for an "element" (an analyzer for temporal position). Indeed, it is hard to imagine how it could be otherwise.

Temporal Extent. Do neurons differ in the temporal extent of their impulse responses (equivalently, the bandwidth of their sensitivity to temporal frequencies) while still having same peak values on the temporal-frequency, spatial-frequency, and spatial-position dimensions? This question is a bit difficult to answer, since neurons' temporal-frequency sensitivity functions are quite broad and do change in shape (from lowpass to bandpass), which makes the exact value of the peak temporal frequency ambiguous. One might perhaps say that two neurons—one with a lowpass temporal-frequency sensitivity function and one with a bandpass function peaking at a medium temporal frequency (see examples in Fig. 15 of Foster et al., 1985, for example) are examples of two analyzers differing in temporal-frequency bandwidth (equivalently, differing in what value they are most sensitive to on the temporal-extent dimension).

Temporal Phase. The existence of different temporal phases (symmetries) of responses from neurons sensitive to the same values on other dimensions (in particular, spatial frequency, temporal frequency, and spatial position) has never been noted as far as I know.

Direction of Motion. The psychophysical evidence for analyzers very selective for direction of movement correlates with the observation reported by Hubel and Wiesel (1962)—and by many others since—that some cortical cells respond well to movement (for a given orientation of stimulus) in one direction but not to movement in the opposite direction (although other cells respond equally well to both directions). In this question of direction selectivity, however, there appears to be a very dramatic species difference that suggests caution in comparing any nonprimate results with human psychophysics. Direction selectivity seems much more pronounced in the cat cortex in general than in the monkey cortex. In the low levels of cortex, only 20 to 30% of monkey V1 cells are directionally selective (by the criterion that they respond twice as well or better to one direction than the opposite) but two thirds of cat area 17 cells are. More important than the overall percentage of directionally selective cells in primate V1 and V2, however, is their distribution within V1 and V2.

Neurons in primate V1 and V2 seem to be segregated into three distinct streams of information processing: (1) The M stream (so called because it receives input from the magnocellular division of the LGN); (2) the P-I stream (so called because it receives input from the parvocellular division of the LGN and contains the neurons in the regions known as "interblobs" in V1 and "interstripes" in V2); and (3) the P-B stream (because it also receives input from the parvocellular LGN but contains the neurons in the V1 "blobs"). According to current evidence (see the overview in DeYoe and Van Essen 1988 and references therein), the great majority of directionally selective V1 and V2 cells are in the M stream! (It is this stream that goes up the higher area MT and from there to parietal cortex as in Fig. 1.4.) There may be few or no directionally selective cells in either of the P streams. Orientation selectivity occurs in both the M stream and the P-I stream but not in the P-B stream. (The P streams go up to area V4 and hence to inferotemporal cortex as in Fig. 1.4.)

Little is known yet about the spatial-frequency and temporal-frequency selectivity of neurons in these three streams. (The studies referred to above have not

identified the locations of the neurons at that fine-grained a level.) But one wonders if the M stream neurons serve as the physiological substrate for the direc-
tionally-selective analyzers sensitive at high velocities (the "motion" analyzers
to use an older term) and the P-I stream for the nondirectionally selective analyzers sensitive at low velocities (the "pattern" analyzers). (The psychophysical
evidence for such analyzers is summarized in sections 12.3.1 and 12.3.5.) If one
considers together the cells in both areas V1 and V2 of the monkey, the cells
preferring higher velocities do tend to be most directionally selective (Foster et
al., 1985).

The higher level cortical area MT in the primate contains predominantly
directionally selective cells. The cells in MT seem to respond to the overall direction of movement of a two-dimensional plaid pattern (a pattern containing two
orientations of grating) rather than to the direction of its components, whereas
lower level cortical cells are known to respond to the direction of movement of
components of complex patterns (Movshon et al., 1984; K. De Valois, De
Valois, & Yund, 1979). Since the directionally selective effect of adaptation in
human psychophysics depends on the direction of the components rather than
on the overall pattern (Adelson & Movshon, 1981), the low-level V1 or V2 neurons rather than the higher level MT neurons may be the substrates for the directionally selective analyzers of near-threshold psychophysics.

Degree of Directional Selectivity. As already stated, neurons in the primate
(and cat) low-level cortex differ a good deal from one another in how directionally selective they are, with some not being directionally selective at all.

12.7.3   The Other Dimensions and Miscellaneous Properties

Contrast. Section 1.9.1 discusses the possibility that neurons with different
sensitivites along the contrast dimension exist.

Mean Luminance. I know of no evidence that some cortical neurons respond
to contrast variation only at some mean luminances and not at others (as they
might if they were totally rod driven or totally cone driven, for example).

Eye and Degree of Monocularity. It has been known since Hubel and Wiesel
that low-level cortical neurons differ from one another in whether they are
responsive to the left eye, the right eye, or various proportions of both (various
degrees of monocularity or ocular dominance), which is quite consistent with
near-threshold psychophysics. Recent studies attempt to understand the mechanism of the summation between the two eyes (e.g., Ohzawa & Freeman, 1986a,
1986b; Skottun & Freeman, 1984).

Linearity. Simple Versus Complex Cells. The spatial (and temporal) tuning
characteristics of simple and complex cells are very similar (e.g., Foster et al.,
1985) and both simple and complex cells tend to respond to the harmonic content of certain complicated patterns as a completely linear system would (e.g.,

Albrecht & De Valois, 1981; K. De Valois et al., 1979; Pollen & Ronner, 1982). Their linearity characteristics are actually very different, however. (Note that, although the prototypical simple and complex cells are indeed very different, many simple and complex cells share more characteristics than is sometimes thought. See, for example, Dean & Tolhurst, 1983.) Simple cells are indeed very linear (at a constant mean luminance), although some exhibit some nonlinear spatial summation (e.g., Tolhurst & Dean, 1987): complex cells are not linear. The nonlinearity of complex cells may involve a summation of rectified outputs from other more linear cells (B. Andrews & Pollen, 1979; R. De Valois, Albrecht, & Thorell, 1982; Pollen & Ronner, 1982; Hochstein & Spitzer, 1985; Movshon, Thompson, & Tolhurst, 1978a, 1978b; Spitzer & Hochstein, 1985a, 1985b). Presumably, therefore, simple and complex cells play rather different roles in visual information processing.

Linearity (The Transducer Function). Discussed in sections 1.9.4 and 3.6.1.

Inhibition. Discussed in sections 1.9.4 and 3.7.8.

Variability. Discussed in sections 1.9.4, 5.4.4, and 8.7.

Adaptability. Discussed in sections 1.9.4 and 3.6.2.

12.8 SUMMARY

Results from the four kinds of near-threshold analyzer-revealing psychophysical experiments were summarized in this chapter, dimension by dimension.

These results can be explained by assuming that analyzers selectively sensitive to different ranges of value and having labeled outputs exist along four of the spatial dimensions—spatial-frequency, orientation, and two spatial-position dimensions.

For the spatial-extent dimensions, there is no evidence from these experiments for multiple analyzers and some evidence against them.

For the spatial-phase dimension, there is little if any evidence from these experiments that can answer the question of whether multiple analyzers exist.

For the temporal-frequency dimension (at any fixed spatial frequency and fixed spatial position), the results suggest that there are not narrowly tuned analyzers but there may be several broadly tuned ones and their outputs may be labeled.

For the temporal-position dimension, the experimental results (which are analogous to those on the spatial-position dimension) are explained by assuming that each mechanism's output at a particular time depends on the recent past and is labeled.

For the temporal-extent and temporal-phase dimensions, there is little information available and/or applicable.

For the direction-of-motion dimension, the results at high velocities are consistent with analyzers that have labeled outputs and are sensitive to one direction but not its opposite. At low velocities, however, there is less direction selectivity. It is not clear from these results whether, at any particular spatial-frequency and temporal-frequency values, analyzers exist having different degrees of direction selectivity.

For the eye-of-origin dimension, although the results are consistent with analyzers differentially sensitive to the two eyes, the outputs of these analyzers are not labeled. It is not clear from these results whether analyzers differing in degree of monocularity exist.

Neurons in cortical areas V1 and V2 in the monkey (17 and 18 in the cat) do show selective sensitivities that agree quite well with the more definitive conclusions about analyzers inferred from near-threshold psychophysical experiments, namely, the conclusions about spatial-frequency, orientation, spatial-position, temporal-frequency, direction-of-motion, and eye.

In addition, these physiological results show multiple spatial-frequency and orientation bandwidths (multiple spatial-extent analyzers)—which is in some disagreement with properties of analyzers inferred from near-threshold psychophysics—as well as multiple analyzers on several dimensions about which near-threshold psychophysics has little to say: symmetries of receptive fields (the more interesting kind of spatial-phase channel), degrees-of-direction selectivity, and multiple degrees of monocularity.

12.9   DESCRIPTION OF LIST OF REFERENCES TO ANALYZER-REVEALING EXPERIMENTS

The last section of this chapter (section 12.10) is an organized list of references to analyzer-revealing experiments in pattern vision. The last portion of Chapter 13 is a similar list for parametric experiments. These lists give only authors and years. The full citation is given in the bibliography at the end of the book.

The pattern dimensions and miscellaneous factors will be used in these lists in the standard order shown in Table 12.1, where they will be referred to frequently by number rather than name (to save space).

12.9.1   Organization by Pattern Dimension

There are 13 major sections of the list corresponding to the first 13 rows of Table 12.1; each major section lists studies done on one (or sometimes two) of the pattern dimensions.

The headings used in the list are illustrated in Table 12.2 and are described here. The top-level headings dividing the chapter into 13 major sections begin with a number, indicating the dimension in question (followed by decimal point and zero) and are capitalized (e.g., **1.0** SPATIAL-FREQUENCY EXPERIMENTS at the beginning of the example in Table 12.2.)

TABLE 12.1. Standard Order of Pattern
Dimensions and Miscellaneous Factors

Number	Dimension or Factor
1	Spatial frequency
2	Orientation
3	Spatial position (two dimensions)
4	Spatial extent (two dimensions)
5	Spatial phase
6	Temporal frequency
7	Temporal position
8	Temporal extent
9	Temporal phase
10	Direction of motion (two dimensions)
11	Contrast
12	Mean luminance
13	Eye of origin (two dimensions)
14	Viewing distance/accommodation
15	Psychophysical procedure
16	Eye movements/stabilizing image
17	Age, species, pathology of observer
18	Color

TABLE 12.2. Example of Headings Used in Reference List

1.0 SPATIAL-FREQUENCY EXPERIMENTS
1.1 Spatial frequency as auxiliary
1.1a Adaptation
　　Appearance threshold
　　Facilitation at far-away values
1.1b Summation
1.1c Uncertainty
1.1d Identification

1.2 Orientation as auxiliary
1.2a Adaptation
1.2c Uncertainty

1.2′ Joint spatial frequency and orientation
1.2′a Adaptation
　　Two-dimensional patterns
1.2′d Identification

Each of the 13 major sections of the table is divided into subsections by second-level headings that indicate an auxiliary or joint dimension. Again, the auxiliary or joint dimensions are gone through in the standard order of Table 12.1. (Second-level headings under which there would be no entries, however, are omitted.) Examples are "**1.2** Orientation as Auxiliary" and "**1.2′** Joint Spatial Frequency and Orientation" in Table 12.2. The numbers to the left and right of the decimal point indicate the experimental and auxiliary/joint dimensions respectively. The prime after a number (e.g., 1.2′ in the example) is used to distinguish cases where one dimension is actually an auxiliary dimension (no prime) from cases where an experiment was done jointly on two dimensions (with a prime).

The third-level headings indicate the type of experiment. They begin with the numbers indicating experimental and auxiliary/joint dimensions followed by a letter a, b, c, or d indicating adaptation, summation, uncertainty, or identification, respectively.

Occasionally other information (e.g., distinguishing between kinds of stimuli used in a type of experiment) appears in a fourth-level heading, which is lowercase and indented four spaces from the left margin.

Still other information is occasionally added as a parenthetical comment after the reference.

12.9.2   Notes About Conventions in List

Auxiliary Dimensions. In some cases, the studies listed under an auxiliary dimension did not actually vary the value on the auxiliary dimension but instead used a value on the auxiliary dimension that is different from that used by the majority of experiments. Thus, comparing the listed study with other studies will provide information about the effect of value on the auxiliary dimension on results from the experimental dimension. (These comparisons should be treated with caution, of course, since not only did value on the auxiliary dimension but also observers and frequently many other factors differed between the experiments.)

When the Experimental and Auxiliary Dimension Are the Same. Studies that have systematically explored various parts of the dimension under consideration (giving information about bandwidth in different parts of that dimension for example) and/or did not use any other auxiliary dimension are listed under the second-level heading having the same dimension as the top-level heading, for example, "**1.1** Spatial Frequency as Auxiliary" under the top-level heading **1.0** SPATIAL-FREQUENCY EXPERIMENTS. This produces some awkwardness. If I had it to do over again I would probably choose another convention, in particular, putting all these studies at the beginning of the main section.

Appearance Thresholds. Studies measuring appearance thresholds rather than detection thresholds are indicated by a fourth-level heading or a parenthetical comment. In some cases marked "appearance thresholds," the two kinds of appearance thresholds were not explicitly measured, but sufficient information is given about the appearance of the patterns at detection threshold that one knows whether the measured detection thresholds were equivalent to spatial or to temporal appearance thresholds.

Joint Experiments. The second-level heading "Joint dimension A and dimension B" will appear twice, once under the top-level heading DIMENSION A EXPERIMENTS and once under the top-level heading DIMENSION B EXPERIMENTS. The references will be given only under the first listing, however, and the second listing will simply direct the reader back to the first.

Embedded Auxiliary Dimensions. Even more occasionally, a study may suggest an embedded dependence (that is, a second auxiliary dimension's effect on a first auxiliary dimension's effect on the experimental dimension).

Color. This heading includes both studies varying the wavelength of monochromatic stimuli and studies using isoluminant wavelength-varying stimuli.

Increments/Decrements. The difference between increments and decrements could be considered a difference of spatial phase or temporal phase (or contrast if negative contrasts are allowed). Most are listed under "temporal phase," although some are under "spatial phase."

Aperiodic Stimuli. Studies varying the spatial or temporal extent of aperiodic stimuli are listed under the spatial-extent and temporal-extent dimensions, respectively (although, as discussed in the text, their values on the frequency and position dimensions were also being varied significantly).

Reanalyses. Articles that have analyzed experimental results from other studies are listed along with the original studies.

12.9.3 Disclaimers and Cautions

This list is certainly not exhaustive, as I did no systematic literature search after deciding to make such a list. Rather I worked from my notes (which had been made with other purposes in mind), because the time involved in going back to the original literature was prohibitive. Such a procedure undoubtedly introduced errors of omission and of misplacement. I apologize for errors introduced this way or any other.

Certain factors (in particular 14, 17, and 18) are rather sparsely covered.

Occasionally an article I wanted to include did not fit logically into any category. So I inserted it into some not too unreasonable category.

A number of the articles in this list reach conclusions different from those I have given in my text. In such cases, I have generally decided that the apparent discrepancy—if not the result of noisy data—was the result of one of the factors described elsewhere in the text. Some discrepancies I cannot resolve remain, however; the ones that seemed most important to me are discussed in the text.

12.10   REFERENCES TO ANALYZER-REVEALING EXPERIMENTS

1.0 SPATIAL FREQUENCY EXPERIMENTS

1.1 Spatial frequency as auxiliary

1.1a Adaptation

Blakemore and Campbell 1969
Bowker and Tulunay-Keesey 1983
Burton 1973
Cavanagh 1978
De Valois 1977
Georgeson and Harris 1984
Graham 1972
Jones and Tulunay-Keesey 1975
Movshon and Blakemore 1973
Pantle and Sekuler 1968a
Regan and Beverly 1983
Stromeyer, Klein, Dawson, and Spillman 1982
Swift and Smith 1982
Tolhurst 1973
Wilson and Regan 1984

Appearance threshold
Tolhurst 1973

Facilitation at far-away values
De Valois 1977b
Tolhurst and Barfield 1978
Williams and Wilson 1983
Williams, Wilson, and Cowan 1982

Compound-stimulus adapting effect
Klein and Stromeyer 1980
Nachmias, Sansbury, Vassilev, and Weber 1973
Stecher, Sigel, and Lange 1973b
Tolhurst 1972a
Tolhurst and Barfield 1978

Missing-fundamental adapting stimulus:
Greenlee and Magnussen 1987
Levinson in Sekuler 1974 p. 217

Afterimages
Burbeck and Kelly 1984
Corwin, Volpe, and Tyler 1976
Koenderink 1972
Leguire and Blake 1982
Long and Kling 1983
Virsu and Laurinen 1979

1.1b Summation

Arend and Lange 1979, 1980
Bergen, Wilson, and Cowan 1979
Blake and Levinson 1977

Graham and Nachmias 1971
Graham and Robson 1987
Graham and Rogowitz 1976
King-Smith and Kulikowski 1975a
Kramer, Graham, and Yager, 1985
Kulikowski and King-Smith 1973
Pantle 1973
Quick and Reichert 1975
Quick, Mullins, and Reichert 1978
Ross and Johnstone 1980
Sachs, Nachmias, and Robson 1971
Stecher, Sigel, and Lange 1973
Stromeyer and Klein 1975
Watson 1982a, 1983

With narrowband noise
Kersten 1987
Mostafavi and Sakrison 1976

Very low spatial frequencies
Wilson 1980
Bergen, Wilson, and Cowan 1979

When compound is square-wave, sawtooth, aperiodic, etc:
Campbell, Carpenter, and Levinson 1969
Campbell and Robson 1964, 1968
Campbell, Howell, and Johnstone 1978
Campbell, Johnstone, and Ross 1981
Green, Corwin, and Schor 1981
Jaschinski-Kruza and Cavonius 1984
Kulikowski and King-Smith 1973
MacLeod and Rosenfeld 1974
Shapley and Tolhurst 1973

Effect of adaptation on summation
Lange, Sigel, and Stecher 1973

1.1c Uncertainty

Cormack and Blake 1980
Davis 1981
Davis and Graham 1981
Davis, Kramer, and Graham 1983
Graham, Robson, and Nachmias 1978
Kramer, Graham, and Yager 1985
Sekuler and Tynan 1978
Yager, Kramer, Graham, and Shaw 1984

1.1d Identification

Barker 1979
Furchner, Thomas, and Campbell 1977
Graham, Kramer, and Haber 1985

Hirsch, Hylton, and Graham 1982
Klein 1985
Lennie 1980
Nachmias 1974
Olzak 1985
Olzak 1986
Olzak and Thomas 1981
Olzak and Wickens 1983
Thomas, Gille, and Barker 1982
Thomas and Gille 1979
Thomas 1983, 1985
Watson and Robson 1981
Wilson and Gelb 1984
Yager, Kramer, Graham, and Shaw 1984

1.2′ Joint spatial frequency and orientation

1.2′a Adaptation

Blakemore and Nachmias 1971

Two-dimensional patterns (e.g., checkerboards, random dots, geometric figures)
De Valois and Switkes 1980
Green 1980
Vassilev 1973
Wright 1982

1.2′d Identification

Barker 1978

1.3 Spatial position as auxiliary

1.3a Adaptation

Peripheral
Sharpe and Tolhurst 1973b
Rose 1983

1.3b Summation

Graham, Robson, and Nachmias, 1978
Graham and Robson 1987
Limb and Rubenstein 1977

1.3d Identification

Thomas 1987

1.4 Spatial extent as auxiliary

1.4a Adaptation

Tolhurst 1973 (lowest adaptable)
Bowker and Tulunay-Keesey 1983

1.4b Summation

Vary effective extent by varying retinal position:
Graham and Robson 1987

1.4d Identification

2 × 2 paradigm
Thomas, Gille, and Barker 1982
Watson 1983

1.4′ Joint spatial frequency and spatial extent

1.4′a Adaptation

Varying spatial extent of aperiodic stimuli
Bagrash, 1973
Heeley (1978) Ch. 7
Legge, 1976
Sullivan, Georgeson, and Oatley 1972

1.5′ Joint spatial frequency and spatial phase

1.5′a Adaptation

Jones and Tulunay-Keesey 1980

1.5′b Summation

Graham and Nachmias 1971
Graham, Robson, and Nachmias 1978
Henning, Derrington, and Madden 1983
Ross and Johnstone 1980
Wilson 1980a

1.6 Temporal frequency as auxiliary

1.6a Adaptation

Bowker and Tulunay-Keesey 1983
Graham 1972
Tolhurst 1973

Appearance thresholds
Green 1981
Harris 1986

Shadows of retinal blood vessels
Sharpe 1972

1.6b Summation

Pantle 1973
Thompson 1981
Wilson 1980

1.6d Identification

Burbeck 1981
Watson and Robson 1981

1.6′ Joint spatial frequency and temporal frequency

1.6′a Adaptation

Not velocity channels
Tolhurst, 1973, Fig. 4
Kelly and Burbeck 1980, Fig. 7

Adapt to 'frequency-doubled' stimulus
Parker 1981
Thompson and Murphy, 1980

1.7 Temporal position as auxiliary

1.7a Adaptation

Experiments varying delay between adapt and test stimuli are in section 7.7 of this list

1.7′ Joint temporal frequency and temporal position

1.7′b Summation

Watson and Nachmias 1980
Limb 1981
Watson 1981

1.8 Temporal extent as auxiliary

1.8a Adaptation

Experiments varying temporal extent of adapting stimulus are listed in section 8.

1.8b Summation

Arend and Lange 1979a
Green, Corwin, and Schor 1981

1.8d Identification

Gorea 1986

1.10′ Joint spatial frequency and direction of motion

1.10′a Adaptation

Tolhurst 1973

1.11 Contrast as auxiliary

1.11a Adaptation

Contrast of adapting stimulus
Blakemore and Campbell 1969
Dealy and Tolhurst 1974
Georgeson and Harris 1984
Graham 1972
Stecher, Sigel, and Lange 1973a
Swift and Smith 1982

Contrast of test stimulus
Stromeyer, Klein, and Sternheim 1977
Williams and Wilson 1983

1.12 Mean luminance as auxiliary

1.12a Adaptation

Graham 1972

1.12b Summation

Early ones done at lower values than later

1.13 Eye-of-origin as auxiliary

1.13a Adaptation

Many studies binocular

Monocular
Sharpe and Tolhurst 1973b

Rivalrous adapting stimuli
Blake and Fox, 1974a

Dichoptic adapting stimuli
Ruddock, Waterfield, and Wigley 1979

1.13′ Joint spatial frequency and eye-of-origin

1.13′a Adaptation

Bjorklund and Magnussen 1981

1.13′b Summation

Bacon 1976
Blake and Levinson 1977

1.14 Effect of viewing distance

1.14a Adaptation depends on retinal not distal spatial frequency:

Blakemore, Garner, and Sweet 1972

1.15 Effect of psychophysical procedure

3.0 SPATIAL POSITION EXPERIMENTS (2 DIMENSIONS)

3.1 Spatial frequency as auxiliary

3.1a Adaptation

Ejima and Takahashi 1984, 1985
Perizonius, Schill, Geiger, and Rohler 1985

3.1b Summation

Vary number of cycles in grating
Anderson and Burr 1987
Estevez and Cavonius 1976
Glezer and Kostelyanets 1975
Hoekstra, van der Goot, van den Brink, and Bilsen 1974
Hess and Howell 1978a
Jamar, Kwakman, and Koenderink 1984
Kelly 1984b
Kersten 1984
Koenderink, Bouman, De Mesquita, and Slappendel 1978
Kroon, Rijsdijk, and van der Wildt 1980
Kroon and van der Wildt 1980
Legge 1978b
Mayer and Tyler 1986
McCann, Savoy, Hall, and Scarpetti 1974
Robson and Graham 1981
Savoy and McCann 1975

Vary length of bars in gratings
Bacon and King-Smith 1977
Howell and Hess 1978
Kulikowski 1966, 1969
Wright 1982

Vary width of sharp versus soft-edged bars
Shapley 1974

3.3 Spatial position as auxiliary

3.3a Adaptation

Perizonius, Schill, Geiger, and Rohler 1985

Facilitation at far-apart values
Ejima and Takahashi 1984, 1985

3.3b Summation

Patches of grating at different positions
Cannon and Fullenkamp 1987

Halter in Mostafavi and Sakrison 1976
Mayer and Tyler 1986

Aperiodic stimuli at different spatial positions
Blommaert and Roufs 1981
Bouman and van den Brink 1952
Cohn and Lasley 1975
Fiorentini 1972
Glezer, Kostelyanets, and Cooperman 1977
Hines 1976
King-Smith and Kulikowski 1975a,b
Kulikowski and King-Smith 1973
Limb and Rubenstein 1977
Rentschler and Fiorentini 1974
Sakitt 1971
Wickelgren 1967
Wilson 1978a,b
Wilson and Bergen 1979
Wilson, Phillips, Rentschler and Hilz 1979

Vary number of cycles or length of bars in grating
Listed in 3.1

Varying spatial extent of aperiodic stimuli
Barlow 1958
Blackwell 1963
Blommaert and Roufs 1981
Graham, Brown, and Mote 1939
Kincaid, Blackwell, and Kristofferson 1960
Lie 1980, 1981
Thomas 1970, 1978
Wilson 1970
Wilson 1978b
Wilson and Bergen 1979

Classical 'areal summation'

3.3b' Effect of adaptation on summation

Vary number of cycles
Williams and Wilson 1983

3.3c Uncertainty

With grating patches
Cormack and Blake 1980 (mention)
Davis, Kramer, and Graham 1983

With aperiodic stimuli
Barlow, Kaushal, Hawken, and Parker 1987
Cohn and Lasley 1974
Cohn and Wardlaw 1985

4.4 Spatial extent as auxiliary

4.4a Adaptation

Bar length
Burton and Ruddock 1978
Nagshineh and Ruddock 1978
Nakayama and Roberts 1972
Wright 1982

Number of cycles in test grating (adapt large)
Williams and Wilson 1983

4.4b Summation

Two aperiodic stimuli of differing spatial extents
Bagrash, Kerr and Thomas 1971
Thomas and Kerr 1971
Thomas, Bagrash, and Kerr 1969
Thomas, Padilla, and Rourke 1969
Thomas 1970

Aperiodic + sine (perhaps masking rather than summation)
Graham 1977, 1980
Hauske 1981
Hauske, Wolfe, and Lupp 1976
Kulikowski and King-Smith 1973
Shapley and Tolhurst 1973

4.4c Uncertainty

Spatially aperiodic stimuli of differing spatial extents
Howarth and Lowe 1966

4.4d Identification

Spatially aperiodic stimuli of different spatial extents
Bagrash, Thomas, and Shimamura 1974
Thomas 1985
Thomas, Gille, and Barker 1982
Thomas and Shimamura 1974
Watson 1983

4.5' Joint spatial extent and spatial phase

4.5'b Summation

Kulikowski and King-Smith 1973
Shapley and Tolhurst 1973

4.13' Joint spatial extent and eye-of-origin

4.13'a Adaptation

Fiorentini, Sireteanu, and Spinelli 1976

4.17 Pathology of observer

4.17b Summation

Vary extent of stationary grating
Hess and Campbell 1980 (amblyopes)

5.0 SPATIAL PHASE EXPERIMENTS

5.1 Spatial frequency as auxiliary

5.1a Adaptation

Jones and Tulunay-Keesey 1980

5.1c Uncertainty

Gratings masked by noise
Kersten 1982

5.1d Identification

Tyler and Gorea 1986

5.1' Joint spatial phase and spatial frequency

Listed in 1.5'

5.5 Spatial phase as auxiliary

5.5a Adaptation

Stationary gratings
Bowker and Tulunay-Keesey 1983
Smith 1977

Flickering gratings
Jones and Tulunay-Keesey 1980
Stromeyer, Klein, Dawson, and Spillman 1982

Black versus white bars
De Valois 1977
Georgeson and Reddin 1981

Compound gratings (relative phase of components)
Tolhurst 1972

5.5c Uncertainty

Kersten 1983

Gratings masked by noise
Burgess and Ghanderian 1984
Howard and Richardson 1988
Kersten 1982, 1983

Drifting gratings
 Pantle and Sekuler 1968b
 Tolhurst, Sharpe, and Hart 1973

Facilitation at far-away values
 Bowker and Tulunay-Keesey 1983

Appearance thresholds
 Tolhurst, Sharpe and Hart 1973

6.6b Summation

Flickering spatially aperiodic stimuli
 Bergen and Wilson 1985
 Levinson 1959, 1960, 1964

Complex temporal waveforms
 See summary in C. Graham 1966 p.
  277–288

Flickering gratings
 Watson 1977, 1979

Comparing flickering or drifting to on-off gratings
 Kulikowski 1971a
 Kulikowski and Tolhurst 1973 (also
  appearance thresholds)
 Sharpe and Tolhurst 1973b

6.6c Uncertainty

Varying velocity of random-dot patterns
 Ball and Sekuler 1980 (Exp. 7)
 Sekuler and Ball 1977

6.6d Identification

Flickering spatially aperiodic
 Mandler and Makous 1984

Gratings
 Hess and Plant 1985
 Rothblum 1982
 Thompson 1981, 1983, 1984
 Watson and Robson 1981

6.10′ Joint temporal frequency and direction of motion

6.10′a Adaptation

 Pantle and Sekuler 1968

6.10′b Summation

 Blake and Rush 1980 (also with aux. =
 sp. freq)

6.12 Mean luminance as auxiliary

6.12a Adaptation

 Nygard and Frumkes 1985—scotopic

6.13′ Joint temporal frequency and eye of origin

6.13′a Adaptation

 Moulden, Renshaw, and Mather 1984

6.14 Effect of optics

 Charman and Walsh 1985

6.16 Effect of eye movements

6.16a Adaptation

 Tolhurst and Hart 1972

6.17 Effect of species of observer

6.17c Uncertainty

 Martens and Blake 1980 (gratings)

7.0 TEMPORAL POSITION EXPERIMENTS

7.1 Spatial frequency as auxiliary

7.1b Summation

Vary duration of stationary gratings
 Arend 1976b
 Breitmeyer and Ganz 1977
 Brown and Black 1976
 Gorea and Tyler 1986
 Kelly 1977
 Kelly and Savoie 1978
 Legge 1978a
 Marx and May 1983
 Nachmias 1967
 Nagano 1980 (duration thresholds)
 Schober and Hilz 1965
 Spitzberg and Richards 1975
 Tolhurst 1975a
 Tulunay-Keesey and Jones 1976
 Tynan and Sekuler 1974
 Watanabe, Mori, Nagata, and Hiwa-
  tashi 1968

Vary duration of blurred versus sharp-edged targets
 Hood 1973

Vary temporal separation between pulses of spatial pattern
Bergen and Wilson 1985
Breitmeyer and Ganz 1977
Georgeson 1987
Green and Blake 1981
Ohtani and Ejima 1988
Watson and Nachmias 1977

Vary duration of moving dot or gratings
Burr 1981

7.1′ Joint temporal position and spatial frequency

Listed in 1.7′

7.3 Spatial position as auxiliary

7.3b Summation

Two spatially separated flashes
Vrolijk and van der Wildt 1985

7.3′ Joint temporal position and spatial position

Listed in 3.7′

7.5 Spatial phase as auxiliary

7.5b Summation

Green and Blake 1981
Watson and Nachmias 1977

7.6 Temporal frequency as auxiliary

7.6b Summation

Vary number of cycles of temporal flicker
Watson 1979

Vary duration comparing abrupt versus gradual onsets-offsets
Breitmeyer and Julesz 1975

7.7 Temporal position as auxiliary

7.7a Adaptation

Vary temporal separation between adapting and test stimulus
Albrecht, Farrar and Hamilton 1984
Blakemore and Campbell 1969
Lorenceau 1987
Magnussen and Greenlee 1985

Magnussen and Greenlee 1986
Rose and Evans 1983
Rose and Lowe 1982

7.7b Summation

Vary temporal separation between brief stimuli
Bergen and Wilson 1985
Broekhuijsen, Rashbass, and Veringa 1976
Green and Blake 1981
Ikeda 1985, 1986
Ikeda and Boynton 1965
Rashbass 1970, 1976
Roufs and Blommaert 1981
Roufs 1973, 1974
Watson 1982b
Watson and Nachmias 1977

Vary number of cycles of temporal flicker
van der Wildt and Rijsdijk 1979
Watson 1979

Vary temporal extent of stationary grating
Listed under 7.1

Vary temporal extent of temporally and spatially aperiodic stimuli
Barlow 1958
Blackwell 1963
Ejima and Takahashi 1988
Krauskopf 1980
Matin 1968
Roufs 1972a
Sperling and Sondhi 1968
Zacks 1970
Other classical temporal summation experiments

Vary temporal extent of temporal noise
Koenderink and van Doorn 1978b

7.7c Uncertainty

Earle and Lowe 1971
Lasley and Cohn 1981a,b
Lowe 1967
Pelli 1981

7.8′ Joint temporal position and temporal extent

7.8′b Summation

Vary relative temporal positions of a long-duration and a short-duration stimulus
Battersby and Schuckman 1970
Tolhurst 1975b (gratings)

7.9 Temporal phase as auxiliary

7.9a Summation

Vary duration of increments versus decrements
Krauskopf 1980

7.12 Mean luminance as auxiliary

7.12b Summation

Vary duration of spatially & temporally aperiodic stimulus
Graham and Kemp 1938
Herrick 1956
Keller 1941
Roufs 1972a,b

Vary temporal separation between two flashes
Vrolijk and van der Wildt 1985

7.13′ Joint temporal position and eye of origin

7.13′b Summation

Vary temporal separation between pulses in two eyes
Green and Blake 1981 (vary phase)
Matin 1962

7.16 Effect of eye movements and stabilized images

7.16b Summation

Vary exposure duration of stationary grating
Tulunay-Keesey and Jones 1976

7.17 Age, species and pathology of observer

7.17a Adaptation

Vary separation between adapt and test stimulus
Hess 1980 (amblyopes)

7.17b Summation

Vary exposure duration of gratings
Harwerth, Boltz, and Smith 1980 (monkeys)
Levi and Harwerth (1977)

8.0 TEMPORAL EXTENT EXPERIMENTS

8.1 Spatial frequency as auxiliary

8.1a Adaptation

Vary duration of adapting stimulus
Stromeyer, Kronauer, and Madsen 1984

8.8 Temporal extent as auxiliary

8.8a Adaptation

Vary duration of adapting stimulus
Albrecht, Farrar, and Hamilton 1984
Bjorklund and Magnussen 1981
Blakemore and Campbell 1969
Bodinger 1978
Daugman and Mansfield 1979
Magnussen and Greenlee 1985, 1986
Rose and Evans 1983
Rose and Lowe 1982
Stromeyer, Kronauer, and Madsen 1984

8.8d Identification

Vary duration of temporally aperiodic stimuli
Casson and Wandell 1984
Maloney and Wandell 1984
Zacks 1970

Discriminating durations
Allan 1979
Creelman 1962
Getty 1975
Rousseau, Poirier, and Lemyre 1983

8.17 Pathology of observer

8.17a Adaptation

Vary duration of adapting stimulus
Hess 1980 (amblyopes)

9.0 TEMPORAL PHASE EXPERIMENTS

9.8 Temporal extent as auxiliary

9.8d Identification

Increments from decrements
Anderson, Lasley, and Cohn 1982
Krauskopf 1980

9.9 Temporal phase as auxiliary

10.6a Adaptation

Stromeyer, Madsen, and Klein 1979
Stromeyer, Madsen, Klein, and Zeevi 1978

10.6b Summation

Arditi, Anderson, and Movshon 1981
Gorea and Lorenceau 1984
Stromeyer, Madsen, Klein, and Zeevi 1978
Watson, Thompson, Murphy, and Nachmias 1980

10.6d Identification

Gratings
Burr and Ross 1982
van der Glas, Orban, Joris, and Verhoeven 1981
Gorea 1985
Green 1983
Lennie 1980
Mansfield and Nachmias 1981
Thompson 1984
Watson, Thompson, Murphy, and Nachmias 1980

10.6′ Joint direction of motion and temporal frequency

Listed in 6.10′

10.8 Temporal extent as auxiliary

10.8d Identification

Green 1983
Thompson 1984

10.10 Direction of motion as auxiliary

10.10a Adaptation

Drifting gratings
Levinson and Sekuler 1975a,b
Pantle and Sekuler 1968b, 1969
Sekuler and Ganz 1963
Sekuler and Levinson 1974, 1977
Sekuler, Rubin, and Cushman 1968
Sharpe and Tolhurst 1973 a,b
Stromeyer, Madsen, Klein, and Zeevi 1978
Random dots
Levinson and Sekuler 1980

No facilitation at far-away values
Levinson and Sekuler 1980
Compound-stimulus effect (yes)
Levinson and Sekuler 1975b
Sekuler and Levinson 1974
Appearance thresholds
Levinson and Sekuler 1980
Levinson and Sekuler 1975a, p. 363

10.10b Summation

Gorea 1979 (movement vs. flicker appearance)
Levinson and Sekuler 1975a
Sekuler and Levinson 1974, 1977
Tolhurst 1973
Wilson 1985 (line plus grating)

10.10c Uncertainty

Random dots
Ball and Sekuler 1980 (exp. 6 and 7), 1981a,b
Lappin and Staller 1981 (masked by dots)
Sekuler and Ball 1977

10.10d Identification

Gratings
Listed under 10.1
Random dots
Ball, Sekuler, and Machamer 1983

10.11 Contrast as auxiliary

10.11a Adaptation

Pantle and Sekuler 1969
Pantle, Lehmkuhle, and Caudill 1968

10.13 Eye-of-origin as auxiliary

10.13a Adaptation

Smith 1983 (color)

10.13′ Joint direction of motion and eye of origin

10.13′b Summation

Arditi, Anderson, and Movshon 1981

10.15 Effect of psychophysical procedure

10.15b Summation

Arditi, Anderson, and Movshon 1981

10.16 Effect of eye movements and stabilized images

10.16a Adaptation

Bipartite fields to discourage tracking
Pantle and Sekuler 1969
Stromeyer et al 1979

10.16b Summation

Stabilized images
Kelly 1979b

10.16d Identification

Stabilized images
Mansfield and Nachmias 1981

10.17 Effect of age, species, and pathology of observer

10.17b Summation

Pasternak 1986 (normal and strobe-reared cats)
Wood and Kulikowski 1978 (on/off gratings, appearance thresholds, amblyopes, retrobulbar neuritis)

10.17d Identification

Pasternak and Leinen 1986
Pasternak, Schumer, Gizzi, and Movshon 1985

11.0 CONTRAST EXPERIMENTS

11.0a Adaptation

See 'contrast as an auxiliary dimension' in other sections

11.0b Summation

See discussion in text

11.0c Uncertainty

Blackwell 1952
Davis, Kramer, and Graham 1983

11.0d Identification

Contrast discrimination with gratings
Barlow, Kaushal, Hawken and Parker 1987

Baro, Lehmkuhle and Applegate 1988
Foley and Legge 1981
Georgeson and Georgeson 1987
Legge and Kersten 1983, 1987
Legge 1984a
Nachmias and Sansbury 1974
Pelli 1985, 1986/7
Stromeyer and Klein 1974
Swanson, Wilson, and Giese 1984
Swift and Smith 1984
Wilson 1980b

With aperiodic stimuli
Nachmias and Kocher 1970
Whittle 1986

Effect of adaptation on
Greenlee and Heitger 1988

12.0 MEAN LUMINANCE EXPERIMENTS

See discussion in text

13.0 EYE-OF-ORIGIN EXPERIMENTS

Adaptation experiments = interocular transfer of adaptation
Summation experiments = binocular summation
Identification experiments = utrocular identification
Joint eye-of-origin and x-dimension experiments are sometimes called dichoptic experiments on the x-dimension. They are given in section on the x-dimension.

13.1 Spatial frequency as auxiliary

13.1a Adaptation

Bjorkland and Magnussen 1981
Blake and Cormack 1979b
Cormack and Blake 1980
Maudarbocus and Ruddock 1973
Selby and Woodhouse 1981

13.1b Summation

Arditi, Anderson, and Movshon 1981
Blake and Cormack 1979b
Holopigian, Blake, and Greenwald 1986
Rose 1978

13.1d Identification

Arditi, Anderson, and Movshon 1981, p. 331
Blake and Cormack 1979a,b

13.1′ Joint eye of origin and spatial frequency

Listed in 1.13′

13.2 Orientation as auxiliary

13.2a Adaptation

Maudarbocus and Ruddock 1973

13.2d Identification

Blake and Cormack 1979b

13.2′ Joint eye and orientation

Listed in 2.13′

13.3 Spatial position as auxiliary

13.3a Adaptation

Sireteanu, Fronius, and Singer 1981

13.3b Summation

Matin 1962 (peripheral)
Sireteanu, Fronius, and Singer 1981

13.3d Identification

Blake and Cormack 1979b

13.4′ Joint eye of origin and spatial extent

Listed in 4.13′

13.5′ Joint eye of origin and spatial phase

Listed in 5.13′

13.6 Temporal frequency as auxiliary

13.6a Adaptation

Moulden, Renshaw, and Mather 1984

13.6b Summation

Arditi, Anderson, and Movshon 1981
Rose 1978

13.6d Identification

Arditi, Anderson, and Movshon 1981
Blake and Cormack 1979a,b

13.6′ Joint eye of origin and temporal frequency

Listed in 6.13′

13.7 Joint eye of origin and temporal position

Listed in 7.13′

13.8 Temporal extent as auxiliary

13.8a Adaptation

Varying duration of adapting stimulus
Bjorklund and Magnussen 1981

13.11 Contrast as auxiliary

13.11a Adaptation

Maudarbocus and Ruddock 1973
Sloane 1982

13.11b Summation

Legge 1984a,b
Anderson and Movshon (in press)

13.11b′ Effect of adaptation on summation

Anderson and Movshon (in press)

13.12 Mean luminance as auxiliary

13.12a Adaptation

Maudarbocus and Ruddock 1973

13.12b Summation

Gilchrist and McIver (1985)

13.13 Eye-of-origin as auxiliary

13.13a Adaptation

Blake, Overton, and Lema-Stern 1981 (review)
Blakemore and Campbell 1969
Stromeyer, Kronauer, Madsen, and Cohen 1980

13.13b Summation

Blake and Fox 1973 (review)
Blake, Sloane, and Fox 1981 (review)
Cambell and Green 1965
Cohn and Lasley 1976
Home 1978
Legge 1984a,b
Westendorf, Blake, Sloane, and Chambers 1982
Classical 'binocular summation' experiments

13.13b′ Effect of adaptation on summation

Anderson and Movshon 1986

13.13c Uncertainty

Cormack and Blake 1980

13.13d Identification

Arditi, Anderson, and Movshon 1981, p. 331
Blake and Cormack 1979a,b
Cohn, Leong, and Lasley 1981
Enoch, Goldman, and Sunga 1969
Martens, Blake, Sloane, and Cormack 1981
Ono and Barbeito 1985

13.17 Age, species, and pathology of observer

13.17a Adaptation

Anderson, Mitchell, and Timney 1980 (stereoblind)
Hess 1978
Sireteanu, Fronius, and Singer 1981 (amblyopes)

13.17b Summation

Crawford, Von Noorden Meharg, Rhodes, Harwerth, Smith, and Miller 1983 (monkeys and children)
Holopigian, Blake, and Greenwald 1986
Lema and Blake 1977 (stereoblindness)
Levi, Harwerth, and Smith 1979 (strabismus)
Sireteanu, Fronius, and Singer 1981 (amblyopes)
Westendorf, Langston, Chambers, and Allegretti (1978)

13.17c Uncertainty

Cormack and Blake 1980 (steroblind)

13.17d Identification

Blake and Cormack 1979a (stereoblind)

Notes

1. *Number of possible experiments.* As mentioned in section 12.1.4, a very large number of experiments might be done. Each of the five kinds of experiment we are considering might be done on each of the 17 pattern dimensions; however, some of these 85 possibilities are problematic to interpret or are essentially equivalent to each other (see, in particular, sections 11.5.3, 11.8.5, 11.8.9, 11.8.12, 11.8.13). At least 60 or 65 of the 85 experiments are distinct and sensible experiments to do. To get complete information about pattern vision, each of these 60 or 65 (e.g., adaptation on the spatial-frequency dimension) ought to be done at all possible combinations of values on the nonexperimental dimensions (orientation, spatial position, spatial extent, etc.). (For parametric experiments, the roles of two dimensions are not distinct, so the number of distinct experiments is less; but this is more than compensated for by the conservative approximations made subsequently in this argument.) Thus, even if there were only two values of interest on each dimension (which is a vast underestimate for most dimensions), the total number of experiments would be more than a million. The number of near-threshold pattern-vision experiments that has been done is large (see reference lists that follow) but not that large. We obviously do not yet know what happens in all regions of pattern-vision's parameter space. (The regions we do know most about are summarized in section 12.1.4.) And we

probably never would if we had to learn about it by doing a complete factorial set of experiments and reporting the results piecemeal. Not only would such an enterprise be boring, but we would not be able to encode or remember the results. As it happens, however, we do know a good deal about pattern vision, because the experiments that have been done have been guided by theory and the results are adding up to a coherent model of near-threshold pattern vision.

2. *Sustained (lowpass) versus transient (bandpass).* An analyzer is called *lowpass* if its sensitivity is maximal at a frequency of zero and (although the sensitivity may stay high over a range of relatively low frequencies) declines at higher frequencies. In other words, a lowpass analyzer only responds to ("passes") relatively low frequencies. The psychophysical analyzer indicated by the lefthand function of Fig. 12.1—discussed in sections 12.3.1 and 12.3.2—is lowpass for temporal frequency; some neurons that are lowpass for temporal frequency are mentioned in section 12.7.2.

The weighting function and impulse response of a lowpass analyzer are monophasic, containing only a positive lobe, for example, the impulse response to 3 c/deg in Fig. 12.3.

A *step stimulus* is one for which the luminance profile looks like a step; in the case of one-dimensional functions of time, the luminance profile is an instantaneous change of intensity from an old steady level to a new steady level. A *step response* is an output to a step stimulus.

The step response of a lowpass analyzer is a (usually gradual) increase to a new higher level of output where this new higher level is sustained as long as the stimulus intensity remains at its higher level. This is why lowpass analyzers have sometimes been called *sustained* analyzers.

An analyzer is called *bandpass* if its sensitivity is maximal at a medium frequency with declining sensitivities for both lower and higher frequencies. The righthand analyzers in Fig. 12.1 are bandpass for temporal frequency, and analogous neurons are discussed in section 12.7.2.

The weighting function and impulse response of a bandpass analyzer contain at least two lobes (of opposite polarity) as in the impulse responses to a 7-degree-wide uniform field in Fig. 12.3, particularly at high mean luminances.

The step response of a bandpass analyzer is a (usually gradual) increase to a maximum followed by a decline to a steady level of output. This new steady level is maintained as long as the stimulus remains at the higher intensity. The new steady level will equal (respectively, be greater than) the level before the stimulus step if the analyzer's sensitivity at a temporal frequency of zero is equal to (respectively, greater than) zero. Since the maximal response to the step occurs only transiently, bandpass analyzers are sometimes called *transient* analyzers.

The transient versus sustained difference in the step responses of bandpass and lowpass analyzers has tempted some to ascribe different functions to them. The function of detecting changes is ascribed to bandpass (transient) analyzers and that of detecting steady levels to lowpass (sustained) analyzers (see some of the early references given in section 1.8.2).

Notice, however, that a lowpass (sustained) analyzer can be sensitive out to higher temporal frequencies than is some bandpass (transient) analyzer. In that case, the lowpass analyzer would actually have a faster rise in its step response than would the bandpass analyzer and thus might be better suited for detecting changes. Alternately, a bandpass analyzer can respond differentially to different steady levels as long as it has some sensitivity to zero temporal frequency. In short, the "rise time" in a step response is not logically dependent on the sustained versus transient nature of the response.

Similarly, the latency from the abrupt step in a stimulus to the maximum in an analyzer's step response is not logically dependent on either the rise time or on the sustained versus transient nature of the step response. For example, an analyzer that has a sustained step response with a slow rise to the maximum (i.e., lowpass and sensitive only out to very low temporal frequencies) may have a much shorter latency to the maximum than does a second analyzer, even though that second analyzer is transient with a fast rise time (i.e., bandpass and maximally sensitive to high temporal frequencies). This difference in latencies can happen when the second analyzer has a built in "delay" before its step response starts rising at all (a delay that is reflected in the analyzers' phase characteristics rather than in the amplitude characteristic, that is, sensitivity).

In fact, however, such cases are not suggested by available psychophysical and physiological studies. Instead, lowpass (sustained) seems to go with lower temporal-frequency ranges (slower rise times) and with longer delays (longer latencies), and bandpass (transient) to go with higher temporal-frequency ranges (faster rise times) and shorter delays (shorter latencies). However, the evidence about temporal-frequency analyzers' properties is still sparse, so it would be premature to say there are no analyzers that, for example, are bandpass (transient) but sensitive only to very low temporal frequencies (slow rise time).

In pattern vision, three other properties seem to be correlated with sensitivity to lower temporal frequencies (and lowpass) versus sensitivity to higher temporal frequencies (and bandpass): (a) pattern versus motion appearances (particularly described in sections 13.2.2 and 13.6.3); (b) directional selectivity versus none (section 12.3.5); and (c) high versus low best spatial frequency (section 12.3.2). It is velocity rather than temporal or spatial frequency per se that is the better predictor of appearance and direction selectivity, however, as indicated in the lower left drawing of Fig. 12.2 and discussed in sections 12.3.5 and 13.6.3.

Further, sensitivity to color may be a property of lowpass (sustained) rather than bandpass (transient) analyzers. See, for example, the reaction-time distributions of Schwartz and Loop (1982, 1983), as well as the contrast-sensitivity references in subsections 1.18 and 6.18 of the list at the end of Chapter 13 (section 13.10).

Auditory psychophysical evidence has suggested that "change" (sustained) versus "level" (transient) analyzers may exist for auditory stimuli (Burbeck & Luce, 1982; Macmillan 1971, 1973) that are rather analogous to the suggestion of transient versus sustained systems for vision.

Note that spatial-frequency analyzers could, in principle, also be lowpass rather than bandpass, that is, have only a a single region in their weighting functions. Such analyzers' outputs would carry upstream information about the space-average luminance (the component at 0 cpd), information to which analyzers having several regions in their weighting functions—where the total excitation approximately balances the total inhibition—are quite insensitive.

3. Random-dot patterns and direction-of-motion uncertainty effects. Random dot patterns contain a wider range of orientations and spatial frequencies than grating patterns. Thus, when monitoring for just one direction of motion, the observer should be monitoring mechanisms sensitive to many more different spatial frequencies and orientations (and that direction of motion) when the stimulus is random dots than when it is a grating. (To put it another way, the composite analyzer or stimulus-defined channel for a moving random-dot pattern contains many more mechanisms than that for a moving grating.) However, the uncertainty effect when going from one to two (far-apart) directions of motion, as predicted by the independent-analyzers models here, is little affected by this difference. It is affected only to the extent that the probability distribution describing the output of the stimulus-defined channel is affected, and that should be revealed in the shapes of the ROC curves for the simple-alone condition. (See section 7.3.6.) I know of no results suggesting that there is a difference between simple-alone ROC curves for random-dot versus grating patterns. Thus one would expect (on the basis of these models) that the direction-of-motion uncertainty effect for random-dot patterns would be no bigger than that for gratings (but see experimental results discussed at end of section 12.3.5).

13

Results of Parametric Experiments

13.1 INTRODUCTION

Parametric experiments measure detection performance as a function of value. The measure of performance is often the intensity at detection threshold or its reciprocal, sensitivity. In the case of pattern vision, the appropriate intensity dimension is contrast, so the performance measures are typically contrast threshold or contrast sensitivity. The logic of interpreting the results of such experiments was discussed in section 11.5.

In this chapter parametric contrast sensitivity on each pattern dimension is summarized and its implications for the parameter values of a full model of low-level pattern analyzers are discussed.

Two issues in this chapter of particular theoretical interest are the description of sensitivity changes with spatial position (size-scaling models and the cortical magnification factors—sections 13.4.2, 13.6.4, 13.6.5, and 13.9.3) and with mean luminance (adaptation, constant-flux models; see section 13.9).

Let me say once more that the generalizations in this kind of summary are inevitably misleading. *Read them with caution!*

13.1.1 Organization of Chapter

The organization of this chapter is by pattern dimension in the standard order (see Table 12.1 in section 12.9) where each major section will discuss sensitivity as a function of value on that one dimension (the primary dimension). Within each major section, subsections will discuss how sensitivity on the primary dimension is influenced by value on other dimensions (as secondary dimensions); the secondary dimensions will be gone through in standard order as well. The discussion of why sensitivity changes the way it does with, for example, spatial position will appear in the section where spatial position is the primary dimension, although some effects of spatial position (as a secondary dimension) will have been described earlier.

At the end of this chapter is a list of references to parametric experiments in pattern vision.

Details. Two of the full 17 dimensions (degree of direction selectivity and degree of monocularity) are little discussed in this chapter, since parametric experiments on these two dimensions are essentially the same as summation experiments on the direction-of-motion and eye dimensions correspondingly and were thus discussed in Chapter 12.

504

Six of the other 15 pattern dimensions are not present in this chapter as secondary dimensions. For five of these—spatial phase, temporal phase, temporal position, direction of motion, and eye of origin—an observer's sensitivity is always approximately uniform (or is on the average; observers certainly show individual differences in sensitivities to the two eyes or to different directions of motion). Thus each of these dimensions has (or is presumed to have) little effect on parametric contrast sensitivity plotted as a value on any other dimension. These five are briefly mentioned as primary dimensions for the sake of completeness.

The sixth—contrast—does not appear as a secondary dimension because contrast is varied to find thresholds (which are what is generally measured). There is a section on contrast as a primary dimension, however, and here studies measuring detection performance as a function of contrast (psychometric functions) are briefly reviewed.

Aperiodic stimuli are primarily discussed under the spatial-extent and temporal-extent dimensions.

When comments are made unqualifed by values on unmentioned dimensions, the values on the unmentioned dimensions are usually the ones given in the list of typical values on auxiliary dimensions that appeared in section 12.1.4.

13.1.2 Precision

It might be well to say something about the standards of precision implied in any summary statement in this chapter, for they are quite different from the standards of the previous chapter (and of the data summaries in the theoretical chapters as well). In one way, the precision of these summaries about parametric contrast sensitivity is much lower: In this chapter, a factor of 2 difference between thresholds will be considered negligible in almost all contexts. (In the previous sections of this book summarizing results from analyzer-revealing experiments, almost all the effects looked at were smaller than a factor of 2!)

In another way, however, the standard of precision in these summaries about parametric contrast sensitivity is much more stringent. For in parametric experiments, the investigator must determine the physical contrast of each stimulus (at least within a factor of 2 or so), whereas in analyzer-revealing experiments the experimenter need only determine the contrast setting on his or her equipment that elicits some desired performance level and then have an accurate reading of relative contrast for that one stimulus in two different situations (e.g., before and after adaptation).

13.2 SENSITIVITY AS A FUNCTION OF SPATIAL FREQUENCY

13.2.1 Low and High Spatial-Frequency Declines

An observer's sensitivity is maximal in a middle range of spatial frequencies, with a gradual decrease toward low spatial frequencies and a precipitous

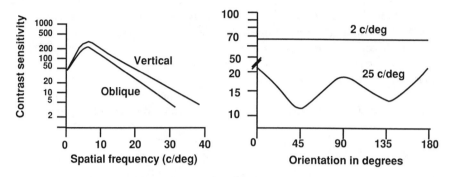

FIG. 13.1 Sensitivity as a function of spatial frequency for two orientations (left). The same results (with an expanded vertical scale) replotted as a function of orientation for two spatial frequencies (right). (Idealized from results in Fig. 2 of Campbell, Kulikowski, and Levinson, 1966).

decrease at high spatial frequencies (eg., Fig. 13.1). This sensitivity function is approximately the envelope of the sensitivity functions of the multiple spatial-frequency analyzers (at any one orientation, spatial position, etc.).

The dramatic high spatial-frequency decline derives from: (1) blurring by the optics; (2) integration across the spatial extent of each individual receptor; and (3) postreceptoral neural factors (e.g., differential effects of photon noise for different sizes of weighting functions, spatial uncertainty in the mapping from receptors to higher levels, decision rules). The second factor may make little contribution in any circumstance, and the third factor seems substantial only for extrafoveal vision; the first factor seems most important for foveal vision (Banks, Geisler, and Bennett, 1987; Williams, 1986; Williams & Coletta, 1987; Williams, D'Zmura, & Lennie, 1984). This high spatial-frequency decline is often straight when plotted as log sensitivity versus linear spatial frequency as in Fig. 13.1; given the problematic nature of calibrations of contrast at high spatial frequencies (see section on effect of equipment problems below), however, this may be an artifact.

The main limitation resulting from the spacing and arrangement of receptors is not the filtering out of high spatial frequencies but aliasing and ambiguity (see Williams 1986 for an introduction).

The low spatial-frequency decline is not present in all conditions, but it does remain after stabilization (see section 3.11.3). It is not yet clear what stage(s) of visual processing is primarily responsible for this low spatial-frequency decline.

13.2.2   *Appearances*

Grating patterns at detection threshold tend to look either spatially patterned or temporally patterned, depending on whether the ratio of temporal frequency to spatial frequency (velocity for drifting gratings) is less than or greater than about 0.5 to 2.0 degrees/second. See section 13.6.3 for further information.

13.2.3 Effect of Other Dimensions and Factors on Spatial-Frequency Sensitivity

Orientation. Figure 13.1 (idealized from Campbell, Kulikowski, & Levinson, 1966) illustrates the slight effect of orientation on sensitivity as a function of spatial frequency. Notice that the effect of orientation occurs only for high spatial frequencies. It slightly changes the slope of the high-spatial-frequency cutoff when sensitivity is plotted against linear spatial frequency and horizontally translates the high spatial-frequency end when sensitivity is plotted against logarithmic spatial frequency.

Spatial Position. The left panel of Fig. 13.2 shows some of the data originally plotted in Fig. 5.6. The right panel of Fig. 13.2 is derived from the results in the left panel and shows sensitivity versus spatial frequency at different spatial positions. Note that the sensitivity function in the right panel moves to the left (to lower spatial frequencies) as eccentricity increases, a direct result of the fact that decrease in sensitivity with eccentricity is faster for high spatial frequencies than for low. (See reference list for many published results.)

Spatial Extent. Figure 13.3 shows some of the data originally plotted in Fig. 5.7 for gratings of different spatial extent centered at the fovea. In the left panel of Fig. 13.3 these data are replotted with spatial extent measured in degrees of

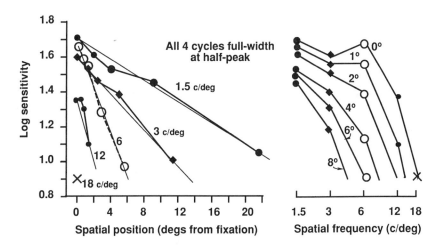

FIG. 13.2 Log sensitivity as a function of spatial position (measured in degrees from the fixation point) for five spatial frequencies (left). The same results plotted as a function of spatial frequency (for six spatial positions) (right). The straight lines drawn in the left panel illustrate the fact that log sensitivity tends to decrease linearly with eccentricity measured in number of periods. (These results were collected with patches having gradual edges and containing four periods (at half-peak contrast) and are some of the results plotted in Fig. 5.6. The points in the right panel were derived from the points in the left by interpolation.)

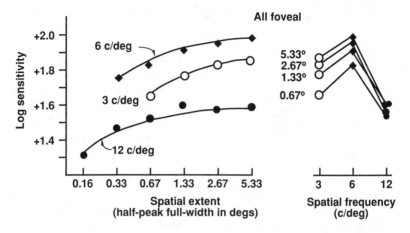

FIG. 13.3 Sensitivity as a function of spatial extent in degrees of visual angle for gratings of three spatial frequencies (left). The same results plotted as a function of spatial frequency for four spatial extents (right). The curves in the left panel are identical except for translations. [These results (some of those in Fig. 5.7) were collected with patches having gradual edges and centered on the fovea.]

visual angle. In the right panel of Fig. 13.3 these data are again replotted as a function of spatial frequency (on the horizontal axis) at different spatial extents (in degrees of visual angle labeling the curves). Notice that the helpful effect of spatial extent is considerably greater for low spatial frequencies than for high; the functions meet at high spatial frequencies, although differing at low.

This is the typical result of the many published measurements of effect of field size on sensitivity as a function of spatial frequency. This effect of spatial extent per se is intermixed in the published reports with effects of sharp edges and surround that are presumably greater in small field sizes than in large (see section 13.12.2).

If spatial extent is measured in periods of the grating (i.e., if sensitivity as a function of spatial frequency is measured for a constant number of cycles in the grating as it was in Fig. 13.2 right panel) or if the whole experiment is repeated peripherally (see Fig. 5.7), the effect of spatial extent on sensitivity as a function of spatial frequency will be different than that shown in Fig. 13.3.

Temporal Frequency. When temporal frequency is increased, spatial-frequency sensitivity as a function of spatial frequency moves lower and to the left and loses its low-spatial-frequency decline (e.g., Fig 3.6 left). (Many references are given in reference list.) Manipulating temporal-frequency content by using abrupt versus gradual onsets of stationary gratings produces analogous effects on spatial-frequency sensitivity (K. Higgins, Caruso, Coletta, & de Monasterio 1983; Tulunay-Keesey & Bennis, 1979).

The effect of temporal frequency can be rephrased as an effect of velocity (of temporal to spatial frequency ratio). See section 13.6.2, which further discusses the interaction between spatial and temporal frequency in determining sensitivity.

Temporal Extent. As temporal extent decreases, the high-temporal-frequency content decreases. Accordingly, the spatial-frequency sensitivity function (in a constant field size) moves lower and to the left and loses its low-spatial-frequency decline (e.g., Nachmias, 1967; Schober & Hilz, 1965).

Mean Luminance. As mean luminance is decreased, the spatial-frequency sensitivity function typically moves lower and to the left and loses its low-spatial-frequency decline (e.g., Fig. 13.11 upper right). See further discussion in section 13.9.

Effects of Eye Movements/Stabilization. Eye movements do produce some spatial-frequency-dependent effects (as judged by a comparison of stabilized with unstabilized viewing) but do not seem responsible for the major qualitative trends in sensitivity described above. See section 13.11.3.

Optics/Accommodation. Improper refraction and accommodation errors tend to decrease sensitivity at high spatial frequencies more than they do at low. See section 13.11.1.

Species of Observer. The spatial-frequency sensitivity of other primates is known to be quite similar to that of humans, but cats' high-spatial-frequency cutoff occurs at much lower spatial frequencies. See section 13.11.4.

13.3 SENSITIVITY AS A FUNCTION OF ORIENTATION

13.3.1 Almost Uniform

Sensitivity is almost flat as a function of orientation, at least approximately. Small anisotropies (nonuniformities in sensitivity as a function of orientation) do exist, but they are very small in typical conditions.

In the so-called oblique effect, which occurs at high spatial frequencies (e.g., Fig. 13.1), sensitivity is somewhat less (a factor of 2 or 3) at the oblique than at the vertical and horizontal orientations.

Many individuals show other anisotropies, being more sensitive, for example, to the vertical or horizontal than to any other meridian. In general, there seem to be substantial individual differences (M. Mayer, 1983b; R. Williams, Boothe, Kiorpes, & Teller, 1981).

Retinal orientation, not gravitational orientation, is the determiner (Lennie, 1974).

Since there are multiple orientation analyzers (at any single spatial frequency, spatial position, etc.), this function is approximately the envelope of the sensitivities of these multiple analyzers.

Appearance Thresholds. The oblique effect has been reported to be larger with spatial-appearance thresholds than with temporal-appearance thresholds (Camisa, Blake, & Lema, 1977; Essock & Lehmkuhle, 1982).

13.3.2   Effect of Other Dimensions/Factors on Orientation Sensitivity

Spatial Frequency. As mentioned previously, the oblique effect is found only at high spatial frequencies, not at low, as is shown in Fig. 13.1.

Spatial Position. The oblique effect is not reported in the periphery; but in the periphery observers are not sensitive to the high spatial frequencies at which the oblique effect occurs (in the fovea). That is, the extent of the oblique effect may be entirely predictable from spatial frequency without any consideration of spatial position (Berkley, Kitterle, & Watkins, 1975).

At large eccentricities (20 degrees or greater), there seems to be a different effect of orientation: Sensitivity is greatest (at least at high spatial frequencies) for gratings in which the bars are meridionally oriented (pointed toward the fovea) and worst (by about a factor of 2) for perpendicular gratings (Rovamo, Virsu, Laurinen, & Hyvarinen, 1982). These meridional effects were present even after correction for peripheral astigmatic refractive errors (which by themselves would produce effects of this sort).

At least for some individuals (with "normal vision" or corrected for acuity at the fovea), there seem to be very large effects of orientation—as large as a log unit—in localized patches at peripheral eccentricities (Koenderink, Bouman, de Mesquita, & Slappendel, 1978b; Regan & Beverly, 1983a; my own eyes corrected with contact lenses showed a 0.5 log unit advantage for horizontal over vertical grating patches located 7 degrees above the fovea for 6 c/deg but not for 2 c/deg). These effects may be optically correctable.

Spatial Extent. The oblique effect has been found for a range of spatial extents (at high spatial frequencies; Quinn & Lehmkuhle, 1983; Tootle & Berkley, 1983).

Temporal Frequency. It is unclear whether the oblique effect disappears at higher temporal frequencies (Camisa et al., 1977; M. Green, 1983).

Temporal Extent. The oblique effect has been reported to exist at 1 millisecond exposure durations (G. Higgins & Stultz, 1950) which, among other implications, makes it unlikely that biased eye movements are the sole cause. (On that issue, also see Nachmias, 1960.)

Optical Effects. These anisotropies remain for many observers even after optical correction of any astigmatism or when gratings are generated on the retina by interference fringes bypassing any astigmatism in the optics (Campbell et al., 1966; Rovamo et al., 1982). These optical deficits may, however, have contributed earlier in the observer's lifetime to the formation of the anisotropies (D. Mitchell, Freeman, Millodot, & Haegerstrom, 1973).

Age of Observer. The oblique effect may be more common in adults than in young children (e.g., M. Mayer, 1983b). The possibility that the oblique effect is a result of a "carpentered environment" (Annis & Frost, 1973; Segal, Campbell, & Herskovits, 1966; Timney & Muir, 1976) has run into difficulties (Ross & Woodhouse, 1979; Switkes, Mayer, & Sloan, 1978).

Practice. Practice may improve sensitivity on the obliques while not affecting sensitivity on the more-sensitive orientations (M. Mayer, 1983a).

13.4 SENSITIVITY AS A FUNCTION OF SPATIAL POSITION

13.4.1 *Usually Highest in Fovea*

Sensitivity is greatest at the foveal center for most stimuli. Grating acuity (the high-spatial-frequency cutoff) is highest at the fovea at all mean luminances (Johnson, Keltner, & Balestrery, 1978; Kerr, 1971).

Sensitivity is often found to be approximately an exponential function of distance from the fovea; that is, log sensitivity versus distance is approximately a straight line (e.g., Robson & Graham, 1981; Koenderink et al., 1978a, 1978b). As there are multiple spatial-position analyzers, this function is approximately the envelope of the sensitivities of these multiple analyzers (at any one spatial frequency, orientation, etc.).

13.4.2 *Spatial-Scaling Models and the Effect of Spatial Frequency on Spatial-Position Sensitivity*

Sensitivity decreases faster (as a function of degrees of visual angle) for higher spatial frequencies than for low. See Fig. 5.6 and Fig. 13.2.

The fall-off in sensitivity for a given spatial frequency may tend to be faster below and above the fovea than to the left and the right, although there are individual differences in this (Regan and Beverly, 1983a; Rijsdijk, Kroon, & van der Wildt, 1980).

Number-of-Periods Rule of Thumb. A useful rule of thumb is that sensitivity tends to decrease approximately linearly as a function of the number of periods away from foveal center with the same constant of proportionality (same slope when logarithmic sensitivity is plotted versus number of periods) for all spatial frequencies at least within the typical parameter ranges listed above. See Fig. 5.6 top panel.

Size-Scaled Models. A question of current interest is whether effects of eccentricity can be explained by simply scaling the size of spatial weighting functions as a function of distance from foveal center. Such scaling would occur if, for example, wiring were identical in different parts of the visual field except for a change of spatial scale (e.g., Anstis, 1974; Drasdo, 1977; Fischer, 1973; Fischer

& May, 1970; Hubel & Wiesel, 1974; Koenderink et al., 1978a, 1978b, 1978c, 1978d; Kretz et al., 1979; Rolls & Cowey, 1970; Rovamo & Virsu, 1979; Rovamo, Virsu, & Nasanen, 1978; Schwartz, 1977, 1980; Watson, 1983). Due to the physiological analogy, the scale factor is sometimes called the *cortical magnification factor*.

Figure 13.4 illustrates such size scaling by showing one of several families of mechanisms in the model of Watson (1983) (described further in section 6.9.2). Each circle represents a mechanism; the diameter of the circle is about two fifths the width (full width at half height) of the mechanism's spatial window function. Notice that in this model the two spatial window functions (parallel and perpendicular to the bars) are taken to be identical. The scaling factor s is set equal to $1 + ke$ where e is eccentricity in degrees and k is a constant (k is about 0.4 for the one observer mentioned in Watson, 1983). This scaling factor s is used to scale not only the width of the window functions but also the spatial frequency of the mechanism, the spatial density of mechanisms at each eccentricity, and the amplitude (gain) of the mechanism's weighting function. Thus if a mechanism at the fovea has a spatial frequency of f, a window width of w, a sampling density (in each dimension) of d, and an amplitude of A, then the related mechanism at eccentricity e will have frequency f/s, width ws, a one-dimensional sampling density of d/s, and an amplitude of A/s^2. These relationships (except for amplitude) are illustrated in Fig. 13.4, which shows the family

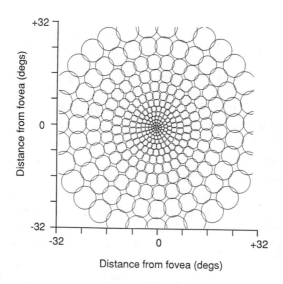

FIG. 13.4 A family of mechanisms from the model of Watson (1983). Each circle represents a mechanism in the family; the diameter of the circle is about two fifths of the full width at half height of the spatial window function of the mechanism. The diameter of the circle increases with eccentricity e according to the function $1 + ke$. The two axes show degrees from the fovea. The mechanism located at the fovea in this family is maximally sensitive to 1 c/deg. (Fig. 6 in Watson 1983; used by permission.)

related to the mechanism for 1 c/deg at the fovea. In Watson's (1983) model, there are eight such families altogether—those related to spatial frequencies at the fovea of 0.25 c/deg to 32 c/deg in octave steps.

Wilson and his colleagues' models (section 6.9.1) include size-scaling of a similar sort. The factor k for scaling width and spatial frequency of their line-spread functions (Fig. 6.13 for example) varied from 0.10 to 0.125 for the three observers in Wilson and Bergen (1979). The scaling factor k used by other authors seems to have varied from about 0.2 to 0.35 (Koenderink et al., 1978c; Rovamo et al., 1978; Virsu, Rovamo, Laurinen, & Nasanen, 1982; Tyler & Silverman, 1983; Kelly, 1984a).

Simple Stimulus-Scaling Hypothesis. An idea related to the above model is the following general prediction (see, e.g., Koenderink et al., 1978c): Two stimuli that are at far-apart spatial positions should be equally detectable if they are identical, except that the spatial scale on two dimensions of one stimulus is expanded relative to that of the other by the proper amount. The proper amount is the ratio of the scale factors—$s(e_1)/s(e_2)$, where s is a monotonically increasing function of eccentricity e. (Mean luminance, temporal profile, depth from the observer, and wavelength distribution of the two stimuli are to be held identical.) I will call this the *simple stimulus-scaling hypothesis.*

When tested, the simple stimulus-scaling hypothesis has held rather well within the limits of imprecision of the experiments (which include considerable psychophysical variability as well as having to specify the scale factor at relevant eccentricities in advance; e.g., Koenderink et al., 1978c; Rovamo et al., 1978; Virsu et al., 1982).

Constant-Number-of-Periods Experiment. Watson (1987) has pointed out that there is a test of the simple stimulus-scaling prediction that does not require specifying the scale factor in advance, namely, to measure sensitivity at different spatial frequencies and spatial positions always using the same number of periods in the sinusoidal patch. For when the number of periods is kept constant throughout an experiment, any two patches (in particular, any two at different eccentricities) are spatially scaled versions of one another (with the relative scale factor equaling the ratio of their spatial frequencies). If the simple stimulus-scaling hypothesis is true, therefore, and all patches in the experiment contain the same number of periods, then the two functions plotting sensitivity versus logarithmic spatial frequency at two different eccentricities will simply be horizontal translations of one another; the horizontal separation between the functions for any two eccentricities is the logarithm of the ratio of the scale factors for those two eccentricities $[s(e_1)/s(e_2)]$.

The functions in the right of Fig. 13.2 are horizontal translations of one another within the precision of the experiment.

Why the Simple Stimulus-Scaling Hypothesis Is Not Quite Consistent with Size-Scaled Models. As Watson (1987) also pointed out, however, size-scaled models do not quite predict the simple stimulus-scaling hypothesis above. For the simple stimulus-scaling hypothesis implicitly assumes that nothing much is changing *within* the area covered by either stimulus, although something (a factor by which the two stimuli are multiplied) is changing between the two locations. But in the size-scaled model, the scaling factor is changing continuously as you move from one receptive field to the next.

For the constant-number-of-periods experiment, therefore, one does not expect the full spatial-frequency functions to be quite horizontal translations of one another. The change of scale factor within the extent of a patch means that the most effective part of peripheral patches is not the centermost part but a part closer to the fovea, and the lower the spatial frequency, the closer it will be. Thus the proper scale factor for a low spatial-frequency patch is actually somewhat less than that for a high spatial-frequency patch centered at the same position. (No such discrepancy is obvious in the right panel of Fig. 13.2, but very low spatial frequencies are not well represented. An example where there is a discrepancy in empirical results—just as predicted by the size-scaled model—is shown in Watson, 1987.)

Size-Scaled Models and the Number-of-Periods Rule of Thumb. Size-scaling models predict that sensitivity will decline with eccentricity (in degrees of visual angle) faster for high spatial frequencies than for low. Are such models consistent (approximately at least) with the number-of-periods rule of thumb described above? Yes, as Fig. 13.5 illustrates. This figure shows hypothetical contrast sensitivity functions at each of two eccentricities (foveal and 5 degrees eccentric) where the stimuli all had a constant number of periods. The functions are horizontal translations of one another on a logarithmic spatial-frequency

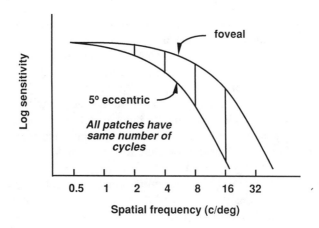

FIG. 13.5 Hypothetical contrast sensitivity functions at two eccentricities where the stimuli all had the same number of periods. The two curves are horizontal translations of one another in accord with a simple stimulus-scaling hypothesis. The drop in logarithmic sensitivity between the two functions is about twice as great for any frequency (e.g., 16 cpd) as for half that frequency (e.g., 8 cpd). This is just the relationship incorporated in the "number-of-periods rule-of-thumb."

axis. (The low spatial frequencies below the peak are ignored here since, as just discussed, size-scaling models do not predict they should be horizontal translations of one another.) Further, and importantly, the functions' high-frequency declines are curved downward on these axes, as is typically found. The four vertical lines represent the drops in sensitivity when going from the fovea to 5 degrees eccentric for four spatial frequencies a factor of 2 apart. Notice that the drop in logarithmic sensitivity is about twice as large for 16 c/deg as for 8 c/deg, which in turn is about twice as large as for 4 c/deg and so on. More generally, the decline in logarithmic sensitivity going from 0 to 5 degrees is about n times as large for any high spatial frequency f as for f/n. It is also true that any given eccentricity is equivalent to n times as many periods for any high spatial frequency f as for f/n (for example, 5 degrees of eccentricity is 80 periods of 16 c/deg but 40 periods of 8 c/deg. Putting these two facts together, the drop in logarithmic sensitivity when going from 0 to 5 degrees is approximately proportional to eccentricity in number of periods—consistent with the number-of-periods rule of thumb.

Why These Effects of Eccentricity? Perhaps it is simply a solution to a problem in the economics of evolution. A high-acuity area extending over more than a degree or so may be too expensive in some sense (too large a proportion of the potential neural tissue a body could support, for example). Yet it may also be too expensive to have a very small visual field (too likely to cause death by a failure to notice danger, for example). A compromise was least expensive. Why the compromise should be a simple linear spatial-scaling scheme is not clear.

Given such a regular scheme as spatial scaling, one is tempted to find some perceptual use for it. Perhaps size constancy under different viewing distances. Several of the references cited here give in to this temptation, at least in passing. The question of why there is (or may be) such simple spatial scaling is not yet convincingly answered.

13.4.3 Effect of Other Dimensions/Factors on Sensitivity as a Function of Spatial Position

Spatial Extent. The decline in sensitivity with eccentricity will tend to be faster with patches of smaller spatial extent than with larger because sensitivity increases more with spatial extent in the periphery than in the fovea. (See Fig. 5.7 and section 13.5.)

Temporal Frequency. The effect of temporal frequency is quite different from that of spatial frequency. If anything, sensitivity for a grating patch (of constant spatial frequency, orientation, etc.) falls faster with eccentricity at low temporal frequencies than at high. For further details, see section 13.6.5

Mean Luminance. The decline in sensitivity with eccentricity is, in general, slower for lower mean luminances than for high. See section 13.9.3.

Optical Factors. Even when an observer is corrected for foveal refractive errors, there remain peripheral ones. Whether proper refraction improves peripheral acuity is still in some dispute, but it undoubtedly improves performance on some tasks. See section 13.11.1.

Further, a number of special optical problems arise in peripheral viewing that bear careful consideration (see, for example, discussions in Alpern & Spencer, 1953; Kerr, 1971; Koenderink et al., 1978d; and Van Meeteren & Dunnewold, 1983).

Local Adaptation. In the periphery, local adaptation (threshold elevation) to stimuli may apparently be quite severe, as has been noted in the flicker literature (e.g., Ginsburg, 1966). One such habituation or adaptation effect—where the threshold rises over a log unit in the course of an hour of testing—has been reported to be size or spatial-frequency specific but not orientation specific (Frome, MacLeod, Buck, & Williams, 1981). Differences in the amount of such adaptation may be one of the reasons that comparison of results across studies of the periphery seem even trickier than in the fovea.

Individual Differences and Practice. In a study of resolution in the periphery (Johnson & Leibowitz, 1979), substantial individual differences were found particularly at the largest peripheries (40–60 degrees eccentric). Then dramatic improvements occurred in peripheral visual resolution over 11 sessions with improvements in acuity of about 40% at 20 to 60 degrees eccentricity compared with 4% at the fovea. This result is somewhat analogous to M. Mayer's (1983a) finding of improvement with practice on the less-sensitive orientations.

13.5   SENSITIVITY AS A FUNCTION OF SPATIAL EXTENT AND SPATIAL PHASE

13.5.1   *Sensitivity Increases With Increasing Spatial Extent*

As spatial extent (either of a grating or an aperiodic stimulus) is increased, sensitivity tends first to increase quickly and then to slow down (e.g., Figs. 5.7 and 13.3).

If there is only a single spatial-extent analyzer (at a given spatial frequency, etc.), this function is approximately the sensitivity of that analyzer as a function of spatial extent (that is, the function giving the effect of integration within the weighting function of a single analyzer). However, changing the spatial extent of a stimulus also changes the spatial positions and spatial frequencies, and there are multiple analyzers on those dimensions. Taking these dimensions into account properly is discussed in section 5.4.

If there really is only a single spatial extent of analyzer (and the rest of the theoretical framework here is at least approximately correct), then all the effects of spatial extent (on sensitivity measured as a function of any dimension) are derivable from the effects of spatial frequency and spatial position. And all of the effects of spatial extent that I know of seem to be consistent with this view. Spatial extent is often a parameter of interest, however—so the effects are summarized here in spite of their derivative nature.

13.5.2 *Effect of Other Dimensions/Factors on Sensitivity as a Function of Spatial Extent*

Spatial Frequency. See Fig. 13.3 and earlier discussion of effect of spatial extent on spatial frequency. In Chapter 5, see Fig. 5.7 and accompanying discussion.

Orientation. A greater increase in sensitivity for vertical than for oblique orientations as number of cycles increased up to 10 has been reported (Quinn & Lehmkuhle, 1983; Tootle & Berkley, 1983). This may result from a slightly different function relating sensitivity to spatial position for those two orientations. (The studies did not measure sensitivity to localized patches, so one does not know.)

Spatial Position. In general, the increase in sensitivity with increasing spatial extent seems more pronounced in the periphery than in the fovea (e.g., Koenderink et al., 1978a, 1978b; Robson & Graham, 1981), just as one would expect from the few existing measurements of sensitivity at local positions (see Fig. 5.7 and discussion there).

Classic Areal Summation Experiments. When the size of an aperiodic stimulus is varied and an observer's sensitivity is measured, sensitivity increases rather rapidly with size initially and then—after reaching a so-called critical size—increases less slowly if at all. This critical size is found to increase progressively with eccentricity (Hallett, Marriott, & Rodger, 1962; M. Wilson, 1970). This may be a result of two factors: (a) the decrease in optimal spatial frequency with eccentricity (which is closer to the original interpretation as increase in excitatory area of a receptive field) and (b) the increase in the area over which spatial probability summation occurs.

Temporal Extent (in Classic Summation Experiments). When spatially and temporally aperiodic stimuli are used, the critical width decreases as the temporal extent of the stimulus increases (Barlow, 1958). This corresponds at least roughly to the move toward higher spatial frequencies when temporal frequency is lowered that one finds with sinusoidal stimuli (e.g., Fig. 13.4). To predict the classic summation effects quantitatively, one has to take into account all the factors mentioned previously for spatial and temporal extent.

Mean Luminance. For spatially aperiodic stimuli, the increase in contrast sensitivity with spatial extent is, in general, greater at low mean luminances than at high. See section 13.9.4.

For gratings, the effect of spatial extent should be predictable from its effect on spatial position. In particular, for foveally fixated gratings, one might find summation over somewhat more periods at low mean luminances than at high, because sensitivity changes more slowly with spatial position at low mean luminances than at high.

13.5.3 *Sensitivity Uniform as a Function of Spatial Phase*

The spatial phase of a sinusoidal patch (values on all other dimensions staying constant) apparently makes little if any difference in the observer's sensitivity except for predictable changes caused when the window is very small relative to the period of the sinusoid.

13.6 SENSITIVITY AS A FUNCTION OF TEMPORAL FREQUENCY

13.6.1 *Greatest Sensitivity at Middle Temporal Frequencies*

In typical conditions sensitivity is greatest at medium temporal frequencies (3–10 c/sec), dropping off slowly toward low temporal frequencies and quickly toward high temporal frequencies, e.g., upper curve in right panel of Fig. 13.6. In fact, sensitivity plotted as a function of temporal frequency looks remarkably like sensitivity plotted as a function of spatial frequency (where cycles per sec-

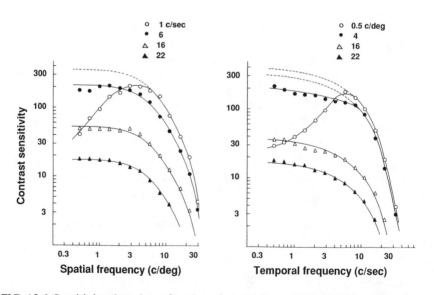

FIG. 13.6 Sensitivity plotted as a function of spatial frequency (left) and as a function of temporal frequency (right). The points are the means of four measurements. The curves in each panel (some with dashed low-frequency sections) are vertical translations of one another. (Figs. 1 and 2 in Robson, 1966; used by permission.)

ond have replaced cycles per degree). This is true for stabilized as well as unstabilized stimuli (e.g., Kelly, 1979b).

Since there are at most only a few broadly tuned analyzers on the temporal-frequency dimension, the middle part of the temporal-frequency sensitivity function probably reflects the envelope of the peaks of the individual analyzers' sensitivity functions while the rest of it reflects the shape of the lowest analyzer's low-frequency end and the highest analyzer's high-frequency end (e.g., Fig. 12.1).

If one assumes that there is only a single temporal-frequency analyzer (at any spatial frequency, etc.), as has often been done, this temporal-frequency sensitivity function can be Fourier inverted (as long as one is willing to make a suitable assumption about phase characteristics) to yield information about the temporal impulse or weighting function, as discussed in Chapter 12 (e.g., Fig. 12.4).

13.6.2 Effect of Spatial Frequency on Sensitivity as a Function of Temporal Frequency

When spatial frequency is increased, the temporal-frequency sensitivity function moves lower and to the left and loses its low temporal-frequency decline (as shown in Fig. 13.6 right panel for foveally centered gratings, moderate mean luminances)—very much like the effect of increasing temporal frequency on spatial-frequency sensitivity shown in the left panel. This general pattern is found with flickering or drifting gratings (e.g., Kelly 1966, 1969; et al., 1967; Koenderink et al., 1978a, 1978b; Watanabe et al., 1968) and is true in stabilized as well as unstabilized viewing (e.g., Kelly, 1979b).

The two-dimensional function giving sensitivity for each temporal frequency and spatial frequency is not separable—that is, it cannot be expressed as the product of two functions, one giving sensitivity at each temporal frequency and one giving sensitivity at each spatial frequency.

Why Do Temporal-Frequency and Spatial-Frequency Parametric Sensitivity Functions Behave So Similarly? Given that analyzer-revealing experiments produce entirely different results for temporal frequency and spatial frequency, it may seem peculiar that the parametric functions for the two behave so similarly with variations in the other (compare, for example, the right and left panels of Fig. 13.6). Also, the effects of increasing mean luminance on either are similar (see relevant sections). Perhaps these parametric contrast sensitivity functions primarily reflect some stage of visual processing other than that of the low-level analyzers whose properties show up in the analyzer-revealing experiments. For example, the shape of the temporal-frequency and spatial-frequency contrast sensitivity functions might be determined by retinal properties, whereas the further wiring up to the visual cortex establishes multiple analyzers without disturbing the relative sensitivities at different frequencies.

The Spatiotemporal Threshold Surface and Contour Map. Figure 13.7 shows two more useful (and slightly idealized) plots—a threshold surface (left) and a contour map (right) illustrating the interaction between spatial frequency and

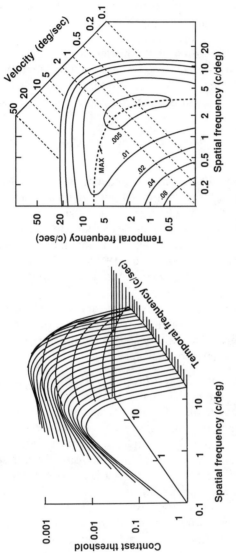

FIG. 13.7 A perspective view of a typical spatiotemporal threshold surface for drifting gratings (left). Each curve represents the spatial frequency response at a fixed temporal frequency. The neighboring curves are separated by a constant increment of about 0.10 log temporal frequency. The hidden part of the surface was not suppressed. [Modified from Fig. 13 in Kelly (1979b); used by permission.]

A contour map of the same surface (right). The contours are labeled by the contrast thresholds to which they correspond. [Fig. 15 in Kelly, 1979b; used by permission.]

temporal frequency in sensitivity for stabilized drifting gratings. The contour map in the right panel shows that there is rather good symmetry around the lines for a velocity of 1 or 2 degrees/second (also visible in Fig. 13.10).

One other published contour map (unstabilized viewing, Koenderink & van Doorn, 1979) is much like those shown here except for a slight dip in sensitivity at the positive diagonal (velocities near 1 degree/second, medium spatial and temporal frequencies) that leads to two peaks, one at high velocities and one at low. No such dips are visible in the (shaded) contour maps of Fig. 13.10.

The drift rate in unstabilized vision may average around 0.15 degrees/second, but is presumably also variable (Kelly, 1979b).

Constant-Velocity Functions. A certain amount of interest has attached to families of curves, where each member of a family shows sensitivity as a function of spatial frequency (or of temporal frequency) for drifting gratings all at the same velocity (e.g., Burr & Ross, 1982, for unstabilized viewing; Kelly, 1979b, for stabilized viewing). The major characteristics of such constant-velocity families can be derived from the contour map in the right of Fig. 13.7; each constant-velocity curve shows sensitivity along a positive diagonal in the contour map plotted as a function of either spatial or temporal frequency (the horizontal or vertical axis, respectively, of the contour map).

First note in the contour map that the contours of equal detectability run quite parallel to the temporal frequency axis at low velocities (less than 0.5 or 1 degree/second) but quite parallel to the spatial frequency axis at high velocities (greater than 1 or 2 degrees/second). Thus, constant-velocity curves for all low velocities should occupy the same range when plotted against spatial frequency (e.g., low-velocity curves in Fig. 6 of Kelly, 1979b) but different ranges when plotted against temporal frequency (no published example I can find but can be plotted from published results). For high velocities, the opposite will hold: Constant-velocity curves should occupy the same range when plotted against temporal frequency (e.g., Fig. 2 of Burr & Ross, 1982) but different ranges when plotted against spatial frequency (Fig. 1 of Burr & Ross and high-velocity curves in Fig. 6 of Kelly, 1979b). [Burr and Ross (1982) measured the identification of direction-of-motion threshold rather than detection threshold. But in the high-velocity region, the identification and detection thresholds are probably much the same as discussed in section 12.4.5.]

Notice also that over quite a wide range of low and high velocities the peak sensitivities along all diagonals in the contour map are rather similar—for example, from about 0.1 to 50 degrees/second in Fig. 13.7 the peak sensitivity is within the contour labeled 0.01. Thus, constant-velocity curves (plotted either against spatial frequency or temporal frequency) will tend to have rather similar peak heights until one gets to very low or very high velocities indeed. In fact, when the spatial extent of the stimulus expands with the velocity studied (as in the study of Burr & Ross, 1982) or presumably when all velocities are studied in a very large field size, the peak sensitivity stays close to constant for velocities from 1 to 800 degrees/second.

13.6.3   Appearance Thresholds

As mentioned earlier, grating patterns at detection threshold tend to look spatially patterned when the ratio of temporal to spatial frequency (velocity in the case of drifting gratings) is greater than 1 or 2 degrees/second or temporally patterned when the ratio is less than 0.5 or 1 degree/second. In addition to the extensive studies of Koenderink and van Doorn (1979), Harris (1980), and Panish, Swift, and Smith (1983), the conglomerate plot in Fig. 13.8 of many other studies shows this trend. The studies compiled in the figure are listed in the figure legend; they differed from one another in many other ways, although in general using values in the typical ranges. There are distinct individual differences in the exact transition (e.g., Harris, 1980).

Figure 13.9 left shows some results when observers were asked to set not only

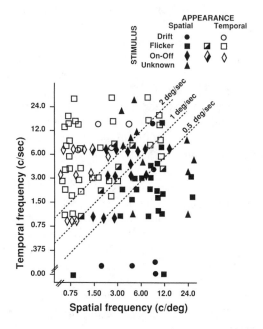

FIG. 13.8 Each point indicates a report of spatial or temporal appearance (closed vs. open symbols) at detection threshold. Several constant-velocity lines are shown. The shape of the symbol indicates the kind of grating. On-off gratings (diamonds) contain a component at 0 c/sec as well as the temporal frequency indicated on the figure; this is probably why some solid diamonds appear above the 2 degree/second line. (The studies contributing points to this figure are: Blake and Mills, 1979; Bodis-Wollner, Harnois, and Bobak, 1983; Brussell, White, Mustillo, and Overbury, 1984; Burbeck, 1981; M. Green, 1981; Kulikowski, 1978; Kulikowski and Tolhurst, 1973; Murray, MacCana, and Kulikowski, 1983; Pantle, 1973; Tolhurst, 1973. Not shown in this figure because each involves too many points are the studies of Harris 1980; Koenderink and van Doorn, 1979; and Panish, Swift, and Smith, 1983. All of the above studies differed from one another in many ways, although in general using values in the typical ranges.)

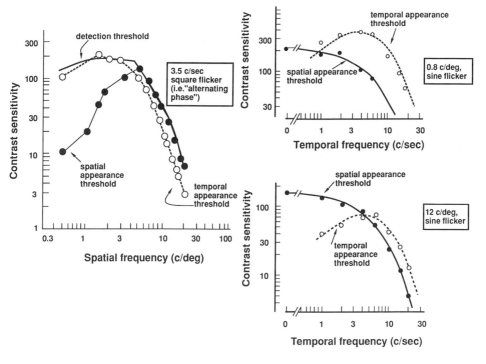

FIG. 13.9 Temporal-appearance thresholds (open symbols), spatial-appearance thresholds (closed symbols), and detection thresholds (solid line). In the left panel, these three thresholds are plotted as a function of spatial frequency for gratings undergoing square-wave flicker at 3.5 c/sec. (Data replotted from Figs. 1 and 3 of Kulikowski & Tolhurst, 1973). The right two panels show the appearance thresholds plotted as a function of temporal frequency for flickering gratings of 0.8 c/deg (top) and 12 c/deg (bottom). (Modified from Figs. 7 and 8 in Kulikowski & Tolhurst, 1973; used by permission.)

detection thresholds (solid heavy line) but also spatial-appearance and temporal-appearance thresholds (see section 1.11.6) at a number of spatial frequencies (all at 3.5 c/sec square-wave flicker).

Figure 13.9 right shows spatial- and temporal-appearance thresholds as a function of temporal frequency of sinusoidally flickering gratings for a low spatial frequency (0.8 c/deg) and a high spatial frequency (12 c/deg). Presumably the detection thresholds would lie on the envelope of the two appearance thresholds.

Notice that spatial-appearance thresholds are bandpass on spatial-frequency (left panel Fig. 13.9) and lowpass on temporal-frequency (right panel) dimensions, whereas the reverse is true for temporal-appearance thresholds.

What this means is unclear, however. To interpret the results at all requires making suitable assumptions linking the outputs of lower level analyzers to the setting of appearance thresholds as well as assumptions about the analyzers themselves. (Are there two essentially different classes of analyzers having different kinds of basic labels, one signaling pattern and one motion, perhaps identical to the nondirectionally selective vs. directionally selective analyzers in Fig. 12.2? Or is there only one class of analyzer, but higher level processing ends up producing different appearances for high-velocity than for low-velocity patterns?)

Further, some investigators have had a good deal of trouble getting observers to set both kinds of thresholds at all (e.g., M. Green, 1980; Murray et al., 1983; Watson, 1977; Watson & Nachmias, 1977); the setting of the less-sensitive one apparently seems quite arbitrary to many observers. Quite possibly the appearance thresholds set in different studies have differed from one another (cf. Panish et al., 1983); it might be worth trying out different kinds of instuctions to observers.

Thresholds based on discriminations between stimuli differing spatially (Burbeck, 1981; Derrington & Henning, 1981; Lennie, 1980a; Virsu et al., 1982) or temporally (Burbeck, 1981; Kulikowski, 1978; and Murray et al., 1983) are certainly not equivalent to the reported spatial- and temporal-appearance thresholds, nor would they be expected to be on many models, even those postulating two classes of analyzers.

13.6.4   *Effect of Orientation on Sensitivity as a Function of Temporal Frequency*

The function for oblique gratings may or may not have a slightly shallower high-temporal-frequency decline than that for horizontal or vertical (that is, the oblique effect may or may not disappear at high temporal frequencies; Camisa et al., 1977; M. Green, 1983).

13.6.5   *Effect of Spatial Position on Sensitivity as a Function of Temporal Frequency—More About Spatially Scaled Models*

To a first approximation, spatial position has little effect on temporal resolution, quite unlike its large deleterious effect on spatial resolution. In fact, for stimuli of high temporal frequency (especially of large spatial extent), the periphery can be slightly more sensitive than the fovea. For example, for some people the flicker in the television screen or fluorescent bulbs may be clearly visible peripherally while quite unobtrusive foveally. For me, a large, bright cathode-ray screen with a sweep rate of 80/second flickers quite disturbingly in the periphery but is steady foveally.

Formally, the critical fusion frequency (CFF) has often been reported to increase initially with eccentricity before decreasing again, at least with relatively large stimuli and high mean luminances (see review in C. Graham's 1966 book; Hartmann, Lachenmayr & Brettel, 1979. See also H. Wilson, 1980a).

Spatial Frequency, Temporal Frequency, and Spatial Position. Figure 13.10 is a plot of the interrelationships among spatial position, temporal frequency,

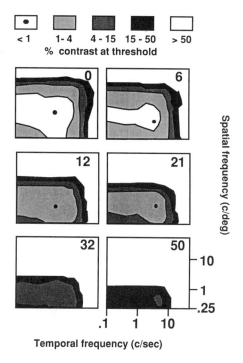

FIG. 13.10 Each panel shows sensitivity (indicated by different kinds of shading; see key) at a different eccentricity, where the number at the upper right of each panel gives eccentricity in degrees. Spatial frequency and temporal frequency are on the vertical and horizontal axes, respectively (opposite to the conventions used in Figs. 13.8 and 12.5 through 12.8). (Modified from Fig. 2.1 Koenderink, Bouman, de Mesquita, & Slappendel, 1978b; used by permission.)

and spatial frequency (from Koenderink, et al., 1978b). Here each panel shows sensitivity (indicated by different kinds of shading, see key) at a different eccentricity; spatial frequency and temporal frequency are on the vertical and horizontal axes, respectively. As eccentricity increases (moving from upper left to lower right panel), the vertical edge (high-temporal-frequency cutoff) of the shaded area changes position very little, although the horizontal edge (high-spatial-frequency cutoff) moves down quite dramatically.

Somewhat oddly, perhaps, in light of the critical flicker fusion studies above, sensitivity in this figure is never better peripherally than foveally (the vertical edge never moves out to higher temporal frequencies). The mean luminance was perhaps too low here; another possibility is that the improvement occurs only for the very highest of the visible temporal frequencies (those visible only near 100% contrast) coupled with even lower spatial frequencies.

As the internal details of Fig. 13.10 show, the pattern of interaction between spatial frequency and temporal frequency is much the same at all spatial positions (and like that shown in Fig. 13.6) except that sensitivity is moved down to lower spatial frequencies but not to lower temporal frequencies as eccentricity is increased.

Size-Scaled Models. Temporal Characteristics Depend on Absolute Spatial Frequency. A priori, the temporal characteristics attached to a particular spatial frequency might stay the same at different eccentricities. Then different mechanisms in a single size-scaled family like that of Fig. 13.4 would have different temporal weighting functions. If this were the case, however, the function plotting sensitivity versus temporal frequency at a given spatial frequency should have the same shape at all eccentricites (be the same up to a multiplicative factor—that is the same except for a vertical shift on the log sensitivity axis). For a given low spatial frequency, however, the low-temporal-frequency decline flattens out at greater eccentricities (as examination of the contour maps in Fig. 13.10 will show or as is plotted directly in Koenderink et al., 1978a, 1978b). Thus, temporal characteristics are probably not determined by absolute spatial frequency.

Size-Scaled Models. Temporal Characteristics Depend on Relative Spatial Frequency. In a second possible version of a spatial-scaling model, the temporal weighting function is assumed to stay the same throughout a scaled family of mechanisms (e.g., throughout the family having the weighting functions in Fig. 13.4), even though the weighting functions are wider and hence the mechanisms are sensitive to lower spatial frequencies at more eccentric positions. Put another way, according to this kind of model, temporal characteristics depend not on the actual spatial frequency but on how high it is relative to the cut-off spatial frequency at that eccentricity. Wilson and his colleague's models make this assumption: The relative sensitivity of any N mechanism, for example, to the two time courses of stimuli they use, are assumed to be the same at all eccentricities (see Fig. 6.13).

The size-scaling experiments, where two stimuli of the same temporal frequency are size scaled as described above (e.g., Koenderink et al, 1978c; Virsu et al., 1983) are tests of this kind of model. Finding the two sensitivities to be equal—as these authors did in many conditions—is support for this model. Similarly, Kelly's (1984a) results using stabilized viewing also seem to be consistent with this kind of model. Indeed this model, although it may not be strictly correct, seems to predict all the large effects of spatial frequency, temporal frequency, and spatial position over large ranges on each dimension and represents an impressive simplification of a large amount of parametric data.

Low Versus High Temporal Frequencies. It is difficult to see, however, how the size-scaled models (even with temporal characteristics depending on relative spatial frequency) could predict an increase in critical flicker frequency at greater eccentricities. Thus such a model cannot be wholly correct throughout the temporal-frequency range. Perhaps the spatial-scaling characteristics for higher temporal frequencies are different from those for the low to medium temporal frequencies most extensively studied. The study described in section 11.5.4 as an example of the "subdivision" argument (Tyler & Silverman, 1983) supports such a conclusion, as does Tyler's 1987 study. Scaling for mean luminance as well as size may partly resolve the discrepancy (see section 13.9.5).

Appearance Thresholds at Different Spatial Positions. Although in the fovea temporal-appearance sensitivity is higher than spatial-appearance sensitivity at velocities greater than about 1 degree/second, at 5 degrees eccentric it is not higher until velocities about 2 degrees/second on the average (Harris, 1980). This result may surprise those who think the periphery is the place for motion. (A somewhat similar result was reported by Murray et al., 1983, although comparison is difficult as all their results show more dependence on spatial frequency per se and less on velocity than do other reports; this may have resulted from their use of on-off gratings, which always have a 0-c/sec component.) Whether a stimulus was shown to the nasal versus temporal retina made no difference in one study (Blake & Mills, 1979).

13.6.6 *Effect of Other Dimensions/Factors on Sensitivity as a Function of Temporal Frequency*

Spatial Extent. Given the usual effects of spatial extent (see main section on spatial extent) one would expect the following: With large spatial extents, the temporal-frequency sensitivity should have a clear low-temporal-frequency decline and a very high CFF. With small spatial extents, the temporal-frequency sensitivity functions might not have a low-temporal-frequency decline (due to the preponderance of high spatial frequencies) and should have a relatively low CFF. This decrease in CFF with spatial extent is well documented at a wide range of spatial positions (Hartmann et al., 1979).

Mean Luminance. At low mean luminances there is no low-temporal-frequency decline even at low spatial frequencies (see section 13.9).

13.7 SENSITIVITY ON THE OTHER TEMPORAL DIMENSIONS

13.7.1 *Sensitivity as a Function of Temporal Position Is Presumably Uniform*

Sensitivity as a function of temporal position (from, for example, the beginning of a trial) is presumably uniform although rarely measured. Assuming that it is completely uniform is probably a mistake, however.

13.7.2 *Sensitivity Increases With Increasing Temporal Extent*

As temporal extent (either of temporally sinusoidal or of temporally aperiodic stimuli) increases, sensitivity increases dramatically at small values and then increases more slowly. The initial dramatic increase is presumably due to temporal integration (characterized by the temporal weighting function) and the more gradual increase is presumably due to independent variability in the outputs at different points in time, that is, to temporal probability summation.

Effect of Spatial Frequency. When gratings are used as stimuli, the increase in sensitivity with increasing temporal extent is greater for high spatial frequencies than for low. See section 13.2.3 on effect of temporal extent on spatial-frequency sensitivity.

Effect of Spatial Extent—Classic Temporal Summation Experiments. When spatially and temporally aperiodic stimuli are used, the critical duration decreases as the spatial extent of the stimulus increases (Barlow, 1958). This corresponds at least roughly to the move toward higher temporal frequencies when spatial frequency is lowered that one finds with sinusoidal stimuli (e.g., Fig. 13.6). To predict the classic summation effects quantitatively, one has to take into account all the factors mentioned previously for spatial and temporal extent.

13.7.3   Temporal Phase (Increments Versus Decrements)

Sensitivity is probably much the same for all temporal phases (everything else being equal), although greater sensitivity has sometimes been reported for on transients than for off (Russell & Wheeler, 1983, very low mean luminances) and for increments than decrements (Krauskopf, 1980).

13.7.4   Sensitivity Is Generally Uniform as a Function of Direction of Motion

Sensitivity is usually reported to be approximately uniform for different directions (with exceptions in some subjects and with possible differences depending on whether the direction is toward or away from the fovea).

13.8   PERFORMANCE AS A FUNCTION OF CONTRAST

13.8.1   Increasing Performance With Increasing Contrast

As contrast increases, detectability increases monotonically. When percent-correct is plotted versus logarithmic contrast, for example, the function is typically S-shaped, going from chance to perfect performance over a range of about 0.3 log units—a factor of 2 of contrast. This function is frequently called the *psychometric function*. As described in Chapter 4, when percent-correct in two-alternative forced-choice experiments or percent-yes in yes-no experiments is plotted against contrast, the function is well described by the Quick psychometric function, with slope parameters reported between 2 and 5. The changes in the horizontal position of this function on the log contrast axis are changes in threshold and are summarized in all the other sections. The question remains to be considered here, however, of whether the slope parameter is consistently affected by variations along any of the pattern dimensions we are considering or by any miscellaneous factors.

13.8.2   Effects on Slope of the Psychometric Function

Careful studies suggest that the slope parameter is remarkably invariant (when measured holding everything else constant) with changes in, at least, spatial frequency and spatial extent, although some small difference between the slope for a bipartite field and for a 12-c/deg grating seemed to appear reliably (Mayer & Tyler, 1986; Nachmias, 1981). I know of no other difference in slope along any of the pattern dimensions we have been considering that has been compellingly demonstrated.

There are, however, consistent differences due to psychophysical procedure. In particular, a yes-no experiment with low false-alarm rates produces steeper slopes (after correction for guessing) than yes-no with higher false-alarm rates or than two-alternative forced-choice (Nachmias, 1981). See sections 4.7.4 and 8.6.2.

There are also differences in slope resulting from the length of time over which data are pooled in order to form a psychometric function. The longer the time, the shallower the slope (e.g., Rashbass, 1970).

Furthermore, there seem to be consistent individual differences (Mayer & Tyler, 1986).

A slope difference in responses to different wavelengths (spatially and temporally aperiodic stimuli) has been reported (Maloney & Wandell, 1983).

13.9   SENSITIVITY AS A FUNCTION OF MEAN LUMINANCE

13.9.1   Increasing, Then Constant, Contrast Sensitivity as Mean Luminance Increases

For a given pattern, contrast sensitivity increases as mean luminance increases, although it may reach an asymptote. Equivalently (and the form shown in the upper left of Fig 13.11), contrast threshold first decreases and then stays constant.

Contrast Versus Amplitude. Effects of mean luminance are best comprehended fully by describing them both in terms of contrast and of a second quantity, amplitude. Remember that amplitude (which we will call ΔL) is the absolute difference between the peak and mean luminance, so that contrast is just amplitude divided by mean luminance. Amplitude thresholds as a function of mean luminance are shown in the lower left of Fig. 13.11. Notice that amplitude

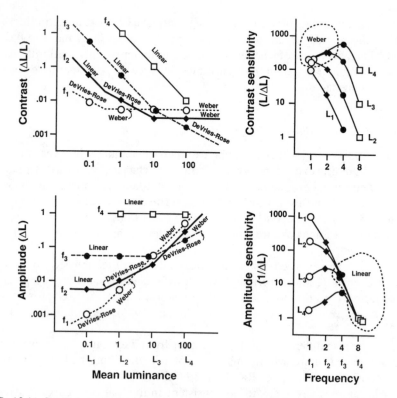

FIG. 13.11 Some hypothetical results, typical of those reported, for the interaction of mean luminance and either temporal or spatial frequency. The same results are plotted in four ways (where the symbols retain their meaning in all four panels): contrast threshold as a function of mean luminance (upper left); amplitude threshold as a function of mean luminance (lower left); contrast sensitivity as a function of frequency (upper right); and amplitude sensitivity as a function of frequency (lower right).

thresholds tend to be constant at low mean luminances and then tend to increase.

A valuable review of the physiological and psychophysical effects of mean luminance, and the models of such effects, including discussion of their perceptual function, can be found in Shapley and Enroth-Cugell (1984). Another valuable review, of the empirical psychophysical literature on "light and dark adaptation" (the effects of mean or background luminance, particularly using aperiodic stimuli), can be found in Hood and Finkelstein (1986).

Linear, Devries-Rose, and Weber Ranges. The changes with mean luminance are often talked about as falling into three regions, although one rarely finds all three regions for the same stimulus. The transitions between these three regions are shown as more abrupt in Fig. 13.11 (left) than in results of experiments. At low mean luminances, there is often a "linear range" where contrast threshold decreases (contrast sensitivity increases) as a linear function of mean luminance; equivalently amplitude threshold remains constant. This is the behavior expected if, for example, an observer's detection threshold is determined by the criterion difference between peak and mean outputs from a deterministic array of mechanisms that act like linear systems. The existence of a linear range is actually rather puzzling (see Shapley & Enroth-Cugell, 1984, pp. 293–294).

At somewhat higher mean luminances, there is a *DeVries-Rose range* (so-called because of theoretical considerations of quantal fluctuations associated with their names) where contrast threshold is decreasing and amplitude threshold is increasing, both as power functions with exponent ½ (therefore as straight lines with slopes $-\frac{1}{2}$ and $+\frac{1}{2}$ respectively on the log-log axes of Fig. 13.11).

At the highest mean luminances, a *Weber range* may appear, where contrast threshold stays constant and amplitude threshold increases in proportion to mean luminance.

Rod-Cone Transitions. Many measures of pattern sensitivity as a function of mean luminance show little obvious evidence of the transition from rod to cone vision, although stimulus situations where wavelengths of background and target are appropriately manipulated clearly do. It is not unreasonable, however, that the visual system should be designed in such a way as to smooth over discontinuities in most situations. The roles of rods and cones are quite extensively discussed in the review by Shapley and Enroth-Cugell (1984), by D'Zmura and Lennie (1986), and by Hood and Finkelstein (1986).

Time Course of Light Adaptation. In this review we have limited ourselves to situations where the mean luminance is constant for a long enough time that the adaptation processes are in a steady state. The steady state is not reached instantaneously, of course. For rod visual pathways, for example, there is a rapid phase that has a time constant of about 100 milliseconds (similar to the adaptation found physiologically; see Shapley & Enroth-Cugell, 1984) followed by a slow phase with a time constant of 30 seconds (e.g., Adelson, 1982). Similarly, for cone vision there is rapid phase (50 milliseconds at onset, 200 milliseconds at offset) followed by a slower phase (e.g., Hayhoe, Benimoff, & Hood, 1987). For further details and references see reviews mentioned earlier. Of course, for stimuli that are changing in time (see 13.9.5) the dynamic properties of light adaptation processes may be important.

13.9.2 The Constant-Flux Hypothesis and the Effect of Spatial Frequency on Sensitivity as a Function of Mean Luminance

The higher the spatial frequency, the higher the mean luminance at which a given transition occurs, as is illustrated in Fig. 13.11. Notice, for example, that the transition between the linear and the DeVries-Rose ranges is lowest (below the range shown) for the lowest frequency f_1, higher for f_2, still higher for f_3, and highest (above the range shown) for the highest frequency f_4.

In the plot of contrast sensitivity as a function of frequency (upper right panel), the low-frequency ends tend to coincide at high mean luminances (reflecting Weber-law behavior). To put this another way, mean luminance has less effect on contrast sensitivity for low frequencies than for high.

In the amplitude-sensitivity plot (lower right panel), however, the high-frequency ends tend to coincide, reflecting linear behavior. There is some disagreement about whether there actually is a completely linear region at high spatial frequencies. This is a tricky question to answer (and certainly depends on whether you are keeping pupil size constant, for example); some studies fail to find a completely linear high-spatial-frequency region (Kelly, 1972, as shown in Fig 3.12; van Nes, 1968) and other studies find such a region (R. De Valois, Morgan, & Snodderly, 1974; Koenderink et al., 1978d).

For nominally stationary gratings at the fovea, the transition from the DeVries-Rose to the Weber region has been reported to occur at a mean luminance that is approximately proportional to the square of the spatial frequency. Or, as the original authors stated it, the square root of the transition luminance multiplied by the reciprocal of the spatial frequency is a constant (van Nes, Koenderink, Nas, & Bouman, 1967; van Nes, 1968). This quantitative relationship is consistent with the *constant-flux hypothesis* (below) and with the closely related *channel hypothesis* of Shapley and Enroth-Cugell (1984).

Constant-Flux Hypothesis. Let's use *flux* to denote the mean luminance summed over the area of the mechanism's excitatory center (i.e., mean luminance multiplied by excitatory center area). Suppose that the mean luminance at which a given transition (e.g., the transition from DeVries-Rose to Weber) occurs for a given spatial frequency is determined by the flux (i.e., the mean luminance times center area) stimulating the relevant mechanisms. The mechanisms sensitive to low spatial frequencies have bigger centers and, therefore, sum luminance over a larger area than do the mechanisms sensitive to high spatial frequencies. Hence, if transitions all occur at the same flux, transitions should occur at lower mean luminances for low spatial frequencies than for high spatial frequencies (as they do in the empirical results).

Quantitatively, if orientation bandwidth in degrees of angular rotation is the same for all spatial frequencies (as it may be, see Chap. 12), then the length of a weighting function's excitatory center is inversely proportional to its best spatial frequency. Since its width is also (by definition), the area will be inversely proportional to its best spatial frequency squared. Hence flux will be proportional to

$$\frac{L_0}{f^2}$$

and therefore the luminance producing a criterion amount of flux will be directly proportional to spatial frequency squared (as observed in experimental results).

Alternatively, rather than the controlling factor being total flux stimulating the pattern-selective mechanisms themselves, it might be total flux at a lower level in the visual system (e.g., the concentric retinal ganglion cells), in which case the above argument is run through for those cells (see the channel hypothesis of Shapley & Enroth-Cugell, 1984). In fact, total flux is known to control cat retinal ganglion cell's light adaptation (Enroth-Cugell & Shapley, 1973).

13.9.3 *More About Spatial-Scaling Models and the Effect of Spatial Position on Sensitivity as a Function of Mean Luminance*

Briefly, the effect of mean luminance on contrast sensitivity has been described as much smaller in the periphery than in the fovea. Equivalently, the Weber region starts at lower mean luminances in the periphery than in the fovea. Indeed, for low spatial frequencies between 0.25 and 1.5 c/deg, Weber's law has been reported in the periphery at the same mean luminance levels where DeVries-Rose behavior is found in the fovea (Koenderink et al., 1978d).

In the periphery (as in the fovea) the transition to Weber's law has been reported to occur at lower mean luminances for low spatial frequencies than for high; at low spatial frequencies Weber's law was found at the lowest mean luminance tested, but for higher spatial frequencies DeVries-Rose behavior was found (Koenderink et al., 1978d).

Crudely speaking, there is a sense in which contrast sensitivity in the periphery at all mean luminances is very much like that in the fovea at low mean luminances: namely, the spatial (acuity) and temporal (CFF) cutoffs occur at quite low frequencies (e.g., Hartmann et al., 1979; Kerr, 1971), and the maximal contrast sensitivity as a function of spatial or temporal frequency is quite low (e.g., Koenderink et al., 1978d).

Size-Scaled Models and the Constant-Flux Hypothesis. There is an important consequence of the interactions between spatial-position and mean-luminance effects: The size-scaled models discussed in sections 13.4.2 and 13.6.5 cannot work at all mean luminances, at least not with the same scaling function. This failure is demonstrated in Figs. 1, 2, and 3 of Koenderink, Bouman, de Mesquita, and Slappendel (1978d). Most tests of the scaling hypothesis have worked with mean luminances in the Weber's law region, where this failure is hidden.

Some extension of the constant-flux hypothesis might work, however. One might consider a modification to the simple stimulus-scaling hypothesis like the following: If two patterns at two different eccentricities are to have the same contrast threshold, not only must the spatial dimensions of the more peripheral pattern be scaled up (relative to the less peripheral pattern), but its mean luminance must also be scaled down by a factor reflecting the greater total flux of the peripheral pattern (cf. Koenderink et al., 1978d; Raninen & Rovamo, 1986; Rovamo & Raninen, 1984, 1988). What this factor should be, whether the same factor applies to both size and mean luminance, whether any such modified scaling hypothesis could be made to work, and what it would imply for the multiple-mechanisms model remain to be seen (and is discussed further in note 1), but it is a very interesting possibility.

13.9.4   *Effect of Spatial Extent on Sensitivity as a Function of Mean Luminance*

For spatially and temporally aperiodic targets, the decrease in contrast sensitivity with mean luminance is faster for large extents than for small because the transition to DeVries-Rose and Weber regions occurs at lower mean luminances (e.g., Barlow, 1958). Presumably the major reason for this dependence on spatial extent is that large-extent aperiodic stimuli contain more lower spatial frequencies than do small-extent aperiodic stimuli.

Whether spatial extent of sinusoidal gratings makes any difference in transition mean luminance is unknown to me; it might make very little difference.

13.9.5   *Effect of Temporal Frequency on Sensitivity as a Function of Mean Luminance*

The effects of temporal frequency on sensitivity as a function of mean luminance are analogous to those of spatial frequency: As temporal frequency gets higher, the transitions move to higher mean luminances. In fact, the transition mean luminances may even be proportional to temporal frequency squared or, as the original authors put it, the square root of the transition luminance times the reciprocal of temporal frequency may be a constant (for flickering spatially aperiodic fields of 2 degrees or less in diameter; data from DeLange, 1958, as analyzed by van Nes et al., 1967).

Why this relationship should hold (if it is confirmed in a larger data base) is less easily related to multiple analyzers than was the spatial-frequency case, as there seem to be only a few broad-band ones (at the most) on the temporal-frequency dimension. This relationship is likely instead to be a result of the dynamics of light adaptation (within analyzers broadband for temporal frequency); and the similarity between the relationship for spatial frequency and that for temporal frequency a coincidence (at least as far as description in terms of multiple mechanisms or neurons is concerned).

Interaction Between Spatial and Temporal Frequency. Figure 13.12 shows the regions of spatial and temporal frequency over which each of the three kinds of behavior hold at two mean luminances (50 trolands on the left and 200 trolands on the right).

Van Nes et al. (1967) suggested that the following quantitative relationship holds for gratings that are neither stationary (of 0 Hz c/sec) nor spatially aperiodic (of 0 c/deg): The transition luminances are proportional to temporal frequency squared times spatial frequency squared, or as they put it, the square root of the transition luminance times the reciprocal of temporal frequency times the reciprocal of spatial frequency is a constant. This relationship held in the small set of experimental results they looked at.

Size-Scaling Models, Temporal Frequency, and Mean Luminance. If stimuli at different eccentricities are scaled not only for size but also for mean luminance

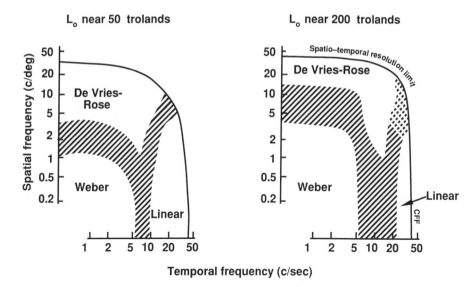

FIG. 13.12 The combinations of spatial frequency and temporal frequency that lead to each of the three kinds of behaviors described in the text, shown at two mean luminances (50 trolands in the left panel and 200 trolands in the right). The hatched areas indicate transition regions. The extra crosshatching in the upper right corner of the right panel shows the region where eye movements made it difficult to obtain a reproducible threshold. (Modified from Figs. 3 and 9 in Kelly, 1972; used by permission.)

(as mentioned at the end of section 13.9.3), the difference between behavior at low and high temporal frequencies (section 13.6.5) may largely disappear. The sensitivities at high temporal frequencies (as well as those at low) may become quite independent of eccentricity. Indeed, the critical flicker fusion frequency has been reported to become independent of eccentricity when size and mean luminance are scaled by slightly different factors (Raninen and Rovamo, 1987; Rovamo and Raninen, 1988—see these studies for motivation for different factors). Remember that low temporal frequencies enter the Weber region at much lower mean luminances than do high temporal frequencies, and therefore are probably in the Weber range at mean luminances typically used in experiments. Whether they are scaled for mean luminance (as well as size) is thus irrelevant as it does not affect contrast sensitivity. In short, scaling for mean luminance as well as for size may make sensitivity at all temporal frequencies quite independent of eccentricity. (It is still difficult to see, however, how a model scaling for both mean luminance and size, as mentioned earlier in section 13.6.5, could actually account for the increases in CFF with eccentricity for some unscaled stimuli, and exactly which scaling factor or factors to use is also quite unclear at this point.)

Rods and High Temporal Frequencies. In plots of high-temporal-frequency cutoffs as a function of mean luminance, there are often rod-cone breaks, that is, two obvious branches with spectral sensitivity measurements verifying that the lower luminance/lower CFF branch is controlled by the rods and the higher luminance/higher CFF branch by the cones. These breaks are particularly obvious at eccentric spatial positions. However, it turns out to be a mistake to assume that rods cannot follow higher temporal frequencies than those at the break. A function isolating the rod CFF as a function of mean luminance still shows two branches oddly enough (with a long plateau in between), and the branch at higher mean luminances that is ordinarily hidden by cone action goes up to quite high temporal frequencies (Conner & MacLeod, 1977).

There is a moral here relevant to the subdivision argument of section 11.5.4. Parametric functions (e.g., pattern sensitivity as a function of mean luminance for many patterns) without any obvious subparts may still reflect the action of two distinct analyzers (e.g., rods and cones), whereas a function with an obvious division into two parts (the rod CFF function of Conner & MacLeod, 1977) may reflect only one analyzer (rod; although the plateau and two branches may reflect two different kinds of action by the rods, this cannot be taken as evidence for the action of both rods and cones).

13.9.6   Effect of Other Dimensions/Factors on Sensitivity as a Function of Mean Luminance

Temporal Extent. For spatially and temporally aperiodic targets, the transition to Weber's law may occur at lower mean luminances for long durations than for short (Barlow, 1958), probably a result of the fact that longer duration stimuli contain more low temporal frequencies than do shorter durations.

Optics. Within many theoretical contexts, it is retinal illuminance rather than the mean luminance of the stimulus that is of importance. An observer's natural pupil contracts to some extent as mean luminance is increased (say from 7 mm diameter to 1 mm diameter). This is not nearly large enough to counteract the many log units of mean luminance over which the visual system adapts. It will, however, partly counteract the effect of increased mean luminances and needs to be considered when natural pupils are used.

Further, at lower mean luminances where the natural pupil is larger, there is more effective spherical aberration, which may make the optimal refractive power different for different spatial frequencies. Placing a small-diameter artificial pupil in front of the eye of the observer overcomes some of these problems, although it introduces other (see references in section 13.4.3).

Species of Observer. Macaque contrast sensitivity as a function of spatial frequency over a range of mean luminances is remarkably like human sensitivity in all respects (R. De Valois et al., 1974). Cat contrast sensitivity, although moved to lower spatial frequencies, changes analogously to that of humans (Pasternak & Merigan, 1981).

Color. Van Nes (1968) measured sensitivity as a function of mean luminance for gratings of several different wavelengths. No important differential effects were observed.

13.10 SENSITIVITY IS GENERALLY THE SAME FOR THE TWO EYES

On average, sensitivity in the right eye is similar to that in the left eye, although many individuals show some differences.

13.11 EFFECTS OF OTHER FACTORS

13.11.1 Optics, Accommodation, and Viewing Distance

Optics. Imperfect focus generally affects high spatial frequencies more than low (e.g., Fig. 12 of Charman & Tucker, 1977; D. Green & Campbell, 1965).

For lenses with spherical aberration (including the human lens, particularly with large pupil sizes), the position of optimal focus varies somewhat with spatial frequency (e.g., Charman & Tucker, 1977; D. Green & Campbell, 1965).

It is interesting to note the following: The optics of the human eye is, to a very good approximation, a linear translation-invariant system. Hence the image of a sinusoidal grating on the retina is still a sinusoidal grating. This kind of invariance is true for no other stimulus. For example, a stimulus that is a point of light is spread out into a fuzzy-edged circle on the retina.

Peripheral Refractive Errors. Even when the eye is corrected for foveal refractive errors, there remain peripheral ones than can be quite substantial. Published examples include the refractions of two observers at various eccentricities in Koenderink et al. (1978a) and of four observers in Millodot et al. (1975).

These imperfect refractions seem not to limit acuity (high-spatial-frequency sensitivity at low temporal frequencies) in the periphery, or at least not very much. Correcting both spherical and astigmatic errors improved acuity little if at all in one study (Millodot et al., 1975; C. Johnson, Leibowitz, Millidot, & Lamont, 1976); but bypassing the optics by using interference-fringe gratings in another study (Frisen & Glansholm, 1975)—thereby eliminating not only the effects of spherical and astigmatic errors but also the effects of oblique chromatic aberration, coma, flatness of field, oblique ray astigmatism, and other optical aberations)—improved acuity more (by somewhat less than a factor of 2). Whether the difference between these two studies is due to the additional optical problems bypassed in the second study or just a reflection of differences among individual observers and practice effects is obviously unclear. In any case, correction of refractive errors might be expected to improve acuity by a factor of 2 or less.

Imperfect refraction does limit performance on other tasks in the periphery, however, including motion thresholds (C. Johnson & Leibowitz, 1974; Leibowitz, Johnson, & Isabelle, 1972) and two tasks using sharp-onset stimuli (peripheral increment thresholds in Fankenhauser & Enoch, 1962, and the Westheimer sensitization paradigm in Enoch, Sunga, & Bachman 1970, and Sunga & Enoch, 1970). In short, imperfect refraction may be a limiting factor only in tasks that the periphery does rather well but not in tasks it does poorly (see discussion in C. Johnson et al., 1976).

Accommodation. Sinusoidal gratings are not a particularly good stimulus for accommodation, at least not within a full log unit of threshold (e.g., Charman & Tucker, 1977; Raymond, Lindblad, & Leibowitz, 1984). There seems to be something like a natural resting position that accommodation will return to given insufficient stimulation (e.g., Baker, Brown, & Garner, 1983; Owens, 1979). Accommodative accuracy (and therefore contrast sensitivity) is generally maximal when viewing distance corresponds to this resting position (e.g., C. Johnson, 1976; Raymond & Leibowitz, 1985).

To make matters more complicated, there are dynamic fluctuations in accommodative response (e.g., Kotulak & Schor, 1986). And the initial accommodation onto a target (bringing it into focus) may well be controlled by different factors from those involved in keeping it in focus (e.g., Charman & Tucker, 1977; Bour, 1981).

Thus, variations in accommodative accuracy may well affect contrast sensitivity measurements substantially, which is particularly important for relatively high spatial frequencies.

Viewing Distance. All patterns producing the same pattern on the retina, no matter from what distance they are viewed, are equally detectable. All reported effects of "viewing distance" seem to be effects of having changed the pattern on the retina (usually by changing at least its spatial extent) or else effects due to inadequate accommodation (e.g., Howell & Hess, 1978).

In spite of this, casual observation in a laboratory immediately demonstrates the usual "size constancy"—as you move away from the display the perceived size of the bars in the gratings stays the same.

13.11.2   Psychophysical Procedure

The exact values of thresholds measured by various procedures (e.g., adjustment, forced-choice, yes-no) will not be the same, although for most purposes they come quite close. A completely adequate theory relating yes-no to forced-choice results has not yet been developed in any sensory/perceptual domain, however (sections 4.7.4, 8.6.2, and 13.8).

Practice Effects. Practice effects on contrast sensitivity are usually minimal: Particularly in forced-choice procedures, observer thresholds will be quite stable from the first session on. However, there are several combinations of stimulus parameters for which substantial practice effects have been reported (e.g., oblique orientations, see section 13.3; peripheral locations, see section 13.4.3; and discriminations involving complex gratings, see section 10.6.3).

Between- and Within-Session Variability. Between-session variability is almost always substantially greater than within-session variability. Thus, for example, variability measures calculated within a session can badly mislead one about conclusions from comparisons across sessions. Some of this between-session variability takes the form of sensitivity shifts (multiplication of all thresholds by a given factor).

13.11.3 Eye Movements, Stabilized Images

A number of studies have now compared contrast sensitivity in stabilized viewing with that in unstabilized viewing. At long durations, sensitivity as a function of spatial frequency has a low-frequency decline even in stabilized vision (Burbeck & Kelly, 1982; Tulunay-Keesey & Bennis, 1979; Tulunay-Keesey & Jones, 1976). This result argues against the possibility (particularly well described in Arend, 1976a) that eye movements might be the only cause of increased sensitivity to middle spatial frequencies relative to low. Though probably not the only cause, eye movements may well contribute to the peak that occurs with nominally stationary gratings in unstabilized viewing.

The spatial-frequency dependent effect of changing from abrupt onsets and offsets to gradual onsets and offsets also remains after stabilization, although there is some spatial-frequency dependent effect of stabilization (Higgins et al., 1983; Tulunay-Keesey & Bennis, 1979).

All the effects in stabilized experiments as well as the effects of introduced eye movements (e.g., Arend, 1976a; Kulikowski, 1971b) seem understandable on the following assumption: Contrast sensitivity is completely explainable by the spatiotemporal characteristics of the retinal image (rather than by those of the stimulus in the world or by some interaction of the two). To a first approximation at least, one can think of eye movements as introducing about an average 0.15 deg/sec velocity into a nominally stationary grating in unstabilized viewing (Kelly 1979b).

In short, although undoubtedly important, eye movements have not turned out to be a devastating artifact in interpreting the near-threshold investigations that are covered in this book.

13.11.4 Age, Species, and Pathology of Observer

Effects of Age. In near-threshold psychophysics as in so much else, the developmental effects are easy to summarize: things get better before they get worse. In particular, contrast sensitivity for almost any pattern shows an increase in infancy and perhaps in early childhood, followed by a plateau for the rest of childhood and most of adulthood, and then perhaps a decline in old age (perhaps due to disease).

The investigation of infants' and young childrens' vision is very difficult and only recently undertaken with rigorous psychophysics. Although there have been a number of studies of acuity, exactly how fast acuity grows with age is still in some dispute as different measures have suggested different answers (e.g., Hainline, Camenzuli, Abramov, Rawlick, and Lemerise, 1986; Teller, Morse, Borton, and Regal, 1974—consult the reference list).

Sensitivity for high spatial and temporal frequencies may be impaired starting in late middle-age (e.g., Owsley, Sekuler, and Siemsen, 1983—see reference list).

Species. Primate contrast sensitivity seems remarkably similar to that of humans studied in the same situations (e.g., R. De Valois et al., 1974; Harwerth et al., 1980; R. Williams et al., 1981). Cat contrast sensitivity seems to act much like that of humans except to be moved to lower spatial frequencies (e.g., Pasternak & Merigan, 1981). Consult the reference list.

Pathology. Consult the reference list. Note that substantial individual differences exist even among observers with no known abnormality (e.g., Ginsburg & Cannon, 1983; M. Mayer, 1983b).

13.11.5   Color

Although not extensively studied, wavelength composition seems to have only relatively small effects as long as it is homogeneous across the grating (e.g., Campbell & Green, 1965; van Nes, 1968; and a number of cross-study comparisons). Using gratings in which wavelength composition is not homogeneous, however, can produce very different results, which are beyond the scope of this book. Briefly, however, the spatial- and temporal-frequency sensitivity for gratings defined by color differences (with no luminance differences) seems coarser than that with luminance gratings; in particular, it has lower high-frequency cutoffs but (sometimes in any case) higher sensitivities at low frequencies. Consult the reference list for a sampling of such studies.

13.12   EQUIPMENT INCLUDING SURROUNDS

13.12.1   *Cathode-Ray Tube (CRT) Displays*

Most recent studies of contrast sensitivity have generated the patterns on cathode-ray tube displays (televisions or monitors). The luminance profile of the patterns is controlled by an input voltage signal generated either by hardware (e.g., a waveform generator) or more frequently, now, by computer. Using a computer to calculate the luminance profiles makes it extremely easy to generate any desired spatiotemporal pattern, as well as to switch patterns between trials, record observers' responses, and so forth.

The linearity between the voltage into a CRT's intensity control (as produced by the hardware or the computer) and the luminance displayed on the CRT face is typically quite good, although far from perfect. Thus, particularly in supra-threshold patterns, considerable distortions may exist if the nonlinearity is not corrected for. In setups where the voltage signal is generated by a computer, it is extremely easy to compensate for the remaining nonlinearity by appropriately distorting the input signal (see description in Williams, Booth, Kiorpes, & Teller, 1981, for example).

Although there are many advantages to these cathode-ray tube displays, there are limitations, several of which are described briefly here. Further discussion of the limitations and of appropriate calibration procedures can be found in a number of places, including Williams, Booth, Kiorpes, & Teller (1981), Morgan and Watt (1982); and Westheimer (1985).

Limited Brightness. It is difficult to get bright enough CRT displays for many purposes.

Limited Display Size. The available field size on a CRT display is limited. The available surface varies from a few centimeters to about 30 centimeters (and soon presumably even larger). The available resolution is limited by the size of the electronic beam's spot and speed of the electronics (see some calibrations and discussion in Morgan & Watt, 1982). Together, these factors typically and severely limit the maximal number of cycles one can put on a screen to about 100.

To study relatively high spatial frequencies, therefore, the viewing distance has to be arranged so that the display size on the retina is only a few degrees. This in turn puts a lower limit on the spatial frequency that can be shown with 3, 4, or more cycles at that same viewing distance.

If only one spatial frequency is studied at a time, viewing distance can be varied between spatial frequencies and a full range of spatial frequencies can be studied (but see section 13.11.1 about viewing distance). In many experiments, however, it is not possible to vary viewing distance between different spatial frequencies.

That the maximum number of cycles is about 100 limits the extent of the visual field that can be studied simultaneously.

Limited Sweep Rate. Each presentation of a stimulus is actually a number of sweeps of the electron beam across the screen. On each sweep the stimulus is painted across the screen, from one side to the other. Typically the number of sweeps per second is between about 60 and 200; thus each sweep takes from 5 to 15 milliseconds. Difficulties arise when fast temporal changes, for example, very short stimulus presentations or quickly moving or flickering patterns, are desired; the fastest they can be is one sweep. Also, for at least some neurons in the visual system, a sweep rate of over 100 c/sec is still not effectively identical to a continuously present stimulus (e.g., Frishman, Freeman, Troy, Schweitzer-Tong & Enroth-Cugell, 1987). This observation raises the worrying possibility that even for psychophysics, where the flicker fusion rate is traditionally thought to be much lower than that, stimuli generated with sweep rates of less than a couple hundred may act differently from steadily presented stimuli. But trying to use higher sweep rates quickly overtaxes the electronics.

Calibrating the Contrast for High Spatial Frequencies. The contrast at high spatial frequencies is not trivial to calibrate on cathode-ray tube displays. When it has been estimated as equal to the contrast at low spatial frequencies produced by the same input voltage, it has undoubtedly been overestimated. (See Williams et al., 1981, for further discussion.)

13.12.2 Surround

Ideally the experimenter would surround the stimulus patterns with a large patternless area exactly matched to the pattern in mean luminance and hue and with no discernible breaks between the pattern and the surrounding area. This ideal is what is assumed implicitly in most theoretical discussions (qualitative and quantitative). In practice, however, the ideal is never met. As we have just noted, available cathode-ray tubes have rather small displays, and placing the observer too close to the display reduces the available resolution range to rather coarse patterns and also makes "natural" viewing impossible for observers (particularly the older ones!).

Consequently, the CRT display is often surrounded with a wider area of a different material (often of illuminated cardboard) that is at least approximately matched in mean luminance and hue to the display. Although there is a clearly discernible boundary between the cathode-ray tube and such a surround (which may well have effects—see below), the use of this surround makes the observer more comfortable than a dark surround by reducing glare and afterimages too close to the fovea. (See review of such effects in earlier studies of flicker in C. Graham, 1966, p. 256.)

A second advantage to the use of cardboard or similar surrounds is that the discernible boundary between the CRT and the surround may be a much better stimulus for accommodation than the pattern itself or than small fixation marks.

Some studies have used a mask made of cardboard with a hole in it to diminish the size of the stimulus for some reason (e.g., to study gratings with different numbers of cycles). This will produce a discernible edge that may cause troubles, as discussed below.

Effects of Surround. A number of studies (Estevez & Cavonius, 1976a; Howell & Hess, 1978; McCann & Hall, 1980; McCann, Savoy, & Hall, 1978; Savoy & McCann, 1975) have shown that, particularly for small numbers of cycles or small heights at low spatial frequencies, the effect of the surround can be significant. The effect that is usually seen is that sensitivity is less (up to a factor of 3 at least) with a dark surround than with a bright surround (when the bright surround is part of the CRT screen and thus there is no discernible boundary).

Indeed, even a relatively thin (12-minute wide) dark line between the grating and an average-luminance surround can decrease sensitivity relative to that in the average-luminance surround, and the effect of a thin interposed line may be as large as that of an edge (Estevez & Cavonius, 1976a; van der Wildt & Waarts, 1983).

When the area of the surround is varied (and the surround as well as the grating are all on the CRT face so there is no discernible border as there is with cardboard surrounds), the surround to some extent mimics the effect of having extra periods of the grating; thus it is the width of the surround in periods that matters (McCann & Hall, 1980). Similarly, van der Wildt and Waarts (1983) found that the depressing effect of luminance discontinuities (dark lines, dark edges) on contrast sensitivity depends on the distance between them and the edge of the grating measured in periods, at least approximately.

The Surround Rule of Thumb. I find the following rule of thumb (suggested by the discussion in Estevez & Cavonius, 1976a) of considerable use: Any discernible edge (including that between, say, cardboard and the CRT face—and certainly that between a CRT and a dark surround) seems to produce a small bordering region on the CRT face in which sensitivity is greatly depressed. This region is of fixed extent—perhaps half a degree wide in typical situations (but don't take this figure seriously). Not only should you avoid putting anything in your own experiments into this region of depressed sensitivity, but correct interpretation of published experiments probably requires trying to discount any part of the stimulus that is in this region.

The size of this depressed-sensitivity boundary does not depend on the size of the field itself (therefore occupying a much larger proportion of small fields than of large) but it probably does depend on spatial frequency, being greater for lower spatial frequencies.

With foveal fixation and relatively large field sizes, the nonuniformity of the visual field often assures there is nothing in that border of depressed sensitivity that is of any significant visibility anyway. But once there are relatively few periods in a grating or the grating's height measured in periods is small (as sometimes happens with the lowest spatial frequencies used in a study or when spatial extent is being varied by cardboard apertures), this depressed-sensitivity region around the edge can matter a good deal.

Edges Caused by Abrupt Transitions. Even when there is a large enough cathode-ray tube that both the grating patch and a sizeable surround can be displayed on it, the use of a rectangular window function (producing abrupt edges on the pattern rather than the gradual edges of a Gaussian window, for example) will introduce difficulties in interpretation, particularly when the abrupt edges are close to the fixation point. For the edge may then be what is detected by the observer. A particularly dramatic example of possible effects is theoretically calculated in Kretz, Scarabin, and Bourguignat (1979). Kelly (1970) also discussed expected effects at the edges of sharply truncated sinusoidal gratings.

13.13   AN ASIDE ABOUT PHYSIOLOGY: POSSIBLE SUBSTRATES FOR PARAMETRIC SENSITIVITY

This section mentions some physiological evidence particularly relevant to parametric sensitivity experiments rather than to analyzer-revealing experiments and thus not included in the physiology described in section 12.7.

The observer's contrast sensitivity along any dimension on which there are multiple analyzers, for example, spatial frequency and orientation, is approximately the envelope of the sensitivity functions of the multiple analyzers. (It will be somewhat higher than the envelope if probability summation among analyzers is considered, as it probably should be.) To explain nonuniform sensitivity along any such dimension, therefore, in terms of the possible physiological substrate, one could assume that (a) the neurons sensitive to some values have lower peak sensitivities than those sensitive to others, (b) fewer neurons are sensitive to some values than to others (although all the neurons have equal peak sensitivity), or (c) some combination of a and b. We will refer to these possibilities as the *greater-sensitivity, greater-number,* and *combination* explanations, respectively.

Along any dimension on which there is only a single analyzer (at given values on the other dimensions, e.g., spatial extent at a given spatial frequency and spatial position), the observer's contrast sensitivity equals the sensitivity of that one analyzer. If cortical neurons in V1 and V2 are candidates for the neurophysiological substrate of these analyzers, therefore, the observer's contrast sensitivity function on such a dimension might have the same form as that of a single neuron. (Even if more than one neuron is actually the substrate for the single analyzer, as seems likely, the forms of the functions relating sensitivity to value should be much the same, even if absolute sensitivity is not.)

13.13.1   Spatial Frequency, Orientation, and Spatial Position

Spatial Frequency. The number of V1 neurons in the monkey tuned to each spatial-frequency range corresponds, roughly at least, to the overall behavioral contrast sensitivity of the macaque in these same conditions (R. De Valois et al., 1982). Thus, greater numbers (explanation b) rather than greater sensitivities (explanation a) may be the explanation of the differing sensitivities along the spatial-frequency dimension.

Orientation. Similarly, current physiological evidence from monkeys (which may show oblique effects much like humans) suggests that the oblique effect is explained by greater numbers (explanation b), although the evidence certainly cannot rule out greater sensitivity (explanation a) as another factor. In the macaque fovea, there seem to be more cortical cells (about 35% more) sensitive to orientations near vertical or horizontal than to those near either oblique (R. De Valois et al., 1982), with a greater trend in this direction for foveal cells tuned to high spatial frequencies than to low (although this latter trend did not reach significance in these relatively small samples). In a sample of parafoveal cells, the number of cells near each of the four orientations was practically identical. Similar results have been reported by Mansfield (1974) and by Mansfield and Ronner (1978), although neither Schiller, Finlay, and Volman (1976b) nor Poggio, Doty, and Talbot (1977) found any significant differences in cells tuned to different orientations.

Given the differences among individual observers (including monkey observers; R. Williams et al., 1981) in displaying the traditional oblique effect, it is somewhat surprising that such total-cell counts reveal as much information as they seem to.

Spatial Position. That the spatial scale of neurons increases with distance from foveal center has been known for a long time (e.g., Linsenmeier, Frishman, Jakiela, & Enroth-Cugell, 1982, and references therein). This physiological evidence was part of the inspiration for the spatially scaled psychophysical models that explain the changes in observer's sensitivity with spatial position quite nicely (see sections 13.4.2, 13.6.5, 13.9.3, and references therein). In the spatially scaled models of section 6.9, it is the greater sensitivity rather than greater numbers possibility that is taken to explain the decrease in sensitivity with increase in distance from foveal center. One could probably substitute greater numbers with little difficulty, since the probability summation (or pooling) across different mechanisms allows number of mechanisms to compensate for sensitivity.

There is probably more than one physiological scaling factor (different ones being associated with different kinds of neurons; e.g., see Lennie, 1977) and more than one psychophysical scaling factor (different ones for different tasks). Which if any of these map into each other is as yet unknown.

13.13.2   Temporal Frequency

The spatial-frequency and temporal-frequency sensitivity functions of retinal ganglion cells and lateral geniculate neurons are not separable. Qualitatively, in any case, the inseparability is of the same form as the human observer's overall contrast sensitivity: At high temporal frequencies, the spatial-frequency contrast sensitivity function loses its low spatial-frequency decline. (And the same is true with spatial and temporal interchanged).

A recent study of macaques in which there was severe damage to the parvocellular-projecting retinal ganglion cells suggests that the parvocellular-projecting pathway (the medium-cell pathway) is involved primarily in the detection of higher spatial and lower temporal frequencies, whereas the magnocellular-projecting pathway (the large-cell pathway) is involved primarily in the detection of lower spatial and higher temporal frequencies (Merigan & Eskin, 1986).

But it is the temporal properties of macaque cortical (V1 and V2) neurons rather than of geniculate neurons that match the overall temporal-frequency sensitivity of human observers, with the peak temporal frequencies of cortical cells falling most often in the 3- to 8-c/sec range (Foster et al., 1985), whereas peak temporal frequencies in macaque geniculate neurons fall between 10 and 20 c/ sec (Hicks, Lee, & Vidyasagar, 1983).

13.13.3 Mean Luminance

The dependence of retinal ganglion cells on constant flux was briefly referred to in section 13.9.2. See the review by Shapley and Enroth-Cugell (1984) for coverage of much of our knowledge about neuronal changes with mean luminance and for references. A more recent definitive study of cat retinal ganglion cells' (both x and y) spatiotemporal sensitivity at different mean luminances is Frishman, Freeman, Troy, Schweitzer-Tong, and Enroth-Cugell (1987).

13.14 SUMMARY

Results from parametric sensitivity experiments were summarized in this chapter dimension by dimension.

Sensitivity as a function along the spatial-frequency dimension peaks at middle values, steeply declines toward higher values, and shallowly declines toward lower. It depends very strongly on value along several other dimensions, in particular, spatial position, temporal frequency, and mean luminance.

Sensitivity as a function of orientation is close to uniform although, at high spatial frequencies, it tends to be slightly greater for vertical and horizontal than for oblique.

Sensitivity as a function of spatial position is generally greatest at foveal center (with some possible exceptions at low spatial frequencies and high temporal frequencies). Sensitivity falls off faster for high spatial frequencies than for low (when distance from foveal center is measured in degrees of visual angle, and when typical values on the other dimensions are used); in fact, sensitivity falls off at about the same rate for all different spatial frequencies when distance from foveal center is measured in number of periods of the spatial frequency under consideration. This pattern of sensitivity may be explainable by simple spatial-scaling models in which the sets of receptive fields at any given position are simply larger versions of the sets of receptive fields at the fovea.

Sensitivity tends to increase with increases in spatial extent in the manner one would expect from spatial probability summation and the nonuniformity of sensitivity at different spatial positions.

Sensitivity is probably the same for all spatial phases and all temporal phases, although greater sensitivity has sometimes been reported for onsets than offsets or for increments than decrements.

Sensitivity as a function of temporal frequency is remarkably similar to that as a function of spatial frequency.

The effect of spatial position on temporal-frequency sensitivity is much less than that on spatial-frequency sensitivity, however.

Across observers, sensitivity to different directions of motion is about flat, although some individuals show rather dramatic non-uniformities (as is also true for orientation).

Contrast sensitivity typically increases with increasing mean luminance, first linearly (the *linear range*) and then as a square root function (the *DeVries-Rose range*), before asymptoting as high mean luminances (the *Weber range*). The ranges of luminances over which these changes occur depend dramatically on spatial and temporal frequency.

Available physiological evidence suggests that it is greater number of neurons of a given type rather than greater sensitivity of neurons of a given type that correlates with greater psychophysical sensitivity.

13.15 DESCRIPTION OF LIST OF REFERENCES TO PARAMETRIC EXPERIMENTS

The purpose and organization of the list of references to parametric experiments (given in section 13.16) are exactly analogous to those for the list of references to analyzer-revealing experiments (section 12.13), except for the following slight differences in details.

The experimental and auxiliary dimensions for analyzer-revealing experiments are replaced by "primary" and "secondary" dimensions for parametric experiments.

If a parametric study measured an observer's sensitivity at many combinations of values on two dimensions, it is listed in section 13.16 in the major sections for each of the two dimensions (under the second-level heading for the other dimension).

If a parametric study investigated many values on one dimension and only a few on a second, it is listed under the major heading for the first dimension (and under the second-level heading corresponding to the second dimension) but not under the major heading for the second dimension.

If a parametric study measured sensitivity at different values on one dimension only (e.g., dimension two, orientation), it is usually listed in the subsection where the secondary and primary dimensions are the same. Occasionally, such a study is listed under a different secondary dimension, however, because it used an unusual value on that dimension (one outside the ranges given in the list of typical values in Chap. 12).

Many of the analyzer-revealing studies listed in the previous chapter are not repeated here, although they might have been. (They might have been because they happened to report several threshold values. Notice that an analyzer-revealing experiment need not report any threshold values at all, and some do not. An adaptation experiment might simply report the difference between before and after thresholds, for example, without reporting the threshold itself.)

Five of the 15 pattern dimensions—spatial phase, temporal phase, temporal position, direction of motion, and eye—are not well represented in the list of parametric experiments (either as primary or secondary dimensions). These have been little studied, since an observer's sensitivity is approximately uniform on each of these dimensions (or is on the average; observers certainly show individual differences in sensitivities to the two eyes or to different directions of motion); and further each of these dimensions has (or is presumed to have) little effect on parametric contrast sensitivity measured on every other dimension.

Contrast does not appear as a secondary dimension in the following list because contrast is varied to find thresholds (which are what is generally measured). Contrast does appear as a primary dimension, however, and here studies measuring detection performance as a function of contrast (psychometric functions) are tabulated.

This list of parametric references is even less exhaustive than the list of analyzer-revealing experiments.

13.16   REFERENCES TO PARAMETRIC EXPERIMENTS

1.0 SPATIAL FREQUENCY PARAMETRIC EXPERIMENTS

1.1 Spatial frequency as secondary

DePalma and Lowry 1962
Fry 1969
Kelly and Burbeck 1984 (review)
Sekuler, Wilson, and Owsley 1984
Watson, Barlow, and Robson 1983

1.2 Orientation as secondary

Campbell, Kulikowski, and Levinson 1966
Carlson, Cohen, and Gorog 1977
Higgins and Stultz 1948 (acuity)
Koenderink, Bouman, de Mesquita, and Slappendel 1978a,b
Mitchell 1976 (filtered noise)
Williams, Boothe, Kiorpes, and Teller 1981

1.3 Spatial position as secondary

Daitch and Green 1969
Deeley and Drasdo 1987
Guzman and Steinbach 1985
Higgins, Caruso, Coletta, and de Monasterio 1983
Hilz and Cavonius 1974
Johnston 1987
Kelly 1978 1984a,b
Koenderink, Bouman, de Mesquita, and Slappendel 1978a,b,c,d

Robson and Graham 1981
Ronchi and Fidanzati 1972
Rovamo, Leinonen, Laurinen, and Virsu 1984
Rovamo, Raninen, and Virsu 1985
Rovamo, Virsu, and Nasanen 1978
van Doorn and Koenderink 1972
van Ness and Bouman 1967
Wright and Johnston 1983

1.4 Spatial extent as secondary

Cohen, Carlson, and Cody 1976 (in Kelly 1977)
Hoekstra, van der Goot, van den Brink, and Bilsen 1974
Koenderink, Bouman, de Mesquita, and Slappendel 1978c,d
Kulikowski 1969
Rovamo, Leinonen, Laurinen, and Virsu 1984
Savoy and McCann 1975
Spitzberg and Richards 1975
van Ness 1968
Wright 1982
Wright and Johnston 1983

1.6 Temporal frequency as secondary

Ginsburg, Evans, Cannon, Owsley, and Mulvanny 1984
Gorea and Lorenceau 1984
Graham 1972
Kelly 1979b

Koenderink, Bouman, de Mesquita, and Slappendel 1978a,b
Robson 1966
Watanabe, Mori, Nagata, and Hiwatashi 1968

Sharp vs. gradual temporal edges
Breitmeyer and Julesz 1975
Budrikis and Lukas 1979
Tulunay-Keesey and Bennis 1979
Wilson and Bergen 1979

Also appearance thresholds
Blake and Mills 1979
Bodis-Wollner, Harnois, and Bobak 1983
Brussell, White, Mustillo, and Overbury 1984
Burbeck 1981
Green 1981
Harris 1980
Koenderink and van Doorn 1979
Kulikowski 1978
Kulikowski and Tolhurst 1973
Murray, MacCana and Kulikowski 1983
Panish, Swift, and Smith 1983
Pantle 1973
Tolhurst 1973

1.8 Temporal extent as secondary

Nachmias 1967
Rovamo, Leinonen, Laurinen, and Virsu 1984
Schober and Hilz 1965
Tulunay-Keesey and Bennis 1979
Tulunay-Keesey and Jones 1976
Watanabe, Mori, Nagata, and Hiwatashi 1968

1.12 Mean luminance as secondary

Banks, Geisler, and Bennett 1987
Blake, Breitmeyer, and Green 1980 (dichoptic)
Burr, Ross, and Morrone 1985 (local)
Burton 1973
Campbell, Kulikowski, and Levinson 1966
Cornsweet and Yellott 1985
De Valois, Morgan, and Snodderly 1974
D'Zmura and Lennie 1986
Graham 1972

Kelly 1972
Koenderink, Bouman, de Mesquita, and Slappendel 1978d
Meeteren and Vos 1972
Pasternak and Merigan 1981
Patel 1966
Schade 1956
van Ness 1968
van Ness and Bouman 1967
van Ness, Koenderink, Nas, and Bouman 1967
Watanabe, Mori, Nagata, and Hiwatashi 1968

1.14 Effect of optics, the retinal mosaic, accommodation and viewing distance

Baker, Brown, and Garner 1983
Banks, Geisler, and Bennett 1987
Campbell and Green 1965
Campbell and Gubisch 1966, 1967
Campbell, Kulikowski, and Levinson 1966
Charman and Tucker 1977
Cuiffreda and Hokoda 1983 (normals and amblyopes)
Green and Campbell 1965
Gu and Legge 1987
Johnson 1976
Kiorpes and Boothe 1984 (amblyopic monkeys)
Legge, Mullen, Woo, and Campbell 1987
Miller 1978
Miller, Pigion, Wesner, and Patterson 1983
Owens 1980
Raymond, Lindblad, and Leibowitz 1984
Raymond and Leibowitz 1985
Regan, Raymond, Ginsburg, and Murray 1981
Robson and Enroth-Cugell 1978
Smith and Harwerth 1984 (monkeys and humans)
Snyder and Srinivasan 1979
Tucker, Charman, and Ward 1986
van Meeteren and Dunnewold 1983
Williams 1985b

Retinal mosaic (sampling) effects
Banks, Geisler, and Bennett 1987
Bossomaier, Snyder, and Hughes 1985
Coletta and Williams 1987

Geisler and Hamilton 1986
Hirsch and Hylton 1984
Jacobs and Blakemore 1988
Miller and Bernard 1983
Smith and Cass 1987
Thibos, Walsh, and Cheyney 1987
Yellott 1982, 1983, 1984
Williams 1985a,b, 1986, 1988
Williams and Coletta 1987
Williams and Collier 1983

1.15 Effects of Psychophysical
Procedure

Banks, Stephens, and Dannemiller
1982
Ginsburg and Cannon 1983, 1984
Kelly and Savoie 1973
Teller, Mayer, Makous, and Allen 1982
Wolfe, Gwiazda, and Held 1983

1.16 Effect of eye movements and
stabilization

Arend 1976
Arend and Skavenski 1979
Arend and Timberlake 1986
Burbeck and Kelly 1982, 1984
Higgins, Caruso, Coletta, and de
Monasterio 1983
Kelly 1979a,b, 1981a, 1983
Kulikowski 1981
Murphy 1978
Tulunay-Keesey and Bennis 1979
Tulunay-Keesey and Jones 1976, 1980
Volkmann, Riggs, White, and Moore
1978
Watanabe, Mori, Nagata, and Hiwa-
tashi 1968

1.17 Effect of age, species, pathology of
observer

Cats
Lehmkuhle, Kratz, and Sherman 1982
Pasternak and Merigan 1981
Pasternak, Merigan, Flood, and Zehl
1983
Pasternak 1986
Sireteanu 1985 (kitten acuity)

Cats with deficits
Blake and di Gianfilippo 1982
Frascella and Lehmkuhle 1982

Holopgian and Blake 1983, 1984
Lehmkuhle, Kratz, and Sherman 1982
Merigan, Pasternak, and Zehl 1981
Pasternak, Merigan, Flood, and Zehl
1983
Pasternak 1986

Nonhuman primates
Boothe, Dobson, and Teller 1985
Boothe, Kiorpes, Williams, and Teller
1988
Boothe, Williams, Kiorpes, and Teller
1980
Crawford, von Noorden, Meharg,
Rhodes, Harwerth, Smith, and
Miller 1983 (also strabismic
monkeys)
De Valois, Morgan, and Snodderly
1974
Harwerth, Boltz, and Smith 1980
Harwerth, Smith, Boltz, Crawford, and
von Noorden 1983a (also abnor-
mally reared)
Jacobs and Blakemore 1988
Langston, Casagrande, and Fox 1986
(galago)
Lee and Boothe 1981
Merigan and Eskin 1986 (loss of P gan-
glion cells)
Miller, Pasik, and Pasik 1980 (also with
cortical ablation)
Smith, Harwerth, and Crawford 1985
(also abnormally reared)
Williams, Boothe, Kiorpes, and Teller
1981

Miscellaneous species
Birch and Jacobs 1979 (rat)
Hirsch 1982, 1983 (falcon)
Legg 1984 (rat)
Petry, Fox, and Casagrande 1982 (tree
shrew)
Reymond and Wolfe 1981 (eagle)
Reymond 1987 (falcon)
Ulrich, Essock, and Lehmkuhle 1981

Human children
Atkinson and Braddick 1981, 1983
Atkinson, Braddick, and Moar 1977a,b
Atkinson, French, and Braddick 1981
Atkinson, Pimm-Smith, Evans, and
Braddick 1983
Banks and Salapatek 1978, 1983
Banks, Stephens, and Dannemiller
1982
Boothe, Dobson, and Teller 1985

Bradley and Freeman 1982
Crawford et al. 1983
Dobson, Salem, and Carson 1983
Dobson and Teller 1978
Dobson, Teller, and Belgum 1978
Dobson, Mayer, and Lee 1980
Gwiazda, Brill, Mohindra, and Held 1980
Hainline, Camenzuli, Abramov, Rawlick, and Lemerise 1986
Harris, Hansen, and Fulton 1984
Held 1979
Mayer and Dobson 1982
Mayer, Fulton, and Hansen 1982
Powers and Dobson 1982
Salapatek and Banks 1978
Sebris, Dobson, and Hartman 1984
van Hof-van, Duin, and Mohn 1986
Teller 1979
Teller, Mayer, Makous and Allen 1982
Teller and Movshon 1986
Wilson, 1988
Wolfe, Gwiazeda, and Held 1983

Human elderly
Morrison and McGrath 1985
Owsley, Sekuler, and Siemsen 1983
Schlotterer, Moscovitch, and Crapper-McLachlan 1983
Sekuler, Wilson, and Owsley 1984
Weale 1986 (Also see Alzeheimer's section)

Humans with visual deficits
• *Alzheimer's*
Nissen, Corkin, Buonanno, Growdon, Wray, and Bauer 1985
Schlotter, Moscovitch, and Crapper-McLachlan 1983
• *Amblyopes*
Bradley and Freeman 1981, 1985
Cuiffreda and Hokoda 1983
Cuiffreda and Rumpf 1985 (accommodation)
Ginsburg 1981
Gstabler and Green 1971
Hess 1977
Hess and Baker 1984
Hess and Howell 1977, 1978a,b
Hess and Pointer 1985
Hess and Smith 1977
Howell, Mitchell, and Keith 1983
Levi and Harwerth 1977
Levi and Klein 1982a,b

MacCana, Cuthbert, and Lovegrove 1986
Rentschler, Hilz, and Brettel 1980, 1981
Thomas 1978 (appearance thresholds)
Wood and Kulikowski 1978
• *Cerebral lesions*
Bodis-Wollner 1972, 1976
Bodis-Wollner and Diamond 1976
• *Diabetes*
Hirsch and Puklin 1983
King-Smith and Kulikowski 1980
King-Smith, Rosen, Alvarez, and Bhargava 1980
Rovamo, Hyvarinen, and Hari 1982
• *Multiple sclerosis*
Bodis-Wollner, Hendley, Mylin, and Thornton 1979
Brussell, White, Mustillo, and Overbury 1984
Ginsburg 1981
Kupersmith, Seiple, Nelson, and Carr 1984
Regan, Raymond, Ginsburg, and Murray 1981
Regan, Silver, and Murray 1977
Regan, Whitlock, Murray, and Beverly 1980
• *Other*
Atkin, Bodis-Wollner, Wolkstein, Moss, and Podos 1979 (glaucoma)
Fiorentini and Maffei 1976 (myopes)
Ginsburg 1981 (congenital coloboma)
Hertz 1986 (nonverbal children)
Lovegrove, Bowling, Badcock, and Blackwood 1980 (reading disabled)
Virsu, Lehtio, and Rovamo 1981 (miscellaneous)
Wilson, Mets, Nagy, and Kreisel 1988 (albino)
Wolkstein, Atkin, and Bodis-Wollner 1977 (tapetoretinal degeneration)

Other factors in humans
Brabyn and McGuiness 1979 (gender)

1.18 Color as secondary

D'Zmura and Lennie 1986
Estevez and Cavonius 1976b
Granger and Hartley 1973
Green 1968
Ingling and Martinez-Uriegas 1983
Kelly 1981a, 1983

Noorlander, Heuts, and Koenderink 1981
Rovamo, Hyvarinen, and Hari 1982
Schade 1958
Stromeyer, Kronauer, and Madsen 1984
Stromeyer and Sternheim 1981
Takahashi and Ejima 1986
van Nes et al. 1967
van Nes 1968
van der Horst 1969
van der Horst, de Weert, and Bouman 1967
van der Horst and Bouman 1969
Williams, Collier, and Thompson 1983

1.19 Effect of surround and other equipment features

Surround
Estevez and Cavonius 1976
Howell and Hess 1978
Marrocco, Carpenter, and Wright 1985
McCann and Hall 1980
McCann, Savoy, and Hall 1978
Savoy and McCann 1975
van der Wildt and Waarts 1983

Figure/ground
Wong and Weisstein 1982, 1983

Other equipment features
Morgan and Watt 1982
Westheimer 1985
Williams, Boothe, Kiorpes, and Teller 1981

2.0 ORIENTATION PARAMETRIC EXPERIMENTS

2.1 Spatial frequency as secondary

Campbell, Kulikowski, and Levinson 1966
Carlson, Cohen, and Gorog 1977
Green 1983
Lennie 1974 (gravity)
Watanabe, Mori, Naga, and Hiwatashi 1968
Williams, Boothe, Kiorpes, and Teller 1981

2.2 Orientation as secondary

Appelle 1972
Banks and Stolarz 1975 (gravity?)
Mayer 1983a,b
Mitchell, Freeman, Millidot, and Haegerstrom 1973
Watanabe, Mori, Nagata, and Hiwatashi 1968

Appearance thresholds
Camisa, Blake, and Lema 1979
Essock and Lehmkuhle 1983

2.3 Spatial position as secondary

Berkley, Kitterle, and Watkins 1975
Koenderink, Bouman, de Mesquita, and Slappendel 1978a,b
Regan and Beverly 1983
Rovamo, Virsu, Laurinen, and Hyvarinen 1982

2.4 Spatial extent as secondary

Quinn and Lehmkuhle 1983
Tootle and Berkley 1983

2.6 Temporal frequency as secondary

Camisa, Blake, and Lema 1977
Green 1983

2.8 Temporal extent as secondary

1 millisecond exposures
Higgins and Stultz 1950

2.14 Effect of optics, accommodation, and viewing distance

Campbell 1958
Dobson, Howland, Moss, and Banks 1983
Freeman 1975
Freeman, Mitchell, and Millodot 1972
Kerr 1971 discusses
Mitchell, Freeman, Millidot, and Haegerstrom 1973

Interference-fringe gratings
Campbell, Kulikowski, and Levinson 1966
Mitchell, Freeman, Millidot, and Haegerstrom 1973
Mitchell, Freeman, and Westheimer 1967

2.15 Effect of psychophysical procedure

Effect of practice
Mayer 1983a

2.16 Effect of eye movements and stabilization

Nachmias 1960

2.17 Effect of age, species, pathology of observer

Monkeys
Boothe and Teller 1982
Williams, Boothe, Kiorpes, and Teller 1981
Boltz, Harwerth, and Smith 1979

Human children
Atkinson and French 1979
Beazley, O'Conner, and Illingsworth 1982
Birch, Gwiazda, Bauer, Naegele, and Held 1983
Gwiazda, Scheiman, and Held 1984
Leehey, Moskowitz-Cook, Brill, and Held 1975
Mayer 1977, 1983b
Mitchell 1980
Teller, Morse, Borton, and Regal 1974

Humans with visual deficits
● *Multiple sclerosis*
Kupersmith, Seiple, Nelson, and Carr 1984
Regan, Whitlock, Murray, and Beverly 1980

Different human populations
Annis and Frost 1973
Ross and Woodhouse 1979
Timney and Muir 1976

Other factors in humans
Brabyn and McGuiness 1979 (gender)

3.0 SPATIAL POSITION PARAMETRIC EXPERIMENTS (2 DIMENSIONS)

3.1 Spatial frequency as secondary

Guzman and Steinbach 1985
Hilz and Cavonius 1974
Klopfenstein and Carlson 1984
Koenderink, Bouman, de Mesquita, and Slappendel 1978a,b

Regan and Beverly 1983
Rijsdijk, Kroon, and van der Wildt 1980
Robson and Graham 1981
Rovamo, Virsu, and Nasanen 1978
Rovamo, Leinonen, Laurinen, and Virsu 1984
Virsu, Rovamo, Laurinen, and Nasanen 1982 (also orientation and direction discrimination)
Wright and Johnston 1983
See also "spatial-scaling" in subsections 3.3 and 3.4

Appearance thresholds
Harris 1980
Murray, MacCana, and Kulikowski 1983

3.3 Spatial position as secondary

Johnson, Keltner, and Balestrery 1978
Appearance thresholds
Blake and Mills 1979
Regan and Neima 1984

Spatial-scaling ideas
Anstis 1974
Carlson, Klopfenstein, and Anderson 1981
Drasdo 1977
Fischer and May 1970
Hubel and Wiesel 1974
Johnston 1987
Kelly 1985a,b,c
Klopfenstein and Carlson 1984
Kretz, Scarbin, and Bourguignet 1979
Koenderink, Bouman, de Mesquita, and Slappendel 1978a,b,c,d
Koenderink and van Doorn 1978, 1982
Rolls and Cowey 1970
Rovamo, Virsu, and Nasanen 1978
Rovamo and Virsu 1984
Schwartz 1977, 1980
Watson 1983
Wilson 1980

3.4 Spatial extent as secondary

Johnson, Keltner, and Balestrery 1978
Size-scaled stimuli (spatial frequency and extent vary):
Koenderink, Bouman, de Mesquita, and Slappendel 1978c,d
Rovamo, Virsu, and Nasanen 1978
Virsu and Rovamo 1979

Virsu, Rovamo, Laurinen, and Nasanen 1982

3.6 Temporal frequency as secondary

Guzman and Steinbach 1985
Koenderink, Bouman, de Mesquita, and Slappendel 1978a,b
Virsu, Rovamo, Laurinen, and Nasanen 1982
Wright and Johnston 1983

Appearance thresholds
Harris 1980
Murray, MacCana, and Kulikowski 1983

CFF studies
Hartmann, Lachenmayr, and Brettel 1979
Hylkema 1942
Reviewed in C. Graham 1965
See also "spatial-scaling ideas" in subsection 3.3.

3.8 Temporal extent as secondary

Rovamo, Leinonen, Laurinen, and Virsu 1984

3.12 Mean luminance as secondary

Hartmann, Lachenmary, and Brettel 1979
Kerr 1971 acuity
Koenderink, Bouman, de Mesquita, and Slappendel 1978d

3.14 Effect of optics, accommodation, and viewing distance

Effect of peripheral optics
Enoch, Sunga, and Bachman 1970
Fankenhauser and Enoch 1962
Frisen and Glansholm 1975
Johnson and Leibowitz 1974
Kerr 1971 (acuity)
Leibowitz, Johnson, and Isabelle 1972
Millidot, Johnson, Lamont, and Leibowitz 1975
Snyder 1982 (sampling considerations)
Sunga and Enoch 1970
van Meeteren and Dunnewold 1983
Wang, Pomerantzeff, and Pankratov 1983

3.15 Effect of psychophysical procedure

Large peripheral adaptation effects
Ginsburg 1966
Frome, MacLeod, Buck, and Williams 1981
Practice effects in periphery
Johnson and Leibowitz 1974, 1979

3.17 Effect of age, species, pathology of observer

Humans with visual deficits
Regan and Neima 1984 (glaucoma, ocular hypertension, multiple sclerosis)
Amblyopes
Bradley, Freeman, and Applegate 1985
Hess and Jacobs 1979
Hess and Pointer 1985
Sireteanu and Fronius 1981

4.0 SPATIAL EXTENT PARAMETRIC EXPERIMENTS (2 DIMENSIONS)

(Also see spatial-position summation experiments in the List of References to Analyzer-Revealing experiments in sect. 12.10. They will appear in subsections 3.xb where x is a number.)

4.1 Spatial frequency as secondary

Estevez and Cavonius 1975
Hoekstra, van der Goot, van den Brink, and Bilsen 1974
Koenderink, Bouman, de Mesquita, and Slappendel 1978c
Robson and Graham 1981
Wright and Johnston 1983

4.2 Orientation as secondary

Findlay 1969
Quinn and Lehmkuhle 1983
Tootle and Berkley 1983

4.3 Spatial position as secondary

Johnson, Keltner, and Balestrery 1978
Koenderink, Bouman, de Mesquita, and Slappendel 1978c
Robson and Graham 1981

Spatially aperiodic stimuli
Hallett 1962
Hallett, Marriott, and Rodger 1962
Wilson 1970

4.4 Spatial extent as secondary

Mayer and Tyler 1986
Watson, Barlow, and Robson 1983

4.6 Temporal frequency as secondary

deLange 1952, 1954, 1958
Wright and Johnston 1983
On-off versus flickering bars
Stromeyer, Zeevi, and Klein 1979

4.12 Mean luminance as secondary

See subsection 12.4

4.17 Effect of age, species, and pathology of observer
Amblyopes
Hess and Campbell 1980
Hagemans and Wildt 1979

Human infants
Lewis, Maurer, and Blackburn 1985

4.18 Color as secondary

Findlay 1969
Pokorny 1968 (acuity)

5.0 SPATIAL PHASE PARAMETRIC
EXPERIMENTS

For thresholds of increments versus decrements, see section 9.0

6.0 TEMPORAL FREQUENCY PARAMETRIC
EXPERIMENTS

6.1 Spatial frequency as secondary

Burr and Ross 1982
Georgeson 1987
Gorea and Lorenceau 1984
Kelly 1979b
Koenderink, Bouman, de Mesquita,
   and Slappendel 1978a,b
Koenderink and van Doorn 1978b
Nakayama 1985

Robson 1966
Virsu, Rovamo, Laurinen, and Nasanen 1982
Also appearance thresholds
Brussell, White, Mustillo, and Overbury 1984
Burbeck 1981
Foster 1969, 1971 (CFF-radial gratings)
Green 1981
Harris 1980
Harris 1984a,b (low and high temporal-
   frequency cutoffs)
Harris 1986
Johnston and Wright 1986
Koenderink and van Doorn 1979
Kulikowski and Tolhurst 1973
Murray, MacCana, and Kulikowski
   1983
Panish, Swift, and Smith 1983
Pantle 1973
Watanabe, Mori, Nagata, and Hiwatashi 1968
Abrupt versus gradual transitions
Stromeyer, Zeevi, and Klein 1979

6.2 Orientation as secondary

Camisa, Blake, and Lema 1977
Green, M. 1983

6.3 Spatial position as secondary

Guzman and Steinbach 1985
Hartmann, Lachenmary, and Brettel
   1979 (CFF only)
Kelly 1984a
Koenderink, Bouman, de Mesquita,
   and Slappendel 1978a,b
Raninen and Rovamo 1986, 1987
Rovamo and Raninen 1984, 1988
   (CFF)
Rovamo, Raninen, and Virsu 1985
   (CFF)

*Scaled stimuli (vary in spatial position,
and in spatial frequency and/or spatial
extent)*
Johnston and Wright 1986 (appearance
   CFF)
Kelly 1984a
Raninen and Rovamo 1986 (CFF)
Rovamo and Raninen 1984 (CFF)
Tyler 1985
Tyler and Silverman 1983

Virsu, Rovamo, Laurinen, and Nasanen 1982

Spatial parameters and mean luminance scaled
Raninen and Rovamo 1986 (CFF)
Rovamo and Raninen 1984 (CFF)

6.4 Spatial extent as secondary

Foster 1971 (radial gratings)
Measure CFF
Foster 1969, 1971 (radial gratings, also appearance ths.)
Harris 1984a,b (low and high temporal–frequency cutoffs—appearance thresholds)
Hartmann, Lachenmayr, and Brettel 1979
Wolf and Vincent 1963

6.6 Temporal frequency as secondary

Corwin and Dunlap 1987
deLange 1952, 1954
Kelly, Boynton, and Baron 1976
Sperling 1964
Sperling and Sondhi 1968
Watson, Barlow, and Robson 1983
Appearance thresholds also
Tulunay-Keesey 1972
van Ness, Koenderink, Nas and Bouman 1967
Watanabe, Mori, Nagata, and Hiwatashi 1968

6.12 Mean luminance as secondary

Burr, Ross, and Morrone 1985
Coletta and Adams 1986a,b
deLange 1958
Frumkes, Naarendorp, and Goldberg 1986 (CFF)
Hartmann, Lachenmary, and Brettel 1979 (CFF only)
Hayhoe and Chen 1986
Ives 1922 (scotopic CFF)
Kelly 1971a,b 1972
Kelly and Savoie 1978
Lennie 1984
Rovamo and Raninen 1988 (CFF)
Stork and Falk 1987
Swanson, Ueno, Smith, and Pokorny 1987

van Nes 1968
van Nes, Koenderink, Nas, and Bouman 1967

6.14 Effect of optics, accommodation and viewing distance

Flitcroft 1988

6.16 Effect of eye movements and stabilization

Kelly 1979b
Kelly 1981, 1983
Murphy 1978

6.17 Effect of age, species, and pathology of observer

Cats
Blake and Camisa 1977
Lehmkuhle, Kratz, and Sherman 1982
Pasternak 1986
Cats with deficits
Blake and di Gianfilippo 1980
Frascella and Lehmkuhle 1982
Holopgian and Blake 1983
Lehmkuhle, Kratz, and Sherman 1982
Merigan, Pasternak, and Zehl 1981
Monkeys
Harwerth, Smith, Boltz, Crawford, and von Noorden 1983b (also abnormally reared)
Merigan and Eskin 1986 (loss of P retinal ganglion cells)
Human children
Regal 1981
Humans with visual deficits
• *Amblyopes*
Bradley and Freeman 1985
Hess, France, and Tulunay-Keesey 1981
Manny and Levi 1982a,b (also appearance thresholds)
van der Tweel and Estevez 1974
Wesson and Loop 1982
• *Other*
Brussell, White, Mustillo, and Overbury 1984 (multiple sclerosis)
Hess, Howell, and Kitchin 1978 (amblyopes)

Tyler 1981 (glaucoma and ocular hypertension)
Tyler 1984 (retinitis pigmentosa)
Tyler, Ryu, and Stamper 1984 (interocular pressure)
Tyler, Ernst, and Lyness 1984 (retinitis pigmentosa)
Wilson, Mets, Nagy, and Kressel 1988

6.18 Color as secondary

Cicerone and Green 1978
Coletta and Adams 1984, 1986a,b
de Lange 1958
Estevez and Cavonius 1975
Estevez and Spekreijse 1974
Frumkes, Naarendorp, and Goldberg 1986 (CFF)
Green 1969
Ingling and Martinez-Uriegas 1985
Kelly 1973, 1974, 1975, 1981, 1983
Kelly and van Norren 1977
Noorlander, Heuts, and Koenderink 1981
Piantanida 1985
Raninen and Rovamo 1986
Raninen and Rovamo 1986 (CFF)
Swanson, Ueno, Smith, and Pokorny 1987
van Ness et al 1967
Wisowaty and Boynton 1980

8.0 TEMPORAL EXTENT PARAMETRIC EXPERIMENTS

(Also see temporal-position summation experiments in List of References to Analyzer-Revealing experiments in sect 12.10. They will be in subsections 7.xb where x is a number.)

8.1 Spatial frequency as secondary

Georgeson 1987
Gorea and Tyler 1986
Harris and Georgeson 1986
Hood 1973 (sharp vs. blurred edges—also appearance ths.)
Kelly and Savoie 1978
Rovamo, Leinonen, Laurinen, and Virsu 1984
Tyler and Gorea 1986

8.3 Spatial position as secondary

Rovamo, Leinonen, Laurinen, and Virsu 1984

8.4 Spatial extent as secondary

Barlow 1958
Harris and Georgeson 1986

8.8 Temporal extent as secondary

Roufs 1974-IV

8.12 Mean luminance as secondary

See subsection 12.8

8.17 Effect of age, species, and pathology of observer

Monkeys
Harwerth, Boltz, and Smith 1980
Amblyopic humans
Levi and Harwerth 1977

8.18 Color as secondary

Mitsuboshi, Funakawa, Kawabata, and Aiba 1987
Mitsuboshi, Kawabata and Aiba 1987

9.0 TEMPORAL PHASE PARAMETRIC EXPERIMENTS

9.4 Spatial extent as secondary

Increments vs. decrements
Legge and Kersten 1983

9.8 Temporal extent as secondary

Increments vs. decrements
Krauskopf 1980
Legge and Kersten 1983

9.9 Temporal phase as secondary

Increments versus decrements
Patel and Jones 1968
Rashbass 1970
Roufs 1974-IV
Short 1966

9.12 Mean luminance as secondary

Cohn 1974

11.0 CONTRAST PARAMETRIC EXPERI-
MENTS—PSYCHOMETRIC FUNCTIONS

This section lists some recent studies in
which detectability is plotted as a
function of contrast. A review of
older studies can be found in Green
and Swets 1966.

11.1 Spatial frequency as secondary

Foley and Legge 1981
Mayer and Tyler 1986
Miller, Pasik, and Pasik 1980
Nachmias 1981
Robson and Graham in Graham 1980
Sachs, Nachmias, and Robson 1971
Thomas 1983

11.3 Spatial position as secondary

Robson and Graham 1981

11.4 Spatial extent as secondary

Mayer and Tyler 1986

11.6 Temporal frequency as secondary

Hess and Plant 1985
Watson 1979

11.11 Contrast as secondary

Pelli 1985

11.13 Eye as secondary

Legge 1984a (monocular vs. binocular)

11.15 Effect   of   psychophysical
procedure

Hallett 1969
Nachmias 1981

11.17 Effect of age, species, and pathology of observer

Monkeys
Boothe, Kiorpes, Williams and Teller
1988
Merigan and Eskin 1986 (loss of P ganglion cells)
Miller, Pasik, and Pasik 1980 (also with
ablations)

11.18 Color as secondary

Maloney and Wandell 1983

12.0 MEAN LUMINANCE PARAMETRIC
EXPERIMENTS

See reviews in Shapley and Enroth-
Cugell 1984 and in Hood and Finkelstein 1986

12.1 Spatial frequency as secondary

Cornsweet and Yellott 1985
Daitch and Green 1969
D'Zmura and Lennie 1986
Hess and Nordby 1986
Jamar and Koenderink 1984
Kelly 1972
Kerr 1971 (acuity)
Koenderink, Bouman, de Mesquita,
and Slappendel 1978d
Patel 1966
Pinter 1985
Schade 1956
Sperling 1970
van Nes 1968
van Nes and Bouman 1967
van Nes, Koenderink, Nas, and Bou-
man 1967
Yellott 1987

12.3 Spatial position as secondary

Daitch and Green 1969 (periph.)
Hartmann, Lachenmayr, and Brettel
1979 (CFF)
Kerr 1971 (acuity)
van Nes 1968

*Scaled stimuli (spatial position and spa-
tial extent varied)*
Koenderink, Bouman, de Mesquita,
and Slappendel 1978d

12.4 Spatial extent as secondary

Pokorny 1968 (acuity)

Spatially aperiodic targets
Barlow 1958
Blackwell 1946, 1963
Chen, MacLeod, and Stockman 1987
Cornsweet and Yellott 1985
Hamer and Schneck 1984
Lie 1980, 1981
Wilson 1970

Of background or surround
Coletta and Adams 1986

12.6 Temporal frequency as secondary

Conner and MacLeod 1977 (CFF)
Cornsweet and Reuman 1986
deLange 1958
Hess and Nordby 1986
Kelly 1971a, b 1972
Sperling and Sondhi 1968
Tyler 1975
van Nes 1968
van Nes, Koenderink, Nas, and Bouman 1967

12.8 Temporal extent as secondary

Vary duration of spatially and temporally aperiodic stimulus
Barlow 1958
Graham and Kemp 1938
Herrick 1956
Keller 1941
Roufs 1972a, b

12.9 Temporal phase as auxiliary

Russell and Wheeler 1983

12.12 Mean luminance as secondary

Barlow 1956, 1957
Daitch and Green 1969 (scotopic)
DeVries 1943
Green D 1986
van Nes and Bouman 1967 (scotopic)

12.17 Effect of age, species, and pathology of observer

Cats
Pasternak and Merigan 1981
Pasternak, Merigan, Flood, and Zehl 1983
Monkey
De Valois, Morgan, and Snodderly 1974
Human children
Brown, Dobson, and Maier 1987
Dannemiller and Banks 1983
Dobson, Salem, and Carson 1983
Hansen, Fulton, and Harris 1986
Howell, Mitchell, and Keith 1983
Human adults
Ginsburg and Cannon 1983
Owsley, Sekuler, and Siemsen 1983
Humans with visual deficits
Hess and Howell 1978b
Howell, Mitchell, and Keith 1983

12.18 Color as secondary

D'Zmura and Lennie 1986
Pokorny 1968 (acuity)

Spatially/temporally aperiodic
Stiles and all the many studies following Stiles

Note

1. The suggestion in section 13.9.3 for extending the simple stimulus-scaling hypothesis to include effects of mean luminance was that mean luminance be scaled down peripherally (as spatial dimensions are scaled up) so that total flux of the pattern remains constant. To incorporate this suggestion into the spatially scaled models, one might assume that total flux for any given transition point is constant across all mechanisms in a family.

In the initial presentation of the constant-flux hypothesis (section 13.9.2), we implicitly limited our discussion to mechanisms at one position (foveal) having excitatory centers of different sizes (being in different families). That is, we were assuming that total flux for any given transition point is constant across foveal mechanisms in different families.

Putting the above two paragraphs together implies that total flux (for any given transition point) is constant across all mechanisms in all families. But then what does this predict? In particular, suppose total flux equals center size times mean luminance (as in the main text). Then, although the transition mean luminance at a given eccentricity will depend on spatial frequency (indeed be proportional to spatial-frequency squared, as argued in section 13.9.2), the transition mean luminance for a given spatial frequency should *not* depend on eccentricity because, for a given spatial frequency, the size of the relevant mechanism's excitatory center will be the same (or almost the same) at all eccentricities. (The sizes may not be exactly the same, if, for example, orientation bandwidth changed with eccentricity, but they will be nearly so.)

Yet, as mentioned above, the transition mean luminance for a given spatial frequency seems to be lower peripherally than foveally (Koenderink et al., 1978d).

Suppose we try to mend matters by using *weighted flux* defined as the integral of the weighting function's excitatory center times the mean luminance. Then, since sensitivity for a given spatial frequency declines with eccentricity (and therefore, the appropriately sized weighting function's height must decline with eccentricity), the luminance necessary to produce a criterion flux for that spatial frequency should actually *increase* with eccentricity. Thus, transition luminance should increase. This seems to be exactly the wrong direction to correct our problem (see beginning section 13.9.3).

In short, it is not clear to me at present how the effects of mean luminance should be included in spatially scaled models.

Appendix

ASSUMPTIONS ACCORDING TO FUNCTION IN MULTIPLE ANALYZERS MODELS

From Stimulus to an Individual Analyzer's Output

Form of Output	*Sections*
Assumption 25. Single-Number Analyzer Output	4.2, 4.4.1, 6.4.2, 7.3.3, 9.3
Assumption 26. Variable Analyzer Output	4.2, 6.4.2 (& whenever Assmpts. 38 or 52 used)
Assumption 30. Output Is a Two-Dimensional Function	4.3.1
Assumption 31. Translation-Invariance	4.3.1
Assumption 32. Deterministic Analyzer Output (No Variability)	4.3.1, 4.4.1
Assumption 33. Peak-in-Output-Profile Rule	4.3.1 (5.2.1)
Assumption 39. High-Threshold Analyzers	4.7.1
Assumption 44. Independent Variability at Different Positions	5.3.3
Assumption 54. Identical Probability Distribution Families	7.3.3, 9.3
Assumption 55. High-Threshold Family	7.3.4, 9.3
Assumption 56. Spread Exponentials Family	7.3.4, 9.3
Assumption 57. Increasing-Variance Gaussians ($r = \frac{1}{8}$) Family	7.3.4, 9.3
Assumption 58. Increasing-Variance Gaussians ($r = \frac{1}{4}$) Family	7.3.4, 9.3
Assumption 59. Constant-Variance Gaussians Family	7.3.4, 9.3
Assumption 60. Shifted Double-Exponentials Family	7.3.4, 9.3

Assumption 66. Intrinsic-Uncertainty   8.1.1
                 Probability Distribution Family

Assumptions not numbered in book:
   Correlated Variability at Each Point in
   Analyzer Output

Transducer Function	*Sections*
Assumption 1. Intensity-Sensitivity Product	3.2.2
Assumption 9. Linear Transducer	3.5.2, 4.2, 4.3.1 (4.8.2, 4.8.5, 5.2.1)
Assumption 16. Monotonic Transducer	3.6.1
Assumption 43. Quick Psychometric Function	4.8.1 (5.3)
Assumption 68. Quick Function With Interdependent Parameters	8.5
Assumption 69. Linear Transducer Functions for Microanalyzers	8.6.1
Assumption 92. Power Function Transducer	10.8.1 (4.8.2, 4.8.5, 8.4)

Sensitivity Functions	*Sections*
Assumption 11. Very Rounded	3.5.2
Assumption 12. Very Peaked	3.5.2
Assumption 35. Nonoverlapping for Far-Apart Values	4.4.1, 7.3.3, 9.3
Assumptions not numbered in book: Triangular	(10.3.4, Table 10.1)
Half-cosine-cycle	(10.3.4, Table 10.1)
Gaussian Sensitivity Function	(6.9.2, 10.3.4, Table 10.1)
DOG Sensitivity Function	(6.9.1)

Additivity or No?	*Sections*
Assumption 27. Additivity to a Compound	4.2, 4.3.1, 6.2.1 (9.5.5, 10.4.2, 10.5.3)
Assumption 29. Additivity of Sensitivities	4.2
Assumption 36. Ineffective Stimulus Rule	4.4.1, 7.3.3, 9.3 (5.2.2, 11.8.10)

Assumption 47. Additive (Linear-System) Analyzers	6.4.2 (5.2.1, 10.5.3)
Assumptions not numbered in book: Nothing Is Assumed About Additivity	Implicit in many sections

Properites of Groups of Analyzers

Number and Spacing of Analyzers	*Sections*
Assumption 13. Close Spacing	3.5.2 (6.4.3)
Assumption 14. Intermediate Spacing	3.5.2
Assumption 15. Sparse Spacing	3.5.2
Assumption 24. One Analyzer	4.2
Assumption 34. Multiple Analyzers	4.4.1, 6.4.2, 7.3.3, 9.3
Assumption 45. Two Relevant Analyzers	6.2.1 (10.3.5, 10.10.3)
Assumption 53. One Analyzer per Stimulus	7.3.3, 9.3
Assumptions not numbered in book: Indefinite Number of Analyzers per Simple Stimulus	(See composite analyzers in 4.7.5, 7.3.6, 9.6)
Arbitrarily Close Spacing of Analyzers (an Effective Continuum)	Frequent in calculations where other spacing assmpt. not specific

Interaction/Independence	*Sections*
Assumption 37. Noninteracting Analyzers	4.4.1, 6.4.2, 7.3.3, 9.3
Assumption 38. Probabilistically Independent Analyzers	4.7.1, 6.3.1, 7.3.3, 9.3
Assumption 52. Probabilistically Independent Trials	7.3.3, 9.3

Relationships Among Analyzers' Sensitivity Functions	*Sections*
Assumption 8. Uniform Peak Sensitivities	3.5.2
Assumption 48. Only One Spatial-Frequency Bandwidth of Analyzer	6.4.2
Assumptions not numbered in book: Possible Selectivity on Other Dimensions Ignored	(6.4: orientation & temporal frequency)

Phase Selectivity Irrelevant	(6.4)
Doubly Selective Along Two Dimensions of Interest	(6.4: spatial position & frequency)
Specified Peak Sensitivities	(6.4, 6.9)

About Adaptation

Assumption 2.	Same Factor for All Test Stimuli	3.2.3
Assumption 3.	Depends Only on Output to Adapting Stimulus	3.2.4
Assumption 5.	Same Most Sensitive Analyzer	3.2.6
Assumption 6.	Most Sensitive Analyzer May Change	3.3.1
Assumption 10.	Power Adaptation Functions	3.5.2
Assumption 17.	Not Selective for Value	3.6.2

About Inhibition

Assumption 18.	Output-Dependent Inhibition Among Analyzers	3.7.2
Assumption 19.	Tonic Inhibition and Excitation	3.7.2
Assumption 20.	Inhibition Effective on Threshold and Below	3.7.2
Assumption 21.	Inhibitory Functions Unaffected by Adaptation	3.7.2
Assumption 22.	Short-acting Inhibition	3.7.2
Assumption 23.	Input-dependent Inhibition of Analyzers	3.7.6

Detection Rules

Relating the Observer's Sensitivity to Analyzers' Sensitivities   *Sections*

Assumption 4.	Most Sensitive Analyzer Rule	3.2.5, 4.2, 4.4.1 (5.2.2), 6.2.1
Assumption 7.	Quick Pooling	3.5.1, 6.4.2
Assumption 28.	Only Analyzer Rule	4.2

Relating the Observer's Decision Variable on Each Trial to Analyzers' Outputs on Each Trial	*Sections*
Assumption 40. Maximum-Output Detection Rule	4.7.1, 6.2.1, 7.3.3, 9.3 (5.2.2, 7.3.2)
Assumption 61. Sum-of-Outputs Detection Rule	7.3.3, 9.3
Assumption 63. Hybrid Decision Rule	7.3.5, 7.4.7, 9.3
Assumption 64. Likelihood-Ratio Decision Rule	7.3.5, 9.3
Assumption 79. Generalized Sum-of-Outputs Detection Rule	9.5.4

Relating the Observer's Decision Variable to the Observer's Responses	*Sections*
Assumption 41. Yes-No Rule	4.7.1, 7.3.3, 9.3
Assumption 42. Forced-Choice Rule	4.7.1, 7.3.3, 9.3
Assumption 62. No Criterion Variance	7.3.3, 9.3

Monitoring Assumptions

Assumption 49. Switching Single-Band Model	7.2.1
Assumption 50. Stationary Single-Band Model	7.2.2
Assumption 51. Perfect Monitoring (Selective and Unlimited)	7.3.1, 9.3
Assumption 65. Monitoring Too Many in Intermixed Conditions	7.4.8
Assumption 67. Monitoring Insensitive Analyzers	8.1.4 (10.7.3, 10.8.2)

Assumption not numbered in book: Monitors All Analyzers All the Time	Used by implication until Chapter 7

Identification Rules

For Classification, Discrimination, and Simple Detection and Identification Paradigms	*Sections*
Assumption 70. Closest Stimulus Classification Rule	9.4.1
Assumption 71. Maximum-Likelihood Classification Rule	9.4.2

DEFINITIONS OF ASSUMPTIONS
IN SEQUENTIAL ORDER

Assumption 1. Intensity-Sensitivity Product

An analyzer's output to a stimulus is a function of the product of its sensitivity for that stimulus (the reciprocal of its threshold for that stimulus) and the stimulus intensity.

Assumption 2. Same Factor for All Test Stimuli

For all test stimuli, an analyzer's threshold is elevated after adaptation by the same factor. This implies Stiles's vertical displacement rule.

Assumption 3. Threshold Elevation Depends Only on Output to Adapting Stimulus

An analyzer's threshold elevation after adaptation depends only on its output to adapting stimulus. This, when coupled with Assumption 1, implies Stiles's horizontal displacement rule.

Assumption 4. Most Sensitive Analyzer Rule

The observer's threshold for a stimulus equals the threshold of the one analyzer (of all the monitored, relevant analyzers) most sensitive to that stimulus.

Assumption 5. Same Most Sensitive Analyzer

A particular analyzer is always the one most sensitive to a given test stimulus no matter what adapting stimulus has been viewed.

Assumption 6. Most Sensitive Analyzer May Change

The negation of Assumption 5.

Assumption 7. Quick Pooling

An observer's sensitivity to a stimulus is determined by probability summation across all analyzers or by equivalent nonlinear pooling as embodied in the following formula:

$$S_{\text{obs}}(\text{stim}) = \left| \sum_{i=1}^{M'} S_i(\text{stim})^k \right|^{1/k}$$

Exponents from 3 to 5 are usually used.

Assumption 8. Uniform Peak Sensitivities

The peak sensitivities of analyzers are assumed to be equal.

Assumption 9. Linear Transducer Function

The expected output of an analyzer to a stimulus is proportional to stimulus intensity. The constant of proportionality is the sensitivity of the analyzer to that stimulus S_i (stim), that is, the reciprocal of the intensity necessary to produce an output of magnitude 1.0.

Assumption 10. Power Adaptation Function

Threshold elevation is a power function of above-threshold adapting contrast.

Assumption 11. Sensitivity Function Is Very Rounded

The individual analyzer's sensitivity function is very rounded. In particular, it equals

$$S_i(v) = \exp\left[-\left(\frac{|v - v_i|}{k} \right)^Q \right]$$

where v_i is the best value of analyzer i, the parameter k determines the bandwidth, and Q is 3.0.

Assumption 12. Sensitivity Function Is Very Peaked

The individual analyzer's sensitivity function is triangular when plotted as log-sensitivity versus linear value on the dimension of interest. The same equation as for Assumption 11 except $Q = 1$.

Assumption 13. Close Spacing of Analyzers

Analyzers are closely spaced relative to the bandwidth of the analyzer (i.e. more than 10 per half-peak full-bandwidth).

Assumption 14. Intermediate Spacing of Analyzers

Analyzers are spaced so that there are several per half-peak full-bandwidth.

Assumption 15. Sparse Spacing of Analyzers

The analyzers are sparsely spaced along the dimension of interest, that is, are widely spaced relative to the bandwidth of the analyzers (i.e. one or less per half-peak full-bandwidth).

Assumption 16. Monotonic Transducer Function

An analyzer's expected output is a monotonic function of sensitivity (at a given intensity) and a monotonic function of intensity (at a given sensitivity).

Assumption 17. Threshold Elevation Not Selective for Value

An analyzer's threshold elevation after adaptation is not selective for value.

Assumption 18. Output-Dependent Inhibition Among Analyzers

There is output-dependent (recurrent, feedback) inhibition among analyzers. That is, the amount of inhibition exerted by one analyzer on another is a function of the total output of the inhibiting analyzer.

Assumption 19. Tonic Inhibition and Excitation

Some inhibition is exerted by an analyzer even when there is no stimulus present to which it is sensitive; this tonic inhibition is the result of tonic excitation.

Assumption 20. Inhibition Effective at Threshold and Below

Inhibition lowers an analyzer's output even when that output is at threshold or below.

Assumption 21. Inhibitory Functions Unaffected by Adaptation

When a test stimulus is presented after an adapting stimulus, the function relating the amount of inhibition exerted by the analyzer to the magnitude of its output is the same as before adaptation.

Assumption 22. Short-acting Inhibition

The excitation and inhibition both have short enough time courses that the response to one stimulus (e.g., the adapting stimulus) is over by the time the next stimulus in the experiment (e.g., the test stimulus) arrives.

Assumption 23. Input-Dependent Inhibition

There is direct inhibition exerted by stimuli on analyzers (nonrecurrent, feed-forward, stimulus-dependent inhibition). The amount of inhibition is a monotonic function of the intensity of the stimulus.

Assumption 24. One Analyzer

Only a single analyzer is on the dimension of interest; thus that single analyzer is sensitive to the entire visible range on that dimension.

Assumption 25. Single-Number Output

To each presentation of a stimulus, the output of the analyzer can be represented as a single number.

Analyzer 26. Variable Analyzer Output

The output of an analyzer to presentations of the same stimulus is variable.

Assumption 27. Additivity to a Compound

The expected output of an analyzer to a compound stimulus is the sum of its outputs to the components by themselves. (This assumption is a very important part of Assumption 47. The two have been separated only for ease of exposition.)

Assumption 28. Only Analyzer Detection Rule

The observer's sensitivity equals the sensitivity of the only analyzer. A stimulus is at (or above) the observer's threshold if and only if the analyzer's output is equal to (or greater than) 1.0.

Assumption 29. Additivity of Sensitivities

The sensitivity of an analyzer to a compound equals the sum of its sensitivities to the components.

Assumption 30. Output Is a Two-Dimensional Function

The analyzer output is a two-dimensional function of spatial coordinates x and y.

Assumption 31. Translation-Invariance (applicable when output is a function)

If one stimulus is just a translation of another (a shifted version), the output to the first stimulus equals the output to the second version shifted by the same amount.

Assumption 32. Deterministic Output (No Variability)

The output of an analyzer in a given state of adaptation to a given stimulus is always the same.

Assumption 33. Peak-in-Output-Profile Rule (applicable when output is a function)

An analyzer's output is above threshold if and only if the maximum of the function representing the output is greater than some criterion level *T*.

Assumption 34. Multiple Analyzers

There are *N'* multiple analyzers having different sensitivity functions along the dimension of interest.

Assumption 35. Nonoverlapping for Far-Apart Values

For values far enough apart on a dimension of interest, no analyzer is sensitive to both values.

Assumption 36. Ineffective-Stimulus Rule (Weak Additivity)

If a stimulus presented alone has no effect on an analyzer, then that stimulus will have no effect when presented in a compound: The analyzer's expected output to the compound (indeed the whole probability distribution of the output) will be exactly like the expected output when the compound has had the one ineffective stimulus removed.

Assumption 37. Noninteracting Analyzers

The outputs of one analyzer have no effects (excitatory or inhibitory) on any other analyzer. The output of each analyzer can always be calculated directly from the stimulus regardless of what other analyzers may or may not be doing.

Assumption 38. Probabilistically Independent Analyzers

The output of each analyzer is variable, and the outputs of different analyzers are probabilistically independent of one another.

Assumption 39. High-Threshold Analyzers

The probability of an analyzer being in the detect state is zero on every trial of the blank stimulus; it is also zero on every trial of any stimulus to which the analyzer is sensitive. (See also Assumption 55.)

Assumption 40. Maximum-Output Detection Rule

In all conditions, the observer's response is based on the maximum of the outputs from the monitored analyzers. In symbols

$$R = \overset{M'}{\underset{i=1}{\text{MAX}}}\ R_i$$

Assumption 41. Yes-No Rule

When the decision variable R is above a criterion, the observer says yes. Otherwise the observer says no. In the high-threshold case, when the observer detects a stimulus, the observer says yes. When the observer does not detect the stimulus, he or she says no and sometimes guesses yes. More generally, for discrete probability distributions, mixture strategies are allowed.

Assumption 42. Forced-choice Rule

The observer indicates the interval during which the decision variable was greater. If there is a tie (as there may be in the high-threshold case), the observer guesses.

Assumption 43. Quick Psychometric Function

The probability that the ith analyzer has an output that exceeds criterion (for the high-threshold case, is in the detect state) equals

$$P_i(\text{stim}) = 1 - 2^{-[c(\text{stim})Si(\text{stim})]k} \tag{Eq. 4.7}$$

where k is a parameter determining the steepness of the psychometric function.

Assumption 44. Independent Variability at Different Positions (applicable when analyzer is a channel and its output, therefore, is a function)

The probability that output at one position exceeds any level is independent of the probability that the output at any other position does.

Assumption 45. Two Relevant Analyzers

There are only two relevant analyzers—one most sensitive to the value of one component and the other most sensitive to the value of the other component.

Assumption 46. Most Sensitive Analyzer Detection Rule

An observer's threshold for the compound equals the threshold of the most sensitive of the two analyzers. (This is a particular application of Assumption 4.)

Assumption 47. Additive (Linear-System) Analyzers

If the expected output of the (linear-system) analyzer is a single number, the expected output can be calculated as the product of a weighting function and the luminance profile of the stimulus. The expected output can be a function (see Assumption 27).

Assumption 48. Only One Spatial-Frequency Bandwidth of Analyzer

Although there may be multiple analyzers along some dimensions of interest, there is only one bandwidth of analyzer at any position along that dimension (e.g., there is not both a narrow-band and a broad-band analyzer having peak sensitivity at 3 cpd).

Assumption 49. Switching Single-Band Model

The observer monitors only one analyzer on each trial, but which analyzer it is switches from trial to trial if more than one stimulus is possible on a trial.

Assumption 50. Stationary Single-Band Model

The observer monitors the same single analyzer on every trial of an intermixed block.

Assumption 51. Perfect Monitoring (Selective and Unlimited)

On each trial the observer monitors all the relevant analyzers and only the relevant analyzers, where the relevant analyzers are those sensitive to any stimulus the observer thinks might be presented on that trial. The probability distribution of the random variable representing the analyzer output is not affected by whether the analyzer is being monitored.

Assumption 52. Probabilistically Independent Trials

The outputs of an analyzer on different trials (or different intervals of a two-alternative forced-choice trial) are probabilistically independent of each other.

Assumption 53. One Analyzer per Stimulus

For any set of far-apart simple stimuli, there is exactly one (and only one) analyzer that is sensitive to each simple stimulus.

Assumption 54. Identical Probability Distribution Families

All analyzers' noise distributions are identical. Further, if any two far-apart simple stimuli are equally detectable when measured in alone conditions, the signal distributions of the corresponding two analyzers are identical.

Assumption 55. High-Threshold Family

The density function describing an analyzer's output to a particular stimulus is a discrete two-state (the detect and non-detect states) function. The signal-strength parameter p is the probability of being in the detect state. Its value is 0.0 for the blank stimulus (noise). (See also Assumption 39.)

Assumption 56. Spread-Exponentials Family

The density function describing an analyzer's output to a particular stimulus has the form

$$f_i(z) = 0 \qquad \text{for } z \leq 0$$
$$= k_i \cdot \exp(-k_i \cdot z) \qquad \text{for } z > 0$$

where $0 < k \leq 1$ and $k = 1$ for the noise stimulus. The signal strength parameter is $k' = 2 \cdot \log_{10}(1/k)$. It is zero for the blank stimulus and increases with increasing intensity.

Assumption 57. Increasing Variance Gaussians ($r = \frac{1}{3}$)

The density function describing an analyzer's output is Gaussian. The signal strength parameter d' is the difference between the means in response to signal and to the blank (noise) divided by the standard deviation in response to the blank. The ratio of the standard deviations in response to a signal and in response to noise is $1 + \frac{1}{3}d'$.

Assumption 58. Increasing-Variance Gaussians ($r = \frac{1}{4}$)

Like Assumption 57 but the ratio of the signal to the noise standard deviations is $1 + \frac{1}{4}d'$.

Assumption 59. Constant-Variance Gaussians ($r = 0$)

Like Assumption 57 but the ratio of the signal to the noise standard deviations is 1.0.

Assumption 60. Shifted Double-Exponentials Family

The density function describing an analyzer's output has the form

$$f_i(z) = \exp(z - U_i) \cdot \exp\{-\exp[-(z + U_i)]\}$$

The signal-strength parameter is U. Its value is zero for the blank stimulus.

Assumption 61. Sum-of-Outputs Detection Rule

In all conditions, the observer's response is based on the sum of the outputs from the monitored analyzers:

$$R = \sum_{i=1}^{M'} R_i$$

Assumption 62. No Criterion Variance

The criterion λ (or, in the high-threshold case, the guessing parameter g) is assumed to be constant throughout the block of trials from which results are pooled to get an empirical measurement.

Assumption 63. Hybrid Decision Rule

In different conditions, the observer uses whichever of the maximum-output or sum-of-outputs decision rule is better.

Assumption 64. Likelihood-Ratio Decision Rule

The observer's decision variable is the likelihood given the signal divided by the likelihood given the blank:

$$\frac{\Pr(R_1, R_2, \ldots, R_{M'} | \text{signal})}{\Pr(R_1, R_2, \ldots, R_{M'} | \text{blank})}$$

Assumption 65. Monitoring Too Many Analyzers in Intermixed Conditions

When $M = 1$, $M' = 1$. As M increases from 1 to 2 or 3, M' increases faster (perhaps to 4 or 5) so the ratio M'/M becomes substantially greater than 1.0. For higher values of M, the increase in M' slows down so the ratio M'/M becomes approximately equal to 1.0 again.

Assumption 66. Intrinsic-Uncertainty Probability Distribution Family

The distribution of an analyzer's output is the distribution of the random variable

$$R_j = \overset{M'_j}{\underset{i=1}{\text{MAX}}} \, R_{ji}(\text{stim})$$

where the R_{ji} ($i = 1, M'_j$) are independent and have Gaussian distributions all of the same variance. The means of the first P'_j of the R_{ji} increase with detectability level but the means of the other $M'_j - P'_j$ remain at zero.

Assumption 67. Monitoring Insensitive Analyzers

For each far-apart simple stimulus in an alone condition, the observer monitors not only the one analyzer sensitive to that stimulus but also a number of insensitive analyzers with the following conditions: (a) The same number of insensitive analyzers must be monitored for each simple stimulus. (b) The sets monitored for different far-apart stimuli are disjoint (i.e., no analyzer monitored in the alone condition for one of the far-apart stimuli is also monitored in the alone condition for another). (c) The analyzers monitored in an intermixed condition or in a compound condition are the union of the analyzers monitored in the alone conditions for the relevant simple stimuli.

Assumption 68. Quick Function With Interdependent Parameters

The probability that the ith analyzer's output is less than criterion is given by

$$\Pr[R_i(\text{stim}) < \lambda] = [1 - g_i(\lambda)] \cdot 2^{-[c(\text{stim}) \cdot S_i(\text{stim}, \lambda)]k(\lambda)}$$

where the three parameters of the Quick function—the sensitivity parameter S, the false-alarm rate parameter g, and the steepness k—depend on the criterion λ. S and g also depend on i (i.e., on which analyzer is under consideration).

Assumption 69. Linear Transducer Functions for Microanalyzers

The mean of the Gaussian distribution characterizing any microanalyzer's output is proportional to stimulus intensity.

Assumption 70. Closest Stimulus Classification Rule

The observer's response on each trial is the stimulus that is closest (as measured by Euclidean distance) in analyzer-output space to the observed analyzer outputs on that trial.

Assumption 71. Maximum-Likelihood Classification Rule

The observer's identification response is the stimulus (indexed by k) for which the likelihood that the observed analyzer outputs were produced is greatest, that is, the k for which the following quantity is greatest:

$$\Pr[R_i(\text{stimulus } k), i = 1, M'] = \Pr(R_1, R_2, \ldots R_{M'} \mid \text{stimulus } k)$$

Assumption 72. Maximum-Output Identification Rule for Simple Stimuli

The observer's response corresponds to the one stimulus (of the N stimuli used in the experiment) to which the maximally responding analyzer is most sensitive.

Assumption 73. Bisector Rule

The observer says whichever stimulus is on the same side of the bisector as the observed point (the point representing the analyzer outputs on that trial).

Assumption 74. Difference-of-Outputs Discrimination Rule

For the case of discrimination between two simple stimuli, the observer uses the difference between the two analyzers' outputs, $R_1 - R_2$, as the decision variable in the way dictated by standard signal-detection theory, where larger (positive) values favor a response of stimulus 1.

Assumption 75. Generalized Difference-of-Outputs Discrimination Rule

The decision variable used by the observer is

$$\mathbf{R} \cdot (\mathbf{A} - \mathbf{B}) = \sum_{i=1}^{M'} R_i \cdot (A_i - B_i)$$

It is used in the standard manner of signal-detection theory, where large values of this decision variable are taken to favor the first stimulus (stimulus A).

Assumption 76. Decision Variables in Single-Interval Discrimination

The observer says that stimulus 1 (rather than stimulus 2) was presented if and only if the decision variable was greater than some criterion.

Assumption 77. Decision Variables in Rating-Scale Discrimination

The greater the value of the decision variable, the more confident the observer is that stimulus 1 (rather than stimulus 2) has been presented.

Assumption 78. Decision Variables in Forced-Choice Discrimination

The observer says that stimulus 1 was presented in the first interval if and only if the decision variable in the first interval minus that in the second interval is greater than a criterion. A criterion of zero is the "unbiased" or "no interval bias" criterion.

Assumption 79. Generalized Sum-of-Outputs Detection Rule

The decision variable is

$$\mathbf{R} \cdot (\mathbf{A} + \mathbf{B})$$

where high values favor the presence of a signal rather than a blank.

Assumption 80. Discriminability of Two Stimuli Determined by Distance

Two pairs of stimuli—one pair A and B and the other C and D—are equally discriminable if the distance between the points representing one pair equals the distance between the two points representing the other pair, that is, if

$$d(\mathbf{A}, \mathbf{B}) = d(\mathbf{C}, \mathbf{D})$$

where d is some distance measure. Generally, discriminability between two stimuli A and B is assumed to be a monotonic function of distance in the analyzer-output space.

Assumption 81. The Minkowski Metric

Like Assumption 80 except that the distance between the points for two stimuli A and B is explicitly given by:

$$d(\mathbf{A}, \mathbf{B}) = \left| \sum_{i=1}^{M'} |A_i - B_i|^k \right|^{1/k}$$

and discriminability is determined by distance.

Assumption 82. The City-Block (Sum-of-Absolute-Differences) Metric

The Minkowski metric with $k = 1$, or

$$d(\mathbf{A}, \mathbf{B}) = \sum_{i=1}^{M'} |A_i - B_i|$$

and discriminability is determined by distance.

Assumption 83. The Euclidean Metric

The Minkowski metric with an exponent of 2, in which case the distance equals the length of the difference vector, or

$$d(\mathbf{A}, \mathbf{B}) = |\mathbf{A} - \mathbf{B}|$$

and discriminability is determined by distance.

Assumption 84. Maximum-of-Absolute-Differences Metric

The Minkowski metric with an exponent of infinity; equivalently, the distance equals the largest absolute difference between individual analyzer's responses to the two stimuli, that is,

$$d(\mathbf{A}, \mathbf{B}) = \mathop{\text{MAX}}_{i=1}^{M'} |A_i - B_i|$$

and discriminability is determined by distance.

Assumption 85. Closest Pattern × Interval 2 × 2 Decision Rule

The stimulus (the pattern and interval combination) for which the expected M' × 2 outputs (M' analyzers in two intervals) are closest (euclidian distance) to the observed outputs on a trial dictates both the detection response (the interval the observer says contains the nonblank pattern) and the identification response (the nonblank pattern the observer says was presented).

Assumption 86. Maximum-Output 2 × 2 Decision Rule

If the maximum of the M' × 2 outputs occurs during the first interval, the observer's detection response is "interval one"; otherwise it is "interval two." If the maximum output is from an analyzer that is more sensitive to stimulus A than to stimulus B, the observer's identification response is "stimulus A"; otherwise it is "stimulus B."

Assumption 87. Maximizing Detection and Identification Independently in the 2 × 2 Paradigm

The rules for detection and identification are stated independently of each other. Let "observed outputs" mean the M' × 2 outputs produced by all analyzers on both intervals of the trial in question.

Detection Subrule. The observer's detection response is the interval ($i = 1$ or 2) for which the value of the following probability is bigger:

Pr(observed outputs | nonblank pattern in interval i)

Identification Subrule. The observer's identification response is the nonblank pattern ($k = A$ or B) for which the value of the following probability is bigger:

Pr(observed outputs | nonblank pattern k)

Assumption 88. Sum-Detection and Difference-Identification in the 2 × 2 Paradigm

The rules for detection and identification are independent of each other.

Detection Subrule. The observer responds "interval one" if and only if the generalized sum-of-outputs in interval one was greater than in interval two, that is, if and only if

$$(\mathbf{A} + \mathbf{B}) \cdot \mathbf{R}(\text{interval 1}) - (\mathbf{A} + \mathbf{B}) \cdot \mathbf{R}(\text{interval 2}) > 0$$

Identification Subrule. The observer responds "pattern A" if and only if the generalized difference of outputs in the first plus that in the second intervals is greater than zero, that is,

$$(\mathbf{A} - \mathbf{B}) \cdot \mathbf{R}(\text{interval } 1) + (\mathbf{A} - \mathbf{B}) \cdot \mathbf{R}(\text{interval } 2) > 0$$

Assumption 89. Direct Reports of Analyzers' Outputs

The decision variable that the observer uses in giving a confidence rating about one component is the maximum of the outputs from the analyzers sensitive to that component.

Assumption 90. Direct Reports of the Relevant Analyzer's Output

The decision variable used by the observer in rating his or her confidence about one component is the output of the one analyzer sensitive to that component.

Assumption 91. Direct Reports Using Perpendicular Criteria

The criterion planes for the decision variable used by the observer in giving a confidence rating about one component in a concurrent experiment are perpendicular to the criterion planes for the other decision variable(s) used to give the confidence rating(s) about the other component(s).

Assumption 92. Power Function Transducer

The mean output of each analyzer is a power function of the stimulus intensity times sensitivity (used in sections 4.8.2, 4.8.5, 8.4, and 10.8.1):

$$E[R_i(c)] = (c \cdot S_i)^b$$

References

Adelson, E. (1982) Saturation and adaptation in the rod system. *Vision Research*, 22, 1299–1312.

Adelson, E. H. & Bergen, J. R. (1985) Spatiotemporal energy models for the perception of motion. *Journal of the Optical Society of America A*, 2, 284–299.

Adelson, E. H. & Movshon, J. A. (1981) Two kinds of adaptation to moving patterns. *Supplement to Investigative Ophthalmology and Visual Science*, 20, 17.

Adelson, E. H. & Movshon, J. A. (1982) Phenomenal coherence of moving visual patterns. *Nature*, 300, 523–525.

Ahumada, A. J. Jr. & Watson, A. B. (1985) Equivalent-noise model for contrast detection and discrimination. *Journal of the Optical Society of America A*, 2, 1133–1139.

Albrecht, D. G. & De Valois, R. L. (1981) Striate cortex responses to periodic patterns with and without the fundamental harmonics. *Journal of Physiology*, 319, 497–514.

Albrecht, D. G., Farrar, S. B., & Hamilton, D. B. (1984) Spatial contrast adaptation characteristics of neurons recorded in cat's visual cortex. *Journal of Physiology*, 347, 713–739.

Albrecht, D. G. & Hamilton, D. B. (1982) Striate cortex of monkey and cat: Contrast response function. *Journal of Neurophysiology*, 48, 217–237.

Allan, L. G. (1979) The perception of time. *Perception and Psychophysics*, 26, 340–354.

Alpern, M. & Spencer, R. W. (1953) Variation of critical flicker frequency in the nasal visual field. *American Archives of Ophthalmology*, 50, 50–63.

Anderson, J., Lasley, D., & Cohn, T. (1982) Discrimination of increment and decrement luminance changes. *Supplement to Investigative Ophthalmology and Visual Science*, 22, 127.

Anderson, P. A., Mitchell, D. E., & Timney, B. (1980) Residual binocular interaction in stereoblind humans. *Vision Research*, 20, 603–611.

Anderson, P. A. & Movshon, J. A. (In press) Binocular combination of contrast signals. *Vision Research*.

Anderson, S. J. & Burr, D. C. (1987) Receptive field size of human motion detection units. *Vision Research*, 27, 621–635.

Andrews, B. W. & Pollen, D. A. (1979) Relationship between spatial frequency selectivity and receptive field profile of simple cells. *Journal of Physiology*, 287, 163–176.

Andrews, D. P. (1967a) Perception of contour orientation in the central fovea. Part I: Short lines. *Vision Research*, 7, 975–997.

Andrews, D. P. (1967b) Perception of contour orientation in the central fovea. Part II: Spatial integration. *Vision Research*, 7, 999–1013.

Annis, R. C. & Frost, B. (1973) Human visual ecology and orientation anisotropies in acuity. *Science*, 182, 729–731.

Anstis, S. M. (1974) A chart demonstrating variations in acuity with retinal position. *Vision Research*, 14, 589–592.

Appelle, S. (1972) Pattern and discrimination as a function of stimulus orientation: The "oblique effect" in man and animals. *Psychological Bulletin*, 78, 266–278.

Arditi, A. R., Anderson, P. A., & Movshon, J. A. (1981) Monocular and binocular detection of moving sinusoidal gratings. *Vision Research*, 21, 329–336.

Arend, L. E. (1976a) Temporal determinants of the form of the spatial contrast threshold MTF. *Vision Research*, 16, 1035–1042.

Arend, L. E. (1976b) Response of the human eye to spatially sinusoidal gratings at various exposure durations. *Vision Research*, 16, 1311–1313.

Arend, L. E. & Lange, R. V. (1979a) Influence of exposure duration on the tuning of spatial channels. *Vision Research,* 19, 195–200.

Arend, L. E. & Lange, R. V. (1979b) Phase-dependent interaction of widely separated spatial frequencies in pattern discrimination. *Vision Research,* 19, 1089–1092.

Arend, L. E. & Lange, R. V. (1980) Narrow-band spatial mechanisms in apparent contrast matching. *Vision Research,* 20, 143–148.

Arend, L. E. & Skavenski, A. A. (1979) Free scanning of gratings produces patterned retinal exposure. *Vision Research,* 19, 1413–1420.

Arend, L. E. & Timberlake, G. T. (1986) What is psychophysically perfect image stabilization? Do perfectly stabilized images always disappear? *Journal of the Optical Society of America A,* 3, 235–241.

Ashby, F. G. (1988) Estimating the parameters of multidimensional signal detection theory from simultaneous ratings on separate stimulus components. *Perception and Psychophysics,* 44, 195–204.

Ashby, F. G. & Townsend, J. T. (1986) Varieties of perceptual independence. *Psychological Review,* 93, 154–179.

Atkin, A., Bodis-Wollner, I., Wolkstein, M., Moss, A., & Podos, S. M. (1979) Abnormalities of central contrast sensitivity in glaucoma. *American Journal of Ophthalmology,* 88, 205–211.

Atkinson, J. & Braddick, O. (1981) Acuity, contrast sensitivity and accommodation in infancy. In *Development of Perception. Vol. 2. The Visual System* (R. M. Aslin, J. R. Alberts, and M. R. Petersen, Eds.). New York: Academic Press.

Atkinson, J. & Braddick, O. (1983) Assessment of visual acuity in infancy and early childhood. *Acta Ophthalmologica Supplementum,* 157, 18–26.

Atkinson, J., Braddick, O., & Moar, K. (1977a) Development of contrast sensitivity over the first three months of life in the human infant. *Vision Research,* 17, 1037–1044.

Atkinson, J., Braddick, O., & Moar, K. (1977b) Contrast sensitivity of the human infant for moving and static patterns. *Vision Research,* 17, 1045–1047.

Atkinson, J. & French, J. (1979) Astigmatism and orientation preference in human infants. *Vision Research,* 19, 1315–1318.

Atkinson, J., French, J., & Braddick, O. (1981) Contrast sensitivity function of preschool children. *British Journal of Ophthalmology,* 65, 525–529.

Atkinson, J., Pimm-Smith, E., & Braddick, O. J. (1983) The effects of screen size and eccentricity on acuity estimates in infants using preferential looking. *Vision Research,* 23, 1479–1483.

Bacon, J. & King-Smith, P. E. (1977) The detection of line segments. *Perception,* 6, 125–131.

Bacon, J. H. (1976) The interaction of dichoptically presented spatial gratings. *Vision Research,* 16, 337–344.

Badcock, D. R. (1984a) Spatial phase or luminance profile discrimination? *Vision Research,* 24, 613–623.

Badcock, D. R. (1984b) How do we discriminate relative spatial phase? *Vision Research,* 24, 1847–1857.

Bagrash, F. M. (1973) Size-selective adaptation: Psychophysical evidence for size-tuning and the effects of stimulus contour and adapting flux. *Vision Research,* 13, 575–598.

Bagrash, F. M., Kerr, L. G., & Thomas, J. P. (1971) Patterns of spatial integration in the detection of compound visual stimuli. *Vision Research,* 11, 635–645.

Bagrash, F. M., Thomas, J. P., & Shimamura, K. K. (1974) Size-tuned mechanisms: Correlation of data on detection and apparent size. *Vision Research,* 14, 937–942.

Baker, R., Brown, B., & Garner, L. (1983) Time course and variability of dark focus. *Investigative Ophthalmology and Visual Science,* 24, 1528–1531.

Ball, K. & Sekuler, R. (1980) Models of stimulus uncertainty in motion perception. *Psychological Review,* 87, 435–469.

Ball, K. & Sekuler, R. (1981a) Adaptive processing of visual motion. *Journal of Experimental Psychology: Human Perception and Performance,* 7, 780–794.

Ball, K. & Sekuler, R. (1981b) Cues reduce direction uncertainty and enhance motion detection. *Perception and Psychophysics,* 30, 119–128.

Ball, K. & Sekuler, R. (1982) A specific and enduring improvement in visual motion discrimination. *Science,* 218, 697–698.

Ball, K., Sekuler, R., & Machamer, J. (1983) Detection and identification of moving targets. *Vision Research,* 23, 229–238.

Banks, M. S., Geisler, W. S., & Bennett, P. J. (1987) The physical limits of grating visibility. *Vision Research,* 27, 1915–1929.

Banks, M. S. & Salapatek, P. (1978) Acuity and contrast sensitivity in 1-, 2-, and 3-month-old human infants. *Investigative Ophthalmology and Visual Science,* 17, 361–365.

Banks, M. S. & Salapatek, P. (1983) Infant visual perception. In *Handbook of Child Psychology* (P. Mussen, Ed.). New York: Wiley.

Banks, M. S., Stephens, B. R., & Dannemiller, J. L. (1982) A failure to observe negative preference in infant acuity testing. *Vision Research,* 22, 1025–1031.

Banks, M. S., Stephens, B. R., & Hartmann, E. E. (1985) The development of basic mechanisms of pattern vision: Spatial frequency channels. *Journal of Experimental Child Psychology,* 40, 501–527.

Banks, M. S. & Stolarz, S. J. (1975) The effect of head tilt on meridional differences in acuity: Implications for orientation constancy. *Perception and Psychophysics,* 17, 17–22.

Barker, R. A. (1978a) Comparison of effects of multiple cues in detection and discrimination. *Supplement to Investigative Ophthalmology and Visual Science,* 17, 221.

Barker, R. A. (1978b) Detection and discrimination of compound gratings. *Journal of the Optical Society of America,* 68, 1379a.

Barker, R. A. (1979) *A vector space model of detection and discrimination of visual patterns.* Ph.D. Thesis, University of California, Los Angeles.

Barlow, H. B. (1953) Summation and inhibition in the frog's retina. *Journal of Physiology,* 119, 69–88.

Barlow, H. B. (1956) Retinal noise and absolute threshold. *Journal of the Optical Society of America,* 46, 634–639.

Barlow, H. B. (1957) Increment thresholds at low intensities considered as signal/noise discriminations. *Journal of Physiology,* 136, 469–488.

Barlow, H. B. (1958) Temporal and spatial summation in human vision at different background intensities. *Journal of Physiology,* 141, 337–350.

Barlow, H. B. & Hill, R. M. (1963) Evidence for a physiological explanation of the waterfall phenomenon and figural after-effects. *Nature,* 20, 1345–1347.

Barlow, H. B., Hill, R. M., & Levick, W. R. (1964) Retinal ganglion cells responding selectively to direction and speed of image motion in the rabbit. *Journal of Physiology,* 173, 377–407.

Barlow, H. B., Kaushal, T. P., Hawken, M., & Parker, A. J. (1987) Human contrast discrimination and the threshold of cortical neurons. *Journal of the Optical Society of America A,* 4, 2366–2371.

Barlow, H. B. & Levick, W. R. (1969) Three factors limiting the reliable detection of light by retinal ganglion cells of the cat. *Journal of Physiology,* 200, 1–24.

Barlow, H. B., Macleod, D. I. A., & van Meeteren, A. (1976) Adaptation to gratings: No compensatory advantages found. *Vision Research,* 16, 1043–1045.

Baro, J. A., Lehmkuhle, S., & Applegate, R. A. (1988) Contrast-increment thresholds are related to variability in the apparent contrast function. *Perception and Psychophysics,* 44, 463–472.

Bartlett, N. R. & Doty, R. W. (1974) Response of units in striate cortex of squirrel monkeys to visual and electrical stimuli. *Journal of Neurophysiology,* 37, 621–641.

Battersby, W. S. & Schuckman, H. (1970) The time-course of temporal summation. *Vision Research,* 10, 263–273.

Baumgartner, G. (1960) Indirekte Grossenbestimmung der receptiven Felder der Retina beim Menschen mittels der Hermannschen Gittertäuschung. *Pfluegers Archiv der gesammten Physiologie,* 272, 21–22.

Beaton, A. & Blakemore, C. (1981) Orientation selectivity of the human visual system as a function of retinal eccentricity and visual hemifield. *Perception,* 10, 273–282.

Beazley, L. D., O'Conner, W. M., & Illingsworth, D. J. (1982) Adult levels of meridional anisotropy and contrast threshold in 5-yr olds. *Vision Research,* 22, 135–138.

Benzschawel, T. & Cohn, T. E. (1981) The theory of signal detectability (TSD) for visual resolution. *Supplement to Investigative Ophthalmology and Visual Science,* 20, 51.

Bergen, J. R. & Wilson, H. R. (1985) Prediction of flicker sensitivities from temporal three-pulse data. *Vision Research,* 25, 577–582.

Bergen, J. R., Wilson, H. R. & Cowan, J. D. (1979) Further evidence for four mechanisms mediating vision at threshold: Sensitivities to complex gratings and aperiodic stimuli. *Journal of the Optical Society of America,* 69, 1580–1587.

Berkley, M. A., Kitterle, F., & Watkins, D. W. (1975) Grating visibility as a function of orientation and retinal eccentricity. *Vision Research,* 15, 239–244.

Biederman, I. (1985) Human image understanding: Recent research and a theory. *Computer Vision, Graphics, and Image Processing,* 32, 29–73.

Birch, D. & Jacobs, G. H. (1979) Spatial contrast sensitivity in albino and pigmented rats. *Vision Research,* 19, 933–938.

Birch, E. E., Gwiazda, J., Bauer, J. A., Jr., Naegele, J., & Held, R. (1983) Visual acuity and its meridional variations in children aged 7–60 months. *Vision Research,* 23, 1019–1025.

Bishop, P. O., Coombs, J. S., & Henry, G. H. (1971) Interaction effects of visual contours on the discharge frequency of simple striate neurones. *Journal of Physiology,* 219, 659–687.

Bishop, P. O., Coombs, J. S., & Henry, G. H. (1973) Receptive fields of simple cells in the cat striate cortex. *Journal of Physiology,* 231, 31–60.

Bjorklund, R. A. & Magnussen, S. (1981) A study of interocular transfer of spatial adaptation. *Perception,* 10, 511–518.

Blackwell, H. R. (1946) Contrast thresholds of the human eye. *Journal of the Optical Society of America,* 36, 624–643.

Blackwell, H. R. (1952) Studies of psychophysical methods for measuring visual thresholds. *Journal of the Optical Society of America,* 42, 606–616.

Blackwell, H. R. (1963) Neural theories of simple visual discriminations. *Journal of the Optical Society of America,* 53, 129–160.

Blackwell, H. R. (1972) Luminance difference thresholds. In *Handbook of Sensory Physiology. Vol. VII/4* (D. Jameson & L. Hurvich, Eds.). Berlin: Springer-Verlag, pp. 78–101.

Blake, R., Breitmeyer, B., & Green, M. (1980) Contrast sensitivity and binocular brightness: Dioptic and dichoptic luminance conditions. *Perception and Psychophysics,* 27, 180–181.

Blake, R. & Camisa, J. M. (1977) Temporal aspects of spatial vision in the cat. *Experimental Brain Research,* 28, 325–333.

Blake, R. & Cormack, R. H. (1979a) Psychophysical evidence for a monocular visual cortex in stereoblind humans. *Science,* 230, 274–275.

Blake, R. & Cormack, R. H. (1979b) On utrocular discrimination. *Perception and Psychophysics,* 26, 53–68.

Blake, R. & Di Gianfilippo, A. (1980) Spatial vision in cats with selective neural deficits. *Journal of Neurophysiology,* 43, 1197–1205.

Blake, R. & Fox, R. (1973) The psychophysical inquiry into binocular summation. *Perception and Psychophysics,* 14, 161–185.

Blake, R. & Fox, R. (1974) Adaptation to invisible gratings and the site of binocular rivalry suppression. *Nature,* 249, 488–490.

Blake, R. & Levinson, E. (1977) Spatial properties of binocular neurones in the human visual system. *Experimental Brain Research,* 27, 221–232.

Blake, R. & Mills, J. (1979) Pattern and flicker detection examined in terms of the nasal-temporal division of the retina. *Perception,* 8, 549–555.

Blake, R., Overton, R., & Lema-Stern, S. (1981) Interocular transfer of visual aftereffects. *Journal of Experimental Psychology: Human Perception and Performance,* 7, 367–381.

Blake, R. & Rush, C. (1980) Temporal properties of binocular mechanisms in the human visual system. *Experimental Brain Research,* 38, 333–340.

Blake, R., Sloane, M., & Fox, F. (1981) Further developments in binocular summation. *Perception and Psychophysics,* 30, 266–276.

Blakemore, C. & Campbell, F. W. (1969) On the existence of neurones in the human visual system selectively sensitive to the orientation and size of retinal images. *Journal of Physiology,* 203, 237–260.

Blakemore, C., Carpenter, R. H. S., & Georgeson, M. A. (1970) Lateral inhibition between orientation detectors in the human visual system. *Nature,* 228, 37–39.

Blakemore, C., Carpenter, R. H. S., & Georgeson, M. A. (1971) Lateral thinking about lateral inhibition. *Nature,* 234, 418–419.

Blakemore, C., Garner, E. T., & Sweet, J. A. (1972) The site of size constancy. *Perception,* 1, 111–119.

Blakemore, C., Muncey, J. P. J., & Ridley, R. M. (1971) Perceptual fading of a stabilized cortical image. *Nature,* 233, 204–205.

Blakemore, C., Muncey, J. P. J., & Ridley, R. M. (1973) Stimulus specificity in the human visual system. *Vision Research,* 13, 1915–1931.

Blakemore, C. & Nachmias, J. (1971) The orientation specificity of two visual after-effects. *Journal of Physiology,* 213, 157–174.

Blakemore, C. & Tobin, E. A. (1972) Lateral inhibition between orientation detectors in the cat's visual cortex. *Experimental Brain Research,* 15, 439–440.

Blommaert, F. J. J. & Roufs, J. A. J. (1981) The foveal point spread function as a determinant for detail vision. *Vision Research,* 21, 1223–1234.

Bodinger, D. M. (1978) The decay of grating adaptation. *Vision Research,* 18, 89–92.

Bodis-Wollner, I. (1972) Visual acuity and contrast sensitivity in patients with cerebral lesions. *Science,* 178, 769–771.

Bodis-Wollner, I. (1976) Vulnerability of spatial frequency channels in cerebral lesions. *Nature,* 261, 309–311.

Bodis-Wollner, I. & Diamond, S. P. (1976) The measurement of spatial contrast sensitivity in cases of blurred vision associated with cerebral lesions. *Brain,* 99, 695–710.

Bodis-Wollner, I., Harnois, C., & Bobak, P. (1983) Psychophysical and electrophysiological correlates for pattern and flicker detection. *Supplement to Investigative Ophthalmology and Visual Science,* 24, 188.

Bodis-Wollner, I., Hendley, C. D., Mylin, L. H., & Thornton, J. (1979) Visual evoked potentials and the visuogram in multiple sclerosis. *Annals of Neurology,* 5, 40–47.

Boltz, R. L., Harwerth, R. S., & Smith, E. L. (1979) Orientation anisotropy of visual stimuli in rhesus monkey: A behavioral study. *Science,* 205, 511–513.

Bonds, A. B. (1983) Inhibitory contribution to the spatial selectivity of single cells in cat striate cortex. *Supplement to Investigative Ophthalmology and Visual Science,* 24, 229.

Boothe, R. G., Dobson, V., & Teller, D. Y. (1985) Postnatal development of vision in human and nonhuman primates. *Annual Review of Neurosciences,* 8, 495–545.

Boothe, R. G., Kiorpes, L., Williams, R. A., & Teller, D. Y. (1988) Operant measurements of contrast sensitivity in infant macaque monkeys during normal development. *Vision Research,* 28, 387–396.

Boothe, R. G. & Teller, D. Y. (1982) Meridional variations in acuity and CSF's in monkeys (Macaca nemestrina) reared with externally applied astigmatism. *Vision Research,* 22, 801–810.

Boothe, R. G., Williams, R. A., Kiorpes, L., & Teller, D. Y. (1980) Development of contrast sensitivity in infant Macaca nemestrina monkeys. *Science,* 208, 1290–1292.

Bossomaier, T. & Snyder, A. W. (1986) Why spatial frequency processing in the visual cortex? *Vision Research,* 26, 1307–1309.

Bossomaier, T. R. J., Snyder, A. W., & Hughes, A. (1985) Irregularity and aliasing: Solution? *Vision Research,* 25, 145–147.

Bouman, M. A. & van den Brink, G. (1952) On the integrative capacity in time and space of the human peripheral retina. *Journal of the Optical Society of America,* 42, 617–620.

Bour, L. J. (1981) The influence of the spatial distribution of a target on the dynamic fluctuations of the accommodation of the human eye. *Vision Research*, 21, 1287–1296.

Bowker, D. O. & Tulunay-Keesey, U. (1983) Sensitivity to countermodulating gratings following spatiotemporal adaptation. *Journal of the Optical Society of America*, 73, 427–435.

Boynton, R. M. (1979) *Human Color Vision.* New York: Holt, Rinehart, and Winston.

Brabyn, L. B. & McGuinness, D. (1979) Gender differences in response to spatial frequency and stimulus orientation. *Perception and Psychophysics*, 26, 319–324.

Bracewell, R. (1965) *The Fourier Transform and its Applications.* New York: McGraw-Hill.

Braddick, O., Campbell, F. W., & Atkinson, J. (1978) Channels in vision: Basic aspects. In *Handbook of Sensory Physiology, Vol. VIII: Perception* (R. Held, H. W. Leibowitz, & H. L. Teuber, Eds.). Springer-Verlag, pp. 3–38.

Braddick, O. J., Atkinson, J., & Wattam-Bell, J. R. (1986) Development of discrimination of spatial phase in infancy. *Vision Research*, 26, 1223–1239.

Bradley, A. & Freeman, R. D. (1981) Contrast sensitivity in anisometropic amblyopia. *Investigative Ophthalmology and Visual Science*, 21, 467–476.

Bradley, A. & Freeman, R. D. (1982) Contrast sensitivity in children. *Vision Research*, 22, 953–959.

Bradley, A. & Freeman, R. D. (1985) Temporal sensitivity in amblyopia: An explanation of conflicting reports. *Vision Research*, 25, 39–46.

Bradley, A., Freeman, R. D., & Applegate, R. (1985) Is amblyopia spatial frequency or retinal locus specific? *Vision Research*, 25, 47–54.

Bradley, A., Switkes, E., & De Valois, K. (1988) Orientation and spatial frequency selectivity of adaptation to color and luminance gratings. *Vision Research*, 28, 841–856.

Breitmeyer, B. G. & Ganz, L. (1976) Implications of sustained and transient channels for theories of visual pattern making, saccadic suppression, and information processing. *Psychological Review*, 83, 1–36.

Breitmeyer, B. G. & Ganz, L. (1977) Temporal studies with flashed gratings: Inferences about human transient and sustained channels. *Vision Research*, 17, 861–865.

Breitmeyer, B. & Julesz, B. (1975) The role of on and off transients in determining the psychophysical spatial frequency response. *Vision Research*, 15, 411–415.

Brindley, G. S. (1960a) *Physiology of the Retina and Visual Pathway.* London: Arnold.

Brindley, G. S. (1960b) Two more visual theorems. *Quarterly Journal of Experimental Psychology*, 12, 110–112.

Broekhuijsen, M., Rashbass, C., & Veringa, F. (1976) The threshold of visual transients. *Vision Research*, 16, 1285–1289.

Brown, A. M., Dobson, V., & Maier, J. (1987) Visual acuity of human infants at scotopic, mesopic and photopic luminances. *Vision Research*, 27, 1845–1858.

Brown, J. L. & Black, J. (1976) Critical duration for resolution of acuity targets. *Vision Research*, 16, 309–315.

Brussell, E. M., White, C. W., Mustillo, P., & Overbury, O. (1984) Inferences about mechanisms that mediate pattern and flicker sensitivity. *Perception and Psychophysics*, 35, 301–304.

Bryngdahl, O. (1964) Characteristics of the visual system: Psychophysical measurements of the response to spatial sine-wave stimuli in the mesopic region. *Journal of the Optical Society of America*, 54, 1152–1160.

Budrikis, Z. L. & Lukas, F. X. (1979) Phase response of the visual system. *Supplement to Investigative Ophthalmology and Visual Science*, 18, 92.

Burbeck, C. A. (1981) Criterion-free pattern and flicker thresholds. *Journal of the Optical Society of America*, 71, 1343–1350.

Burbeck, C. A. & Kelly, D. H. (1982) Eliminating transient artifacts in stabilized-image contrast thresholds. *Journal of the Optical Society of America*, 72, 1238–1243.

Burbeck, C. A. & Kelly, D. H. (1984) Role of local adaptation in the fading of stabilized images. *Journal of the Optical Society of America*, 1, 216–220.

Burbeck, C. A. & Regan, D. (1983) Independence of orientation and size in spatial discriminations. *Journal of the Optical Society of America*, 73, 1691–1694.

Burbeck, S. L. & Luce, R. D. (1982) Evidence from auditory simple reaction times for both change and level detectors. *Perception and Psychophysics,* 32, 117–133.

Burgess, A. & Ghanderian, H. (1984) Visual signal detection. I. Ability to use phase information. *Journal of the Optical Society of America,* 1, 900–905.

Burr, D. C. (1980) Sensitivity to spatial phase. *Vision Research,* 20, 391–396.

Burr, D. C. (1981) Temporal summation of moving images by the human visual system. *Proceedings of the Royal Society of London B,* 211, 321–339.

Burr, D. C., Morrone, M. C., & Maffei, L. (1981) Intracortical inhibition prevents simple cells from responding to textured visual patterns. *Experimental Brain Research,* 43, 455–458.

Burr, D. C. & Ross, J. (1982) Contrast sensitivity at high velocities. *Vision Research,* 22, 479–484.

Burr, D. C., Ross, J., & Morrone, M. C. (1985) Local regulation of luminance gain. *Vision Research,* 25, 717–727.

Burt, P. & Sperling, G. (1981) Time, distance, and feature trade-offs in visual apparent motion. *Psychological Review,* 88, 171–195.

Burton, G. J. (1973) Evidence for nonlinear response processes in the human visual system from measurements on the thresholds of spatial beat frequencies. *Vision Research,* 13, 1211–1225.

Burton, G. J. (1976) Visual detection of patterns periodic in two dimensions. *Vision Research,* 16, 991–998.

Burton, G. J. & Ruddock, K. H. (1978) Visual adaptation to patterns containing two dimensional spatial structure. *Vision Research,* 18, 93–100.

Bush, R., Galanter, E., & Luce, R. D. (1963) Characterization and classification of choice experiments. In *Handbook of Mathematical Psychology* (R. D. Luce, R. Bush, & E. Galanter, Eds.). New York: Wiley.

Camisa, J. M., Blake, R., & Lema, S. (1977) The effects of temporal modulation on the oblique effect in humans. *Perception,* 6, 165–171.

Campbell, F. W. (1958) A retinal acuity direction effect. *Journal of Physiology,* 144, 25–26.

Campbell, F. W., Carpenter, R. H. S., & Levinson, J. Z. (1969) Visibility of aperiodic patterns compared with that of sinusoidal gratings. *Journal of Physiology,* 204, 283–298.

Campbell, F. W., Cooper, G. F., & Enroth-Cugell, C. (1969) The spatial selectivity of the visual cells of the cat. *Journal of Physiology,* 203, 223–235.

Campbell, F. W. & Green, D. G. (1965) Optical and retinal factors affecting visual resolution. *Journal of Physiology,* 181, 576–593.

Campbell, F. W. & Gubisch, R. W. (1966) Optical quality of the human eye. *Journal of Physiology,* 186, 558–578.

Campbell, F. W. & Gubisch, R. W. (1967) The effect of chromatic aberration on visual acuity. *Journal of Physiology,* 192, 345–358.

Campbell, F. W., Howell, E. R., & Johnstone, J. R. (1978) A comparison of threshold and suprathreshold appearance of gratings with components in the low and high spatial frequency range. *Journal of Physiology,* 284, 193–201.

Campbell, F. W., Johnston, J. R., and Ross, J. (1981) An explanation for the visibility of low frequency gratings. *Vision Research,* 21, 723–730.

Campbell, F. W. & Kulikowski, J. J. (1966) Orientation selectivity of the human visual system. *Journal of Physiology,* 187, 437–445.

Campbell, F. W., Kulikowski, J. J., & Levinson, J. (1966) The effect of orientation on the visual resolution of gratings. *Journal of Physiology,* 187, 427–436.

Campbell, F. W., Nachmias, J., & Jukes, J. (1970) Spatial-frequency discrimination in human vision. *Journal of the Optical Society of America,* 60, 555–559.

Campbell, F. W. & Robson, J. G. (1964) Application of Fourier analysis to the modulation response of the eye. *Journal of the Optical Society of America,* 54, 581 (abstract).

Campbell, F. W. & Robson, J. G. (1968) Application of Fourier analysis to the visibility of gratings. *Journal of Physiology,* 197, 551–566.

Cannon, M. W. & Fullenkamp, S. C. (1987) Probability summation among spatially separated stimuli is less than predicted. *Supplement to Investigative Ophthalmology and Visual Science,* 28, 357.

Carlson, C. R., Cohen, R. W., & Gorog, I. (1977) Visual processing of simple two-dimensional sine-wave luminance gratings. *Vision Research, 17,* 351–358.

Carlson, C. R., Klopfenstein, R. W., & Anderson, C. H. (1981) Spatially inhomogeneous scaled transforms for vision and pattern recognition. *Optics Letters, 6,* 386–388.

Carpenter, R. H. S. & Blakemore, C. (1973) Interactions between orientations in human vision. *Experimental Brain Research, 18,* 287–303.

Casson, E. J. & Wandell, B. A. (1984) Duration discrimination between weak test lights. *Vision Research, 24,* 641–645.

Cavanagh, P. (1978) Subharmonics in adaptation to sine wave gratings. *Vision Research, 18,* 741–742.

Cavonius, C. R. (1979) Binocular interactions in flicker. *Quarterly Journal of Experimental Psychology, 31,* 273–280.

Charman, W. N. & Tucker, J. (1977) Dependence of accommodation response on the spatial frequency spectrum of the observed object. *Vision Research, 17,* 129–139.

Charman, W. N. & Walsh, G. (1985) The optical phase transfer function of the eye and the perception of spatial phase. *Vision Research, 25,* 619–623.

Chen, B., MacLeod, D. I. A., & Stockman, A. (1987) Improvement in human vision under bright light: Grain or gain? *Journal of Physiology, 394,* 41.

Cicerone, C. M. & Green, D. G. (1978) Relative modulation sensitivities of the red and green color mechanisms. *Vision Research, 18,* 1593–1598.

Cleland, B. G., Dubin, M. W., & Levick, W. R. (1971) Sustained and transient neurons in the cat's retina and lateral geniculate nucleus. *Journal of Physiology, 217,* 473–497.

Cohen, R. W., Carlson, C. R., & Cody, G. (1976) *Image Descriptors for Displays.* Princeton, N.J.: RCA Laboratories.

Cohn, T. E. (1974) A new hypothesis to explain why the increment threshold exceeds the decrement threshold. *Vision Research, 14,* 1277–1279.

Cohn, T. E. (1978) Detection of 1-of-M orthogonal signals: Asymptotic equivalence of likelihood ratio and multiband models. *Optics Letters, 3,* 22–23.

Cohn, T. E. (1981) Absolute threshold: Analysis in terms of uncertainty. *Journal of the Optical Society of America, 71,* 783–785.

Cohn, T. E. & Lasley, D. J. (1974) Detectability of a luminance increment: Effect of spatial uncertainty. *Journal of the Optical Society of America, 64,* 1715–1719.

Cohn, T. E. & Lasley, D. J. (1975) Spatial summation of foveal increments and decrements. *Vision Research, 15,* 389–399.

Cohn, T. E. & Lasley, D. J. (1976) Binocular vision: Two possible central interactions between signals from two eyes. *Science, 192,* 561–563.

Cohn, T. E., Leong, H., & Lasley, D. J. (1981) Binocular luminance detection: Availability of more than one central interaction. *Vision Research, 21,* 1017–1023.

Cohn, T. E., Thibos, L. N., & Kleinstein, R. N. (1974) Detectability of a luminance increment. *Journal of the Optical Society of America, 64,* 1321–1327.

Cohn, T. E. & Wardlaw, J. C. (1985) Effect of large spatial uncertainty on foveal luminance increment detectability. *Journal of the Optical Society of America A, 2,* 820–825.

Coletta, N. J. & Adams, A. J. (1984) Rod-cone interaction in flicker detection. *Vision Research, 24,* 1333–1340.

Coletta, N. J. & Adams, A. J. (1986a) Spatial extent of rod-cone and cone-cone interactions for flicker detection. *Vision Research, 26,* 917–925.

Coletta, N. J. & Adams, A. J. (1986b) Adaptation of a color-opponent mechanism increases parafoveal sensitivity to luminance flicker. *Vision Research, 26,* 1241–1248.

Coletta, N. J. & Williams, D. R. (1987) Psychophysical estimate of extrafoveal cone spacing. *Journal of the Optical Society of America A, 4,* 1503–1513.

Collins, J. F. (1973) Independence of sensitivity on different foveal areas. *Perception and Psychophysics, 13,* 212–216.

Conner, J. D. & MacLeod, D. I. A. (1977) Rod photoreceptors detect rapid flicker. *Science, 195,* 698–699.

Coombs, C., Dawes, R., & Tversky, A. (1970) *Mathematical Psychology*. Englewood Cliffs, N.J.: Prentice-Hall.

Cormack, R. H. & Blake, R. (1980) Do the two eyes constitute separate visual channels? *Science, 207*, 1100–1102.

Cornsweet, T. N. (1970) *Visual Perception*. New York: Academic Press.

Cornsweet, T. N. & Reuman, S. (1986) CVIDS—A new model for spatio-temporal retinal interaction. *Supplement to Investigative Ophthalmology and Visual Science, 27*, 226.

Cornsweet, T. N. & Yellott, J. I. (1985) Intensity-dependent spatial summation. *Journal of the Optical Society of America A, 2*, 1769–1786. (Errata: *Journal of the Optical Society of America A, 1986, 3*, 165)

Corwin, T. R. & Dunlap, W. P. (1987) The shape of the high frequency flicker sensitivity curve. *Vision Research, 27*, 2119–2123.

Corwin, T. R., Volpe, L. C., & Tyler, C. W. (1976) Images and afterimages of sinusoidal gratings. *Vision Research, 16*, 345–350.

Cowey, A. (1985) Aspects of cortical organization related to selective attention and selective impairments of visual perception. In *Mechanisms of Attention: Attention and Performance XI* (M. I. Posner & O. S. M. Marin, Eds.). Hillsdale, N.J.: Lawrence Erlbaum.

Crawford, M. L. J., von Noorden, G. K., Meharg, L. S., Rhodes, J. W., Harwerth, R. S., Smith, E. L. III, & Miller, D. D. (1983) Binocular neurons and binocular function in monkeys and children. *Investigative Ophthalmology and Visual Science, 24*, 491–495.

Creelman, C. D. (1962) Human discrimination of auditory duration. *Journal of the Acoustical Society of America, 34*, 582–593.

Creelman, C. D. & Macmillan, N. A. (1979) Auditory phase and frequency discrimination: A comparison of nine procedures. *Journal of Experimental Psychology: Human Perception and Performance, 5*, 146–156.

Cuiffreda, K. J. & Hokoda, S. C. (1983) Spatial frequency dependence of accommodative responses in amblyopia eyes. *Vision Research, 23*, 1585–1594.

Cuiffreda, K. J. & Rumpf, D. (1985) Contrast and accommodation in amblyopia. *Vision Research, 25*, 1445–1457.

Daitch, J. M. & Green, D. G. (1969) Contrast sensitivity of the human peripheral retina. *Vision Research, 9*, 947–952.

Dannemiller, J. L. & Banks, M. S. (1983) The development of light adaptation in human infants. *Vision Research, 23*, 599–609.

Daugman, J. G. (1980) Two-dimensional spectral analysis of cortical receptive field profiles. *Vision Research, 20*, 847–856.

Daugman, J. G. (1984) Spatial visual channels in the Fourier plane. *Vision Research, 24*, 891–910.

Daugman, J. G. (1985) Uncertainty relation for resolution in space, spatial frequency, and orientation optimized by two-dimensional visual cortical filters. *Journal of the Optical Society of America A, 2*, 1160–1169.

Daugman, J. G. & Manfield, R. J. (1979) Adaptation of spatial channels in human vision. *Supplement to Investigative Ophthalmology and Visual Science, 18*, 91.

Davidson, M. (1968) Perturbation approach to spatial brightness interaction in human vision. *Journal of the Optical Society of America, 58*, 1300–1308.

Davis, E. T. (1981) Allocation of attention: Uncertainty effects when monitoring one or two visual gratings of noncontiguous spatial frequencies. *Perception and Psychophysics, 29*, 618–622.

Davis, E. T. & Graham, N. (1981) Spatial frequency uncertainty effects in the detection of visual sinusoidal gratings. *Vision Research, 21*, 705–712.

Davis, E. T., Kramer, P., & Graham, N. (1983) Uncertainty about spatial frequency, spatial position, or contrast of visual patterns. *Perception and Psychophysics, 33*, 20–28.

Dealy, R. S. & Tolhurst, D. J. (1974) Is spatial adaptation an after-effect of prolonged inhibition? *Journal of Physiology, 241*, 261–270.

Dean, A. F. (1981a) The relationship between response amplitude and contrast for cat striate cortical neurons. *Journal of Physiology, 318*, 413–427.

Dean, A. F. (1981b) The variability of discharge of simple cells in the cat striate cortex. *Experimental Brain Research,* 44, 437–440.

Dean, A. F. (1983) Adaptation-induced alteration of the relation between response amplitude and contrast in cat striate cortical neurons. *Vision Research,* 23, 249–256.

Dean, A. F. & Tolhurst, D. J. (1983) On the distinctness of simple and complex cells in the visual cortex of the cat. *Journal of Physiology,* 344, 305–325.

Deeley, R. J. & Drasdo, N. (1987) The effect of optical degradation on the contrast sensitivity function measured at the fovea and in the periphery. *Vision Research,* 27, 1179–1186.

DeLange, H. (1952) Experiments on flicker and some calculations on an electrical analogue of the fovea. *Physica,* 28, 935–950.

DeLange, H. (1954) Relationship between critical flicker-frequency and a set of low-frequency characteristics of the eye. *Journal of the Optical Society of America,* 44, 380–389.

DeLange, H. (1958) Research into the dynamic nature of the human fovea-cortex systems with intermittent and modulated light. *Journal of the Optical Society of America,* 48, 771–789.

DePalma, J. J. & Lowry, E. M. (1962) Sine-wave response of the visual system. II. Sine-wave and square-wave contrast sensitivity. *Journal of the Optical Society of America,* 52, 328–335.

Derrington, A. M. & Henning, G. B. (1981) Pattern discrimination with flickering stimuli. *Vision Research,* 21, 597–602.

De Valois, K. K. (1977a) Independence of black and white: Phase-specific adaptation. *Vision Research,* 17, 209–215.

De Valois, K. K. (1977b) Spatial frequency adaptation can enhance contrast sensitivity. *Vision Research,* 17, 1057–1066.

De Valois, R. L. & De Valois, K. K. (1988) *Spatial Vision.* New York: Oxford University Press.

De Valois, K. K., De Valois, R. L., & Yund, E. W. (1979) Responses of striate cortex cells to grating and checkerboard patterns. *Journal of Physiology,* 291, 483–505.

De Valois, K. K. & Switkes, E. (1980) Spatial frequency specific interaction of dot patterns and gratings. *Proceedings of the National Academy of Sciences USA,* 77, 662–665.

De Valois, K. K. & Tootell, R. B. H. (1983) Spatial-frequency-specific inhibition in cat striate cortex cells. *Journal of Physiology,* 336, 339–376.

De Valois, R. L., Albrecht, D. G., & Thorell, L. G. (1982) Spatial frequency selectivity of cells in macaque visual cortex. *Vision Research,* 22, 545–559.

De Valois, R. L., Morgan, H., & Snodderly, D. M. (1974) Psychophysical studies of monkey vision. III. Spatial luminance contrast sensitivity tests of macaque and human observers. *Vision Research,* 14, 75–81.

De Valois, R. L., Yund, E. W., & Hepler, N. (1982) The orientation and direction selectivity of cells in macaque visual cortex. *Vision Research,* 22, 531–544.

DeVries, H. (1943) The quantum character of light and its bearing upon the threshold of vision, the differential sensitivity and the visual acuity of the eye. *Physica,* 10, 533–564.

DeYoe, E. A. & Van Essen, D. C. (1988) Concurrent processing streams in monkey visual cortex. *Trends in Neurosciences,* 11, 219–226.

Dobson, V., Howland, H. C., Moss, C., & Banks, M. S. (1983) Photorefraction of normal and astigmatic infants during viewing of patterned stimuli. *Vision Research,* 23, 1043–1052.

Dobson, V., Mayer, D. L., & Lee, C. P. (1980) Visual acuity screening of preterm infants. *Investigative Ophthalmology and Visual Science,* 19, 1498–1505.

Dobson, V., Salem, D., & Carson, J. B. (1983) Visual acuity in infants: The effect of variations in stimulus luminance within the photopic range. *Investigative Ophthalmology and Visual Science,* 24, 519–522.

Dobson, V. & Teller, D. Y. (1978) Visual acuity in human infants: A review and comparison of behavioral and electrophysiological studies. *Vision Research,* 18, 1469–1483.

Dobson, V., Teller, D. Y., & Belgum, J. (1978) Visual acuity in human infants assessed with stationary stripes and phase-alternated checkerboards. *Vision Research,* 18, 1233–1238.

Doehrman, S. (1974) The effect of visual orientation uncertainty in a simultaneous detection-recognition task. *Perception and Psychophysics,* 15, 519–523.

Doorn, A. J. van, Koenderink, J. J., & Bouman, M. A. (1972) The influence of the retinal inhomogeneity on the perception of spatial patterns. *Kybernetik,* 10, 223–230.

Drasdo, N. (1977) The neural representation of visual space. *Nature,* 266, 554–556.

Durlach, N. I. & Braida, L. D. (1969) Intensity perception. I. Preliminary theory of intensity resolution. *Journal of the Acoustical Society of America,* 46, 372–383.

D'Zmura, M. & Lennie, P. (1986) Shared pathways for rod and cone vision. *Vision Research,* 26, 1273–1280.

Earle, D. C. & Lowe, G. (1971) Channel, temporal, and composite uncertainty in the detection and recognition of auditory and visual signals. *Perception and Psychophysics,* 9, 177–181.

Edwards, D. H. Jr. (1983) Response vs. excitation in response-dependent and stimulus-dependent lateral inhibitory networks. *Vision Research,* 23, 469–472.

Egan, J. (1975) *Signal Detection Theory and ROC Analysis.* New York: Academic Press.

Egeth, H. (1977) Attention and preattention. In *The Psychology of Learning and Motivation. Vol. II* (G. H. Bower, Ed.). New York: Academic Press.

Ejima, Y. & Takahashi, S. (1984) Facility and inhibitory after-effect of spatially localized grating adaptation. *Vision Research,* 24, 979–985.

Ejima, Y. & Takahashi, S. (1985) Effect of localized grating adaptation as a function of separation along the length axis between test and adaptation areas. *Vision Research,* 25, 1701–1708.

Ejima, Y. & Takahashi, S. (1988) Temporal integration of stimulus increments under chromatic adaptation: Effects of adaptation level, wavelength, and target size. *Vision Research,* 28, 157–170.

Enoch, J. M., Sunga, R., & Bachman, E. (1970) A static perimetric technique believed to test receptive field properties. 1. Extension of the Westheimer experiments on spatial interaction. *American Journal of Ophthalmology,* 70, 113–126.

Enroth-Cugell, C. (1952) The mechanism of flicker and fusion studied on single retinal elements in the dark-adapted eye of the cat. *Acta Physiologica Scandinavia,* 27 (Suppl), 100.

Enroth-Cugell, C. & Robson, J. G. (1966) The contrast sensitivity of retinal ganglion cells of the cat. *Journal of Physiology,* 187, 517–552.

Enroth-Cugell, C. & Robson, J. G. (1984) Functional characteristics and diversity of cat retinal ganglion cells. *Investigative Ophthalmology and Visual Science,* 25, 250–267.

Enroth-Cugell, C. & Shapley, R. M. (1973) Flux, not illumination, is what cat retinal ganglion cells really care about. *Journal of Physiology,* 233, 311–319.

Essock, E. & Lehmkuhle, S. (1982) The oblique effects of pattern and flicker sensitivity: Implications for mixed physiological input. *Perception,* 11, 441–455.

Estevez, O. & Cavonius, C. R. (1975) Flicker sensitivity of the human red and green color mechanisms. *Vision Research,* 15, 879–881.

Estevez, O. & Cavonius, C. R. (1976a) Low frequency attenuation in the detection of gratings: Sorting out the artefacts. *Vision Research,* 16, 497–500.

Estevez, O. & Cavonius, C. R. (1976b) Modulation sensitivity of human color mechanisms. *Journal of the Optical Society of America,* 66, 1436–1438.

Estevez, O. & Spekreijse, H. (1974) A spectral compensation method for determining the flicker characteristics of the human colour mechanisms. *Vision Research,* 14, 823–830.

Falmagne, J. C. (1986) Psychophysical measurement and theory. In *Handbook of Perception and Human Performance. Vol. I* (K. Boff, L. Kaufman, & J. Thomas, Eds.). New York: Wiley.

Fankenhauser, F. & Enoch, J. M. (1962) The effects of blur on perimetric thresholds. *American Medical Association Archives of Ophthalmology,* 68, 240–251.

Feller, W. (1966) *An Introduction to Probability Theory and Its Applications. Vol. II.* New York: Wiley.

Field, D. (1987) Relations between the statistics of natural images and the response properties of cortical cells. *Journal of the Optical Society of America A,* 4, 2379–2394.

Field, D. J. & Nachmias, J. (1984) Phase reversal discrimination. *Vision Research,* 24, 333–340.

Field, D. & Tolhurst, D. (1986) The structure and symmetry of simple-cell receptive-field profiles in the cat's visual cortex. *Proceedings of the Royal Society of London B,* 228, 379–400.

Findlay, J. M. (1969) A spatial integration effect in visual acuity. *Vision Research,* 9, 157–166.

Fiorentini, A. (1972) Mach band phenomena. In *Handbook of Sensory Physiology. Vol. VII/4.* (D. Jameson & L. Hurvich, Eds.). Berlin: Springer-Verlag.

Fiorentini, A. & Berardi, N. (1981) Learning in grating waveform discrimination: Specificity for orientation and spatial frequency. *Vision Research,* 21, 1149–1158.

Fiorentini, A. & Maffei, L. (1976) Spatial contrast sensitivity of myopic subjects. *Vision Research,* 16, 437–438.

Fiorentini, A., Sireteanu, R., & Spinelli, D. (1976) Lines and gratings: Different interocular aftereffects. *Vision Research,* 16, 1303–1320.

Fischer, B. (1973) Overlap of receptive field centers and representation of the visual field in the cat's optic tract. *Vision Research,* 13, 2113–2120.

Fischer, B. & May, H. V. (1970) Invarianzen in der Katzenretina: Gesetzmassige Beziehungen zwischen Empfindlichkeit, Grosse und Lag receptiver Felder von Ganglienzellen. *Experimental Brain Research,* 11, 448–464.

Flitcroft, D. I. (1988) Effects of temporal frequency on the contrast sensitivity of the human accommodation system. *Vision Research,* 28, 269–278.

Foley, J. M. & Legge, G. E. (1981) Contrast detection and near-threshold discrimination in human vision. *Vision Research,* 21, 1041–1053.

Foster, D. H. (1969) The response of the human visual system to moving spatially periodic patterns. *Vision Research,* 9, 577–590.

Foster, D. H. (1971) The response of the human visual system to moving spatially periodic patterns: Further analysis. *Vision Research,* 11, 57–81.

Foster, K. H., Gaska, J. P., Nagler, M., & Pollen, D. A. (1985) Spatial and temporal frequency selectivity of neurons in visual cortical areas V1 and V2 of the macaque monkey. *Journal of Physiology,* 365, 331–363.

Frascella, J. & Lehmkuhle, S. (1982) An electrophysiological and behavioral assessment of X- and Y-cells as neural substrates of pattern and flicker mechanisms. *Supplement to Investigative Ophthalmology and Visual Science,* 22, 252.

Freeman, R. D. (1975) Asymmetries in human accommodation and visual experience. *Vision Research,* 15, 483–492.

Freeman, R. D., Mitchell, D. E., & Millodot, M. (1972) A neural effect of partial visual deprivation in humans. *Science,* 175, 1384–1386.

Frisby, J. P. & Mayhew, J. E. W. (1980) Spatial frequency tuned channels: Implications for structure and function from psychophysical and computational studies of stereopsis. In *The Psychology of Vision* (H. C. Longuet-Higgins & N. S. Sutherland, Eds.). London: The Royal Society, pp. 95–116.

Frisen, L. & Glansholm, A. (1975) Optical and neural resolution in peripheral vision. *Investigative Ophthalmology,* 14, 528–536.

Frishman, L. J., Freeman, A. W., Troy, S. B., Schweitzer-Tong, D. E., & Enroth-Cugell, C. (1987) Spatio-temporal frequency responses of cat retinal ganglion cells. *Journal of General Physiology,* 89, 599–628.

Frome, F. S., MacLeod, D. I. A., Buck, S. L., & Williams, D. R. (1981) Large loss of visual sensitivity to flashed peripheral targets. *Vision Research,* 21, 1323–1328.

Frumkes, T. E., Naarendorp, F., & Goldberg, S. H. (1986) The influence of cone adaptation upon rod mediated flicker. *Vision Research,* 26, 1167–1176.

Fry, G. A. (1969) Visibility of sine-wave gratings. *Journal of the Optical Society of America,* 59, 610–617.

Furcher, C. S., Thomas, J., & Campbell, F. (1977) Detection and discrimination of simple and complex patterns at low spatial frequencies. *Vision Research,* 17, 827–836.

Furman, G. G. (1965) Comparison of models for subtractive and shunting inhibition in receptor-neuron fields. *Kybernetik,* 2, 257–274.

Gabor, D. (1946) Theory of Communication. *Journal of the Institution of Electrical Engineers,* 93, 429–457.

Gaskill, J. D. (1978) *Linear Systems, Fourier Transforms, and Optics.* New York: Wiley & Sons.

Geisler, W. S. & Hamilton, D. B. (1984) Discrimination, identification, and the cortical sampling lattice. *Journal of the Optical Society of America,* 21A, 1231.

Geisler, W. S. & Hamilton, D. B. (1986) Sampling-theory analysis of spatial vision. *Journal of the Optical Society of America A,* 3, 62–70.

Georgeson, M. A. (1975) *Mechanisms of visual image processing: Studies on pattern interaction and selective channels in human vision.* Ph.D. Thesis, University of Sussex, Brighton, England.

Georgeson, M. A. (1976) Psychophysical hallucinations of orientation and spatial frequency. *Perception,* 5, 99–111.

Georgeson, M. A. (1980) The perceived spatial frequency, contrast, and orientation of illusory gratings. *Perception,* 9, 695–712.

Georgeson, M. A. (1985) The effect of spatial adaptation on perceived contrast. *Spatial Vision,* 1, 103–112.

Georgeson, M. A. (1987) Temporal properties of spatial contrast vision. *Vision Research,* 27, 765–780.

Georgeson, M. A. & Georgeson, J. M. (1987) Facilitation and masking of briefly-presented gratings: Time-course and contrast dependence. *Vision Research,* 27, 369–379.

Georgeson, M. A. & Harris, M. G. (1984) Spatial selectivity of contrast adaptation: Models and data. *Vision Research,* 24, 729–742.

Georgeson, M. A. & Reddin, S. K. (1981) Adaptation to gratings: Equal spatial selectivity for light and dark bar width variation. *Vision Research,* 21, 419–421.

Georgeson, M. A. & Turner, R. S. E. (1985) Afterimages of sinusoidal, square-wave and compound gratings. *Vision Research,* 25, 1709–1720.

Gescheider, G. (1976) *Psychophysics, Method, and Theory.* Hillsdale, N.J.: Lawrence Erlbaum.

Getty, D. J. (1975) Discrimination of short temporal intervals: A comparison of two models. *Perception and Psychophysics,* 18, 1–8.

Gibson, J. J. & Radner, M. (1937) Adaptation, aftereffect, and contrast in the perception of tilted lines. I. Quantitative studies. *Journal of Experimental Psychology,* 20, 453–467.

Gilchrist, J. & McIver, C. (1985) Fechner's paradox in binocular contrast sensitivity. *Vision Research,* 25, 609–613.

Gilinsky, A. S. (1968) Orientation-specific effects of patterns of adapting light on visual acuity. *Journal of the Optical Society of America,* 58, 13–18.

Gilinsky, A. S. & Mayo, T. H. (1971) Inhibitory effects of orientational adaptation. *Journal of the Optical Society of America,* 61, 1710–1714.

Gilliom, J. D. & Mills, W. M. (1976) Information extraction from contralateral cues in the detection of signals of uncertain frequency. *Journal of the Acoustical Society of America,* 59, 1428–1433.

Ginsburg, A. P. (1981) Spatial filtering and vision: Implications for normal and abnormal vision. In *Clinical Application of Visual Psychophysics,* (L. M. Proenza, J. M. Enoch, & A. Jampolsky, Eds.). New York: Cambridge University Press, pp. 70–106.

Ginsburg, A. P. & Cannon, M. W. (1983) Comparison of three methods for rapid determination of threshold contrast sensitivity. *Investigative Ophthalmology and Visual Science,* 24, 798–802.

Ginsburg, A. P. & Cannon, M. W. (1984) Comments on variability in contrast sensitivity methodology (letter to editor). *Vision Research,* 24, 287.

Ginsburg, A. P., Evans, D. W., Cannon, M. W. Jr., Owsley, C., & Mulvanny, P. (1984) Large-sample norms for contrast sensitivity. *American Journal of Optometry and Physiological Optics,* 61, 80–84.

Ginsburg, N. (1966) Local adaptation to intermittent light as a function of frequency and eccentricity. *American Journal of Psychology,* 79, 296–300.

Glas, H. W. van der, Orban, G. A., Joris, P. X., & Verhoeven, F. J. (1981) Direction selectivity in human visual perception investigated with low contrast gratings. *Acta Psychologia,* 48, 15–23.

Glezer, V. D. & Kostelyanets, N. B. (1975) The dependence of threshold for perception of rectangular grating upon the stimulus size. *Vision Research,* 15, 753–756.

Glezer, V. D., Kostelyanets, N. B., & Cooperman, A. M. (1977) Composite stimuli are detected by grating detectors rather than line detectors. *Vision Research,* 17, 1067–1070.

Gorea, A. (1979) Directional and nondirectional coding of a spatio-temporal modulated stimulus. *Vision Research,* 19, 545–549.

Gorea, A. (1985) Spatial integration characteristics in motion detection and direction identification. *Spatial Vision,* 1, 185–204.

Gorea, A. (1986) Temporal integration characteristics in spatial frequency identification. *Vision Research,* 26, 511–515.

Gorea, A. & Lorenceau, J. (1984) Perceptual bistability with counterphase gratings. *Vision Research,* 24, 1321–1331.

Gouled-Smith, B. (1986) *The psychometric function for contrast discrimination.* Ph.D. thesis, University of California, Los Angeles.

Graham, C. (Ed.) (1966) *Vision and Visual Perception.* New York: Wiley.

Graham, C. H., Brown, R. H., & Mote, F. A. Jr. (1939) The relation of size of stimulus and intensity in the human eye. I. Intensity thresholds for white light. *Journal of Experimental Psychology,* 24, 555–573.

Graham, C. H. & Kemp, E. H. (1938) Brightness discrimination as a function of the duration of the increment intensity. *Journal of General Physiology,* 21, 635–650.

Graham, N. (1970) *Spatial frequency channels in the human visual system: Effects of luminance and pattern drift rate.* Ph.D. thesis, University of Pennsylvania, Philadelphia.

Graham, N. (1972) Spatial frequency channels in the human visual system: Effects of luminance and pattern drift rate. *Vision Research,* 12, 53–68.

Graham, N. (1977) Visual detection of aperiodic spatial stimuli by probability summation among narrow band channels. *Vision Research,* 17, 637–652.

Graham, N. (1980) Spatial frequency channels in human vision: Detecting edges without edge detectors. In *Visual Coding and Adaptability* (C. Harris, Ed.). Hillsdale, N.J.: Lawrence Erlbaum, pp. 215–262.

Graham, N. (1981) Psychophysics of spatial-frequency channels. In *Perceptual Organization* (M. Kubovy & J. Pomerantz, Eds.). Hillsdale, N.J.: Lawrence Erlbaum, pp. 1–26.

Graham, N. (1985) Detection and identification of near-threshold visual patterns. *Journal of the Optical Society of America A,* 2, 1468–1482.

Graham, N., Kramer, P., & Haber, N. (1985) Attending to the spatial frequency and spatial position of near-threshold visual patterns. In *Attention and Performance XI* (M. I. Posner & O. S. M. Marin, Eds.). Hillsdale, N.J.: Lawrence Erlbaum, pp. 269–284.

Graham, N., Kramer, P., & Yager, D. (1987) Signal-detection models for multidimensional stimuli: Probability distributions and combination rules. *Journal of Mathematical Psychology,* 31, 366–409.

Graham, N. & Nachmias, J. (1971) Detection of grating patterns containing two spatial frequencies: A comparison of single-channel and multiple-channels models. *Vision Research,* 11, 251–259.

Graham, N. & Robson, J. G. (1987) Summation of very close spatial frequencies: The importance of spatial probability summation. *Vision Research,* 27, 1997–2007.

Graham, N., Robson, J. G., & Nachmias, J. (1978) Grating summation in fovea and periphery. *Vision Research,* 18, 815–826.

Graham, N. & Rogowitz, B. (1976) Spatial pooling properties deduced from the detectability of FM and quasi-AM gratings: A reanalysis. *Vision Research,* 16, 1021–1026.

Granger, E. (1973) An alternative model for grating detection. Paper presented at the spring meeting of the Association for Research in Vision and Ophthalmology, Sarasota, Florida.

Granger, E. M. & Heurtley, J. C. (1973) Visual chromaticity-modulation transfer function. *Journal of the Optical Society of America,* 63, 1173–1174.

Green, D. G. (1968) The contrast sensitivity of the colour mechanisms of the human eye. *Journal of Physiology,* 196, 415–429.

Green, D. G. (1969) Sinusoidal flicker characteristics of the color-sensitive mechanisms of the eye. *Vision Research,* 9, 591–601.

Green, D. G. (1986) The search for the site of visual adaptation. *Vision Research,* 26, 1417–1430.

Green, D. G. & Campbell, F. W. (1965) Effect of focus on the visual response to a sinusoidally modulated spatial stimulus. *Journal of the Optical Society of America,* 55, 1154–1157.

Green, D. M. & Birdsall, T. G. (1978) Detection and recognition. *Psychological Review,* 85, 192–206.

Green, D. M. & Swets, J. A. (1966, 1974) *Signal Detection Theory and Psychophysics.* New York: Wiley. Reprinted with corrections. Huntington, N.Y.: Krieger.

Green, D. M. & Weber, D. L. (1980) Detection of temporally uncertain signals. *Journal of the Acoustical Society of America,* 67, 1304–1311.

Green, M. (1980) Orientation-specific adaptation: Effects of checkerboards on the detectability of gratings. *Perception,* 9, 369–377.

Green, M. (1981) Psychophysical relationships among mechanisms sensitive to pattern, motion, and flicker. *Vision Research,* 21, 971–983.

Green, M. (1983) Contrast detection and direction discrimination of drifting gratings. *Vision Research,* 23, 281–289.

Green, M. (1984) Masking by light and the sustained-transient dichotomy. *Perception and Psychophysics,* 35, 519–535.

Green, M. & Blake, R. (1981) Phase effects in monoptic and dichoptic temporal integration: Flicker and motion detection. *Vision Research,* 21, 365–372.

Green, M., Corwin, T., & Schor, C. (1981) Spatiotemporal variations in the square/sine ratio: Evidence of independent channels at low spatial frequencies. *Vision Research,* 21, 423–425.

Greenberg, G. Z. & Larkin, W. D. (1968) Frequency-response characteristics of auditory observers detecting signals of a single frequency in noise: The probe-signal method, *Journal of the Acoustical Society of America,* 44, 1513–1523.

Greenlee, M. W. & Magnussen, S. (1987) Higher-harmonic adaptation and the detection of square-wave grating. *Vision Research,* 27, 249–255.

Greenlee, M. W. & Heitger, F. (1988) The functional role of contrast adaptation. *Vision Research,* 28, 791–797.

Grossberg, S. (1983) The quantized geometry of visual space: The coherent computation of depth, form, and lightness. *The Behavioral and Brain Sciences,* 6, 625–692.

Gstabler, R. J. & Green, D. G. (1971) Laser interferometric acuity in amblyopia. *Journal of Pediatric Ophthalmology,* 8, 251–256.

Gu, Y. & Legge, G. E. (1987) Accommodation to stimuli in peripheral vision. *Journal of the Optical Society of America A,* 4, 1681–1687.

Guzman, O. & Steinbach, M. J. (1985) Contrast sensitivity to drifting low spatial frequency gratings in central and peripheral retinal areas. *Vision Research,* 25, 137–140.

Gwiazda, J., Brill, S., Mohindra, I., & Held, R. (1980) Preferential looking acuity in infants from two to fifty-eight weeks of age. *American Journal of Optometry and Physiological Optics,* 57, 428–432.

Gwiazda, J., Scheiman, M., & Held, R. (1984) Anisotropic resolution in children's vision. *Vision Research,* 24, 527–531.

Haber, N. (1976) *Correlation of noise sources and bandwidth estimates: An analysis of a multiple-channels model of visual form perception.* Master's thesis, Columbia University, New York.

Hacker, M. J. & Ratcliff, R. (1979) A revised table of d' for M-alternative forced choice. *Perception and Psychophysics,* 26, 168–170.

Hagemans, K. H., & Wildt, G. J. van der, (1979) The influence of the stimulus width on the contrast sensitivity function in amblyopia. *Investigative Ophthalmology and Visual Science,* 18, 842–847.

Hainline, L., Camenzuli, C., Abramov, I., Rawlick, L., & Lemerise, E. (1986) A forced-choice method for deriving infant spatial contrast sensitivity functions from optokinetic nystagmus. *Supplement to Investigative Ophthalmology and Visual Science,* 27, 266.

Hall, J. L. & Sondhi, M. M. (1977) Detection threshold for a two-tone complex. *Journal of the Acoustical Society of America,* 62, 636–640.

Hallett, P. E. (1962) Scotopic acuity and absolute threshold in brief flashes. *Journal of Physiology,* 163, 175–189.

Hallett, P. E. (1969) The variations in visual threshold measurement. *Journal of Physiology,* 202, 403–419.

Hallett, P. E., Marriott, F. H. C., & Rodger, F. C. (1962) The relationship of visual threshold to retinal position and area. *Journal of Physiology,* 160, 364–373.

Hamer, R. D. & Schneck, M. E. (1984) Spatial summation in dark-adapted infants. *Vision Research,* 24, 77–86.

Hansen, R. H., Fulton, A. B., & Harris, S. J. (1986) Background adaptation in human infants. *Vision Research,* 26, 771–779.

Harris, M. G. (1980) Velocity specificity of the flicker to pattern sensitivity ratio in human vision. *Vision Research,* 20, 687–691.

Harris, M. G. (1984a) The role of pattern and flicker mechanisms in determining the spatiotemporal limits of velocity perception. 1. Upper movement thresholds. *Perception,* 13, 401–407.

Harris, M. G. (1984b) The role of pattern and flicker mechanisms in determining the spatiotemporal limits of velocity perception. 2. The lower movement threshold. *Perception,* 13, 409–415.

Harris, M. G. (1986) The perception of moving stimuli: A model of spatiotemporal coding in human vision. *Vision Research,* 26, 1281–1287.

Harris, M. G. & Georgeson, M. A. (1986) Sustained and transient temporal integration functions depend on spatial frequency, not grating area. *Vision Research,* 26, 1779–1782.

Harris, S. J., Hansen, R. M., & Fulton, A. B. (1984) Assessment of acuity in human infants using face and grating stimuli. *Investigative Ophthalmology and Visual Science,* 25, 782–786.

Hartline, H. K. (1938) The response of single optic nerve fibers of the vertebrate eye to illumination of the retina. *American Journal of Physiology,* 121, 400–415.

Hartmann, E., Lachenmayr, B., & Brettel, H. (1979) The peripheral critical flicker frequency. *Vision Research,* 19, 1019–1023.

Harwerth, R. S., Boltz, R. L., & Smith, E. L. III (1980) Psychophysical evidence for sustained and transient channels in the monkey visual system. *Vision Research,* 20, 15–22.

Harwerth, R. S., Smith, E. L. III, Boltz, R. L., Crawford, M. L. J., & Noorden, G. K. von (1983a) Behavioral studies on the effect of abnormal early visual experience in monkeys: Spatial modulation sensitivity. *Vision Research,* 23, 1501–1510, 1511–1517.

Hauske, G. (1981) Superposition of edges and gratings: Interaction between central and peripheral regions. *Vision Research,* 21, 373–384.

Hauske, G., Wolf, W, & Lupp, U. (1976) Matched filters in human vision. *Biological Cybernetics,* 22, 181–188.

Hawken, M. J. & Parker, A. J. (1987) Spatial properties of neurons in the monkey striate cortex. *Proceedings of the Royal Society of London B,* 231, 251–288.

Hayhoe, M. M., Benimoff, N. I., & Hood, D. C. (1987) The time-course of multiplicative and subtractive adaptation processes. *Vision Research,* 27, 1981–1996.

Hayhoe, M. M. & Chen, B. (1986) Temporal modulation sensitivity in cone dark adaptation. *Vision Research,* 26, 1715–1725.

Heeley, D. W. (1978) *Mechanisms for the perception of size and texture.* Ph.D. thesis, University of Cambridge, Cambridge, England.

Heeley, D. W. (1979a) Spatial frequency shifts independent of contrast threshold elevation: Adaptation to broad-band stimuli. *Supplement to Investigative Ophthalmology and Visual Science,* 18, 60.

Heeley, D. W. (1979b) A perceived spatial frequency shift at orientations orthogonal to adapting gratings. *Vision Research,* 19, 1229–1236.

Heggelund, P. & Hohmann, A. (1976) Long-term retention of the "Gilinsky-effect." *Vision Research,* 16, 1015–1017.

Held, R. (1979) Development of visual resolution. *Canadian Journal of Psychology,* 33, 213–221.

Henning, G. B., Derrington, A. M., & Madden, B. C. (1983) Detectability of several ideal spatial patterns. *Journal of the Optical Society of America,* 73, 851–854.

Henning, G. B., Hertz, B. G., & Broadbent, D. E. (1975) Some experiments bearing on the hypothesis that the visual system analyzes spatial patterns in independent bands of spatial frequency. *Vision Research,* 15, 887–899.

Herrick, R. M. (1956) Foveal luminance discrimination as a function of the duration of the decrement or increment in luminance. *Journal of Comparative and Physiological Psychology,* 49, 437–443.

Hertz, B. G. (1973) *Frequency-adaptation in the human visual system: Effects on perceived contrast of suprathreshold gratings.* Ph.D. thesis, University of Pennsylvania, Philadelphia.

Hertz, B. G. (1986) Visual acuity tests for non-verbal children: Preferential looking: *Ugeskrift for Laeger (Journal of the Danish Medical Association),* 148, 574–576.

Hess, R. F. (1977) Eye movements and grating acuity in strabismic amblyopia. Ophthalmology Research, 9, 225–237.

Hess, R. F. (1978) Interocular transfer in individuals with strabismic amblyopia: A cautionary note. *Perception,* 7, 201–205.

Hess, R. F. (1980) A preliminary investigation on neural function and dysfunction in amblyopia. I. Size-selective channels. *Vision Research,* 20, 749–754.

Hess, R. & Baker, C. L. Jr. (1984) Assessment of retinal function in severely amblyopic individuals. *Vision Research,* 24, 1367–1376.

Hess, R. F. & Campbell, F. M. (1980) A preliminary investigation of neural function and dysfunction in amblyopia. II. Activity within an amblyopic "channel." *Vision Research,* 20, 755–756.

Hess, R. F., France, T. D., & Tulunay-Keesey, U. (1981) Residual vision in humans who have been monocularly deprived of pattern stimulation in early life. *Experimental Brain Research,* 44, 295–311.

Hess, R. F. & Howell, E. R. (1977) The threshold contrast sensitivity function in strabismic amblyopia: Evidence for a two-type classification. *Vision Research,* 17, 1049–1055.

Hess, R. F. & Howell, E. R. (1978a) The influence of field size for a periodic stimulus in strabismic amblyopia. *Vision Research,* 18, 501–503.

Hess, R. F. & Howell, E. R. (1978b) The luminance-dependent nature of the visual abnormality in strabismic amblyopia. *Vision Research,* 18, 931–936.

Hess, R. F., Howell, E. R., & Kitchin, J. E. (1978) On the relationship between pattern and movement perception in strabismic amblyopia. *Vision Research,* 18, 375–377.

Hess, R. F. & Jacobs, R. J. (1979) A preliminary report of acuity and contour interactions across the amblyope's visual field. *Vision Research,* 19, 1403–1408.

Hess, R. F. & Nordby, K. (1986) Spatial and temporal limits of vision in the achromat. *Journal of Physiology,* 371, 365–385.

Hess, R. F. & Plant, G. T. (1985) Temporal frequency discrimination in human vision: Evidence for an additional mechanism in the low spatial and high temporal frequency region. *Vision Research,* 25, 1493–1500.

Hess, R. F. & Pointer, J. S. (1985) Differences in the neural basis of human amblyopia: The distribution of the anomaly across the visual field. *Vision Research,* 25, 1577–1594.

Hess, R. F. & Smith, G. (1977) Do optical alienations contribute to visual loss in strabismic amblyopia? *American Journal of Optometry,* 54, 627–633.

Hicks, T. P., Lee, B. B., & Vidyasagar, T. R. (1983) The responses of cells in macaque lateral geniculate nucleus to sinusoidal grating. *Journal of Physiology,* 337, 183–200.

Higgins, G. C. & Stultz, K. (1948) Visual acuity as measured with various orientations of a parallel-line test object. *Journal of the Optical Society of America,* 38, 756–758.

Higgins, G. C. & Stultz, K. (1950) Variation of visual acuity with various test-object orientations and viewing conditions. *Journal of the Optical Society of America,* 40, 135–137.

Higgins, K. E., Caruso, R. C., Coletta, N. J., & de Monasterio, F. M. (1983) Effect of artificial central scotoma on spatial contrast sensitivity in normal subjects. *Investigative Ophthalmology and Visual Science,* 24, 1131–1138.

Hilz, R. & Cavonius, C. R. (1974) Functional organization of the peripheral retina: Sensitivity to periodic stimuli. *Vision Research,* 14, 1333–1337.

Hines, M. (1976) Line spread function variation near the fovea. *Vision Research,* 16, 567–572.

Hirsch, J. (1977) *Properties of human visual spatial frequency selective systems: A two-frequency two-response recognition paradigm.* Ph.D. thesis, Columbia University, New York.

Hirsch, J. (1982) Falcon visual sensitivty to grating contrast. *Nature,* 300, 57–58.

Hirsch, J. (1983) Reply to factors underlying falcon grating acuity by D. Dvorak, R. Mark, and L. Reyword. *Nature,* 303, 729–730.

Hirsch, J. & Hylton, R. (1984) Quality of the primate photoreceptor lattice and limits of spatial vision. *Vision Research,* 24, 347–355.

Hirsch, J., Hylton, R., & Graham, N. (1982) Simultaneous recognition of two spatial-frequency components. *Vision Research,* 22, 365–375.

Hirsch, J. & Puklin, J. Z. (1983) Reduced contrast sensitivity may precede clinically observable retinopathy in type I diabetes. In *Acta: XXIV International Congress of Ophthalmology,* (P. Henkind, Ed.). Philadelphia: J. B. Lippincott.

Hochberg, J. E. (1978) *Perception.* Englewood Cliffs, N. J.: Prentice-Hall.

Hochstein, S. & Shapley, R. M. (1976a) Quantitative analysis of retinal ganglion cell classifications. *Journal of Physiology,* 262, 237–264.

Hochstein, S. & Shapley, R. (1976b) Linear and nonlinear spatial subunits in Y cat retinal ganglion cells. *Journal of Physiology,* 262, 265–284.

Hochstein, S. & Spitzer, H. (1985) One, few, infinity: Linear and nonlinear processing in the visual cortex. In *Models of the Visual Cortex,* (D. Rose & V. G. Dobson, Eds.). New York: Wiley, pp. 341–350.

Hoekstra, J., Goot, D. P. J. van der, Brink, G. van den, & Bilsen, F. A. (1974) The infuence of the number of cycles upon the visual contrast threshold for spatial sine waves. *Vision Research,* 14, 365–368.

Holopigian, K. & Blake, R. (1983) Spatial vision in strabismic cats. *Journal of Neurophysiology,* 50, 287–296.

Holopigian, K. & Blake, R. (1984) Abnormal spatial frequency channels in esotropic cats. *Vision Research,* 24, 677–687.

Holopigian, K., Blake, R., & Greenwald, M. J. (1986) Selective losses in binocular vision in anisometropic amblyopes. *Vision Research,* 26, 621–630.

Home, R. (1978) Binocular summation: A study of contrast sensitivity, visual acuity, and recognition. *Vision Research,* 18, 579–585.

Hood, D. C. (1973) The effects of edge sharpness and exposure duration on detection threshold. *Vision Research,* 13, 759–766.

Hood, D. C. & Finkelstein, M. A. (1986) Sensitivity to light. In *Handbook of Perception and Human Performance Vol. 1: Sensory Processes and Perception* (K. R. Boff, L. Kaufman, & J. P. Thomas, Eds.). New York: Wiley.

Horst, G. J. C. van der (1969) Fourier analysis and color discrimination. *Journal of the Optical Society of America,* 59, 1670–1676.

Horst, J. C. van der & Bouman, M. A. (1969) Spatiotemporal chromaticity discrimination. *Journal of the Optical Society of America,* 59, 1482–1488.

Horst, J. C. van der, de Wert, C. M. M., & Bouman, M. A. (1967) Transfer of spatial chromaticity-contrast at threshold in the human eye. *Journal of the Optical Society of America,* 57, 1260–1266.

Howard, J. H. & Richardson, K. H. (1988) Absolute phase uncertainty in sinusoidal grating detection. *Perception and Psychophysics,* 43, 38–44.

Howarth, C. I. & Lowe G. (1966) Statistical detection theory of Piper's law. *Nature,* 212, 324–326.

Howell, E. R. & Hess, R. F. (1978) The functional area for summation to threshold for sinusoidal gratings. *Vision Research,* 18, 369–374.

Howell, E. R., Mitchell, D. E., & Keith, C. G. (1983) Contrast thresholds for sine gratings of children with amblyopia. *Investigative Ophthalmology and Visual Science,* 24, 782–787.

Hubel, D. H. & Wiesel, T. N. (1962) Receptive fields, binocular interaction, and functional architecture in the cat's visual cortex. *Journal of Physiology,* 160, 106–123.

Hubel, D. H. & Wiesel, T. N. (1965) Receptive fields and functional architecture in two nonstriate visual areas (18 and 19) of the cat. *Journal of Neurophysiology,* 28, 229–289.

Hubel, D. H. & Wiesel, T. N. (1968) Receptive fields and functional architecture of monkey striate cortex. *Journal of Physiology,* 195, 215–243.

Hubel, D. H. & Wiesel, T. N. (1974) Uniformity of monkey striate cortex: A parallel relationship between field size, scatter, and magnification factor. *Journal of Comparative Neurology,* 158, 295–305.

Hubel, D. H. & Wiesel, T. N. (1977) Ferrier Lecture: Functional architecture of macaque monkey visual cortex. *Proceedings of the Royal Society of London Series B,* 198, 1–59.

Hunter, W. S. & Sigler, M. (1940) The span of visual discrimination as a function of time and intensity of stimulation. *Journal of Experimental Psychology,* 26, 160–179.

Hurvich, L. (1981) *Color Vision.* Sunderland, Mass.: Sinauer Associates.

Hurvich, L. & Jameson, D. (1957) An opponent-process theory of color vision. *Psychological Review,* 64, 384–404.

Hylkema, B. S. (1942) Examination of the visual field by determining the fusion frequency. *Acta Ophthalmologia,* 20, 181.

Ikeda, M. (1965) Temporal summation of positive and negative flashes in the visual system. *Journal of the Optical Society of America,* 55, 1527–1534.

Ikeda, M. (1986) Temporal impulse response. *Vision Research,* 26, 1431–1440.

Ikeda, M. & Boynton, R. M. (1965) Temporal summation of positive and negative flashes in the visual system. *Journal of the Optical Society of America,* 55, 1527–1534.

Ingling, C. R. Jr. & Martinez-Uriegas, E. (1983) The relationship between spectral sensitivity and spatial sensitivity for the primate r-g X-channel. *Vision Research,* 23, 1495–1500.

Ingling, C. R. Jr. & Martinez-Uriegas, E. (1985) The spatiotemporal properties of the r-g X-cell channel. *Vision Research,* 25, 33–38.

Iverson, G. J., Movshon, J. A. & Arditi, A. (1981) Binocular additivity of monocular contrasts. *Supplement to Investigative Ophthalmology and Visual Science,* 20, 224.

Ives, H. E. (1922a) A theory of intermittent vision. *Journal of the Optical Society of America,* 6, 343–361.

Ives, H. E. (1922b) Critical frequency relations in scotopic vision. *Journal of the Optical Society of America and Review of Scientific Instruments,* 6, 254–268.

Jacobs, D. S. & Blakemore, C. (1988) Factors limiting the postnatal development of visual acuity in the monkey. *Vision Research,* 28, 947–958.

Jacobs, G. H. (1986) Cones and opponency. *Vision Research,* 26, 1533–1542.

Jamar, J. H. T. & Koenderink, J. J. (1984) Dependence of contrast detection and independence of AM and FM detection on retinal illuminance. *Vision Research,* 24, 625–629.

Jamar, J. H. T., Kwakman, L. F. T., & Koenderink, J. J. (1984) The sensitivity of the peripheral visual system to amplitude-modulation and frequency-modulation of sine-wave patterns. *Vision Research,* 24, 243–249.

Jaschinski-Kruza, W. & Cavonius, C. R. (1984) A multiple channel model for grating detection. *Vision Research,* 24, 933–942.

Jennison, R. C. (1961) *Fourier Transforms and Convolutions for the Experimentalist.* New York: Pergamon Press.

Johnson, C. (1976) Effects of luminance and stimulus distance on accommodation and visual resolution. *Journal of the Optical Society of America,* 66, 138–142.

Johnson, C. A., Keltner, J. L., & Balestrery, F. (1978) Effects of target size and eccentricity on visual detection and resolution. *Vision Research,* 18, 1217–1222.

Johnson, C. A. & Leibowitz, H. W. (1974) Practice, refractive error, and feedback as factors influencing peripheral motion thresholds. *Perception and Psychophysics,* 15, 276–280.

Johnson, C. A. & Leibowitz, H. W. (1979) Practice effects for visual resolution in the periphery. *Perception and Psychophysics,* 25, 439–442.

Johnson, C. A., Leibowitz, H. W., Millidot, M., & Lamont, A. (1976) Peripheral visual acuity and refractive error: Evidence for "two visual systems"? *Perception and Psychophysics,* 20, 460–462.

Johnson, D. M. & Hafter, E. R. (1980) Uncertain-frequency detection: Cuing and condition of observation. *Perception and Psychophysics,* 28, 143–149.

Johnson, K. O. (1980a) Sensory discrimination: Decision process. *Journal of Neurophysiology,* 43, 1771–1792.

Johnson, K. O. (1980b) Sensory discrimination: Neural processes preceding discrimination decision. *Journal of Neurophysiology,* 43, 1793–1815.

Johnston A. (1987) Spatial scaling of central and peripheral contrast-sensitivity functions. *Journal of the Optical Society of America A,* 4, 1583–1593.

Johnston, A. & Wright, M. J. (1986) Matching velocity in central and peripheral vision. *Vision Research,* 26, 1099–1109.

Jones, J. P. & Palmer, L. A. (1987a) The two-dimensional spatial structure of simple receptive fields in cat striate cortex. *Journal of Neurophysiology,* 58, 1187–1211.

Jones, J. P. & Palmer, L. A. (1987b) An evaluation of the two-dimensional Gabor filter model of simple receptive fields in cat striate cortes. *Journal of Neurophysiology,* 58, 1233–1258.

Jones, J. P., Stepnoski, A., & Palmer, L. A. (1987) The two-dimensional spectral structure of simple receptive fields in cat striate cortex. *Journal of Neurophysiology,* 58, 1212–1232.

Jones, R. M. & Tulunay-Keesey, U. (1975) Local retinal adaptation and spatial frequency channels. *Vision Research,* 15, 1239–1244.

Jones, R. M. & Tulunay-Keesey, U. (1980) Phase selectivity of spatial frequency channels. *Journal of the Optical Society of America,* 70, 66–70.

Kahneman, D. & Treisman, A. M. (1984) Changing views of attention and automaticity. In *Varieties of Attention,* (R. Parasuraman & R. Davies, Eds.). Orlando, Fla.: Academic, pp. 29–61.

Keller, M. (1941) The relation between the critical duration and intensity in brightness discrimination. *Journal of Experimental Psychology,* 28, 407–418.

Kelly, D. H. (1966) Frequency doubling in visual responses. *Journal of the Optical Society of America,* 56, 1628–1633.

Kelly, D. H. (1969) Flickering patterns and lateral inhibition. *Journal of the Optical Society of America,* 59, 1361–1370.

Kelly, D. H. (1970) Effect of sharp edges on the visibility of sinusoidal gratings. *Journal of the Optical Society of America,* 60, 98–103.

Kelly, D. H. (1971a) Theory of flicker and transient responses. I. Uniform fields. *Journal of the Optical Society of America,* 61, 537–546.

Kelly, D. H. (1971b) Theory of flicker and transient responses. II. Counterphase gratings. *Journal of the Optical Society of America,* 61, 632–640.

Kelly, D. H. (1972) Adaptation effects on spatio-temporal sine-wave thresholds. *Vision Research,* 12, 89–101.

Kelly, D. H. (1973) Lateral inhibition in human colour mechanisms. *Journal of Physiology,* 228, 55–72.

Kelly, D. H. (1974) Spatiotemporal frequency characteristics of color-vision mechanisms. *Journal of the Optical Society of America,* 64, 983–990.

Kelly, D. H. (1975) Luminous and chromatic flickering patterns have opposite effects. *Science,* 188, 371–372.

Kelly, D. H. (1976) Pattern detection and the two-dimensional Fourier transform: Flickering checkerboards and chromatic mechanisms. *Vision Research,* 16, 277–287.

Kelly, D. H. (1977) Visual contrast sensitivity. *Optica Acta,* 24, 107–129.

Kelly, D. H. (1978) Photopic contrast sensitivity without foveal vision. *Optics Letters,* 2, 79–81.

Kelly, D. H. (1979a) Motion and vision. I. Stabilized images of stationary gratings. *Journal of the Optical Society of America,* 69, 1266–1273.

Kelly, D. H. (1979b) Motion and vision. II. Stabilized spatiotemporal threshold surface. *Journal of the Optical Society of America,* 69, 1340–1349.

Kelly, D. H. (1981) Disappearance of stabilized chromatic gratings. *Science,* 214, 1257–1258.

Kelly, D. H. (1982a) Motion and vision. IV. Isotropic and anisotropic spatial responses. *Journal of the Optical Society of America,* 72, 432–439.

Kelly, D. H. (1982b) Fourier components of moving gratings. *Behavioral Research Methods and Instrumentation,* 14, 435–437.

Kelly, D. H. (1983) Spatiotemporal variation of chromatic and achromatic contrast thresholds. *Journal of the Optical Society of America,* 73, 742–750.

Kelly, D. H. (1984a) Retinal inhomogeneity. I. Spatiotemporal contrast sensitivity, *Journal of the Optical Society of America A,* 1, 107–113.

Kelly, D. H. (1984b) Retinal inhomogeneity. II. Spatial summation. *Journal of the Optical Society of America A,* 1, 114–119.

Kelly, D. H. (1985a) Visual processing of moving stimuli. *Journal of the Optical Society of America A,* 2, 216–225.

Kelly, D. H. (1985b) Retinal inhomogeneity. III. Circular retina theory. *Journal of the Optical Society of America A,* 2, 810–819.

Kelly, D. H. (1985c) Receptive-field-like functions inferred from large area psychophysical measurements. *Vision Research,* 25, 1895–1900.

Kelly, D. H., Boynton, R. M., & Baron, W. S. (1976) Primate flicker sensitivity: Psychophysics and electrophysiology. *Science,* 194, 1077–1080.

Kelly, D. H. & Burbeck, C. A. (1980) Motion and vision. III. Stabilized patten adaptation. *Journal of the Optical Society of America,* 70, 1283–1289.

Kelly, D. H. & Burbeck, C. A. (1984) Critical problems in spatial vision. *CRC Critical Reviews in Biomedial Engineering,* 10, 125–177.

Kelly, D. H. & Burbeck, C. A. (1987) Further evidence for a broadband isotropic mechanism sensitive to high-velocity stimuli. *Vision Research,* 27, 1527–1537.

Kelly, D. H. & Magnuski, H. S. (1975) Pattern detection and the two-dimensional Fourier transform: Circular targets. *Vision Research,* 15, 911–915.

Kelly, D. H. & Norren, D. van, (1977) Two-band model of heterochromatic flicker. *Journal of the Optical Society of America,* 67, 1081–1091.

Kelly, D. H. & Savoie, R. E. (1973) A study of sine-wave contrast sensitivity by two psychophysical methods. *Perception and Psychophysics,* 14, 313–318.

Kelly, D. H. & Savoie, R. E. (1978) Theory of flicker and transient responses. III. An essential nonlinearity. *Journal of the Optical Society of America,* 68, 1481–1489.

Kerr, J. L. (1971) Visual resolution in the periphery. *Perception and Psychophysics,* 9, 375–378.

Kersten, D. (1982) Phase uncertainty in visual detection. *Supplement to Investigative Ophthalmology and Visual Science,* 22, 206.

Kersten, D. (1983) *A comparison of human and ideal performance for the detection of visual patterns.* Ph.D. thesis, University of Minnesota, Minneapolis.

Kersten, D. (1984) Spatial summation in visual noise. *Vision Research,* 24, 1977–1990.

Kersten, D. (1987) Statistical efficiency for the detection of visual noise. *Vision Research,* 27, 1029–1040.

Kincaid, W. M., Blackwell, H. R., & Kristofferson, A. B. (1960) Neural formulation of the effects of target size and shape upon visual detection. *Journal of the Optical Society of America,* 50, 143–148.

King-Smith, P. E. & Kulikowski, J. J. (1975a) The detection of gratings by independent activation of line detectors. *Journal of Physiology,* 247, 237–271.

King-Smith, P. E. & Kulikowski, J. J. (1975b) Pattern and flicker detection analyzed by subthreshold summation. *Journal of Physiology,* 249, 519–548.

King-Smith, P. E. & Kulikowski, J. J. (1980) Pattern and movement detection in a patient lacking sustained vision. *Journal of Physiology,* 300, 60P.

King-Smith, P. E. & Kulikowski, J. J. (1981) The detection and recognition of two lines, *Vision Research,* 21, 235–250.

King-Smith, P. E., Rosten, J. G. & Bhargava, S. K. (1980) Human vision without tonic ganglion cells? In *Color Vision Deficiencies V.* Adam Hilger, pp. 99–105.

Kiorpes, L. & Boothe, R. G. (1984) Accommodative range in amblyopic monkeys. *Vision Research,* 24, 1829–1834.

Klein, S. A. (1985) Double-judgment psychophysics: Problems and solutions. *Journal of the Optical Society of America A,* 2, 1560–1585.

Klein, S. A. & Levi, D. M. (1985) Hyperacuity thresholds of 1 sec: Theoretical predictions and empirical validations. *Journal of the Optical Society of America A,* 2, 1170–1190.

Klein, S. A. & Stromeyer III, C. F. (1980) On inhibition between spatial frequency channels: Adaptation to complex gratings. *Vision Research,* 20, 459–466.

Klein, S. A., Stromeyer, C. F., & Ganz, L. (1974) The simultaneous spatial frequency shift: A dissociation between the detection and perception of gratings. *Vision Research,* 14, 1421–1432.

Klein, S. A. & Tyler, C. W. (1986) Phase discrimination of compound gratings: Generalized autocorrelation analysis. *Journal of the Optical Society of America A,* 3, 868–879.

Klopfenstein, R. W. & Carlson, C. R. (1984) Theory of shape-invariant imaging systems. *Journal of the Optical Society of America A,* 1, 1040.

Knight, B. W. (1972) Dynamics of encoding in a population of neurons. *Journal of General Physiology,* 59, 734–766.

Knight, B. W., Toyoda, J. I., & Dodge, F. A. (1970) A quantitative description of the dynamics of excitation and inhibition in the eye of *Limulus*. *Journal of General Physiology, 56,* 421–437.

Koenderink, J. J. (1972) Contrast enhancement and the negative afterimage. *Journal of the Optical Society of America, 62,* 685–689.

Koenderink, J. J., Bouman, M. A., de Mesquita, A. E., & Slappendel, S. (1978a) Perimetry of contrast detection thresholds of moving spatial sine wave patterns. I. The near peripheral visual field (eccentricity 0–8 degrees). *Journal of the Optical Society of America, 68,* 845–849.

Koenderink, J. J., Bouman, M. A., de Mesquita, A. E., & Slappendel, S. (1978b) Perimetry of contrast detection thresholds of moving spatial sine wave patterns. II. The far peripheral visual field (eccentricity 0–50 degrees). *Journal of the Optical Society of America, 68,* 850–854.

Koenderink, J. J., Bouman, M. A. de Mesquita, A. E. & Slappendel, S. (1978c) Perimetry of contrast detection thresholds of moving spatial sine wave patterns. III. The target extent as a sensitivity controlling parameter. *Journal of the Optical Society of America, 68,* 854–860.

Koenderink, J. J., Bouman, M. A., de Mesquita, A. E., & Slappendel, S. (1978d) Perimetry of contrast detection thresholds of moving spatial sine wave patterns. IV. The influence of the mean retinal illuminance. *Journal of the Optical Society of America, 68,* 860–865.

Koenderink, J. J. & van Doorn, A. J. (1978a) Visual detection of spatial contrast: Influence of location in the visual field, target extent and illuminance level. *Biological Cybernetics, 30,* 157–167.

Koenderink, J. J. & van Doorn, A. J. (1978b) Detectability of power fluctuations of temporal visual noise. *Vision Research, 18,* 191–195.

Koenderink, J. J., van Doorn, A. J. (1979) Spatiotemporal contrast detection surface is bimodal. *Optics Letters, 4,* 32–34.

Koenderink, J. J. & van Doorn, A. J. (1980) Spatial summation for complex bar patterns. *Vision Research, 20,* 169–176.

Koenderink, J. J. & van Doorn, A. J. (1982) Invariant features of contrast detection: An explanation in terms of self-similar detector arrays. *Journal of the Optical Society of America, 72,* 83–87.

Kotulak, J. C. & Schor, C. M. (1986) Temporal variation in accomodation during steady-state conditions. *Journal of the Optical Society of America A, 3,* 223–227.

Kramer, P. (1984) *Summation and uncertainty effects in the detection of spatial frequency.* Ph.D. thesis, Columbia University, New York.

Kramer, P., Graham, N., & Yager, D. (1985) Simultaneous measurement of spatial-frequency summation and uncertainty effects. *Journal of the Optical Society of America A, 2,* 1533–1542.

Krauskopf, J. (1980) Discrimination and detection of changes in luminance. *Vision Research, 20,* 671–677.

Kretz, F., Scarabin, F., & Bourguignat, E. (1979) Predictions of an inhomogeneous model: Detection of local and extended spatial stimuli. *Journal of the Optical Society of America, 69,* 1635–1648.

Kroom, J. N., Rijsdijk, S. P., & van der Wildt, G. J. (1980) Peripheral contrast sensitivity for sine-wave gratings and single periods. *Vision Research, 20,* 243–252.

Kroom, J. N. & van der Wildt, G. J. (1980) Spatial frequency tuning studies: Weighting as a prerequisite for describing psychometric curves by probability summation. *Vision Research, 20,* 253–264.

Kuffler, S. W. (1953) Discharge pattern and functional organization of mammalian retina. *Journal of Neurophysiology, 16,* 37–68.

Kulikowski, J. J. (1967) Models of the detection of simple patterns by the visual system. *Autometria, 6,* 113–120. (translated from Russian by S. A. Sullivan)

Kulikowski, J. J. (1969) Limiting conditions of visual perception. *Prace instytutu Automatyki Poskiej Akadeji Nauk Warsaw,* 1–133.

Kulikowski, J. J. (1971a) Some stimulus parameters affecting spatial and temporal resolution of human vision. *Vision Research, 11,* 83–93.

Kulikowski, J. J. (1971b) Effect of eye movements on the contrast sensitivity of spatio-temporal patterns. *Vision Research, 11,* 261–273.

Kulikowski, J. J. (1972) Orientational selectivity of human binocular and monocular vision revealed by simultaneous and successive masking. *Journal of Physiology, 226,* 67–69P.

Kulikowski, J. J. (1978) Spatial resolution for the detection of pattern and movement (real and apparent). *Vision Research, 18,* 237–238.

Kulikowski, J. J., Abadi, R., & King-Smith, P. E. (1973) Orientational selectivity of gratings and line detectors in human vision. *Vision Research,* 13, 1479–1486.

Kulikowski, J. J. & Bishop, P. O. (1981) Fourier analysis and spatial representation in the visual cortex. *Experientia,* 37, 160–163.

Kulikowski, J. J. & King-Smith, P. E. (1973) Spatial arrangement of line, edge, and grating detectors revealed by subthreshold summation. *Vision Research,* 13, 1455–1478.

Kulikowski, J. J., Marcelja, S., & Bishop, P. O. (1982) Theory of spatial position and spatial frequency relations in the receptive fields of simple cells in the visual cortex. *Biological Cybernetics,* 43, 187–198.

Kulikowski, J. J. & Tolhurst, D. J. (1973) Psychophysical evidence for sustained and transient detectors in human vision. *Journal of Physiology,* 232, 149–162.

Kupersmith, M. J., Seiple, W. H., Nelson, J. I., & Carr, R. E. (1984) Contrast sensitivity loss in multiple sclerosis. *Investigative Ophthalmology and Visual Science,* 25, 632–639.

Kurtenbach, W. & Magnussen, S. (1979) Summation of tilt illusion and tilt aftereffect. *Supplement to Investigative Ophthalmology and Visual Science,* 18, 251.

Lange, R., Sigel, C., & Stecher, S. (1973) Adapted and unadapted spatial-frequency channels in human vision. *Vision Research,* 13, 2139–2143.

Langston, A., Casagrande, V. A., & Fox, R. (1986) Spatial resolution of the galago. *Vision Research,* 26, 791–796.

Lappin, J. S. & Staller, J. D. (1981) Prior knowledge does not facilitate the perceptual organization of dynamic random-dot patterns. *Perception and Psychophysics,* 29, 445–456.

Lappin, J. S. & Uttal, W. R. (1976) Does prior knowledge facilitate the detection of visual targets in random noise? *Perception and Psychophysics,* 20, 367–374.

Lasley, D. J. & Cohn, T. E. (1981a) Why luminance discrimination may be better then detection. *Vision Research,* 21, 273–278.

Lasley, J. D. & Cohn, T. (1981b) Detection of a luminance increment: Effect of temporal uncertainty. *Journal of the Optical Society of America,* 71, 845–850.

Lawden, M. C. (1983) An investigation of the ability of the human visual system to encode spatial phase relationships. *Vision Research,* 23, 1451–1463.

Lawden, M. C., Hess, R. F. & Campbell, F. W. (1982) The discriminability of spatial phase relationships in amblyopia. *Vision Research,* 22, 1005–1016.

Lee, C. P. & Boothe, R. G. (1981) Visual acuity development in infant monkeys (macaca nemestrina) having known gestational ages. *Vision Research,* 21, 805–809.

Leehey, S. C., Moskowitz-Cook, A., Brill, S., & Held, R. (1975) Orientational anisotropy in infant vision. *Science,* 190, 900–902.

Legg, C. R. (1984) Contrast sensitivity at low spatial frequencies in the hooded rat. *Vision Research,* 24, 159–161.

Legg, G. (1976) Adaptation to a spatial impulse: Implications for Fourier transform models of visual processing. *Vision Research,* 16, 1407–1418.

Legg, G. E. (1978a) Sustained and transient mechanisms in human vision: Temporal and spatial properties. *Vision Research,* 18, 69–81.

Legg, G. E. (1978b) Space domain properties of a spatial frequency channel in human vision. *Vision Research,* 18, 959–969.

Legg, G. E. (1984a) Binocular contrast summation. I. Detection and discrimination. *Vision Research,* 24, 373–383.

Legg, G. E. (1984b) Binocular contrast summation. II. Quadratic summation. *Vision Research,* 24, 385–394.

Legg, G. E. & Kersten, D. (1983) Light and dark bars: Contrast discrimination. *Vision Research,* 23, 473–483.

Legg, G. E. & Kersten, D. (1987) Contrast discrimination in peripheral vision. *Journal of the Optical Society of America A,* 4, 1594–1598.

Legg, G. E., Mullen, K. T., Woo, G. C., and Campbell, F. W. (1987) Tolerance to visual defocus. *Journal of the Optical Society of America A,* 4, 851–863.

Leguire, L. E. & Blake, R. (1982) Role of threshold in afterimage visibility. *Journal of the Optical Society of America,* 72, 1232–1237.

Lehmkuhle, S., Kratz, K. E., & Sherman, S. M. (1982) Spatial and temporal sensitivity of normal and amblyopic cats. *Journal of Neurophysiology,* 48, 372–387.

Leibowitz, H. W., Johnson, C. A., & Isabelle, E. (1972) Peripheral motion detection and refractive error. *Science,* 177, 1207–1208.

Lema, S. A. & Blake, R. (1977) Binocular summation in normal and stereoblind humans. *Vision Research,* 17, 691–695.

Lennie, P. (1971) Distortions of perceived orientation. *Nature New Biology,* 233, 155–157.

Lennie, P. (1972) *Mechanisms underlying the perception of orientation.* Ph.D. thesis, University of Cambridge, Cambridge, England.

Lennie, P. (1974) Head orientation and meridional variations in acuity, *Vision Research,* 14, 107–111.

Lennie, P. (1977) Neuroanatomy of visual acuity. *Nature,* 266, 496.

Lennie, P. (1980a) Perceptual signs of parallel pathways. *Philosophical Transactions of the Royal Society of London B,* 290, 23–37.

Lennie, P. (1980b) Parallel visual pathways: A review. *Vision Research,* 20, 561–594.

Lennie, P. (1984) Temporal modulation sensitivities of red- and green-sensitive cone systems in dichromats. *Vision Research,* 24, 1995–1999.

Lerner, R. M. (1961) Representation of signals. In *Lectures on Communication System Theory* (E. J. Baghdady, Ed.). New York: McGraw-Hill.

Levi, D. M. & Harwerth, R. S. (1977) Spatiotemporal interactions in anisometric and strabismic amblyopia. *Investigative Ophthalmology and Visual Science,* 16, 90–95.

Levi, D. M., Harwerth, R. S. & Smith, E. L. III (1979) Humans deprived of normal binocular vision have binocular interactions tuned to size and orientation. *Science,* 206, 852–854.

Levi, D. M. & Klein, S. (1982a) Differences in vernier discrimination for gratings between strabismic and anisometropic amblyopes. *Investigative Ophthalmology and Visual Science,* 23, 398–407.

Levi, D. M. & Klein, S. (1982b) Hyperacuity and amblyopia. *Nature,* 298, 268–270.

Levinson, E. & Sekuler, R. (1975a) The independence of channels in human vision selective for direction of motion. *Journal of Physiology,* 150, 347–366.

Levinson, E. & Sekuler, R. (1975b) Inhibition and disinhibition of direction-specific mechanisms in human vision. *Nature,* 254, 692–694.

Levinson, E. & Sekuler, R. (1980) A two-dimensional analysis of direction-specific adaptation. *Vision Research,* 20, 103–108.

Levinson, J. (1959) Fusion of complex flicker. *Science,* 130, 919–921.

Levinson, J. (1960) Fusion of complex flicker. II. *Science,* 131, 1438–1440.

Levinson, J. Z. (1964) Nonlinear and spatial effects in the perception of flicker. *Documenta Ophthalmologica,* 18, 36–55.

Lewis, T. L., Maurer, D., & Blackburn, K. (1985) The development of young infant's ability to detect stimuli in the nasal visual field. *Vision Research,* 25, 943–950.

Lie, I. (1980) Visual detection and resolution as a function of retinal locus. *Vision Research,* 20, 967–974.

Lie, I. (1981) Visual detection and resolution as a function of adaptation and glare. *Vision Research,* 21, 1793–1797.

Limb, J. O. (1981) Prediction of the visibility of asynchronous gratings by a single-channel model. *Vision Research,* 21, 1409–1412.

Limb, J. O. & Rubinstein, C. B. (1977) A model of threshold vision incorporating inhomogeneity of the visual field. *Vision Research,* 17, 571–584.

Lindsey, D. T., Pokorny, J., & Smith, V. C. (1986) Phase-dependent sensitivity to heterochromatic flicker. *Journal of the Optical Society of America A,* 3, 921–927.

Linsenmeier, R. A. Frishman. L. J., Jakiela, H. G., & Enroth-Cugell, C. (1982) Receptive field properties of X and Y cells in the cat retina derived from contrast sensitivity measurements. *Vision Research,* 22, 1173–1183.

Logan, J. (1962) *An examination of the relationship between visual illusion and after-effect.* Ph.D. dissertation, University of Sydney, Sydney, Australia.

Long, G. M. & Kling, S. C. (1983) Positive and negative afterimages from brief target gratings. *Vision Research*, 23, 959–964.

Lorenceau, J. (1987) Recovery from contrast adaptation: Effects of spatial and temporal frequency. *Vision Research*, 27, 2185–2191.

Lovegrove, W. (1976) Inhibition in simultaneous and successive contour interactions in human vision. *Vision Research*, 16, 1519–1521.

Lovegrove, W. (1977) Inhibition between channels selective to contour orientation and wavelength in the human visual system. *Perception & Psychophysics*, 22, 49–53.

Lovegrove, W. J., Bowling, A., Badcock, D., & Blackwood, M. (1980) Specific reading disability: Differences in contrast sensitivity as a function of spatial frequency. *Science*, 210, 439–440.

Lowe, G. (1967) Interval of time uncertainty in visual detection. *Perception and Psychophysics*, 2, 278–280.

Luce, R. D. (1963) Detection and recognition. In *Handbook of Mathematical Psychology, Vol. I* (R. D. Luce, R. R. Bush, & E. Galanter, Eds.). New York: Wiley, pp. 103–189.

Luce, R. D. & Green, D. M. (1974) Detection, discrimination, and recognition. In *Handbook of Perception, Vol. II* (E. C. Carterette & M. P. Friedman, Eds.). New York: Academic, pp. 249–342.

MacCana, F., Cuthbert, A., & Lovegrove, W. (1986) Contrast and phase processing in amblyopia. *Vision Research*, 26, 781–789.

MacKay, D. M. (1957) Moving visual images produced by regular stationary patterns. *Nature*, 18, 849–850.

MacLeod, I. D. G. & Rosenfeld, A. (1974) The visibility of gratings: Spatial frequency channels or bar-detecting units? *Vision Research*, 14, 909–915.

Macmillan, N. A. (1971) Detection and recognition of increments and decrements in auditory intensity. *Perception and Psychophysics*, 10, 233–238.

Macmillan, N. A. (1973) Detection and recognition of intensity changes in tone and noise: The detection-recognition disparity. *Perception and Psychophysics*, 13, 65–75.

Macmillan, N. A. (1987) Beyond the categorical/continuous distinction: A psychophysical approach to processing modes. In *Categorical Perception* (S. Harnad, Ed.). Cambridge University Press, Cambridge, England, pp. 53–87.

Macmillan, N. A. & Creelman, C. D. (in press) Detection theory: A User's Guide. New York: Cambridge University Press.

Macmillan, N. A. & Kaplan, H. L. (1985) Detection theory analysis of group data: Estimating sensitivity from average hit and false-alarm rates. *Psychological Bulletin*, 98, 185–199.

Macmillan, N. A., Kaplan, H. L., & Creelman, C. D. (1977) The psychophysics of categorical perception. *Psychological Review*, 84, 452–471.

Macmillan, N. A. & Schwartz, M. (1975) A probe-signal investigation of uncertain-frequency detection. *Journal of the Acoustical Society of America*, 58, 1051–1058.

MacNichol, D. (1972) *A Primer of Signal Detection Theory*. London: George Allen and Unwin.

Maffei, L. & Fiorentini, A. (1973) The visual cortex as a spatial frequency analyzer. *Vision Research*, 13, 1255–1267.

Maffei, L. & Fiorentini, A. (1976) The unresponsive regions of visual cortical receptive fields. *Vision Research*, 16, 1131–1140.

Maffei, L., Fiorentini, A., & Bisti, S. (1973) Neural correlate of perceptual adaptation to gratings. *Science*, 182, 1036–1038.

Magnussen, S. & Greenlee, M. W. (1985) Marathon-adaptation to spatial contrast: Saturation in sight. *Vision Research*, 25, 1409–1411.

Magnussen, S. & Greenlee, M. W. (1986) Contrast threshold elevation following continuous and interrupted adaptation. *Vision Research*, 26, 673–675.

Magnussen, S. & Kurtenbach, W. (1980) Adapting to two orientations: Disinhibition in a visual aftereffect. *Science*, 207, 908–909.

Maloney, L. & Wandell, B. A. (1983) The slope of the psychometric function at different wavelengths. *Supplement to Investigative Ophthalmology and Visual Science*, 24, 183.

Maloney, L. T. & Wandell, B. A. (1984) A model of a single visual channel's response to weak test lights. *Vision Research*, 24, 633–640.

Mandler, M. B. & Makous, W. (1984) A three channel model of temporal frequency perception. *Vision Research,* 24, 1881–1887.

Manny, R. E. & Levi, D. M. (1982a) Psychophysical investigations of the temporal modulation function in amblyopia: Uniform field flicker. *Investigative Ophthalmology and Visual Science,* 22, 515–524.

Manny, R. E. & Levi, D. M. (1982b) Psychophysical investigations of the temporal modulation sensitivity functions in amblyopia: Spatiotemporal interaction. *Investigative Ophthalmology and Visual Science,* 22, 525–534.

Mansfield, R. J. W. (1974) Neural basis of orientation perception in primate vision. *Science,* 186, 133–135.

Mansfield, R. J. W. & Nachmias, J. (1981) Perceived direction of motion under retinal image stabilization. *Vision Research,* 21, 1423–1425.

Mansfield, R. J. W. & Ronner, S. F. (1978) Orientation anisotropy in monkey visual cortex. *Brain Research,* 149, 224–234.

Marcelja, S. (1980) Mathematical description of the responses of simple cortical cells. *Journal of the Optical Society of America,* 70, 1297–1300.

Marr, D. (1982) *Vision.* San Francisco: W. H. Freeman.

Marr, D. & Hildreth, E. (1980) Theory of edge detection. *Proceedings of the Royal Society of London,* 207, 187–217.

Marr, D. & Ullman, S. (1981) Directional selectivity and its use in early visual procession. *Proceedings of the Royal Society of London Series B,* 211, 151–180.

Marrocco, R. T., Carpenter, M. A., & Wright, S. E. (1985) Spatial contrast sensitivity: Effects of peripheral field stimulation during monocular and dichoptic viewing. *Vision Research,* 25, 917–924.

Martens, W. & Blake, R. (1980) Uncertainty impairs grating detection performance in the cat. *Perception and Psychophysics,* 27, 229–231.

Martens, W. & Blake, R. (1982) Spatial tuning in cat vision assessed by subthreshold summation. *Supplement to Investigative Ophthalmology and Visual Science,* 22, 251.

Martens, W., Blake, R., Sloane, M., & Cormack, R. H. (1981) What masks utrocular discrimination. *Perception and Psychophysics,* 30, 521–532.

Marx, M. S. & May, J. G. (1983) The relationship between temporal integration and persistence. *Vision Research,* 23, 1101–1106.

Mastronarde, D. N. (1983a) Correlated firing of cat retinal ganglion cells. I. Spontaneously active inputs to X- and Y-cells. *Journal of Neurophysiology,* 49, 303–324.

Mastronarde, D. N. (1983b) Correlated firing of cat retinal ganglion cells. II. Responses of X- and Y-cells to single quantal events. *Journal of Neurophysiology,* 49, 325–349.

Mastronarde, D. N. (1983c) Interactions between ganglion cells in cat retina. *Journal of Neurophysiology,* 49, 350–365.

Matin, E. (1975) The two-transient (masking) paradigm. *Psychological Review,* 82, 451–461.

Matin, L. (1962) Binocular summation at the absolute threshold of peripheral vision. *Journal of the Optical Society of America,* 52, 1276–1286.

Matin, L. (1968) Critical duration, the differential luminance threshold, critical flicker frequency, and visual adaptation: A theoretical treatment. *Journal of the Optical Society of America,* 58, 404–415.

Maudarbocus, A. Y. & Ruddock, K. H. (1973) Non-linearity of visual signals in relation to shape-sensitive adaptation responses. *Vision Research,* 13, 1713–1737.

Mayer, D. L. & Dobson, V. (1982) Visual acuity development in infants and young children, as assessed by operant preferential looking. *Vision Research,* 22, 1141–1151.

Mayer, D. L., Fulton, A. B., & Hansen, R. M. (1982) Preferential looking acuity obtained with a staircase procedure in pediatric patients. *Investigative Ophthalmology and Visual Science,* 23, 538–542.

Mayer, M. & Tyler, C. W. (1984) Handout and personal communication in connection with: On the slope of the psychometric function. *Supplement to Investigative Ophthalmology and Visual Science,* 25, 295.

Mayer, M. J. (1977) Development of anisotropy in late childhood. *Vision Research,* 17, 703–710.

Mayer, M. J. (1983a) Practice improves adults' sensitivity to diagonals. *Vision Research,* 23, 547–550.

Mayer, M. J. (1983b) Non-astigmatic children's contrast sensitivities differ from anisotropic pattern of adults. *Vision Research,* 23, 551–559.

Mayer, M. J. & Tyler, C. W. (1986) Invariance of the slope of the psychometric function with spatial summation. *Journal of the Optical Society of America A,* 3, 1166.

Mayhew, J. E. W. & Frisby, J. P. (1978) Contrast summation effects and stereopsis. *Perception,* 7, 537–550.

McBurney, D. H. (1978) Psychological dimensions and perceptual analyses of taste. In *Handbook of Perception. Vol. VI A: Tasting and smelling.* (E. C. Carterette & M. P. Friedman, Eds.). New York: Academic.

McCann, J. J. & Hall, J. A. Jr. (1980) Effects of average-luminance surrounds on the visibility of sine-wave gratings. *Journal of the Optical Society of America,* 70, 212–219.

McCann, J. J., Savoy, R. L., & Hall, J. A. Jr. (1978) Visibility of low-frequency sine-wave targets: Dependence on number of cycles and surround parameters. *Vision Research,* 18, 891–894.

McCann, J. J., Savoy, R. L., Hall, J. A. Jr., & Scarpetti, J. J. (1974) Visibility of continuous luminance gradients. *Vision Research,* 14, 917–927.

McCollough, C. (1965) Color adaptation of edge-detectors in the human visual system. *Science,* 149, 1115–1116.

Merigan, W. H. & Eskin, T. A. (1986) Spatio-temporal vision of macaques with severe loss of P-(beta) retinal ganglion cells. *Vision Research,* 26, 1751–1761.

Merigan, W. H., Pasternak, T., & Zehl, D. (1981) Spatial and temporal vision of macaques after central retinal lesions. *Investigative Ophthalmology and Visual Science,* 18, 17–26.

Mertens, J. J. (1956) Influence of knowledge of target location upon the probability of observation of peripherally observable test flashes. *Journal of the Optical Society of America,* 46, 1069–1070.

Miller, M., Pasik, P., & Pasik, T. (1980) Extrageniculostriate vision in the monkey. VII. Contrast sensitivity functions. *Journal of Neurophysiology,* 43, 1510–1526.

Miller, R. J. (1978) Mood changes and the dark focus of accommodation. *Perception and Psychophysics,* 24, 437–443.

Miller, R. J., Pigion, R. G., Wesner, M. F., & Patterson, J. G. (1983) Accommodation fatigue and dark focus: The effects of accommodation-free visual work as assessed by two psychophysical methods. *Perception and Psychophysics,* 34, 532–540.

Miller, W. H. & Bernard, G. D. (1983) Averaging over the foveal receptor aperture curtails aliasing. *Vision Research,* 23, 1365–1369.

Millodot, M., Johnson, C. A., Lamont, A., & Leibowitz, H. W. (1975) Effect of dioptics on peripheral visual acuity. *Vision Research,* 15, 1357–1362.

Mitchell, D. E. (1980) The influence of early visual experience on visual perception. In *Visual Coding and Adaptability* (C. Harris, Ed.). Hillsdale, N.J.: Lawrence Erlbaum, pp. 1–50.

Mitchell, D. E., Freeman, R. D., Millodot, M., & Haegerstrom, G. (1973) Meridional amblyopia: Evidence for modification of the human visual system by early visual experience. *Vision Research,* 13, 535–558.

Mitchell, D. E., Freeman, R. D., & Westheimer, G. (1967) Effect of orientation on the modulation sensitivity for interference fringes on the retina. *Journal of the Optical Society of America,* 57, 246–249.

Mitchell, O. R. (1976) Effect of spatial frequency on the visibility of unstructured patterns. *Journal of the Optical Society of America,* 66, 327–332.

Mitsuboshi, M., Funakawa, M., Kawataba, Y., & Aiba, T. S. (1987) Temporal integration in human vision and the opponent-color systems. *Vision Research,* 27, 1179–1186.

Mitsuboshi, M., Kawataba, Y., and Aiba, T. S. (1987) Color-opponent characteristics revealed in temporal integration time. *Vision Research,* 27, 1187–1196.

Morant, R. B. & Harris, J. R. (1965) Two different aftereffects of exposure to visual tilts. *American Journal of Psychology,* 78, 218–226.

Moray, N., Fitter, M., Ostry, D., Favreau, D., & Nagy, V. (1976) Attention to pure tones. *Quarterly Journal of Experimental Psychology,* 28, 271–283.

Morgan, M. J. (1980a) Analogue models of motion perception. *Philosophical Transactions of the Royal Society of London B,* 290, 117–135.

Morgan, M. J. (1980b) Spatiotemporal filtering and the interpolation effect in apparent motion. *Perception,* 9, 161–174.

Morgan, M. J. & Watt, R. J. (1982) The modulation transfer function of a display oscilloscope: Measurements and comments. *Vision Research,* 22, 1083–1085.

Morgan, M. J. & Watt, R. J. (1983) On the failure of spatiotemporal interpolation: A filtering model. *Vision Research,* 23, 997–1004.

Morrison, J. D. & McGrath, C. (1985) Assessment of the optical contribution to age-related deterioration in vision. *Quarterly Journal of Experimental Physiology,* 70, 249–269.

Morrone, M. C., Burr, D. C., & Maffei, L. (1982) Functional implications of cross-orientation inhibition of cortical visual cells. I. Neurophysiological evidence. *Proceedings of the Royal Society of London B,* 216, 335–354.

Mostafavi, H. & Sakrison, D. J. (1976) Structure and properties of a single channel in the human visual system. *Vision Research,* 16, 957–968.

Moulden, B., Renshaw, J., & Mather, G. (1984) Two channels for flicker in the human visual system. *Perception,* 13, 387–400.

Movshon, J. A., Adelson, E. H., Gizzi, M., & Newsome, W. T. (1984) The analysis of moving visual patterns. In *Pattern Recognition Mechanisms* (C. Chagas, R. Gattass, & C. G. Gross, Eds.). New York: Springer-Verlag.

Movshon, J. A. & Blakemore, C. (1973) Orientation specificity and spatial selectivity in human vision. *Perception,* 2, 53–60.

Movshon, J. A. & Lennie, P. (1979) Pattern-selective adaptation in visual cortical neurons. *Nature,* 278, 850–852.

Movshon, J. A., Thompson, I. D., & Tolhurst, D. J. (1978a) Spatial summation in the receptive fields of simple cells in the cat's striate cortex. *Journal of Physiology,* 283, 53–77.

Movshon, J. A., Thompson, I. D., & Tolhurst, D. J. (1978b) Receptive field organization of complex cells in the cat's striate cortex. *Journal of Physiology,* 283, 79–99.

Movshon, J. A., Thompson, I. D., & Tolhurst, D. J. (1978c) Spatial and temporal contrast sensitivity of neurons in areas 17 and 18 of the cat's visual cortex. *Journal of Physiology,* 283, 101–120.

Mueller, C. G. (1950) Quantum concepts in visual intensity-discrimination. *American Journal of Psychology,* 63, 92–100.

Muir, D. & Over, R. (1970) Tilt aftereffects in central and peripheral vision. *Journal of Experimental Psychology,* 85, 165–170.

Mullikin, W. H., Jones, J. P., & Palmer, L. A. (1984) Periodic simple cells in cat area 17. *Journal of Neurophysiology,* 52, 372–387.

Müller, H. J. & Findley, J. M. (1987) Sensitivity and criterion effects in the spatial cueing of visual attention. *Perception and Psychophysics,* 42, 383–399.

Mullins, W. W. (1978) Convexity theorem for substhreshold stimuli in linear models of visual contrast detection. *Journal of the Optical Society of America,* 68, 456–459.

Murphy, B. J. (1978) Pattern thresholds for moving and stationary gratings during smooth eye movement. *Vision Research,* 18, 521–530.

Murray, I., MacCana, F., & Kulikowski, J. J. (1983) Contribution of two movement detecting mechanisms to central and peripheral vision. *Vision Research,* 23, 151–159.

Nachmias, J. (1960) Meriodional variations in visual acuity and eye-movements during fixation. *Journal of the Optical Society of America,* 50, 569–571.

Nachmias, J. (1967) The effect of exposure duration on visual contrast sensitivity with square-wave gratings. *Journal of the Optical Society of America,* 57, 421–427.

Nachmias, J. (1972) Signal detection theory and its application to problems in vision. In *Handbook of Sensory Physiology. Vol. VII/4* (D. Jameson & L. Hurvich, Eds.). Berlin: Springer-Verlag, pp. 56–78.

Nachmias, J. (1974) A new approach to bandwidth estimation of spatial frequency channels. Paper presented at spring meeting of Association for Research in Vision and Ophthalmology, Sarasota, Fla.

Nachmias, J. (1981) On the psychometric function for contrast detection. *Vision Research,* 21, 215–223.

Nachmias, J. & Kocher, E. C. (1970) Visual detection and discrimination of luminance increments. *Journal of the Optical Society of America,* 60, 382–389.

Nachmias, J. & Rogowitz, B. E. (1983) Masking by spatially modulated gratings. *Vision Research,* 23, 1621–1630.

Nachmias, J. & Sansbury, R. V. (1974) Grating contrast: Discrimination may be better than detection. *Vision Research,* 14, 1039–1042.

Nachmias, J., Sansbury, R., Vassilev, A., & Weber, A. (1973) Adaptation to square-wave gratings: In search of the elusive third harmonic. *Vision Research,* 13, 1335–1342.

Nachmias, J. & Weber, A. (1975) Discrimination of simple and complex gratings. *Vision Research,* 15, 217–224.

Nagano, T. (1980) Temporal sensitivity of the human visual system to sinusoidal gratings. *Journal of the Optical Society of America,* 70, 711–716.

Nagshineh, S. & Ruddock, K. H. (1978) Properties of length-selective and non-length-selective adaptation mechansims in human vision. *Biological Cybernetics,* 31, 37–47.

Nakayama, K. (1985) Biological image motion processing: A review. *Vision Research,* 25, 625–660.

Nakayama, K. & Roberts, D. J. (1972) Line length detectors in the human visual system: Evidence from selective adaptation. *Vision Research,* 12, 1709–1713.

Nes, F. L. van (1968) *Experimental studies in spatiotemporal contrast transfer by the human eye.* Ph.D. thesis, University of Utrecht, The Netherlands.

Nes, F. L. van & Bouman, M. A. (1967) Spatial modulation transfer in the human eye. *Journal of the Optical Society of America,* 57, 401–406.

Nes, F. L. van, Koenderink, J. J., Nas, H., & Bouman, M. A. (1967) Spatiotemporal modulation transfer in the human eye. *Journal of the Optical Society of America,* 57, 1082–1088.

Nielsen, K. R. K. & Wandell, B. A. (1988) Discrete analysis of spatial-sensitivity models. *Journal of the Optical Society of America A,* 5, 743–755.

Nielsen, K. R. K., Watson, A. B., & Ahumada, A. J. Jr. (1985) Application of a computable model of human spatial vision to phase discrimination. *Journal of the Optical Society of America A,* 2, 1600–1606.

Nilsson, T., Richmond, C., & Nelson, T. (1975) Flicker adaptation shows evidence of many visual channels selectively sensitive to temporal frequency. *Vision Research,* 15, 621–623.

Nissen, M. J., Corkin, S., Buonanno, F. S., Growden, J. H., Wray, S. H., & Bauer, M. S. (1985) Spatial vision in Alzheimer's disease: General findings and a case report. *Archives of Neurology,* 42, 667–671.

Nolte, L. W. & Jaarsma, D. (1967) Mone on the detection of one of M orthogonal signals. *Journal of the Acoustical Society of America,* 41, 497–505.

Noorlander, C., Heuts, M. J. G., & Koenderink, J. J. (1981) Sensitivity to spatiotemporal combined luminance and chromaticity contrast. *Journal of the Optical Society of America,* 71, 453–459.

Nordby, K., Greenlee, M. W., & Magnussen, S. (1986) Does experience shape spatial frequency channels? Presented at the Nordita/DIKU meeting on Vision, Copenhagen, August.

Nygaard, R. W. & Frumkes, T. E. (1985) Frequency dependence in scotopic flicker sensitivity. *Vision Research,* 25, 115–128.

O'Toole, B. I. (1979) The tilt illusion: Length and luminance changes of induction line and third (disinhibiting) line. *Perception and Psychophysics,* 25, 487–496.

O'Toole, B. I. & Wenderoth, P. (1977) The tilt illusion: Repulsion and attraction effects in the oblique meridian. *Vision Research,* 17, 367–374.

Ohtani, Y. & Ejima, Y. (1988) Relation between flicker and two-pulse sensitivities for sinusoidal gratings. *Vision Research,* 28, 145–156.

Ohzawa, I. & Freeman, R. D. (1986a) The binocular organization of simple cells in the cat's visual cortex. *Journal of Neurophysiology,* 56, 221–242.

Ohzawa, I. & Freeman, R. D. (1986b) The binocular organization of complex cells in the cat's visual cortex. *Journal of Neurophysiology,* 56, 243–259.

Ohzawa, I., Sclar, G. & Freeman, R. D. (1982) Contrast gain in the cat's visual cortex. *Nature,* 298, 266–268.

Olzak, L. & Kramer, P. (1984) Inhibition between spatially tuned mechanisms: Temporal influences. *Optic News,* 10, 85.

Olzak, L. & Thomas, J. P. (1981) Gratings: Why frequency discrimination is sometimes better than detection. *Journal of the Optical Society of America,* 71, 64–70.

Olzak, L. A. (1981) *Inhibition and stochastic interactions in spatial pattern perception.* Ph.D. thesis, University of California, Los Angeles.

Olzak, L. A. (1985) Interactions between spatially tuned mechanisms: Converging evidence. *Journal of the Optical Society of America A,* 2, 1551–1559.

Olzak, L. A. (1986) Widely separated spatial frequencies: Mechanism interactions. *Vision Research,* 26, 1143–1153.

Olzak, L. A. & Wickens, T. D. (1983) The interpretation of detection data through direct multivariate frequency analysis. *Psychological Bulletin,* 93, 574–585.

Ono, H. & Barbeito, R. (1985) Utrocular discrimination is not sufficient for utrocular identification. *Vision Research,* 25, 289–300.

Ostry, D., Moray, N., & Marks, G. (1976) Attention, practice, and semantic targets. *Journal of Experimental Psychology: Human Perception and Performance,* 2, 326–336.

Over, R., Broerse, J. & Crassini, B. (1972) Orientation illusion and masking in central and peripheral vision. *Journal of Experimental Psychology,* 96, 25–31.

Owens, D. A. (1979) The Mandelbaum effect: Evidence for accommodative bias toward intermediate viewing distances. *Journal of the Optical Society of America,* 69, 646–652.

Owens, D. A. (1980) A comparison of accommodative responsiveness and contrast sensitivity for sinusoidal gratings. *Vision Research,* 20, 159–167.

Owsley, C., Sekuler, R., & Siemsen, D. (1983) Contrast sensitivity throughout adulthood. *Vision Research,* 23, 689–700.

Panish, S. C., Swift, D. J., & Smith, R. A. (1983) Two-criterion threshold techniques: Evidence for separate spatial and temporal mechanisms? *Vision Research,* 23, 1519–1525.

Pantle, A. (1971) Flicker adaptation. I: Effect on visual sensitivity to temporal fluctuations of light intensity. *Vision Research,* 11, 943–952.

Pantle, A. (1973) Visual effects of sinusoidal components of complex gratings: Independent or additive? *Vision Research,* 13, 2195–2205.

Pantle, A. Lehmkuhle, S., & Caudill, M. (1978) On the capacity of directionally selective mechanisms to encode different dimensions on moving stimuli. *Perception,* 7, 261–267.

Pantle, A. & Picciano, L. (1976) A multistable movement display: Evidence for two separate motion systems in human vision. *Science,* 193, 500–502.

Pantle, A. & Sekuler, R. (1968a) Size-detecting mechanisms in human vision. *Science,* 162, 1146–1148.

Pantle, A. & Sekuler, R. (1968b) Velocity-sensitivity elements in human vision: Initial psychophysical evidence. *Vision Research,* 8, 445–450.

Pantle, A. & Sekuler, R. (1969) Contrast response of human visual mechanisms sensitive to orientation and direction of motion. *Vision Research,* 9, 397–406.

Papoulis, A. (1962) *The Fourier integral and its applications.* New York: McGraw-Hill.

Parker, A. (1981) Shifts in perceived periodicity induced by temporal modulation and their influence on the spatial frequency tuning of two aftereffects. *Vision Research,* 21, 1739–1747.

Pass, A. F. & Levi, D. M. (1982) Spatial processing of complex stimuli in the amblyopic visual system. *Investigative Ophthalmology and Visual Science,* 23, 780–786.

Pasternak, T. (1986) The role of cortical directional selectivity in detection of motion and flicker. *Vision Research,* 26, 1187–1194.

Pasternak, T. & Leinen, L. (1986) Pattern and motion vision in cats with selective loss of cortical directional selectivity. *Journal of Neurosciences,* 6, 938–945.

Pasternak, T. & Merigan, W. H. (1981) The luminance dependence of spatial vision in the cat. *Vision Research*, 21, 1333–1339.

Pasternak, T., Merigan, W. H., Flood, D. G., & Zehl, D. (1983) The role of area centralis in the spatial vision of the cat. *Vision Research*, 23, 1409–1416.

Pasternak, T., Schumer, R. A., Gizzi, M. S., & Movshon, J. A. (1985) Abolition of visual direction selectivity affects visual behavior in cats. *Experimental Brain Research*, 61, 214–217.

Patel, A. S. (1966) Spatial resolution by the human visual system: The effect of mean retinal illuminance. *Journal of the Optical Society of America*, 56, 689–694.

Patel, A. S. & Jones, R. W. (1968) Increment and decrement visual thresholds. *Journal of the Optical Society of America*, 58, 696–699.

Pelli, D. (1981a) The effect of uncertainty: Detecting a signal at one of ten-thousand possible times and places. *Supplement to Investigative Ophthalmology and Visual Science*, 20, 178.

Pelli, D. (1981b) *Effects of visual noise.* Ph.D. thesis, Cambridge University, Cambridge, England.

Pelli, D. G. (1985) Uncertainty explains many aspects of visual contrast detection and discrimination. *Journal of the Optical Society of America A*, 2, 1508–1531.

Pelli, D. G. (1987) On the relation between summation and facilitation. *Vision Research*, 27, 119–124.

Perizonius, E., Schill, W., Geiger, H., & Rohler, R. (1985) Evidence on the local character of spatial frequency channels in the human visual system. *Vision Research*, 25, 1233–1240.

Petrov, A. P., Pigarev, I. N., & Zenkin, G. M. (1980) Some evidence against Fourier analysis as a function of the receptive fields in cat's striate cortex. *Vision Research*, 20, 1023–1025.

Petry, H. M., Fox, R., & Casagrande, V. A. (1982) Behavioral measurement of spatial contrast sensitivity in the tree shrew. *Supplement to Investigative Ophthalmology and Visual Science*, 22, 252.

Phillips, G. C. & Wilson, H. R. (1984) Orientation bandwidths of spatial mechanisms measured by masking. *Journal of the Optical Society of America A*, 1, 226–232.

Piantanida, T. P. (1985) Temporal modulation sensitivity of the blue mechanism: Measurments made with extraretinal chromatic adaptation. *Vision Research*, 25, 1439–1444.

Pinter, R. B. (1983) Product term nonlinear lateral inhibition enhances visual selectivity for small objects or edges. *Journal of Theoretical Biology*, 100, 525–531.

Pinter, R. B. (1985) Adaptation of spatial modulation transfer functions via nonlinear lateral inhibition. *Biological Cybernetics*, 51, 285–291.

Poggio, G. F., Doty, R. W., & Talbot, W. H. (1977) Foveal striate cortex of behaving monkey: Single-neuron responses to square-wave gratings during fixation of gaze. *Journal of Neurophysiology*, 40, 1369–1391.

Pohlmann, L. D. & Sorkin, R. D. (1976) Simultaneous three-channel signal detection: Performance and criterion as a function of order of report. *Perception and Psychophysics*, 20, 179–186.

Pokorny, J. (1968) The effect of target area on grating acuity. *Vision Research*, 8, 543–554.

Pollen, D. A., Foster, K. H., & Gaska, J. P. (1985) Phase-dependent response characteristics of visual cortical neurons. In *Models of the Visual Cortex* (D. Rose & V. G. Dobson, Eds.). New York: Wiley.

Pollen, D. A. & Ronner, S. F. (1981) Phase relationships between adjacent simple cells in the visual cortex. *Science*, 212, 1409–1411.

Pollen, D. A. & Ronner, S. F. (1982) Spatial computation performed by simple and complex cells in the visual cortex of the cat. *Vision Research*, 22, 101–118.

Posner, M. I. (1978) *Chronometric Explorations of Mind.* Hillsdale, N.J.: Lawrence Erlbaum.

Powers, M. K. & Dobson, V. (1982) Effect of focus on visual acuity of human infants. *Vision Research*, 22, 521–528.

Quick R. F. (1974) A vector-magnitude model of contrast detection. *Kybernetik*, 16, 65–67.

Quick R. F., Mullins, W. W., & Reichert, T. A. (1978) Spatial summation effects on two-component grating thresholds. *Journal of the Optical Society of America*, 68, 116–121.

Quick R. F. & Reichert, T. A. (1975) Spatial-frequency selectivity in contrast detection. *Vision Research*, 15, 637–643.

Quinn, P. C. & Lehmkuhle, S. (1983) An oblique effect of spatial summation. *Vision Research,* 23, 655–658.

Raninen, A. & Rovamo, J. (1986) Perimetry of critical flicker frequency in human rod and cone vision. *Vision Research,* 26, 1249–1255.

Raninen, A. & Rovamo, J. (1987) Retinal ganglion-cell density and receptive-field size as determinants of photopic flicker sensitivity across the human visual field. *Journal of the Optical Society of America A,* 4, 1620–1626.

Rao, V. M. & Kulikowsi, J. J. (1980) Disinhibition between orientation-specific channels. *Supplement to Neuroscience Letters,* 5, 548.

Rashbass, C. (1970) The visibility of transient changes of luminance. *Journal of Physiology,* 210, 165–186.

Rashbass, C. (1976) Unification of two contrasting models of the visual incremental threshold. *Vision Research,* 16, 1281–1283.

Ratliff, F. (1965) *Mach Bands: Quantitative Studies on Neural Networks in the Retina.* San Francisco: Holden-Day.

Raymond, J. E. & Leibowitz, H. W. (1985) Viewing distance and the sustained detection of high spatial frequency gratings. *Vision Research,* 25, 1655–1659.

Raymond, J. E., Lindblad, I. M., & Leibowitz, H. W. (1984) The effect of contrast on sustained detection. *Vision Research,* 24, 183–188.

Regal, D. M. (1981) Development of critical flicker frequency in human infants. *Vision Research,* 21, 549–556.

Regan, D. & Beverly, K. I. (1983a) Visual fields described by contrast sensitivity, by acuity, and by relative sensitivity to different orientations. *Investigative Ophthalmology and Visual Science,* 24, 754–759.

Regan, D. & Beverly, K. I. (1983b) Spatial frequency discrimination and detection: Comparison of post adaptation thresholds. *Journal of the Optical Society of America,* 73, 1684–1690.

Regan, D. & Beverly, K. I. (1985) Postadaptation orientation discrimination. *Journal of the Optical Society of America A,* 2, 147–155.

Regan, D. & Neima, D. (1984) Balance between pattern and flicker sensitivities in the visual fields of ophthalmological patients. *British Journal of Ophthalmology,* 68, 310–315.

Regan, D., Raymond, J., Ginsburg, A. P., & Murray, T. J. (1981) Contrast sensitivity, visual acuity, and the discrimination of Snellen letters in multiple sclerosis. *Brain,* 104, 333–350.

Regan, D., Silver, R., & Murray, T. J. (1977) Visual acuity and contrast sensitivity in multiple-sclerosis—hidden visual loss. *Brain,* 100, 563–579.

Regan, D., Whitlock, J. A., Murray, T. J. & Beverley, K. I. (1980) Orientation-specific losses of contrast sensitivity in multiple sclerosis. *Investigative Ophthalmology and Visual Science,* 19, 324–328.

Rentschler, I. & Fiorentini, A. (1974) Meridional anisotropy of psychophysical spatial interaction. *Vision Research,* 14, 1467–1473.

Rentschler, I. & Hilz, R. (1976) Evidence for disinhibition in line detectors. *Vision Research,* 16, 1299–1302.

Rentschler, I., Hilz, R., & Brettel, H. (1980) Spatial tuning properties in human amblyopia cannot explain the loss of optotype acuity. *Behavioural Brain Research,* 1, 433–443.

Rentschler, I., Hilz, R., & Brettel, H. (1981) Amblyopic abnormality involves neural mechanisms concerned with movement processing. *Investigative Ophthalmology and Visual Science,* 20, 695–700.

Reymond, L. (1987) Spatial visual acuity of the falcon, Falco berigora: A behavioral, optical and anatomical investigation. *Vision Research,* 27, 1859–1874.

Reymond, L. & Wolfe, J. (1981) Behavioural determination of the contrast sensitivity function of the eagle *Aquila audax. Vision Research,* 21, 263–271.

Rijsdijk, J. P., Kroon, J. N., & van der Wildt, G. J. (1980) Contrast sensitivity as a function of position on the retina. *Vision Research,* 20, 235–241.

Robson, J. G. (1966) Spatial and temporal contrast-sensitivity functions of the visual system. *Journal of the Optical Society of America,* 56, 1141–1142.

Robson, J. G. (1975) Receptive fields: Spatial and intensive representations of the visual image. In *Handbook of Perception. Vol. 5. Seeing,* (E. C. Carterette & M. P. Friedman, Eds.). New York: Academic, pp. 81–116.

Robson, J. G. (1980) Neural images: The physiological basis of spatial vision. In *Visual Coding and Adaptability* (C. Harris, Ed.). Hillsdale, N.J.: Lawrence Erlbaum, pp. 177–214.

Robson, J. G. (1983) Frequency domain in visual processing. In *Physical and Biological Processing of Images* (O. J. Braddick & A. C. Sleigh, Eds.). Berlin: Springer-Verlag, pp. 73–87.

Robson, J. G. & Enroth-Cugell, C. (1978) Light distribution in the cats' retinal image. *Vision Research,* 18, 159–174.

Robson, J. G. & Graham, N. (1981) Probability summation and regional variation in contrast sensitivity across the visual field. *Vision Research,* 21, 409–418.

Rodieck, R. W. (1965) Quantitative analysis of cat retinal ganglion cell response to visual stimuli. *Vision Research,* 5, 583–601.

Rodieck, R. W. & Stone, J. (1965) Analysis of receptive fields of cat retinal ganglion cells. *Journal of Neurophysiology,* 28, 833–849.

Rolls, E. T. & Cowey, A. (1970) Topography of the retina and striate cortex and its relationship to visual acuity in rhesus monkeys and squirrel monkeys. *Experimental Brain Research,* 10, 298–310.

Ronchi, L. & Fidanzati, G. (1972) Changes of psychophysical organization across the light-adapted retina. *Journal of the Optical Society of America,* 62, 912–915.

Rose, D. (1978) Monocular versus binocular contrast thresholds for movement and pattern. *Perception,* 7, 195–200.

Rose, D. (1979) Mechanisms underlying the receptive field properties of neurons in cat visual cortex. *Vision Research,* 19, 533–544.

Rose, D. (1983) An investigation into hemispheric differences in adaptation to contrast. *Perception and Psychophysics,* 34, 89–95.

Rose, D. & Evans, R. (1983) Evidence against saturation of contrast adaptation in the human visual system. *Perception and Psychophysics,* 34, 158–160.

Rose, D. & Lowe, I. (1982) Dynamics of adaptation to contrast. *Perception,* 11, 505–528.

Ross, H. E. & Woodhouse, J. M. (1979) Genetic and environmental factors in orientation anisotropy: A field study in the British Isles. *Perception,* 8, 507–521.

Ross, J. & Johnstone, J. R. (1980) Phase and detection of compound gratings. *Vision Research,* 20, 189–192.

Rothblum, A. M. (1982) Separate detectors for static and counterphase gratings. *Supplement to Investigative Ophthalmology and Visual Science,* 22, 253.

Roufs, J. A. J. (1972a) Dynamic properties of vision. I. Experimental relationships between flicker and flash thresholds. *Vision Research,* 12, 261–278.

Roufs, J. A. J. (1972b) Dynamic properties of vision. II. Theoretical relationships between flicker and flash thresholds. *Vision Research,* 12, 279–292.

Roufs, J. A. J. (1973) Dynamic properties of vision. III. Twin flashes, single flashes and flicker fusion. *Vision Research,* 13, 309–323.

Roufs, J. A. J. (1974a) Dynamic properties of vision. IV. Thresholds of decremental flashes, incremental flashes and doublets in relation to flicker fusion. *Vision Research,* 14, 831–851.

Roufs, J. A. J. (1974b) Dynamic properties of vision. V. Perception lag and reaction time in relation to flicker and flash thresholds. *Vision Research,* 14, 853–869.

Roufs, J. A. J. (1974c) Dynamic properties of vision. VI. Stochastic threshold fluctuations and their effect on flash-to-flicker sensitivity ratio. *Vision Research,* 14, 871–888.

Roufs, J. A. J. & Blommaert, F. J. J. (1981) Temporal impulse and step response of the human eye obtained psychophysically by means of a drift-correcting perturbation technique. *Vision Research,* 21, 1203–1221.

Rousseau, R., Poirier, J., & Lemyre, L. (1983) Duration discrimination of empty time intervals marked by intermodal pulses. *Perception and Psychophysics,* 34, 541–548.

Rovamo, J., Hyvarinen, L., & Hari, R. (1982) Human vision without luminance-contrast system: Selective recovery of the red-green colour-contrast system from acquired blindness. *Docu-*

menta Ophthalmologica Proceeding Series. Vol. 33, (G. Verriest, Ed.). The Hague: Junk, pp. 457–466.

Rovamo, J., Leinonen, L., Laurinen, P., & Virsu, J. (1984) Temporal integration and contrast sensitivity in foveal and peripheral vision. *Perception,* 13, 665–674.

Rovamo, J. & Raninen, A. (1984) Critical flicker frequency and M-scaling of stimulus size and retinal illuminance. *Vision Research,* 24, 1127–1132.

Rovamo, J. & Raninen, A. (1988) Critical flicker frequency as a function of stimulus area and luminance at various eccentricities in human cone vision: a revision of Granit-Harper and Ferry-Porter laws. *Vision Research,* 28, 785–790.

Rovamo, J., Raninen, A., & Virsu, V. (1985) The role of retinal ganglion cell density and receptive field size in photopic perimetry. *Documenta Ophthalmologica Proceedings Series,* Vol. 42, (A. Heijl & E. L. Greve, Eds.). Dordrecht, The Netherlands: Junk, pp 589–594.

Rovamo, J. & Virsu, V. (1979) An estimation and application of the human cortical magnification factor. *Experimental Brain Research,* 37, 495–510.

Rovamo, J. & Virsu, V. (1984) Isotropy of cortical magnification and topography of striate cortex. *Vision Research,* 24, 283–286.

Rovamo, J., Virsu, V., Laurinen, P., & Hyvarinen, L. (1982) Resolution of gratings oriented along and across meridians in peripheral vision. *Investigative Ophthalmology and Visual Science,* 23, 666–670.

Rovamo, J., Virsu, V., & Nasanen, R. (1978) Cortical magnification factor predicts the photopic contrast sensitivity of peripheral vision. *Nature,* 271, 54–56.

Ruddock, K. H., Waterfield, V. A., & Wigley, E. (1979) The response characteristics of an inhibitory binocular interaction in human vision. *Journal of Physiology,* 290, 37–49.

Russell, P. W. & Wheeler, T. G. (1983) Scotopic sensitivity to ON and OFF stimulus transients. *Vision Research,* 23, 525–528.

Sachs, M. B., Nachmias, J., & Robson, J. G. (1971) Spatial-frequency channels in human vision. *Journal of the Optical Society of America,* 61, 1176–1186.

Sagi, D. (1988) The combination of spatial frequency and orientation is effortlessly perceived. *Perception and Psychophysics,* 43, 601–603.

Sakitt, B. (1971) Configuration dependence of scotopic spatial summation. *Journal of Physiology,* 216, 513–529.

Salapateck, P. & Banks, M. S. (1978) Infant sensory assessment: Vision. In *Communicative and Cognitive Abilities: Early Behavioral Assessment* (F. D. Minifie & L. L. Lloyd, Eds.) Baltimore, Md.: University Park Press, pp. 61–106.

Sansbury, R. V. (1974) *Some properties of spatial channels revealed by pulsed simultaneous masking.* Ph.D. thesis. University of Pennsylvania, Philadelphia.

Sansbury, R. V., Distelhorst, J. E., & Moore, S. (1978) A phase-specific adaptation effect of the square-wave grating. *Investigative Ophthalmology and Visual Science,* 17, 442–448.

Sansbury, R. V., Distelhorst, J. E., & Zappala, A. T. (1979) A phase-specific adaptation effect of the sawtooth grating. *Supplement to Investigative Ophthalmology and Visual Science,* 18, 60.

Santen, J. P. H. van & Sperling, G. (1984) Temporal covariance model of human motion perception. *Journal of the Optical Society of America A,* 1, 451–473.

Santen, J. P. H. van & Sperling, G. (1985) Elaborated Reichardt detectors. *Journal of the Optical Society of America A,* 2, 300–321.

Savoy, R. L. & McCann, J. J. (1975) Visibility of low-spatial-frequency sine-wave targets: Dependence on number of cycles. *Journal of the Optical Society of America,* 65, 343–350.

Schade, O. H. (1948) Electro-optical characteristics of television systems. I. Characteristics of vision and visual systems. *RCA Review,* 9, 5–37.

Schade, O. H. (1956) Optical and photelectric analog of the eye. *Journal of the Optical Society of America,* 46, 721–739.

Schade, O. H. (1958) On the quality of color-television images and the perception of color detail. *Journal of the Society of Motion Picture Television Engineers,* 67, 801–819.

Scharf, B., Quigley, S., Aoki, C., Peachey, N., & Reeves, A. (1987) Focused auditory attention and frequency selectivity. *Perception and Psychophysics,* 42, 215–223.

Schiller, P. H. (1986) The central visual system. *Vision Research,* 26, 1351–1388.

Schiller, P. H., Finlay, B. L., & Volman, S. F. (1976a) Quantitative studies of single-cell properties in monkey striate cortex. I. Spatiotemporal organization of receptive fields. *Journal of Neurophysiology,* 39, 1288–1319.

Schiller, P. H., Finlay, B. L., & Volman, S. F. (1976b) Quantitative studies of single-cell properties in monkey striate cortex. II. Orientation specificity and ocular dominance. *Journal of Neurophysiology,* 39, 1320–1333.

Schiller, P. H., Finlay, B. L., & Volman, S. F. (1976c) Quantitative studies of single-cell properties in monkey striate cortex. III. Spatial frequency. *Journal of Neurophysiology,* 39, 1334–1351.

Schlossberg, H. (1948) A probability formulation of the Hunter-Sigler effect. *Journal of Experimental Psychology,* 38, 155–167.

Schlotterer, G., Moscovitch, M., & Crapper-McLachlan, D. (1983) Visual processing deficits as assessed by spatial frequency contrast sensitivity and backward masking in normal aging and Alzheimer's disease. *Brain,* 107, 309–325.

Schneck, M. E., Hamer, R. D., Packer, O. S., & Teller, D. Y. (1984) Area-threshold relations at controlled retinal locations in 1-month-old infants. *Vision Research,* 24, 1753–1764.

Schober, H. A. W. & Hilz, R. (1965) Contrast sensitivity of the human eye for square-wave gratings. *Journal of the Optical Society of America,* 55, 1086–1091.

Schuckman, H. (1963) Attention and visual threshold. *American Journal Optometry Archives American Academy Optometry,* 40, 284–291.

Schwartz, E. (1977) Spatial mapping in the primate sensory projection: Analytic structure and relevance to perception. *Biological Cybernetics,* 25, 181–194.

Schwartz, E. (1980) Computational anatomy and functional architecture of striate cortex: A spatial mapping approach to perpetual coding. *Vision Research,* 20, 645–670.

Schwartz, S. H. & Loop, M. S. (1982) Evidence for transient luminance and quasi-sustained color mechanisms. *Vision Research,* 22, 445–447.

Schwartz, S. H. & Loop, M. S. (1983) Differences in temporal appearance associated with activity in chromatic and achromatic systems. *Perception and Psychophysics,* 33, 388–390.

Sclar, G. & Freeman R. D. (1982) Orientation selectivity in the cat's striate cortex is invariant with stimulus contrast. *Experimental Brain Research,* 46, 457–461.

Sebris, S. L., Dobson, V., & Hartmann, E. E. (1984) Assessment and prediction of visual acuity in 3- to 4-year-old children born prior to term. *Human Neurobiology,* 3, 87–93.

Segal, M. H., Campbell, D. T., & Herskovits, M. J. (1966) *The Influence of Culture on Visual Perception.* Indianapolis, In.: Bobbs-Merrill.

Sekuler, R. (1965) Spatial and temporal determinants of visual backward masking. *Journal of Experimental Psychology,* 70, 401–406.

Sekuler, R. (1974) Spatial vision. *Annual Reviews of Psychology,* 25, 195–232.

Sekular, R. & Ball, K. (1977) Mental set alters visibility of moving targets. *Science,* 198, 60–62.

Sekuler, R. & Ganz, L. (1963) Aftereffect of seen motion with a stabilized retinal image. *Science,* 139, 419–420.

Sekuler, R. & Levinson, E. (1974) Mechanisms of motion perception. *Psychologia (Kyoto),* 17, 38–49.

Sekuler, R. & Levinson, E. (1977) The perception of moving targets. *Scientific American,* 236, 60–73.

Sekuler, R., Pantle, A., & Levinson, E. (1978) Physiological basis of motion perception. In *Handbook of Sensory Physiology. Vol. VIII: Perception* (R. Held, H. W. Leibowitz, & H. L. Teuber, Eds.). Berlin: Springer-Verlag, pp. 67–96.

Sekuler, R., Rubin, E. L., & Cushman, W. H. (1968) Selectivities of human visual mechanisms for direction of movement and contour orientation. *Journal of the Optical Society of America,* 58, 1146–1150.

Sekuler, R. & Tynan, P. (1978) Rapid measurement of contrast-sensitivity functions. *American Journal of Optometry and Physiological Optics,* 54, 573–575.

Sekuler, R., Wilson, H. R., & Owsley, C. (1984) Structural modeling of spatial vision. *Vision Research,* 24, 689–700.

Selby, S. A. & Woodhouse, J. M. (1981) The spatial frequency dependence of interocular transfer in amblyopes. *Vision Research*, 21, 1401–1408.

Shapley, R. M. (1974) Gaussian bars and rectangular bars: The influence of width and gradiant on visibility. *Vision Research*, 14, 1457–1462.

Shapley, R. M. & Enroth-Cugell, C. (1984) Visual adaptation and retinal gain controls. In *Progress in Retinal Research. Vol. 3* (N. N. Osborne & G. J. Chader, Eds.). Oxford: Pergamon, pp. 263–343.

Shapley, R. M. & Lennie, P. (1985) Spatial frequency analysis in the visual system. *Annual Reviews of Neuroscience*, 8, 547–583.

Shapley, R. M. & Tolhurst, D. J. (1973) Edge detectors in human vision. *Journal of Physiology*, 229, 165–183.

Shapley, R. M. & Victor, J. D. (1978) The effect of contrast on the transfer properties of cat retinal ganglion cells. *Journal of Physiology*, 285, 275–298.

Shapley, R. M. & Victor, J. D. (1979) Non-linear spatial summation and the contrast gain control of cat retinal ganglion cells. *Journal of Physiology*, 290, 141–161.

Sharpe, C. R. (1972) The visibility and fading of thin lines visualized by their controlled movement across the retina. *Journal of Physiology*, 222, 113–134.

Sharpe, C. R. & Tolhurst, D. J. (1973a) The effects of temporal modulation on the orientation channels of the human visual system. *Perception*, 2, 23–29.

Sharpe, C. R. & Tolhurst, D. J. (1973b) Orientation and spatial frequency channels in peripheral vision. *Vision Research*, 13, 2103–2112.

Shaw, M. L. (1980) Identifying attentional and decision-making components in information processing. In *Attention and performance VIII* (R. S. Nickerson, Ed.) Hillsdale, New Jersey: Erlbaum, pp. 277–296.

Shaw, M. L. (1982) Attending to multiple sources of information. I. The integration of information in decision making. *Cognitive Psychology*, 14, 353–409.

Shaw, M. L., Mulligan, R. M., & Stone, L. D. (1983) Two-state versus continuous-state stimulus representations: A test based on attentional constraints. *Perception and Psychophysics*, 33, 338–354.

Shiffrin, R. M., McKay, D. P., & Shaffer, W. O. (1976) Attending to forty-nine spatial positions at once. *Journal of Experimental Psychology: Human Perception and Performance*, 2, 14–22.

Shipley, E. F. (1965) Detection and recognition: Experiments and choice models. *Journal of Mathematical Psychology*, 2, 277–311.

Short, A. D. (1966) Decremental and incremental visual thresholds. *Journal of Physiology*, 185, 646–654.

Sillito, A. M. (1977) Inhibitory processes underlying the directional specificity of simple, complex, and hypercomplex cells in the cat's visual cortex. *Journal of Physiology*, 271, 699–720.

Sillito, A. M. & Versiani, V. (1977) The contribution of excitatory and inhibitory inputs to the length preference of hypercomplex cells in layer II and III of the cat's striate cortex. *Journal of Physiology*, 273, 775–790.

Sireteanu, R. (1985) Development of visual acuity in very young kittens: A study with forced-choice preferential looking. *Vision Research*, 25, 781–788.

Sireteanu, R. & Fronius, M. (1981) Naso-temporal asymmetries in human amblyopia: Consequence of long-term interocular suppression. *Vision Research*, 21, 1055–1063.

Sireteanu, R., Fronius, M., & Singer, W. (1981) Binocular interaction in the peripheral visual field of humans with strabismic and anisometropic amblyopia. *Vision Research*, 21, 1065–1074.

Skottun, B. C. & Freeman R. D. (1984) Stimulus specificity of binocular cells in the cat's visual cortex: Ocular dominance and the matching of left and right eyes. *Experimental Brain Research*, 56, 206–216.

Sloane, M. (1982) Binocular interaction assessed by unequal adaptation of the two eyes. *Supplement to Investigative Ophthalmology and Visual Science*, 22, 272.

Smith, A. T. (1983) Interocular transfer of colour-contingent threshold elevation. *Vision Research*, 23, 729–734.

Smith, E. L. III & Harwerth, R. S. (1984) Behavioral measurements of accommodative amplitude in rhesus monkeys. *Vision Research,* 24, 1821–1828.

Smith, E. L. III, Harwerth, R. S., & Crawford, M. L. J. (1985) Spatial contrast sensitivity deficits in monkeys produced by optically induced anisometropia. *Investigative Ophthalmology and Visual Science,* 26, 330–342.

Smith, J. E. K. (1982) Simple algorithms for M-alternative forced-choice calculations. *Perception and Psychophysics,* 31, 95–96.

Smith, R. A. (1970) Adaptation of visual contrast sensitivity to specific temporal frequencies. *Vision Research,* 10, 275–279.

Smith, R. A. (1971) Studies of temporal frequency adaptation in visual contrast sensitivity. *Journal of Physiology,* 216, 531–552.

Smith, R. A. (1977) Spatial-frequency adaptation and afterimages. *Perception,* 6, 153–160.

Smith, R. A. & Cass, P. F. (1987) Aliasing in the parafovea with incoherent light. *Journal of the Optical Society of America A,* 4, 1530–1534.

Smith, R. A. & Swift, D. J. (1986) Towards a general model of spatiotemporal contrast sensitivity. *Supplement to Investigative Ophthalmology and Visual Science,* 27, 342.

Snyder, A. W. (1982) Hyperacuity and interpolation by the visual pathways. *Vision Research,* 22, 1219–1220.

Snyder, A. W. & Srinivasan, M. V. (1979) Human psychophysics: Functional interpretation for contrast sensitivity versus spatial frequency curve. *Biological Cybernetics,* 32, 9–17.

Soodak, R. E. (1986) Two-dimensional modeling of visual receptive fields using Gaussian subunits. *Proceedings of the National Academy of Sciences USA,* 83, 9259–9263.

Sorkin, R. D., Pohlmann, L. D., & Gilliom, J. D. (1973) Simultaneous two-channel signal detection. III. 630 and 1400 Hz signals. *Journal of the Acoustical Society of America,* 53, 1045–1050.

Sorkin, R. D., Pohlmann, L. D., & Woods, D. D. (1976) Decision interaction between auditory channels. *Perception and Psychophysics,* 19, 290–295.

Sperling, G. (1964) Linear theory and psychophysics of flicker. *Documenta Ophthalmologica,* 18, 3–15.

Sperling, G. (1970) Model of visual adaptation and contrast detection. *Perception and Psychophysics,* 8, 143–157.

Sperling, G. (1984) A unified theory of attention and signal detection. In *Varieties of Attention* (R. Parasuraman & D. R. Davis, Eds.). New York: Academic.

Sperling, G. & Dosher, B. A. (1986) Strategy and optimization in human information processing. In *Handbook of Perception and Performance* (K. Boff, L. Kaufman, & J. Thomas, Eds.). New York: Wiley.

Sperling, G. & Sondhi, M. M. (1968) Model for visual luminance discrimination and flicker detection. *Journal of the Optical Society of America,* 58, 1133–1145.

Spitzberg, R. & Richards, W. (1975) Broad band spatial filters in the human visual system. *Vision Research,* 15, 837–841.

Spitzer, H. & Hochstein, S. (1985a) Simple- and complex-cell response dependencies on stimulation parameters. *Journal of Neurophysiology,* 53, 1244–1264.

Spitzer, H. & Hochstein, S. (1985b) A complex-cell receptive-field model. *Journal of Neurophysiology,* 53, 1266–1286.

Starr, S. J., Metz, C. E., Lusted, L. B., & Goodenough, D. J. (1975) Visual detection and localization of radiographic images. *Radiology,* 116, 533–538.

Stecher, S., Sigel, C., & Lange, R. V. (1973a) Spatial frequency channels in human vision and threshold for adaptation. *Vision Research,* 13, 1691–1700.

Stecher, S., Sigel, C., & Lange, R. V. (1973b) Composite adaptation and spatial frequency interactions. *Vision Research,* 13, 2527–2531.

Stein, R. B. (1970) The role of spike trains in transmitting and distorting sensory signals. In *The Neurosciences: Second Study Program* (F. O. Schmitt, Ed.). New York: Rockefeller University Press.

Stephenson, C. & Braddick, O. (1983) Discrimination of relative spatial phase in fovea and periphery. *Supplement to Investigative Ophthalmology and Visual Science,* 24, 146.

Stiles, W. S. (1939) The directional sensitivity of the retina and the spectral sensitivites of the rods and cones. *Proceedings of the Royal Society of London B,* 127, 64–105.

Stiles, W. S. (1967) Mechanism concepts in colour theory. *Journal of the Color Group,* 11, 106–123.

Stork, D. G. & Falk, D. S. (1987) Temporal impulse responses from flicker sensitivities. *Journal of the Optical Society of America A,* 4, 1130–1135.

Stroymeyer, C. F. III & Klein, S. (1974) Spatial frequency channels in human vision as asymmetric (edge) mechanisms. *Vision Research,* 14, 1409–1420.

Stromeyer, C. F. III & Klein, S. (1975) Evidence against narrow-band spatial frequency channels in human vision: The detectability of frequency modulated gratings. *Vision Research,* 15, 899–910.

Stromeyer, C. F. III, Klein, S., Dawson, B. M., & Spillmann, L. (1982) Low spatial-frequency channels in human vision: Adaptation and masking. *Vision Research,* 22, 225–234.

Stromeyer, C. F. III, Klein, S., & Sternheim, C. E. (1977) Is spatial adaptation caused by prolonged inhibition?. *Vision Research,* 17, 603–606.

Stromeyer, C. F. III & Snodderly, D. M. Jr. (1981) Questions about spatial adaptation of short wavelength pathways in humans. *Science,* 214, 471–472.

Stromeyer, C. F. III & Sternheim, C. E. (1981) Visibility of red and green spatial patterns upon spectrally mixed adapting fields. *Vision Research,* 21, 397–407.

Stromeyer, C. F. III, Kronauer, R. E., & Madsen, J. C. (1984) Adaptive processes controlling sensitivity of short-wave cone pathways to different spatial frequencies. *Vision Research,* 24, 827–834.

Stromeyer, C. F. III, Kronauer, R. E., Madsen, J. C., & Cohen, M. A. (1980) Spatial adaptation of short wavelength pathways in humans. *Science,* 207, 555–557.

Stromeyer, C. F. III, Madsen, J. C., & Klein, S. (1979) Direction-selective adaptation with very slow motion. *Journal of the Optical Society of America,* 69, 1039–1041.

Stromeyer, C. F. III, Madsen, J. C., Klein, S., & Zeevi, Y. Y. (1978) Movement-selective mechanisms in human vision sensitive to high spatial frequencies. *Journal of the Optical Society of America,* 68, 1002–1005.

Stromeyer, C. F. III, Zeevi, Y. Y., & Klein, S. (1979) Response of visual mechanisms to stimulus onsets and offsets. *Journal of the Optical Society of America,* 69, 1350–1354.

Stuart, R. D. (1961) *An Introduction to Fourier Analysis.* London: Science Paperbacks, Methuen & Co.

Sullivan, G. D., Georgeson, M. A., & Oatley, K. (1972) Channels for spatial frequency selection and the detection of single bars by the human visual system. *Vision Research,* 12, 383–394.

Sunga, R. N. & Enoch, J. M. (1970) Further perimetric analysis of patients with lesions of the visual pathways. *American Journal of Ophthalmology,* 70, 403–422.

Swanson, W. H., Pokorny, J., & Smith, V. C. (1987) Effects of temporal frequency on phase-dependent sensitivity to heterochromatic flicker. *Journal of the Optical Society of America A,* 4, 2266–2273.

Swanson, W. H., Ueno, T., Smith, V. C. & Pokorny, J. (1987) Temporal modulation sensitivity and pulse-detection thresholds for chromatic and luminance perturbations. *Journal of the Optical Society of America A,* 4, 1992–2005. Errata. *Journal of the Optical Society of America A,* 5, 1525.

Swanson, W. H., Wilson, H. R., & Giese, S. C. (1984) Contrast matching data predicted from contrast increment thresholds. *Vision Research,* 24, 63–75.

Swensson, R. G. & Judy, P. F. (1981) Detection of noisy visual targets: Models for the effects of spatial uncertainty and signal-to-noise ratio. *Perception and Psychophysics,* 29, 521–534.

Swets, J. A. (1964) *Signal Detection and Recognition by Human Observers.* New York: Wiley.

Swets, J. A. & Sewall, S. T. (1961) Stimulus versus response uncertainty in recognition. *Journal of the Acoustical Society of America,* 33, 1586–1592.

Swift, D. J. & Smith, R. A. (1982) An action spectrum for spatial frequency adaptation. *Vision Research,* 22, 235–246.

Swift, D. J. & Smith, R. A. (1983) Spatial frequency masking and Weber's laws. *Vision Research,* 23, 495–506.

Swift, D. J. & Smith, R. A. (1984) An inherent nonlinearity in near-threshold contrast detection. *Vision Research,* 24, 977–978.

Switkes, E., Mayer, M. J., & Sloan, J. (1978) Spatial frequency analysis of the visual environment: Anisotropy and the carpentered environment hypothesis. *Vision Research,* 18, 1393–1399.

Takahashi, S. & Ejima, Y. (1986) Increment spectral sensitivities for spatial periodic grating patterns: Evidence for variable tuning of the chromatic system. *Vision Research,* 26, 1851–1864.

Tanaka, K. (1983) Cross-correlation analysis of geniculostriate neuronal relationships in cats. *Journal of Neurophysiology,* 49, 1303–1318.

Tanner, W. P. (1961) Physiological implications of psychophysical data. *Annals of the New York Academy of Sciences,* 166, 752.

Teller, D. Y. (1979) The forced-choice preferential looking procedure: A psychophysical technique for use with human infants. *Infant Behavior and Development,* 2, 135–153.

Teller, D. Y., Mayer, D. L., Makous, W. L., & Allen, J. L. (1982) Do preferential looking techniques underestimate infant visual acuity? *Vision Research,* 22, 1017–1024.

Teller, D. Y., Morse, R., Borton, R., & Regal, D. (1974) Visual acuity for vertical and diagonal gratings in human infants. *Vision Research,* 14, 1433–1439.

Teller, D. Y. & Movshon, J. A. (1986) Visual development. *Vision Research,* 26, 1483–1506.

Thibos, L. N., Walsh, D. J., & Cheyney, F. E. (1987) Vision beyond the resolution limit: Aliasing in the periphery. *Vision Research,* 27, 2193–2197.

Thomas, J. (1978) Normal and amblyopic contrast sensitivity functions in central and peripheral retinas. *Investigative Ophthalmology and Visual Science,* 17, 746–753.

Thomas, J. P. (1970) Model of the function of receptive fields in human vision. *Psychological Review,* 77, 121–134.

Thomas, J. P. (1978) Spatial summation in the fovea: Asymmetrical effects of longer and shorter dimensions. *Vision Research,* 18, 1023–1029.

Thomas, J. P. (1981) Do channels give symmetrical positive and negative responses? *Supplement to Investigative Ophthalmology and Visual Science,* 20, 124.

Thomas, J. P. (1983) Underlying psychometric function for detecting gratings and identifying spatial frequency. *Journal of the Optical Society of America,* 73, 751–758.

Thomas, J. P. (1985) Detection and identification: How are they related? *Journal of the Optical Society of America* A, 2, 1457–1467.

Thomas, J. P. (1986) Spatial vision then and now. *Vision Research,* 26, 1523–1530.

Thomas, J. P. (1987) Effect of eccentricity on the relationship between detection and identification. *Journal of the Optical Society of America,* 4, 1599–1605.

Thomas, J. P., Bagrash, F. M., & Kerr, L. G. (1969) Selective stimulation of two form-sensitive mechanisms. *Vision Research,* 9, 625–627.

Thomas, J. P., Barker, R. A., & Gille, J. (1979) A multidimensional space model for detection and discrimination of spatial pattern. Paper presented to 10th Pittsburgh Conference on Modeling and Simulation.

Thomas, J. P. & Gille, J. (1979) Bandwidths of orientation channels in human vision. *Journal of the Optical Society of America,* 69, 652–660.

Thomas, J. P., Gille, J., & Barker, R. A. (1982) Simultaneous visual detection and identification: Theory and data. *Journal of the Optical Society of America,* 72, 1642–1651.

Thomas, J. P. & Kerr, L. G. (1971) Evidence of role of size-tuned mechanisms in increment threshold task. *Vision Research,* 11, 647–655.

Thomas, J. P., Padilla, G. J., & Rourke, D. L. (1969) Spatial interactions in identification and detection of compound visual stimuli. *Vision Research,* 9, 283–292.

Thomas, J. P. & Shimamura, K. K. (1974) Perception of size at the detection threshold: Its accuracy and possible mechanisms. *Vision Research,* 14, 535–544.

Thomas, J. P. & Shimamura, K. K. (1975) Inhibitory interaction between visual pathways tuned to different orientations. *Vision Research,* 15, 1373–1380.

Thompson, P. (1981) Detection and discrimination of moving gratings. *Acta Psychologia,* 48, 5–13.

Thompson, P. (1983) Discrimination of moving gratings at and above detection threshold. *Vision Research,* 23, 1533–1538.

Thompson, P. (1984) The coding of velocity of movement in the human visual system. *Vision Research*, 24, 41–45.

Thompson, P. G. & Murphy, B. (1980) Adaptation to a spatial-frequency doubled stimulus. *Perception*, 9, 523–528.

Timney, B. N. & Muir, D. W. (1976) Orientation anisotropy: Incidence and magnitude in Caucasian and Chinese subjects. *Science*, 193, 699–701.

Tolhurst, D. J. (1972a) Adaptation to square-wave gratings: Inhibition between spatial frequency channels in the human visual system. *Journal of Physiology*, 226, 231–248.

Tolhurst, D. J. (1972b) On the possible existence of edge detector neurons in the human visual system. *Vision Research*, 12, 797–804.

Tolhurst, D. J. (1973) Separate channels for the analysis of the shape and movement of a moving visual stimulus. *Journal of Physiology*, 231, 385–402.

Tolhurst, D. J. (1975a) Reaction times in the detection of gratings by human observers: A probabilistic mechanism. *Vision Research*, 15, 1143–1150.

Tolhurst, D. J. (1975b) Sustained and transient channels in human vision. *Vision Research*, 15, 1151–1156.

Tolhurst, D. J. & Barfield, L. P. (1978) Interactions between spatial frequency channels. *Vision Research*, 18, 951–958.

Tolhurst, D. J. & Dealy, R. S. (1975) The detection and identification of lines and edges. *Vision Research*, 15, 1367–1372.

Tolhurst, D. J. & Dean, A. F. (1987) Spatial summation by simple cells in the striate cortex of the cat. *Experimental Brain Research*, 66, 607–620.

Tolhurst, D. J., Dean, A. F., & Thompson, I. D. (1981) Preferred direction of movement as an element in the organization of cat visual cortex. *Experimental Brain Research*, 44, 340–342.

Tolhurst, D. J. & Hart, G. (1972) A psychophysical investigation of the effects of controlled eye movements on the movement detectors of the human visual system. *Vision Research*, 12, 1441–1446.

Tolhurst, D. J. & Movshon, A. J. (1975) Spatial and temporal contrast sensitivity of striate cortical neurons. *Nature*, 257, 674–675.

Tolhurst, D. J., Movshon, J. A., & Dean, A. F. (1983) The statistical reliability of signals in single neurons in cat and monkey visual cortex. *Vision Research*, 23, 775–785.

Tolhurst, D. J., Movshon, J. A., & Thompson, I. D. (1981) The dependence of response amplitude and variance of cat visual cortical neurons on stimulus contrast. *Experimental Brain Research*, 41, 414–419.

Tolhurst, D. J., Sharpe, C. R., & Hart, G. (1973) The analysis of the drift rate of moving sinusoidal gratings. *Vision Research*, 13, 2545–2555.

Tolhurst, D. J. & Thompson, I. D. (1981) On the variety of spatial frequency selectivities shown by neurons in area 17 of the cat. *Proceedings of the Royal Society of London B*, 213, 183–199.

Tolhurst, D. J. & Thompson, P. G. (1975) Orientation illusions and after-effects: Inhibition between channels. *Vision Research*, 15, 967–972.

Tootle, J. S. & Berkley, M. A. (1983) Contrast sensitivity for vertically and obliquely oriented gratings as a function of grating area. *Vision Research*, 23, 907–910.

Townsend, J. T., Hu, G. C., & Ashby, F. G. (1981) Perceptual sampling of orthogonal straight line features. *Psychological Research*, 43, 259–275.

Townsend, J. T., Hu, G. G., & Evans, R. J. (1984) Modeling feature perception in brief displays with evidence for positive interdependencies. *Perception and Psychophysics*, 36, 35–49.

Townsend, J. T., Hu, G. G., & Kadlec, H. (1988) Feature sensitivity, bias, and interdependencies as a function of energy and payoffs. *Perception and Psychophysics*, 43, 575–591.

Toyama, K., Kimura, M., & Tanaka, K. (1981a) Cross-correlation analysis of interneuronal connectivity in cat visual cortex. *Journal of Neurophysiology*, 46, 191–201.

Toyama, K., Kimura, M., & Tanaka, K. (1981b) Organization of cat visual cortex as investigated by cross-correlation technique. *Journal of Neurophysiology*, 46, 202–214.

Treisman, A. (1986) Properties, parts, and objects. In *Handbook of Perception and Human Performance* (K. Boff, L. Kaufman, & J. Thomas, Eds.). New York: Wiley.

Treisman, A. & Gormican, S. (1988) Feature analysis in early vision: Evidence from search asymmetries. *Psychological Review*, 95, 15–48.

Treisman, M. & Williams, T. C. (1984) A theory of criterion setting with an application to sequential dependencies. *Psychological Review*, 91, 68–111.

Tretter, F., Cynader, M., & Singer, W. (1975) Cat parastriate cortex: A primary or secondary visual area? *Journal of Neurophysiology*, 38, 1099–1113.

Tucker, J., Charman, W. N., & Ward, P. A. (1986) Modulation dependence of the accommodation response to sinusoidal gratings. *Vision Research*, 26, 1693–1707.

Tulunay-Keesey, U. (1972) Flicker and pattern detection: A comparison of thresholds. *Journal of the Optical Society of America*, 62, 446–448.

Tulunay-Keesey, U. & Baker, E. D. (1982) Eye movements: Stabilized and normal viewing. *Supplement to Investigative Ophthalmology and Visual Science*, 22, 49.

Tulunay-Keesey, U. & Bennis, B. J. (1979) Effects of stimulus onset and image motion on contrast sensitivity. *Vision Research*, 19, 767–774.

Tulunay-Keesey, U. & Jones, R. B. (1976) The effect of micromovements of the eye and exposure duration on contrast sensitivity. *Vision Research*, 16, 481–488.

Tulunay-Keesey, U. & Jones, R. M. (1980) Contrast sensitivity measures and accuracy of image stabilization systems. *Journal of the Optical Society of America*, 70, 1306–1310.

Tweel, L. H. van der & Estevez, O. (1974) Subjective and objective evaluation of flicker. *Ophthalmologica*, 169, 70–81.

Tyler, C. W. (1975) Analysis of visual modulation sensitivity. II. Two components in flicker perception. *Vision Research*, 15, 843–848.

Tyler, C. W. (1981) Specific deficits of flicker sensitivity in glaucoma and ocular hypertension. *Investigative Ophthalmology and Visual Science*, 20, 204–212.

Tyler, C. W. (1985) Analysis of visual modulation sensitivity: Peripheral retina and the role of photoreceptor dimensions. *Journal of the Optical Society of America A*, 2, 393–398.

Tyler, C. W. (1987) Analysis of visual modulation sensitivity. III. Meridional variations in peripheral flicker sensitivity. *Journal of the Optical Society of America A*, 4, 1612–1619.

Tyler, C. W., Ernst, W., & Lyness, A. L. (1984) Photopic flicker sensitivity losses in simplex and multiplex retinitis pigmentosa. *Investigative Ophthalmology and Visual Science*, 25, 1035–1042.

Tyler, C. W. & Gorea, A. (1986) Different encoding mechanisms for phase and contrast. *Vision Research*, 26, 1073–1082.

Tyler, C. W., Ryu, S., & Stamper, R. (1984) The relation between visual sensitivity and intraocular pressure in normal eyes. *Investigative Ophthalmology and Visual Science*, 25, 103–105.

Tynan, P. & Sekuler, R. (1974) Perceived spatial frequency varies with stimulus duration. *Journal of the Optical Society of America*, 64, 1251–1255.

Tyler, C. W. & Silverman, G. (1983) Mechanisms of flicker sensitivity in peripheral retina. *Supplement to Investigative Ophthalmology and Visual Science*, 24, 145.

Uhlrich, D. J., Essock, E. A., & Lehmkuhle, S. (1981) Cross-species correspondence of spatial contrast sensitivity functions. *Behavior and Brain Research*, 2, 291–299.

Ullman, S. (1984) Maximizing rigidity: The incremental recovery of 3-D structure from rigid and nonrigid motion. *Perception*, 13, 255–274.

Van Essen, D. C. (1985) Functional organization of primate visual cortex. In *Cerebral Cortex. Volume 3* (E. G. Jones & A. Peters, Eds.). New York: Plenum, pp. 259–329.

Van Essen, D. C. & Maunsell, J. H. R. (1983) Hierarchical organization and functional streams in the visual cortex. *Trends in Neurosciences*, 6, 370–375.

van Hof-van Duin, J. & Mohn, G. (1986) The development of visual acuity in normal fullterm and preterm infants. *Vision Research*, 26, 909–916.

Van Meeteren, A. & Dunnewold, C. J. W. (1983) Image quality of the human eye for eccentric entrance pupils. *Vision Research*, 23, 573–579.

Van Meeteren, A. & Vos, J. J. (1972) Resolution and contrast sensitivity at low luminances. *Vision Research*, 12, 825–833.

Varju, D. (1962) Vergleich zweier Modelle fur laterale Inhibiton. *Kybernetik*, 1, 200–208.

Vassilev, A. (1973) Selective changes of sensitivity after adaptation to simple geometrical figures. *Perception and Psychophysics,* 13, 356–360.

Vautin, R. G. & Berkley, M. A. (1977) Responses of single cells in cat visual cortex to prolonged stimulus movement: Neural correlates of visual aftereffects. *Journal of Neurophysiology,* 40, 1051–1065.

Victor, J. D. & Shapley, R. M. (1979a) Receptive field mechanisms of cat X and Y retinal ganglion cells. *Journal of General Physiology,* 74, 275–298.

Victor, J. D. & Shapley, R. M. (1979b) The nonlinear pathway of Y ganglion cells in the cat retina. *Journal of General Physiology,* 74, 671–689.

Virsu, V. & Laurinen, P. (1977) Long-lasting afterimages caused by neural adaptation. *Vision Research,* 17, 853–860.

Virsu, V., Lehtio, P., & Rovamo, J. (1981) Contrast sensitivity in normal and pathological vision. *Documenta Ophthalmologica Proceedings Series, Vol. 30.* (L. Maffei, Ed.). The Hague: Junk, pp. 263–272.

Virsu, V. & Rovamo, J. (1979) Visual resolution, contrast sensitivity, and the cortical magnification factor. *Experimental Brain Research,* 37, 475–494.

Virsu, V., Rovamo, J., Laurinen, P., & Nasanen, R. (1982) Temporal contrast sensitivity and cortical magnification. *Vision Research,* 22, 1211–1217.

Volkmann, F. C., Riggs, L. A., White, K. D., & Moore, R. K. (1978) Contrast sensitivity during saccadic eye movements. *Vision Research,* 18, 1193–1199.

Vrolijk, P. C. & Wildt, G. J. van der (1985) The infuence of the background on the generation of inhibition. *Vision Research,* 25, 1423–1429.

Walters, D., Biederman, I., & Weisstein, N. (1983) The combination of spatial frequency and orientation is not effortless. *Supplement to Investigative Ophthalmology and Visual Science,* 24, 238.

Wandell, B. A. (1982) Measurement of small color differences. *Psychological Review,* 89, 281–302.

Wang, G. J., Pomerantzeff, O., & Pankratov, M. M. (1983) Astigmatism of oblique incidence in the human model eye. *Vision Research,* 23, 1079–1085.

Watanabe, A., Mori, T., Nagata, S., & Hiwatashi, K. (1968) Spatial sine-wave responses of the human visual system. *Vision Research,* 8, 1245–1263.

Watson, A. B. (1977) *The visibility of temporal modulations of a spatial pattern.* Ph.D. thesis, University of Pennsylvania, Philadelphia.

Watson, A. B. (1979) Probability summation over time. *Vision Research,* 19, 515–522.

Watson, A. B. (1981) A single-channel model does not predict visibility of asynchronous gratings. *Vision Research,* 21, 1799–1800.

Watson, A. B. (1982a) Summation of grating patches indicates many types of detector at one retinal location. *Vision Research,* 22, 17–26.

Watson, A. B. (1982b) Derivation of the impulse response: Comments on the method of Roufs and Blommaert. *Vision Research,* 22, 1335–1337.

Watson, A. B. (1983) Detection and recognition of simple spatial forms. In *Physical and Biological Processing of Images* (O. J. Braddick & A. C. Sleigh, Eds.). New York: Springer-Verlag. Also available as NASA Technical Memorandum 84353, April 1983, Ames Research Center, Moffett Field, CA 94035.

Watson, A. B. (1986) Temporal sensitivity. In *Handbook of Perception and Human Performance Vol. I* (K. Boff, L. Kaufman, & J. Thomas, Eds.). New York: Wiley.

Watson, A. B. (1987) Estimation of local spatial scale. *Journal of the Optical Society of America A,* 4, 1579–1582.

Watson, A. B. & Ahumada, A. J. (1985) A model of human visual-motion sensing. *Journal of the Optical Society of America A,* 2, 322–342.

Watson, A. B., Ahumada, A. J. Jr., & Farrell, J. (1986) Window of visibility: A psychophysical theory of fidelity in time-sampled visual motion displays. *Journal of the Optical Society of America A,* 3, 300–307.

Watson, A. B., Barlow, H. B., & Robson, J. G. (1983) What does the eye see best? *Nature,* 302, 419–422.

Watson, A. B. & Nachmias, J. (1977) Patterns of temporal interaction in the detection of gratings. *Vision Research,* 17, 893–902.

Watson, A. B. & Nachmias, J. (1980) Summation of asynchronous gratings. *Vision Research,* 20, 91–94.

Watson, A. B. & Pelli, D. G. (1983) QUEST: A Bayesian adaptive psychometric method. *Perception and Psychophysics,* 33, 113–120.

Watson, A. B. & Robson, J. G. (1981) Discrimination at threshold: Labelled detectors in human vision. *Vision Research,* 21, 1115–1122.

Watson, A. B., Thompson, P. G., Murphy, B. J., & Nachmias, J. (1980) Summation and discrimination of gratings moving in opposite directions. *Vision Research,* 20, 341–348.

Weale, R. A. (1986) Aging and vision. *Vision Research,* 26, 1507–1514.

Webster, M. A. and DeValois, R. L. (1985) Relationship between spatial-frequency and orientation tuning of striate cortex cells. *Journal of the Optical Society of America A,* 2, 1124–1132.

Weibull, W. (1951) A statistical distribution function of wide applicability. *Journal of Applied Mechanics,* 18, 292–297.

Weisstein, N. (1980) The joy of Fourier analysis. In *Visual Coding and Adaptability,* (C. Harris, Ed.). Hillsdale, N.J.: Lawrence Erlbaum.

Weisstein, N., Ozog, G. & Szoc, R. A. (1975) A comparison and elaboration of two models of metacontrast. *Psychological Review,* 82, 325–345.

Wenderoth, P. & Tyler, T. (1979) The role of apparent motion cues in orientation masking. *Perception and Psychophysics,* 25, 413–418.

Wesson, M. D. & Loop, M. S. (1982) Temporal contrast sensitivity in amblyopia. *Investigative Ophthalmology and Visual Science,* 22, 98–102.

Westendorf, D. H., Blake, R., Sloane, M., & Chambers, D. (1982) Binocular summation occurs during interocular suppression. *Journal of Experimental Psychology: Human Perception and Performance,* 8, 81–90.

Westendorf, D. H. & Fox, R. (1974) Binocular detection of positive and negative flashes. *Perception and Psychophysics,* 15, 61–65.

Westendorf, D. H., Langston, A., Chambers, D., & Allegretti, C. (1978) Binocular detection by normal and stereoblind observers. *Perception and Psychophysics,* 24, 209–214.

Westheimer, G. (1965) Spatial interaction in the human retina during scotopic vision. *Journal of Physiology,* 181, 881–894.

Westheimer, G. (1967) Spatial interaction in human cone vision. *Journal of Physiology,* 190, 139–154.

Westheimer, G. (1985) The oscilloscopic view: Retinal illumanance and contrast of point and line targets. *Vision Research,* 25, 1097–1103.

Whittle, P. (1986) Increments and decrements: Luminance discrimination. *Vision Research,* 26, 1677–1691.

Wickelgren, W. A. (1967) Strength theories of disjunctive visual detection. *Perception and Psychophysics,* 2, 331–337.

Wickelgren, W. A. (1968) Unidimensional strength theory and component analysis of noise in absolute and comparative judgments. *Journal of Mathematical Psychology,* 5, 102–122.

Wickelgren, W. A. (1979) *Cognitive Psychology.* Englewood Cliffs, N.J.: Prentice-Hall.

Wildt, G. J. van der & Rijsdijk, J. P. (1979) Flicker sensitivity measured with intermittent stimuli. I. Influence of the stimulus duration on the flicker threshold. *Journal of the Optical Society of America,* 69, 660–665.

Wildt, G. J. van der & Waarts, R. G. (1983) Contrast detection and its dependence on the presence of edges and lines in the stimulus field. *Vision Research,* 23, 821–830.

Williams, D. R. (1985a) Aliasing in human foveal vision. *Vision Research,* 25, 195–206.

Williams, D. R. (1985b) Visibility of interference fringes near the resolution limit. *Journal of the Optical Society of America A,* 2, 1087–1093.

Williams, D. R. (1986) Seeing through the photoreceptor mosaic. *Trends in Neurosciences,* 9, 193–198.

Williams, D. R. (1988) Topography of the foveal cone mosaic in the living human eye. *Vision Research,* 28, 433–454.

Williams, D. R. & Coletta, N. J. (1987) Cone spacing and the visual resolution limit. *Journal of the Optical Society of America A,* 4, 1514–1523.

Williams, D. R. & Collier, R. (1983) Consequences of spatial sampling by a human photoreceptor mosaic. *Science,* 221, 385–387.

Williams, D. R., Collier, R., & Thompson, B. J. (1983) Spatial resolution of the short wavelength mechanism. In *Colour Vision: Physiology and Psychophysics* (J. D. Mollon & L. T. Sharpe, Eds.). New York: Academic.

Williams, D. R., D'Zmura, M., & Lennie, P. (1984) New interferometric estimate of neural contrast sensitivity. *Supplement to Investigative Ophthalmology and Visual Science,* 25, 343.

Williams, D. W. & Wilson, H. R. (1983) Spatial-frequency adaptation affects spatial-probability summation. *Journal of the Optical Society of America,* 73, 1367–1371.

Williams, D. W., Wilson, H. R., & Cowan, J. D. (1982) Localized effects of spatial-frequency adaptation. *Journal of the Optical Soceity of America,* 72, 878–886.

Williams, R. A., Boothe, R. G., Kiorpes, L., & Teller, D. Y. (1981) Oblique effects in normally reared monkeys *(Macaca nemestrina):* Meridional variations in contrast sensitivity measured with operant techniques. *Vision Research,* 21, 1253–1266.

Wilson, H. R. (1975) A synaptic model for spatial frequency adaption. *Journal of Theoretical Biology,* 50, 327–352.

Wilson, H. R. (1978a) Quantitative prediction of line spread function measurements: Implications for channel bandwidths. *Vision Research,* 18, 493–496.

Wilson, H. R. (1978b) Quantitative characterization of two types of line-spread function near the fovea. *Vision Research,* 18, 971–982.

Wilson, H. R. (1980a) Spatiotemporal characterization of a transient mechanism in the human visual system. *Vision Research,* 20, 443–452.

Wilson, H. R. (1980b) A transducer function for threshold and suprathreshold human vision. *Biological Cybernetics,* 38, 171–178.

Wilson, H. R. (1985) A model for direction-selectivity in threshold motion perception. *Biological cybernetics,* 51, 213–222.

Wilson, H. R. (1988) Development of spatiotemporal mechanisms in infant vision. *Vision Research,* 28, 611–628.

Wilson, H. & Bergen, J. (1979) A four-mechanism model for threshold spatial vision. *Vision Research,* 19, 19–32.

Wilson, H. R. & Gelb, D. J. (1984) Modified line-element theory for spatial-frequency and width discrimination. *Journal of the Optical Society of America A,* 1, 124–131.

Wilson, H. R., McFarlane, D. K., & Phillips, G. C. (1983) Spatial frequency tuning of orientation selective units estimated by oblique masking. *Vision Research,* 23, 873–882.

Wilson, H. R., Mets, M. B., Nagy, S. E., & Kressel, A. B. (1988) Albino spatial vision as an instance of arrested development. *Vision Research,* 28, 979–980.

Wilson, H. R., Phillips, G., Rentschler, I., & Hilz, R. (1979) Spatial probability summation and disinhibition in psychophysically measured line-spread functions. *Vision Research,* 19, 593–598.

Wilson, H. R. & Regan, D. (1984) Spatial-frequency adaptation and grating discrimination: Predictions of a line-element model. *Journal of the Optical Society of America A,* 1, 1091–1096.

Wilson, M. E. (1970) Invariant features of spatial summation with changing locus in the visual field. *Journal of Physiology,* 207, 611–622.

Wisowaty, J. J. & Boynton, R. M. (1980) Temporal modulation sensitivity of the blue mechanism: Measurements made without chromatic adaptation. *Vision Research,* 20, 895–909.

Wolf, E. & Vincent, R. J. (1963) Effect of target size on critical flicker frequency in flicker perimetry. *Vision Research,* 3, 523–529.

Wolfe, J. M., Gwiazda, J., & Held, R. (1983) The meaning of non-monotonic psychometric functions in the assessment of infant preferential looking acuity. A reply to Banks et al. (1982) and Teller et al. (1982). *Vision Research,* 23, 917–920.

Wolkstein, M., Atkin, A., & Bodis-Wollner, I. (1977) Grating acuity in two sisters with tapetoretinal degeneration. *Documenta Opthalmologica Proceedings,* 12, 41.

Wong, E. & Weisstein, N. (1983) Sharp targets are detected better against a figure, and blurred targets are detected better against a background. *Journal of Experimental Psychology: Human Perception and Performance,* 9, 194–202.

Wong, E. & Weisstein, N. (1982) A new perceptual context-superiority effect: Line segments are more visible against a figure than against a ground. *Science,* 218, 587–589.

Wood, I. C. J. & Kulikowski, J. J. (1978) Pattern and movement detection in patients with reduced visual acuity. *Vision Research,* 18, 331–334.

Wright, M. J. (1982) Contrast sensitivity and adaptation as a function of grating length. *Vision Research,* 22, 139–149.

Wright, M. J. & Johnston, A. (1983) Spatiotemporal contrast sensitivity and visual field locus. *Vision Research,* 23, 983–989.

Yager, D., Kramer, P., Shaw, M., & Graham, N. (1984) Detection and identification of spatial frequency: Models and data. *Vision Research,* 24, 1021–1035.

Yellott, J. I. (1977) The relationship between Luce's choice axiom, Thurstone's theory of comparative judgment and the double exponential distribution. *Journal of Mathematical Psychology,* 15, 109–144.

Yellott, J. I. (1982) Spectral analysis of spatial sampling by photoreceptors: Topological disorder prevents aliasing. *Vision Research,* 22, 1205–1210.

Yellott, J. I. (1983) Spectral consequences of photoreceptor sampling in the rhesus retina. *Science,* 221, 382–385.

Yellott, J. I. (1984) Image sampling properties of photoreceptors: A reply to Miller and Bernard. *Vision Research,* 24, 281–283.

Yellott, J. I. J. (1987) Photon noise and constant volume operators. *Journal of the Optical Society of America A,* 4, 2418–2446.

Young, R. A. (1987) Gaussian derivative model for spatial vision: I. Retinal mechanisms. *Spatial Vision,* 2, 273–294.

Zachs, J. L. (1970) Temporal summation phenomena at threshold: Their relation to visual mechanisms. *Science,* 170, 197–199.

Index of Assumptions

Note: Numbers in brackets are assumption numbers. Pages on which formal definitions of the assumptions appear are boldface. Pages in the grouping-by-function part of the Appendix are italicized. The assumptions are indexed first by short phrase and then by number.

BY NUMBER

Index

Notes: The abbreviations *asmp., dim.,* and *expt.* are abbreviations for *assumption, dimension* and *experiment* respectively. All symbols starting with a given letter appear at the beginning of that letter's entries. Greek symbols are alphabetized according to their English names (e.g., θ, theta, is under T). An index of assumptions precedes this index.